Handbook of Experimental Pharmacology

Continuation of Handbuch der experimentellen Pharmakologie

Vol. 64

Inhibition
of Folate Metabolism
in Chemotherapy

The Origins and Uses of Co-trimoxazole

Contributors

J. F. Acar · N. Anand · D. W. Barry · R. E. Black · J. J. Burchall
S. R. M. Bushby · M. L. Clements · A. D. Dayan
R. E. Desjardins · F. W. Goldstein · L. T. Gutman · I. Hansen
G. H. Hitchings · D. T. D. Hughes · G. T. Keusch · D. H. Lawson
M. M. Levine · F. O'Grady · K. H. Pattishall · I. M. Rollo
B. Roth · J. K. Seydel · C. W. Sigel · T. A. Stamey · W. E. Stamm
C. M. Wilfert · G. P. Wormser

Editor

G. H. Hitchings

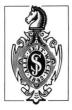

Springer-Verlag Berlin Heidelberg New York 1983

Professor Dr. GEORGE H. HITCHINGS
The Wellcome Research Laboratories, Burroughs Wellcome Co.,
3030 Cornwallis Road, Research Triangle Park, NC 27709/USA

With 51 Figures

ISBN 3-540-11782-2 Springer-Verlag Berlin Heidelberg New York
ISBN 0-387-11782-2 Springer-Verlag New York Heidelberg Berlin

Library of Congress Cataloging in Publication Data. Main entry under title: Inhibition of folate metabolism in chemotherapy. (Handbook of experimental pharmacology; v. 64) Bibliography: p. Includes index. 1. Co-trimoxazole–Physiological effect. 2. Folic acid antagonists. I. Acar, J. F. (Jacques F.) II. Hitchings, George H. (George Herbert), 1905–. III. Series. [DNLM: 1. Folic acid–Metabolism. 2. Sulfamethoxazole–Pharmacodynamics. 3. Trimethoprim–Pharmacodynamics. W1 HA51L v. 64/QV 265 I55]. QP905.H3 vol. 64. 615'.1s [615.5'8]. 82-10641 [RM666.C567]

Typesetting, printing, and bookbinding: Brühlsche Universitätsdruckerei Giessen
2122/3130-543210

Preface

The literature on co-trimoxazole (TMP/SMX) is voluminous, but in the main it consists of research reports. The same can be said of various symposia that have appeared. This volume attempts to present the current status of this antibacterial combination in a series of topical reviews, each of which represents a comprehensive summary of a segment of the field.

The editor acknowledges with appreciation the help provided by JACKIE, JENKS, LEE KUYPER, and particularly, RUTH ROSS in the preparation of the Subject Index, and thanks Burroughs Wellcome Co. for providing access to library and word processing facilities.

Research Triangle Park   GEORGE H. HITCHINGS

List of Authors

Dr. J. F. ACAR, Hospital Saint-Joseph, 7, rue Pierre-Larousse, F-75674 Paris Cedex 14

Dr. N. ANAND, National Information Centre for Drugs and Pharmaceuticals, Central Drug Research Institute, Chattar Manzil, P.O. Box No. 173, Lucknow, 226 001/IND

Dr. D. W. BARRY, The Wellcome Research Laboratories, Burroughs Wellcome Co., 3030 Cornwallis Road, Research Triangle Park, NC 27709/USA

Dr. R. E. BLACK, Center for Vaccine Development, University of Maryland, Division of Infectious Diseases, 29 S. Greene Street, Bressler Building, Room 404, Baltimore, MD 21201/USA

Dr. J. J. BURCHALL, Department of Microbiology, The Wellcome Research Laboratories, Burroughs Wellcome Co., 3030 Cornwallis Road, Research Triangle Park, NC 27709/USA

Dr. S. R. M. BUSHBY, The Wellcome Research Laboratories, Burroughs Wellcome Co., 3030 Cornwallis Road, Research Triangle Park, NC 27709/USA

Dr. M. L. CLEMENTS, Center for Vaccine Development, University of Maryland, Division of Infectious Diseases, 29 S. Greene Street, Bressler Building, Room 404, Baltimore, 21201/USA

Dr. A. D. DAYAN, Department of Pathology. Wellcome Research Laboratories, Langley Court, GB Beckenham, Kent BR3 3BS

Dr. R. E. DESJARDINS, The Wellcome Research Laboratories, Burroughs Wellcome Co., 3030 Cornwallis Road, Research Triangle Park, NC 27709/USA

Dr. F. W. GOLDSTEIN, Hospital Saint-Joseph, 7, rue Pierre-Larousse, F-75674 Paris Cedex 14

Professor Dr. L. T. GUTMAN, Pe 3971, Duke University Medical Center, Durham, NC/USA

Professor Dr. I. HANSEN, Clinic of Occupational Medizine, University Hospital, Rigshospitalet, 9 Bledamsvej, DK 2100 Copenhagen

Professor Dr. G. H. HITCHINGS, The Wellcome Research Laboratories, Burroughs Wellcome Co., 3030 Cornwallis Road, Research Triangle Park, NC 27709/USA

Dr. D. T. D. HUGHES, Department of Clinical Investigations, The Clinical Research Division, The Wellcome Research Laboratories, Langley Court, GB Beckenham, Kent BR3 3BS

Professor Dr. G. T. KEUSCH, Division of Geographic Medicine, Tufts University School of Medicine, 136 Harrison Avenue M & V 304, Boston, MA 02111/USA

Professor Dr. D. H. LAWSON, Glasgow Royal Infirmary, School of Pharmaceutical Sciences, University of Strathclyde, GB Glasgow G4 0SF

Dr. M. M. LEVINE, Center for Vaccine Development, University of Maryland, Division of Infectious Diseases, 29 S. Greene Street, Bressler Building, Room 404, Baltimore, MD 21201/USA

Dr. F. O'GRADY, Department of Microbiology und Public Health Laboratory, University Hospital, Queen's Medical Centre, GB Nottingham NG7 2UH

K. H. PATTISHALL, The Wellcome Research Laboratories, Burroughs Wellcome Co., 3030 Cornwallis Road, Research Triangle Park, NC 27709/USA

Professor Dr. I. M. ROLLO, Department of Pharmacology and Therapeutics, Faculty of Medicine, University of Manitoba, 770 Bannatyne Avenue, Winnipeg, Manitoba, R3T 2N2/CDN

Dr. B. ROTH, Department of Organic Chemistry, The Wellcome Research Laboratories, Burroughs Wellcome Co., 3030 Cornwallis Road, Research Triangle Park, NC 27709/USA

Professor Dr. J. K. SEYDEL, Biochemische Abteilung, Forschungsinstitut Borstel, Institut für Experimentelle Biologie und Medizin, D-2061 Borstel

Dr. C. W. SIGEL, Department of Medicinal Biochemistry, The Wellcome Research Laboratories, Burroughs Wellcome Co., 3030 Cornwallis Road, Research Triangle Park, NC 27709/USA

Professor Dr. T. A. STAMEY, Division of Urology, Stanford University, School of Medizine, Stanford, CA 94305/USA

Professor Dr. W. E. STAMM, Epidemiology, University of Washington, Harborview Medical Center, 325 Ninth Avenue, Seattle, WA 98104/USA

Professor Dr. C. M. WILFERT, Duke University Medical Center, Department of Pediatrics, P.O. Box 2951, Durham, NC 27710/USA

Dr. G P. WORMSER, Division of Infectious Diseases, New York Medical College, Valhalla, NY 10595/USA

Contents

Trimethoprim/Sulfamethoxazole: An Overview. G. P. WORMSER and
G. T. KEUSCH. With 1 Figure

A. Introduction 1
B. Mechanisms of Action 1
C. Resistance 3
    I. Chromosome-Mediated Resistance 3
    II. Plasmid-Mediated Resistance 4
    III. Thymidine Dependence 4
D. Clinical Use of TMP/SMX 5
    I. Approved Indications in the United States 5
    II. Other Important Uses 5
E. Use of TMP or SMX as Single Agents 6
F. Adverse Effects 6
G. Summary 7
References 7

Pharmacology and Biochemistry

CHAPTER 1

**Functions of Tetrahydrofolate and the Role of Dihydrofolate Reductase
in Cellular Metabolism.** G. H. HITCHINGS. With 6 Figures

A. General 11
B. Occurrence of Folates 11
C. Functions of Tetrahydrofolate: Cofactors 12
    I. Formate and Equivalents 12
        1. Purine Biosynthesis 13
    II. Formaldehyde Equivalents, Hydroxymethyl, and Methyl Derivatives 14
        1. Methionine Biosynthesis 14
        2. Thymidylate Synthesis 15
        3. Vitamins and Other Metabolites 16
D. Origins of Cellular Folates 16
E. Transport Systems 17
    I. Selective Rescue 18
F. Mechanism of Action of TMP/SMX 18
    I. Thymineless Death 20

G. Summary 20
References 20

CHAPTER 2

Sulfonamides: Structure-Activity Relationships and Mechanism of Action.
N. ANAND. With 1 Figure

A. Introduction 25
B. Development of Sulfonamides and Sulfones 26
     I. Sulfonamides 26
     II. Sulfones 29
     III. Antimicrobial Spectrum 30
C. Structure and Biological Activity 31
     I. Structure-Activity Relationship 31
     II. Physicochemical Properties and Antimicrobial Activity 32
        1. Water Solubility 34
        2. Lipid Solubility 36
        3. Protein Binding 36
     III. Pharmacokinetics and Metabolism 37
        1. Sulfonamides 37
        2. Sulfones 38
     IV. Half-Life 38
D. Mode of Antimicrobial Action 39
     I. Folic Acid Metabolism 39
     II. Action of Sulfonamides and Sulfones 41
        1. Selectivity of Action 44
     III. Synergism with Dihydrofolate Reductase Inhibitors 45
     IV. Drug Resistance 45
E. Present Status in Therapeutics 46
References 47

CHAPTER 3

Dihydrofolate Reductase. J. J. BURCHALL

A. Introduction 55
B. Assay and Kinetic Studies 56
C. Mechanism of Action 57
D. Basis of Selectivity 58
     I. Kinetic Studies 58
     II. Inhibitor Binding Analysis 59
     III. Enzyme Conformation and Cooperativity 62
     IV. Amino Acid Sequences 63
     V. Three-Dimensional Structures of DHFR 65
E. Plasmid-Coded Reductases 68
F. Genetics of DHFR 69
References 70

CHAPTER 4

Antibacterial Activity. S. R. M. BUSHBY. With 4 Figures

A. Introduction 75
B. In Vitro Activity 75
    I. Effects of Medium and Size of Inoculum 75
    II. Bacteriostatic Activity 77
    III. Bactericidal Activity 80
    IV. Demonstration of Synergy 80
C. Synergy and Sulfonamide-Resistant Strains 86
D. Reversal of Activity of TMP 87
E. Development of Resistance 87
F. Spectrum of Activity of TMP/SMX 90
G. Choice of Sulfonamide 92
H. 2,4-Diaminopyrimidines as Single Agents 94
J. Susceptibility Testing 96
References 99

CHAPTER 5

Selective Inhibitors of Bacterial Dihydrofolate Reductase: Structure-Activity Relationships. B. ROTH. With 2 Figures

A. Introduction 107
B. Historical Perspective 109
C. Some General Requirements for DHFR Inhibition and Antibacterial
    Activity 111
D. Inhibitors of Specific DHFRs 111
    I. The 5-Phenyl Derivatives and Related Compounds 111
    II. 5-Benzyl-2,4-Diaminopyrimidines and Close Relatives 112
        1. The 6-Unsubstituted Derivatives 112
        2. 6-Substituted Derivatives 115
        3. Substitution of a Heterocyclic Ring for the Benzene Moiety . . 116
        4. Variations in the Bridge Between the Pyrimidine and Benzene
          Rings 116
    III. The 1,2-Dihydro-1,3,5-Triazines 117
    IV. Bicyclic Analogs of the Diaminopyrimidines 117
E. Discussion 118
F. Conclusion 121
References 122

CHAPTER 6

Kinetics of Antibacterial Effects. J. K. SEYDEL. With 19 Figures

A. Introduction: Bacterial Growth Kinetics in the Presence of Folate
    Inhibitors 129
B. Sulfonamides (Synthetase Inhibitors) 131
    I. Effect of Sulfonamides on Generation Rates of E. coli 131

C. Trimethoprim (TMP): Dihydrofolate Reductase Inhibitor 133
    I. Effect of TMP on Generation Rates of E. coli 133
    II. Influence of TMP Concentration and Inoculum Size on the
       "Bactericidal" Effect of TMP 135
    III. Reversibility of TMP Action 137
    IV. Influence of Culture Broth Constituents on Biphasic Inhibition . . 138
    V. Development of Resistance Against Dihydrofolic Acid Reductase
       Inhibitors 142
D. Combined Action of Sulfonamides and Trimethoprim (Folate Inhibitors) 143
    I. Effect of TMP/SMX on Generation Rates of E. coli 143
    II. Influence of Inhibitory Power and Concentration of Sulfonamides
       or Sulfones on the Degree of Synergism 145
    III. Influence of Inhibitory Power of TMP Derivatives on the Degree
        of Synergism and Maximal Possible Effect 151
    IV. Selection Criteria for Combination of TMP and TMP Derivatives
       with Sulfonamides 151
    V. Mode of Action of Sulfonamides, TMP, and Their Combinations 155
       1. Sulfonamides 155
       2. TMP 156
       3. Combinations of Sulfonamides and TMP 158
References 158

CHAPTER 7

Disposition and Metabolism of Trimethoprim, Tetroxoprim, Sulfamethoxazole, and Sulfadiazine. C. W. SIGEL. With 4 Figures

A. Introduction 163
B. Drug Disposition 163
    I. Drug Absorption 163
    II. Distribution into Biologic Fluids and Tissues 164
       1. Physicochemical Properties that Influence Distributions 164
       2. Relationship Between Plasma and Tissue Concentrations . . . 164
    III. Excretion 168
    IV. Metabolism 169
       1. Trimethoprim 169
       2. Tetroxoprim 173
       3. Sulfamethoxazole 174
       4. Sulfadiazine 175
C. Drug Assay Methods 177
    I. Trimethoprim and Related Benzylpyrimidines 177
       1. Spectrofluorometric Methods 177
       2. Quantitative Thin Layer Chromatography 177
       3. High Pressure Liquid Chromatographic Methods 178
       4. Gas-Liquid Chromatographic Analysis 178
       5. Microbiologic Procedures 178
       6. Other Methods 179

  II. Sulfonamides . . . .
    1. Spectrophotometric Methods 179
    2. Quantitative Thin Layer Chromatography 179
    3. High Pressure Liquid Chromatography Methods 180
D. Conclusion 180
References 180

CHAPTER 8

**Preclinical Toxicity Testing of Co-trimoxazole and Other Trimethoprim/
Sulfonamide Combinations.** A. D. DAYAN

A. Introduction 185
B. General Pharmacodynamic Actions 185
    I. Trimethoprim 185
   II. Trimethoprim and Sulfamoxole 186
C. Acute Toxicity 186
    I. Trimethoprim, Sulfamethoxazole, and Co-trimoxazole . . . 186
   II. Trimethoprim and Sulfamethoxypyridazine 187
D. Subacute and Chronic Toxicity Tests 188
    I. Trimethoprim 188
    1. Rats 188
    2. Monkeys 189
    3. Other Species 190
   II. Trimethoprim and Sulfamethoxazole 190
    1. Rats 190
    2. Rabbits 192
    3. Monkeys 192
E. Combinations of Trimethoprim and Other Sulfonamides 192
    I. Trimethoprim and Sulfafurazole 192
   II. Trimethoprim and Sulfadiazine 192
  III. Trimethoprim and Sulfamoxole 193
   IV. Trimethoprim and Sulfamethoxypyrazine 194
F. Special Studies of the Thyroid and Trimethoprim/Sulfonamide
   Combinations 194
G. Other Actions of Trimethoprim Alone or Combined with Sulfonamides 195
    I. Co-trimoxazole and Immunosuppression 195
   II. Local Effects of Intramuscular Injection of Trimethoprim and
       Various Sulfonamides 195
  III. Co-trimoxazole and Renal Failure 196
H. Reproductive Toxicology 196
    I. Fetal Toxicity Tests 196
    1. Rats 196
    2. Rabbits 198
   II. Fertility Tests 198
    1. Rats 198
    2. Rabbits 199

    3. Hamsters 199
    4. Conclusions 199
    5. Other Related Information 200
  III. Reproductive Toxicity of Trimethoprim Combined with Other
       Sulfonamides 200
    1. Trimethoprim and Sulfamoxole 200
    2. Trimethoprim and Sulfamethoxypyrazine 201
J. Mutagenicity 201
  I. Point Mutation Tests in Bacteria 201
  II. Human Cytogenetic Studies 201
References 202

Clinical Pharmacology

CHAPTER 9

Adverse Effect of Co-trimoxazole. D. H. LAWSON. With 5 Figures

A. Introduction 207
B. Gastrointestinal Disorders 209
   I. Upper Gastrointestinal Symptoms 209
   II. Lower Gastrointestinal Symptoms 210
C. Skin Disorders 210
   I. Toxic Erythema 214
   II. Other Skin Reactions 215
   III. Sulfamethoxazole or Trimethoprim? 216
D. Renal Disorders 216
E. Haematological Disorders 218
   I. Folic Acid Deficiency 218
   II. Leucopenia/Agranulocytosis 218
   III. Thrombocytopenia 220
   IV. Haemolytic Anaemia 220
F. Jaundice 221
   I. Liver Damage 221
   II. Hyperbilirubinaemia of the Newborn 221
G. Pregnancy 221
H. Miscellaneous 222
J. Drug Interactions 222
   I. Pyrimethamine 222
   II. Azathioprine 223
   III. Warfarin 223
   IV. Phenytoin 223
   V. Hypoglycaemic Agents 224
K. Conclusions 224
References 224

CHAPTER 10

Clinical Pharmacokinetics of Co-trimoxazole. I. HANSEN

A. Introduction 229
B. Absorption and Biologic Half-Lives 229
C. Distribution 231
    I. Plasma 231
    II. Cerebrospinal Fluid 232
    III. Aqueous Humor 232
    IV. Breast Milk 232
    V. Prostatic and Seminal Material 233
    VI. Vaginal Fluid 233
    VII. Placental and Fetal Material 233
    VIII. Bile Fluid 233
    IX. Erythrocytes 234
    X. Bone 234
    XI. Other Tissues and Organs 234
D. Metabolism 234
E. Elimination 235
F. Interactions 238
References 238

CHAPTER 11

Resistance: Genetics and Medical Implications: J. F. ACAR and F. W. GOLDSTEIN

A. Introduction 243
B. Resistance to Sulfonamides 243
    I. Definition 243
    II. Natural Resistance 243
    III. Acquired Resistance 243
C. Resistance to Trimethoprim 243
    I. Definition 243
    II. Natural Resistance 244
    III. Acquired Resistance 244
D. Mechanisms of Acquired Resistance to Sulfonamides 244
    I. Results of Mutations 244
        1. Decreased Permeability 244
        2. Hyperproduction of p-Aminobenzoic Acid 244
        3. Altered Dihydropteroate Synthase 245
    II. Acquisition of R Factors 245
E. Mechanism of Acquired Resistance to Trimethoprim 245
    I. By Mutation 245
        1. Thymineless Organisms 245
        2. Modification of Dihydrofolate Reductase 246
    II. Plasmid-Mediated Resistance 247
        1. Transferable 248
        2. Nontransferable 248

F. Medical Implications 248
    I. Sulfonamide-Resistant Strains 248
    II. Sulfonamide-Sensitive, Trimethoprim-Resistant Strains 249
    III. Emergence of Resistant Strains During Therapy 249
G. Epidemiologic Overview of Resistance to Trimethoprim 250
    I. Gram-Positive Bacteria 250
    II. Gram-Negative Bacteria 250
References 252

Clinical Studies

CHAPTER 12

Trimethoprim Alone: Clinical Uses. D. W. BARRY and K. H. PATTISHALL.
With 2 Figures

A. Introduction 261
B. Microbiologic and Pharmacokinetic Properties 261
C. Relation of Sensitivities and Pharmacokinetics to Therapy of Urinary
   Tract Infections 264
    I. General 264
    II. Uncomplicated Urinary Tract Infections 267
    III. Complicated Urinary Tract Infections 271
D. Prophylaxis 273
    I. Recurring Urinary Infection in Women and Children 273
    II. Immunosuppressed Patients 275
E. Adverse Reactions and Safety 276
    I. General 276
    II. Dermatologic 277
    III. Gastrointestinal 280
    IV. Hematologic 280
F. Bacterial Resistance 281
    I. General 281
    II. Finnish Experience 282
    III. Effect on Fecal Flora 286
G. Conclusion 286
References 287

CHAPTER 13

Inhibitors of Dihydrofolate Reductase as Antiprotozoal Agents. I. M. ROLLO.
With 4 Figures

A. Introduction 293
B. Points of Possible Therapeutic Attack 295

C. Antimalarial Therapeutics 296
    I. Early Trials 297
    II. Clinical Cure with Pyrimethamine 298
    III. Causal Prophylaxis 299
    IV. Suppression and Mass Prophylaxis 300
    V. Gametocyticidal Effects 301
    VI. Radical Cure 302
    VII. Drug Resistance 303
    VIII. Combination with Sulfonamides and Sulfones 303
        1. Suppressive and Clinical Cure 303
        2. Effect on Other Sporozoa 305
References 306

CHAPTER 14

Pediatric Uses of Sulfonamides, Trimethoprim, and the Combination.
L. T. GUTMAN and C. M. WILFERT

A. Introduction 309
B. Hemophilus influenzae Infections 309
    I. Otitis Media 310
        1. Acute 310
        2. Serous and Chronic 311
    II. Sinusitis 311
    III. Prophylaxis to Prevent Secondary Infection 312
C. Meningitis 314
D. Urinary Tract Infections 315
    I. Acute 315
    II. Structural Defects of the Urinary System 315
    III. Prevention 315
    IV. Therapy of Periurethral and Rectal Flora 316
    V. Chlamydial Infections 316
E. Pneumocystis carinii Pneumonia 318
    I. Therapy 318
    II. Prevention 319
F. Enteric Diseases 320
    I. Salmonellosis 320
    II. Shigellosis 321
    III. Yersinia Infections 322
        1. Acute Enteritis 323
        2. Chronic Enteritis 323
        3. Mesenteric Adenitis 323
G. Miscellaneous Conditions 324
    I. Chronic Granulomatous Disease 324
    II. Osteomyelitis 324
    III. Ascending Cholangitis 324
References 325

CHAPTER 15

Use of Co-trimoxazole in Urinary Tract Infection. F. O'GRADY. With 2 Figures

A. Introduction 331
B. Co-trimoxazole in Acute Urinary Tract Infection 331
    I. Epidemiology of Resistance 332
       1. Types of Resistance 332
    II. Effects of Carriage Sites 333
       1. Effect on Gut Flora 333
       2. Effect on Urethral Colonisation 334
    III. Overtreatment 334
C. Control of Recurrent Infection 335
D. Role of the Combination 337
    I. Contrasting Effects of Trimethoprim and Sulfonamide in the Urine 337
    II. Toxicity 339
References 339

CHAPTER 16

Treatment of Genital Infections with Trimethoprim, Sulfonamides, and Combinations. W. E. STAMM

A. Introduction 343
B. Treatment of Gonorrhea with Trimethoprim/Sulfamethoxazole 343
    I. Uncomplicated Anogenital Infection 343
    II. Rectal Infection 348
    III. Pharyngeal Infection 348
    IV. In Vitro Studies and Treatment of Gonorrhea with Trimethoprim/
       Sulfamethoxazole 348
C. Infections Due to Chlamydia trachomatis 350
    I. Postgonococcal Urethritis 350
    II. Nongonococcal Urethritis 351
    III. Lymphogranuloma Venereum 352
D. Chancroid 352
E. Syphilis 354
References 354

CHAPTER 17

Treatment of Enteric Infections and Combinations. M. L. CLEMENTS, R. E. BLACK, and M. M. LEVINE

A. Escherichia coli Diarrhea 357
    I. Introduction 357
    II. Trimethoprim/Sulfamethoxazole Treatment of E. coli Diarrhea . . 357
       1. In Vitro Studies 357
       2. Clinical Studies 358
    III. Summary 358

B. Isospora belli Infections 358
   I. Introduction 358
   II. Trimethoprim/Sulfamethoxazole Treatment of an Isospora belli
      Infection 359
C. Salmonella Infections 359
   I. Introduction 359
      1. Typhoidal and Paratyphoidal Salmonella Infections 359
      2. Non-Typhoidal Salmonella Infections 360
   II. Trimethoprim/Sulfamethoxazole in the Treatment of Salmonella
      typhi Infections 361
      1. Therapeutic Studies in Antibiotic-Sensitive S. typhi Infections . 361
      2. Studies in Infections Due to Chloramphenicol-Resistant S. typhi
        Strains 363
      3. Trimethoprim/Sulfamethoxazole Treatment of Typhoid Carriers 364
      4. Adverse Effects 365
      5. Summary 365
   III. Trimethoprim Alone in Treatment of Enteric Fever 366
   IV. Trimethoprim/Sulfamethoxazole Therapy in Non-Typhoidal
      Salmonellosis 366
      1. In Vitro Studies 366
      2. Clinical Studies 367
      3. Summary 368
D. Shigella 368
   I. Introduction 368
   II. Trimethoprim/Sulfamethoxazole Treatment in Shigellosis 369
      1. In Vitro Studies 369
      2. Clinical Studies 370
      3. Summary 371
E. Vibrio cholerae Infections 371
   I. Introduction 371
   II. Trimethoprim/Sulfamethoxazole Treatment in Cholera 372
      1. In Vitro Studies 372
      2. Clinical Studies 372
      3. Summary 373
F. Yersinia enterocolitica Infections 373
   I. Introduction 373
   II. Trimethoprim/Sulfamethoxazole and Yersinia enterocolitica . . . 374
      1. In Vitro Studies 374
      2. Clinical Report 375
      3. Summary 375
References 375

CHAPTER 18

Prostatitis. T. A. STAMEY. With 1 Figure

A. Introduction 379
B. Classification and Description of Patient Categories 379

C. Acute and Chronic Bacterial Prostatitis 382
    I. Diagnosis 382
    II. Pathology 384
    III. Prostatic Immunoglobulins 384
    IV. The Antibacterial Factor in Prostatic Fluid 385
    V. Treatment 386
D. Nonbacterial Prostatitis 390
References 392

CHAPTER 19

Co-trimoxazole in Chest Infections Including its Long-Term Use in Chest Disease. D. T. D. HUGHES

A. Introduction 397
B. Exacerbations of Chronic Bronchitis 397
    I. Levels of Two Components in Sputum 399
    II. Comparative Trials 400
C. Other Acute Conditions 402
    I. Pneumocystis carinii Pneumonia 403
D. Long-Term Treatment 404
E. Parenteral TMP/SMX 406
F. Alternative Drugs 406
G. Trimethoprim Alone 407
H. Future Developments 408
References 409

CHAPTER 20

Treatment of Miscellaneous and Unusual Infections with Trimethoprim and Trimethoprim/Sulfonamide Combinations. R. E. DESJARDINS

A. Introduction 411
B. Brucellosis 411
C. Toxoplasmosis 414
D. Nocardiosis 417
E. Atypical Mycobacteria 421
F. Mycoses 422
    I. Histoplasmosis 422
    II. Paracoccidioidomycosis 423
    III. Phycomycosis 424
    IV. Chromomycosis 425
G. Pseudomonas Infections 425
    I. Pseudomonas pseudomallei 426
    II. Pseudomonas cepacia and Pseudomonas maltophilia 427
H. Other Infections 428
    I. Bubonic Plague 429

   II. Rickettsiosis 429
       1. Boutonneuse Fever 430
       2. Q Fever 430
  III. Legionella pneumophila and Pittsburgh Pneumonia Agent Infections 430
  IV. Isospora belli Infections 430
   V. Malakoplakia 431
  VI. Pediculosis 431
References 431

Subject Index 441

Trimethoprim/Sulfamethoxazole: An Overview

G.P. WORMSER and G.T. KEUSCH

A. Introduction

The antibacterial chemotherapeutic era, which has dominated much of medicine in the past 50 years, was really initiated by the introduction of the sulfonamides in 1932 (see DOMAGK 1935). After widespread and effective use of sulfonamides in a variety of infectious diseases, resistant organisms began to emerge, at first slowly, but then with frightening rapidity. In Japan, for example, species of *Shigella* were invariably sensitive to sulfonamides in the mid 1940s, but by early 1952 were just as invariably resistant. Fortunately, or so it was naively thought at the time, newer drugs were introduced to which the organisms were susceptible, including tetracycline, chloramphenicol, and streptomycin, and therapy once again became possible. However, over the next 5 years there emerged organisms resistant to each of these agents, and of greater importance, to several of them at the same time. By 1957 it was observed that an initially sulfonamide-resistant but otherwise sensitive isolate in a patient treated with just one of the agents, would suddenly appear with the resistance pattern of sulfonamide, streptomycin, tetracycline, and chloramphenicol. AKIBA et al. (1960) and OCHIAI et al. (1959) independently suggested that the information mediating such one-step resistance might be transferred from bacteria to bacteria, and proceeded to demonstrate this in vitro. In this fashion the world of transferable drug resistance (R factors) and the biology of extrachromosomal deoxyribonucleic acid, plasmids, was opened to the eyes and the minds of scientists. The past two decades of the chemotherapeutic era have been dominated as much by transferable drug resistance as by the introduction of new and potent drugs or combinations such as trimethoprim/sulfamethoxazole (TMP/SMX, Co-trimoxazole, Bactrim, Septrin, Septra). In this chapter, we will present an overview of TMP/SMX as a guide to the detailed information to follow and as a perspective for clinical thinking in current and future use of the drug or its individual components.

B. Mechanisms of Action

Both TMP and sulfonamides are inhibitors of folic acid metabolism (Fig. 1). SMX, as a typical example of the many sulfonamide variants, is a structural analog of p-aminobenzoic acid (pABA) and thus acts as a competitive inhibitor of dihydropteroate synthetase-catalyzed condensation of pABA and pteridine in the pathway to dihydrofolic acid (DHFA) synthesis. TMP, a structural analog of the pteridine portion of DHFA, serves the same competitive inhibitor role in the reduction of

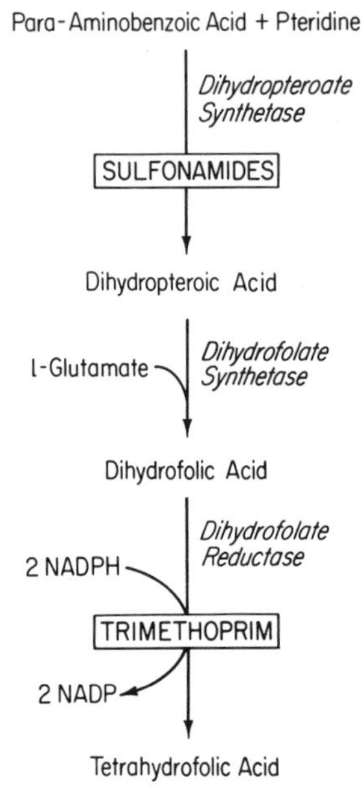

Para-Aminobenzoic Acid + Pteridine

|
Dihydropteroate
Synthetase

[SULFONAMIDES]

↓

Dihydropteroic Acid

L-Glutamate ⟍ | Dihydrofolate
Synthetase

↓

Dihydrofolic Acid

2 NADPH ⟍ | Dihydrofolate
Reductase

[TRIMETHOPRIM]

2 NADP ⟋ |

↓

Tetrahydrofolic Acid

Fig. 1. Site of action of sulfonamides and trimethoprim in the metabolic pathway leading to synthesis of tetrahydrofolic acid

Table 1. Concentration of trimethoprim and sulfamethoxazole in various body tissues and fluids in humans

Tissue or fluid	TMP level in tissue/ TMP level in serum	SMX level in tissue/ SMX level in serum	Approximate ratio TMP: SMX in tissue or fluid
Saliva	2	0.03	3: 1
Middle ear fluid	0.75	0.2	1: 6
Human breast milk	1.25	0.1	1: 2
Prostatic tissue	2	0.35	1: 3
Seminal fluid	0.5	0.3	1:10
Epididymis	2	0.51	1: 5
Sputum	1.5	0.2	1: 3
Lung parenchyma	3.5	(?) 0.3[a]	(?) 1: 2[a]
Vaginal secretions	1.5	0.01	8: 1
Fetal blood	0.6	0.8	1:30
Amniotic fluid	0.8	0.5	1:10
Aqueous humor	0.4	0.25	1:10
Cerebrospinal fluid	0.5	0.4	1:15
Bile	1	0.4	1: 8
Spongy bone	0.67		
Compact bone	0.1		
Synovial fluid	1	1	1:20

[a] Presumptive, based on animal data

DHFA to the biologically active form of folic acid, tetrahydrofolic acid (THFA), catalyzed by the enzyme dihydrofolate reductase.

TMP, however, will increase the concentration of DHFA, which, by the law of mass action, will drive the reaction to the right and produce THFA, partially overcoming the TMP-induced metabolic block. This biologic effect can be minimized by inclusion of a sulfonamide which blocks the synthesis of DHFA. This sequential blockade in the biosynthetic pathway of THFA results in potentiation of the action of the combination of TMP and sulfonamide over the action of each component alone (synergy). The biochemical basis for the actions of TMP/SMX is discussed in detail by HITCHINGS (Chap. 1). Potentiation of antibacterial effects by TMP in combination with SMX has been demonstrated for many microorganisms both in vitro and in in vivo (see Chap. 4).

For most organisms studied in vitro, a ratio of the two drugs equivalent to the ratio of their individual minimal inhibitory concentrations (MIC) produces maximum synergy. This optimal ratio is approximately 1:20 TMP:SMX (BUSHBY 1973). It is for this reason that the ratio of the two drugs in the fixed combination tablet (marketed as Septra, Septrin, or Bactrim) has been set at 1:5 TMP:SMX, for this produces a ratio of approximately 1:20 in serum. For most organisms, however, significant potentiation is observed over a wide range of ratios from 1:20 to 1:1 or thereabout, which is important because the pharmacology of the distribution of the individual components in various tissues does not preserve the 1:20 ratio obtained in plasma (Table 1). See also Chaps. 4 and 6.

C. Resistance

I. Chromosome-Mediated Resistance

Resistance to TMP or SMX is mediated by either chromosomal or plasmid DNA. In the laboratory, chromosomal resistance to TMP can be selected by passage of heavy inocula of bacteria in media containing increasing concentrations of the drug. Selection of TMP-resistant mutants can be delayed or prevented by addition of a sulfonamide, provided the organism is sensitive to the latter. The chance of a double mutation to two drugs occurring in the same organism is vanishingly small, providing a rationale for the use of TMP/SMX combination in clinical practice for the same reason that combined chemotherapy is employed in the therapy of tuberculosis. The biochemical mechanism for resistance in most of these "one-step" TMP resistant mutants is unknown, but their clinical significance seems to be minimal, for the isolates appear to be grossly defective in vitro and have not been observed to emerge during clinical use of TMP as a single agent in humans. In some strains of *Escherichia coli* or *Klebsiella*, resistance has been shown to be due to production of an altered dihydrofolate reductase enzyme with decreased affinity for TMP, while in other instances markedly increased production of the enzyme serves to overcome the block (GREY et al. 1979). In *Pseudomonas aeruginosa*, insensitivity may relate to a relative permeability block to the drug which cannot penetrate the bacterial cell to work (HITCHINGS 1973). See Chaps. 4 and 11.

Clinical isolates with intrinsic or acquired resistance to TMP/SMX are generally (90%) chromosomally determined. Emergence of such organisms during a course of therapy is infrequent, except perhaps in the case of *Streptococcus faecium (faecalis)* (Chattopadhyay 1972). In Europe, where TMP/SMX has been extensively used for 13 years, resistance in nosocomial isolates has slowly increased, particularly in *Klebsiella*, with a disproportionate number showing R factors of late. See also Chap. 4.

II. Plasmid-Mediated Resistance

A number of distinct plasmids, belonging to separate compatibility classes (principally I, P, or W), mediate TMP resistance, principally by coding for at least three different drug resistant DHFA reductase enzymes (Towner et al. 1979; Tennhammer-Ekman and Sköld 1979; Pattishall et al. 1977). These are of different molecular weight, and vary from total insensitivity to the action of TMP to partial susceptibility. The latter type, however, is synthesized in increased (10- to 20-fold) amounts (Stone and Smith 1979; Amyes and Smith 1978; Tennhammer-Ekman and Sköld 1979). A rare type of R factor contains a mutator gene modulating a chromosomally directed permeability barrier (Amyes and Smith 1975). Plasmid-conferred resistance is usually expressed at high concentrations of drug, for example greater than 1,000 µg/ml TMP (Datta and Hedges 1972). Although it appeared initially that such high resistance was a marker for plasmid-mediated resistance, only 75% of such strains can be shown to possess transferable plasmids (Towner et al. 1980; West and White 1979). This does not rule out a plasmid locus for the resistance, for there are classes of nontransferable plasmids that are only mobilizable by other plasmids (cotransfer). Moreover, it has been learned in recent years that genetic information contained in short segments of the circular DNA of a plasmid may jump from plasmid type to type or from plasmid to chromosome. These plasmid segments, called transposons, can thus mediate transferable or nontransferable apparently chromosomal resistance, or other properties such as enterotoxin production in *E. coli*. For this reason, the selective pressures of antibiotic usage may be compressing the evolutionary history of pathogenic bacteria from millenia into minutes on a cosmic scale. R factors for TMP generally confer resistance to sulfonamides, and often, but less frequently, to other drugs as well. While spread of R factor resistance to TMP/SMX has been observed in both humans and animals, given the extensive use of the drug combination and the discovery of transposons (Tn7 and Tn402) mediating TMP resistance, it is surprising how infrequently such isolations occur (Richards et al. 1978; Grüneberg and Bendall 1979). These events, however, do impose a sense of awe for the complexity of nature and introduce a degree of caution in our thinking about and use of antimicrobials. See also Chaps. 4 and 1.

III. Thymidine Dependence

An infrequent (less than 1% of TMP-resistant isolates) but important type of resistance is the example of thymidine-dependent organisms. Such bacteria have lost the ability to synthesize thymidine and instead have a mechanism to utilize exogenous nucleoside. The roles of thymidine and thymidine phosphorylase are discussed in detail by Bushby (Chap. 4).

D. Clinical Use of TMP/SMX

The drug has been employed for a wide variety of infections, including acute and chronic urinary tract infections, prostatitis, upper respiratory illnesses including otitis media, lower respiratory disease such as bronchitis or pneumonitis, venereal diseases, typhoid fever, shigellosis, and other acute diarrheas, *Pneumocystis carinii* infection, toxoplasmosis, malaria, *Isospora belli* infection, gram-negative bacillary sepsis or meningitis, nocardiosis, brucellosis, melioidosis, soft tissue and bone infection, and acne. The evidence for efficacy ranges from impressive and conclusive to anecdotal and suspect. These data have recently been reviewed (WORMSER and KEUSCH 1979) and will be covered in detail in subsequent chapters. See especially Chap. 19.

I. Approved Indications in the United States

In the United States, only five indications for the use of TMP/SMX are presently approved by the Food and Drug Administration: chronic urinary tract infections, childhood otitis media due to susceptible bacteria, acute exacerbations of chronic bronchitis, shigellosis, and pneumocystosis. This is not because other indications are not valid or effectively treatable by TMP/SMX, but rather because there are special aspects to the use of the drug in each of the approved situations that particularly recommend it. In the case of chronic urinary tract infection, TMP/SMX has especially desirable effects on the fecal flora, the usual source of new infecting strains. Even during prolonged administration, the drug will completely eliminate the fecal Enterobacteriaceae without recolonization by resistant organisms; the latter phenomenon is attributed to the preservation of the anaerobic bowel flora (SCHIMPFF 1980; STAMEY et al. 1977; KNOTHE 1973; CATTELL et al. 1976; GRÜNE-BERG et al. 1976; NAFF 1971). In otitis media, the drug is active against *Streptococcus pneumoniae* and ampicillin-sensitive *Hemophilus influenzae* as it is against β-lactamase-producing, ampicillin-resistant strains. In shigellosis, multiply antibiotic-resistant *Shigella sonnei* and *Shigella flexneri* are frequently involved and these are effectively treated with TMP/SMX. For *Pneumocystis carinii* opportunistic infections, TMP/SMX is equal or superior to pentamidine, the agent it has replaced as drug of first choice, and significantly less toxic or productive of undesired side effects. Exacerbations of chronic bronchitis are major causes of morbidity in chronic obstructive pulmonary disease and therefore effective therapy is highly desirable. TMP/SMX has been shown to be as effective as other commonly employed antimicrobial agents. See also Chaps. 15–20.

II. Other Important Uses

A few other indications deserve special mention. One is the use of TMP/SMX in treatment of chloramphenicol–ampicillin-resistant isolates of *Salmonella typhi*. Such strains were isolated in a few patients in the epidemics of typhoid fever due to chloramphenicol-resistant *Salmonella typhi* in Mexico in 1972–1975, and in Vietnam and Korea over the past 5 years. TMP/SMX is of proven value in typhoid fever, irrespective of the chloramphenicol or ampicillin resistance of the isolate and it is therefore also an alternative for treatment of mild typhoid in the penicillin-allergic patient. The drug, with or without rifampin, can eradicate the carrier state in some who are either allergic to or fail on therapy with ampicillin or amoxycillin. See also Chap. 20.

Particularly with parenteral forms of the drug, preliminary data indicate that TMP/SMX may be effective in treating neutropenic cancer patients who fail on carbenicillin–aminoglycoside regimens (Grose and Bodey 1980). Since this is a high risk patient population with high mortality rates, effective antimicrobial regimens are greatly desired. Preliminary evidence of a prophylactic effect of TMP/SMX in such patients through chronic administration to suppress the enterobacteriaceal fecal flora are also encouraging (Gurwith et al. 1979; Schimpff 1980). This needs to be investigated taking into consideration the concerns for selection of resistant nosocomial bacteria discussed in Sect. C.I. For more details see Chap. 19. In these and other clinical situations involving TMP/SMX-sensitive organisms, we believe a controlled and guarded use of the drug is appropriate. This is because of the availability of other effective drugs, combined with the potential risk of emergence and spread in nature of plasmid resistance to TMP/SMX, and through R factor linkage, possibly other antibiotics as well.

E. Use of TMP or SMX as Single Agents

It has been demonstrated that the sulfonamide component of the TMP/SMX formulation is not critical to the efficacy of the combination in treatment of urinary tract infection. Use of regimens with ratios of 1:20, 1:10, or 1:2 TMP:SMX, substitution of sulfadiazine for SMX, or use of TMP alone are equally efficacious in clinical trials (e.g., Brumfitt and Hamilton-Miller 1979). It has been argued, therefore, that TMP be used as a single agent in this, and perhaps other clinical situations, for example in chronic bronchitis (Lacey et al. 1980). For discussion see Chap. 12.

F. Adverse Effects

TMP/SMX is remarkably free of adverse side effects or toxicity, even during long-term administration. This may be due, in part, to the relatively greater affinity of TMP for bacterial DHFA reductase compared with the mammalian enzyme. Hence, abnormalities in folate metabolism in the human host are rarely detected. With long-term use, a few patients may demonstrate an antimetabolite effect, manifested by increased neutrophil lobe counts or forminiminoglutamate excretion in urine, or more significantly, pancytopenia and a megaloblastic marrow (Blackwell et al. 1978; Kahn et al. 1968). Patients with known folate or vitamin B_{12} deficiency are at greater risk of these complications, and therefore, caution is suggested in patients likely to have marginal reserves of either or both of these nutrients (including the elderly), patients with malabsorption syndromes, malnutrition, alcoholism, chronic hemolysis such as homozygous sickle cell hemoglobinopathy, or patients receiving phenytoin, or folic acid antimetabolites such as methotrexate. Administration of folinic acid will reverse the metabolic effects of TMP/SMX without alteration of antimicrobial activity, except for *Streptococcus faecium (faecalis)* (Grüneberg et al. 1970; Bushby 1973). For discussion see Chap. 9.

G. Summary

TMP/SMX has proven to be an effective antimicrobial in many clinical situations without important or frequent toxicity or side effects. The development of this successful drug combination is a highly visible example of the rational and creative use of microbiologic, biochemical, pharmacologic, and clinical data and insight in the conceptualization and production of a valuable therapeutic agent. However, the possibilities and reality of emerging microbial resistance dictate the need for cautious use of the drug. The U.S. Food and Drug Administration approved uses of TMP/SMX and other clinical settings in which the drug may prove to be valuable have been discussed, as a framework for the detailed discussions to follow.

References

Akiba T, Koyama K, Ishiki Y, Kimura S, Fukushima J (1960) On the mechanism of development of multiple drug-resistant clones of *Shigella*. Jpn J Microbiol 4:219–227

Amyes SGB, Smith JT (1975) R-factor conferred ability to mutate to trimethoprim resistance. J Pharm Pharmacol [Suppl 2] 27:44P

Amyes SGB, Smith JT (1978) R-factor mediated dihydrofolate reductases which confer trimethoprim resistance. J Gen Microbiol 107:263–271

Blackwell EA, Hauson CAT, Leer J, Bain B (1978) Acute pancytopenia due to megaloblastic arrest in association with cotrimoxazole. Med J Aust 2:38–41

Brumfitt W, Hamilton-Miller JMT (1979) General survey of trimethoprim combination in the treatment of urinary tract infections. Infection [Suppl 4] 7:388–393

Bushby SRM (1973) Trimethoprim sulfamethoxazole: in vitro microbiological aspects. J Infect Dis [Suppl] 128:442–462

Cattell WR, McSherry MA, Brooks HL, O'Grady FW (1976) The carriage of *Escherichia coli* on the periurethral area and in the feces in patients on long-term low dose cotrimoxazole therapy. Clin Nephrol 6:506–508

Chattopadhyay B (1972) Trimethoprim-sulfamethoxazole in urinary tract infection due to *Streptococcus faecalis*. J Clin Pathol 25:531–533

Datta N, Hedges RW (1972) Trimethoprim resistance conferred by W plasmids in Enterobacteriaceae. J Gen Microbiol 72:349–355

Domagk G (1935) Ein Beitrag zur Chemotherapie der bakteriellen Infektionen. Dt Med Wochenschr 61:250–253

Grey D, Hamilton-Miller JMT, Brumfitt W (1979) Incidence and mechanisms of resistance to trimethoprim in clinically isolated gram-negative bacteria. Chemotherapy 25:147–156

Grose WE, Bodey GP (1980) Intravenous trimethoprim-sulfamethoxazole alone or combined with tobramycin for infections in cancer patients. Am J Med Sci 279:4–13

Grünberg E, Prince HN, DeLorenzo WF (1970) The in vivo effect of folinic acid (citrovorum factor) on the potentiation of the antibacterial activity of sulfisoxazole by trimethoprim. J Clin Pharmacol 10:231–234

Grüneberg RN, Smellie JM, Leakey A, Atkin WS (1976) Long-term, low dose cotrimoxazole in prophylaxis of childhood urinary tract infection. Bacteriological aspects. Br Med J 2:206–208

Grüneberg RN, Bendall MJ (1979) Hospital outbreak of trimethoprim resistance in pathogenic coliform bacteria. Br Med J 2:7–9

Gurwith MJ, Brunton JL, Lank BA, Harding GKM, Ronald AR (1979) A prospective controlled investigation of prophylactic trimethoprim/sulfamethoxazole in hospitalized granulocytopenic patients. Am J Med 66:248–256

Hitchings GH (1973) Biochemical background of trimethoprim-sulfamethoxazole. Med J Aust [Suppl] 1:5–9

Kahn SB, Fein SA, Brodsky I (1968) Effect of trimethoprim on folate metabolism in man. Clin Pharmacol Ther 9:550–560

Knothe H (1973) The effect of a combined preparation of trimethoprim and sulphamethoxazole following short-term and long-term administration on the flora of the human gut. Chemotherapy 18:284–296

Lacey RW, Lord VL, Gunasekera HKW, Lieberman PJ, Luxton DEA (1980) Comparison of trimethoprim alone with trimethoprim-sulphamethoxazole in the treatment of respiratory and urinary infections with particular reference to selection of trimethoprim resistance. Lancet 1:1270–1273

Naff H (1971) On the changes in the intestinal flora induced in man by Bactrim. Pathol Microbiol 37:1–22

Ochiai K, Yamanaka T, Kimura K, Sowada O (1959) Inheritance of drug resistance (and its transfer) between *Shigella* strains and between *Shigella* and *E. coli* strains. Nihon Iji Shimpo 1861:34

Pattishall KH, Acar J, Burchall JJ, Goldstein FW, Harvey RJ (1977) Two distinct types of trimethoprim-resistant dihydrofolate reductase specified by R-plasmids of different compatibility groups. J Biol Chem 252:2319–2323

Richards H, Datta N, Sojka WJ, Wray C (1978) Trimethoprim-resistant plasmids and transposons in salmonella. Lancet 2:1194–1195

Schimpff SC (1980) Infection prevention during profound granulocytopenia. New approaches to alimentary canal microbial suppression. Ann Intern Med 93:358–361

Stamey TA, Condy M, Mihara G (1977) Prophylactic efficacy of nitrofurantoin macrocrystals and trimethoprim-sulfamethoxazole in urinary infections: biologic effects on the vaginal and rectal flora. N Engl J Med 296:780–783

Stone D, Smith SL (1979) The amino acid sequence of the trimethoprim-resistant dihydrofolate reductase specified in *Escherichia coli* by R plasmid R 67. J Biol Chem 254:10857–10861

Tennhammer-Ekman B, Sköld O (1979) Trimethoprim-resistance plasmids of different origin encode different drug-resistant dihydrofolate reductases. Plasmid 2:334–346

Towner KJ, Pearson NJ, Cattell WR, O'Gray F (1979) Trimethoprim R plasmids isolated during long-term treatment of urinary tract infections with cotrimoxazole. J Antimicrob Agents 5:45–52

Towner KJ, Pearson NJ, Pinn PA, O'Grady F (1980) Increasing importance of plasmid-mediated trimethoprim resistance in enterobacteria: two six-month clinical surveys. Br Med J 280:517–519

West B, White G (1979) A survey of trimethoprim resistance in the enteric bacterial flora of farm animals. J Hyg (Lond) 82:481–488

Wormser GP, Keusch GT (1979) Trimethoprim-sulfamethoxazole in the United States. Ann Intern Med 91:420–429

Symposia Reports

1. "The synergy of trimethoprim and sulphonamides" (1969) Postgrad Med J 45: suppl (Editorial Committee: L.P. Garrod, D.G. James, A.A.G. Lewis)

2. "The synergy of trimethoprim and sulphonamides" (1970) S Afr Med J 15

3. "Trimethoprim/sulphamethoxazole in bacterial infections." (Sardinia 1972). In: Bernstein LS, Salter AJ (eds) Churchill Livingstone (1973)

4. "Trimethoprim/sulphonamide conference" (Boston 1972). J Infect Dis 128 (suppl) (1973). Maxwell Finland, Edward H. Kass (eds)

5. "Septrin symposia" (Australia 1973). Med J Aust 1 (suppl) (1973)

6. "Combination chemotherapy of infectious diseases" (Canada 1975). Canad Med Ass J 112 (suppl) (1975). [JR Anderson (Scientific Editor CMAJ)]

7. "Advances in therapy with antibacterial folate inhibitors" (London 1979). J Antimicrob Chemother 5: (suppl B) (1979). Richard Wise and David S. Reeves

8. "Trimethoprim/sulphamethoxazole revisited" (1982). Rev. Infect. Dis. 4:196–618. (M. Finland and E. H. Kass eds)

Pharmacology and Biochemistry

CHAPTER 1

Functions of Tetrahydrofolate
and the Role of Dihydrofolate Reductase
in Cellular Metabolism

G.H. HITCHINGS

A. General

Tetrahydrofolate functions as a one-carbon unit carrier in a variety of biosynthetic reactions. In autotrophic microorganisms, the metabolites produced are wide-ranging indeed, not only those biosynthesized by mammalian organisms, but several vitamins and antibiotics as well. Folate is unique in that it is required for its own biosynthesis. Folates are ubiquitous in distribution, not only in plants and animals, but in rickettsiae and bacteriophages (RABINOWITZ 1960; BLAKLEY 1969). Their determination is not easy because a multiplicity of forms exists, with two levels of oxidation of the pyrazine ring, three levels of oxidation of one-carbon substituents, two possible positions of substitution of these, or indeed bridging the 5,10 positions, and one or several glutamyl residues (Fig. 1). Most of the work described in this chapter has been carried out with monoglutamate forms, but it is becoming quite clear that the bulk of intracellular folates are polyglutamate derivatives (e.g., MACKENZIE and BAUGH 1980).

B. Occurrence of Folates

Until about 1960, microbiologic assays were used for folates. In order to get even good approximations, one had to use three microorganisms, and one or more enzymes to remove "extra" glutamyl residues. The reliability of most literature values is questionable. Somewhat better data have been achieved in recent years through the application of chromatography, but this too has its limitations. As a result of the technical difficulties, comparisons of different sources are difficult to make. Values for human serum cluster around 10 mμg/ml (0.02 μM) but in the rat, the

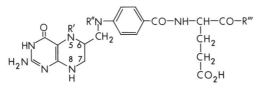

Fig. 1. General formula for tetrahydrofolate and cofactors derived from it. R′ or R″ may be H or –CHO, or together may be –CH$_2$– or –CH=, R′ may be CH$_3$, R″ may be –CH= NH. R‴ may be H or one or more γ-glutamyl residues in peptide linkage. Removal of H$_2$ from positions 5 and 6 leaves 7,8-dihydrofolate; removal of the 7,8 hydrogens from it leaves folic acid (pteroylglutamic acid)

values may be as much as 10-fold greater. Whole blood values reflect the much higher concentrations in erythrocytes. Many foods reach values 100-fold higher than serum (approximately $1-10 \ \mu g/g = 2 \ \mu M$–$0.02 \ mM$) with yeast still higher. Daily intakes have been estimated in the range of 200 µg, which is not much more than an estimated daily requirement. Nevertheless, doses of this order or even lower of calcium leucovorin seem adequate to reserve any tendency toward dyscrasias in long-term therapy with co-trimoxazole (JEWKES et al. 1970).

C. Functions of Tetrahydrofolate: Cofactors

Tetrahydrofolate (FAH_4, Fig. 1) serves as a carrier of one-carbon units (RABINOWITZ and HIMES 1960). It does so through the intermediation of a number of cofactors. Each of these is formed enzymatically from a suitable carbon source and tetrahydrofolate. After reaction with a suitable precursor, again catalyzed by a specific enzyme, a new product and unsubstituted FAH_4 are formed. In most reactions, FAH_4 is thus just a carrier, shuttling back and forth between the loaded and empty state (Fig. 2, center and right-hand side). Thymidylate synthetase, however, requires two atoms of hydrogen in addition to the methylene group to complete the methyl group of deoxythymidylate. These are abstracted from the carrier itself (Fig. 2, left-hand side) producing dihydrofolate (FAH_2). Dihydrofolate reductase (DHFR) thus is required to keep the system running (to return the folate to the tetrahydro state).

It is proposed to discuss the cofactors, their formations and functions in the order of level of oxidation of the one-carbon fragment which they contain. For detailed discussions see FRIEDKIN (1963) and RADER and HUENNEKENS (1973).

I. Formate and Equivalents

A number of cofactors are equivalents of formate. These are:
    10-Formyl-FAH_4
 5,10-Methenyl-FAH_4
        5-Formyl-FAH_4
        5-Formimino-FAH_4

The interrelationships of these are shown in Fig. 3. 5,10-Methylene-FAH_4 is included since it is interconvertible through the action of a dehydrogenase with 5,10-methenyl-FAH_4. Particular interest is attached to the cofactors of Fig. 3. Although these were originally believed to be separate enzymes, a trifunctional protein has now been isolated from a variety of sources that has the enzymatic activities of methylenetetrahydrofolate dehydrogenase, methenyltetrahydrofolate cyclohydrolase, and formyltetrahydrofolate synthetase. Chymotryptic cleavage of the enzyme from pig liver yields a fragment two-thirds the size of the original that has only the synthetase activity, and a smaller fragment with dehydrogenase–cyclohydrolase activities (COHEN and MACKENZIE 1978; TAN and MACKENZIE 1979). The polyfunctional enzyme has been reported from pig (TAN et al. 1977), rabbit (SCHIRCH 1978), and sheep (PAUKERT et al. 1976) liver preparations. In some bacterial sources the enzymes appear to be separate (see PAUKERT et al. 1976), but a

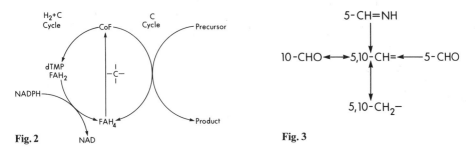

Fig. 2. Functions of folates. FAH_4 is converted to cofactors (CoF) by the addition of one-carbon units. These are donated to precursors to form products and regenerate FAH_4 (right-hand side). In one reaction (left-hand side) thymidylate (dTMP) is formed from deoxyuridylate by reaction with 5,10-methylene-FAH_4, but at the same time FAH_4 is oxidized to FAH_2. To re-form FAH_4, dihydrofolate reductase and nicotinamide adenine dinucleotidephosphate (NADPH) are needed

Fig. 3. Cofactor forms of FAH_4. 5,10-Methylenetetrahydrofolate contains carbon at the level of oxidation of formaldehyde; the others contain carbon equivalent to formate

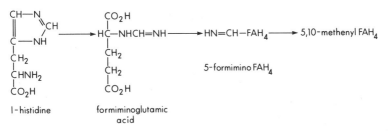

Fig. 4. Formation of 5-formimino-FAH_4 from histidine and FAH_4

multifunctional enzyme has been isolated from *Escherichia coli* (DEV and HARVEY 1978).

The 5-formyl- and 5-forminotetrahydrofolates are outside the mainstream of folate-controlled biosynthetic reactions. Leucovorin, 5-formyltetrahydrofolate, is a chemical synthetic product (ROTH et al. 1952). It is converted to 5,10-methenyl-FAH_4 enzymatically, however, in a reaction requiring ATP (PETERS and GREENBERG 1957). 5-Formimino-FAH_4 arises from formiminoglutamate which in turn is formed by the ring opening of the imidazole ring of histamine (Fig. 4). The transfer of the formimino group from glutamate to FAH_4 is blocked when FAH_4 is depleted following the administration of folate analogs. *Excretion of formiminoglutamate is thus a sensitive clinical test for impaired folate metabolism* (HIATT et al. 1958). Formimino FAH_4 in turn is cyclized to 5,10-methenyl-FAH_4 with elimination of ammonia (TABOR and RABINOWITZ 1956; TABOR and WYNGAARDEN 1959).

1. Purine Biosynthesis

The cofactor participation in purine biosynthesis is shown in Fig. 5. The cofactor for glycinamide ribonucleotide transformylase was shown by HARTMAN and

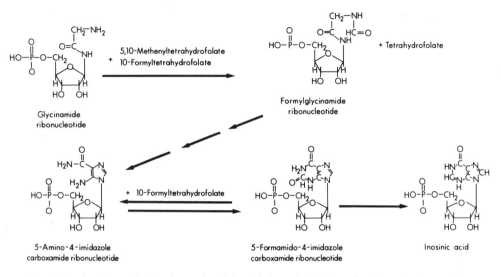

Fig. 5. Purine biosynthetic scheme involving 10-formyl-FAH$_4$ and 5,10-methylene-FAH$_4$

BUCHANAN (1959), using a preparation of pigeon liver enzyme, to be 5,10-methenyltetrahydrofolate. When DEV and HARVEY (1978) examined the same system in preparations of *E. coli*, the cofactor was found unequivocally to be N^{10}-formyltetrahydrofolate. This seems to be a real species difference. Consequently, both cofactors are shown in the diagram in Fig. 5. There seem to be no differences with respect to the cofactor for formylation of aminoimidazole carboxamide ribonucleotide (AICAR) the second reaction in Fig. 5. AICAR, of course, is the penultimate precursor of inosinic acid (hypoxanthine ribonucleotide) the first purine produced in the de novo biosynthetic pathway.

II. Formaldehyde Equivalents, Hydroxymethyl, and Methyl Derivatives

5,10-Methylenetetrahydrofolate is one of the more important cofactors. Its oxidative conversion to 5,10-methenyltetrahydrofolate (and *thence* to 10-formyltetrahydrofolate) has been mentioned (Fig. 3). 5,10-Methylene-FAH$_4$ arises mainly by the transfer of the hydroxymethyl group of serine to FAH$_4$, accompanied by cyclization.

$$\text{L-serine} + \text{FAH}_4 \rightleftharpoons \text{glycine} + 5,10\text{-CH}_2\text{FAH}_4. \tag{1}$$

It is the precursor of methyl groups in two ways. The methylene group may be reduced to form 5-methyltetrahydrofolate.

$$5,10\text{-methylene FAH}_4 + \text{NADPH} + \text{H}^+ \text{ (FAD)} \rightarrow 5\text{-methyl-FAH}_4 + \text{NADP}. \tag{2}$$

1. Methionine Biosynthesis

Some confusing complications have arisen regarding this reaction and apparent roles have been assigned to flavin adenine dinucleotide (FAD) and nicotinamide adenine dinucleotide (NAD) as well as cobalamine (BLAKLEY 1969; FRIEDKIN

1963). 5-Methyl-FAH_4 is important not only as the principal reservoir of FAH_4 in the mammal (BLAKLEY 1969) but as a precursor of methionine by transfer of the methyl group to homocysteine (Hycs) (BUCHANAN et al. 1964; FINKELSTEIN 1979). Methionine in turn is not only a building block for proteins, but also a precursor of the important metabolite, S-adenosylmethionine (Ado-Met) (TURNER 1979; TAYLOR and WEISSBACH 1973):

$$CH_3FAH_4 \xrightarrow[FAH_4]{Hcys} Methionine \xrightarrow[PPi+Pi]{ATP} S\text{-adenosylmethionine} \qquad (3)$$

5,10-Methylene FAH_4 is a precursor of another methyl group, that of thymine and thymidylate (dTMP), where its role is vital and unique. (Other routes to the methyl group of methionine are available from foods, as methionine itself, and labile methyl groups from choline).

2. Thymidylate Synthesis

Thymidylate synthesis is unique among the biosynthetic reactions that employ FAH_4 as catalyst in that it involves not only the transfer of a one-carbon moiety, but also the oxidation of the carrier:

$$\text{Deoxyuridylate} + 5,10\text{-methylenetetrahydrofolate} \rightarrow \text{deoxythymidylate} + \text{dihydrofolate} \qquad (4)$$

Synthesis de novo of dTMP by this route is nearly ubiquitous. Most organisms also possess a thymidine kinase:

$$\text{Thymidine} + \text{adenosine triphosphate} \rightarrow \text{deoxythymidylate} + \text{adenosine diphosphate.} \qquad (5)$$

Uptake and incorporation of thymidine are important to mammalian cells, and thymidine ^3H has become a much-used tracer for cellular DNA synthesis and replication in studies of cellular kinetics, especially of malignant cells (CLEAVER 1967).

The enzymatic synthesis of thymidylate (Eq. 4) has been the subject of a large volume of detailed work (FRIEDKIN 1973). After establishment of $5,10\text{-}CH_2FAH_4$ as the source of the carbon, the identification of the reducing hydrogen atoms was next undertaken. The most probable mechanism is the intermediate formation of a methylene bridge between the tetrahydrofolate moiety and the 5 position of the deoxyuridine monophosphate (dUMP). Rearrangement results in completion of the methyl group of thymidylate by transfer of a hydrogen atom from the A side of the pyrazine ring of the tetrahydrofolate. Further work on the stereochemistry of folate derivatives is occurring in some volume, accelerated, no doubt, by the X-ray conformational studies of dihydrofolate reductases (e.g., MATTHEWS et al. 1978). These and other data led to the conclusion that FAH_2 and methotrexate (MTX) have opposite configurations in the enzyme about the C-6–C-9 bond (HITCHINGS and ROTH 1980; HITCHINGS and SMITH 1980). This and other work on absolute configurations may eventually lead to the modeling of superior inhibitors.

The reactions discussed are the principal and most vital reactions. The important reaction from the standpoint of the present volume is that of thymidylate synthetase, because in the presence of an inhibitor of dihydrofolate reductase all folates eventually become trapped in the functionally inactive FAH_2 form. The biosynthetic reaction that is first to suffer from depletion of the FAH_4 pool is not necessarily the same in all circumstances, since it depends on the relative demands of the reactions bonding FAH_4 and the various one-carbon units (HITCHINGS 1975).

3. Vitamins and Other Metabolites

Folate metabolism in the mammal encompasses a number of vital reactions, but in autotrophic microorganisms the number of vital reactions dependent on folate catalysis is very much larger. Many of these derive from guanosine triphosphate (GTP) through expulsion of the C-8 atom, e.g., riboflavin (MAILÄNDER and BACHER 1976; MITSUDA et al. 1977), folic acid itself (REYNOLDS and BROWN 1964), xanthopterin, and more exotic antibiotics such as toxoflavin and dimethylbenzimidazole antibiotics (ELSTNER and SUHADOLINIK 1971). Folate derivatives catalyze essential steps in pantothenate biosynthesis (TELLER et al. 1976) and an intermediate in purine biosynthesis (4-aminoimidazole ribonucleotide, AIR) is the precursor for the pyrimidine moiety of thiamin (WHITE and RUDOLPH 1979). One could pursue this theme to more exotic products such as the carbon monoxide of the gas gland of the Portuguese man-of-war (FRIEDKIN 1963), but if one enlarges the field of view to encompass all purine nucleotides, including adenosine triphosphate (ATP) then the scope of folate-catalyzed reactions indeed becomes enormous. In higher species, many of the products produced in autotrophic organisms have become essential nutritional elements, e.g. folic acid, riboflavin, and pantothenic acid. Many of the products of the reactions surviving evolutionary change are known, and also can be assimilated preformed (e.g., methionine, purines, and thymidine). In spite of this knowledge, however, no one has yet succeeded in maintaining a mammal using end products alone; it has not yet been possible to bypass completely a block of dihydrofolate reductase maintained with excess methotrexate, although this is possible in cultured cells (PINEDO et al. 1976; SEMON and GRINDEY 1978).

D. Origins of Cellular Folates

Folates arise in two different ways in higher and lower organisms, as has been stated in the preceeding sections. This difference has profound implications for chemotherapy, especially for the action of sulfonamides. The biosynthesis of folates in microorganisms and the inhibitory activity of sulfonamides are dealt with in Chap. 2, and have been described in a number of articles on trimethoprim sulfamethoxazole (TMP/SMX) synergism (HITCHINGS 1962; BUSHBY and HITCHINGS 1968; HITCHINGS and ROTH 1980). Equally, or perhaps even more fundamentally important for the action of sulfonamides, is the fact that most pathogens are unable to utilize preformed folates. Perhaps the strangest case of all is that of plasmodia, which engulf folate-rich erythrocyte substance, but are unable to utilize the preformed folate present and synthesize dihydrofolate de novo from p-aminobenzoic acid (pABA) (HITCHINGS 1978). Pathogenic bacteria are no better. They live in an environment that contains ample folic acid for their growth, but are unable to use it. They do use pABA and synthesize folates from it, but pteroylglutamate (PGA) will not substitute for its precursor in organisms like *E. coli* and *Staphylococcus aureus* (LASCELLES and WOODS 1952; LAMPEN et al. 1946). The problem may very well lie in the difficulty of transporting the p-aminobenzoylglutamate (pABG) moiety since it was found very early that pABG could not reverse the effects of sulfanilamide in a number of pathogenic microorganisms in which pABA was active (WILLIAMS 1944). Since RICHEY and BROWN (1969) later found pABG to be converted to PGA by extracts of some of the same organisms, a failure of uptake is indicated.

Folate transport systems exist, not only in eukaryotic cells, but in a few prokaryotes as well. With the exception of some streptococci, these generally are not pathogens, and generally the utilization of exogenous folates and synthesis de novo are alternatives. In the course of evolution, deletion of the biosynthetic pathway necessarily would have occurred only when ample folates were available preformed, and the means for their utilization had developed. Such utilization seems to depend in the first instance on the occurrence of active transport mechanisms.

E. Transport Systems

The folate transport systems of prokaryotes were recognized first and have provided models for studies of the transport in eukaryotic cells (HUENNEKENS et al. 1978). *Lactobacillus casei* factor (SNELL and PETERSON 1940) was recognized later as pteroylglutamic acid. The ability of the organism to grow on low concentrations of the vitamin became the basis for a variety of assay (BLAKLEY 1969) and testing (HITCHINGS et al. 1950) procedures, and presumptive evidence for concentrative uptake of the vitamin. This was first examined carefully with the analogous *Streptococcus faecalis* (now *faecium*). WOOD and HITCHINGS (1959) compared the uptake of folic acid, folinic acid, aminopterin, and pyrimethamine. The vitamins and aminopterin were shown to be assimilated by an active transport mechanism which is dependent on glucose, whereas pyrimethamine entered the bacterial cells by passive diffusion (WOOD et al. 1961). Trimethoprim, like its relative pyrimethamine, seems to enter cells by passive diffusion. Its concentration in the cytosol of *E. coli*, for example, approximates that in the medium (P. RAY, personal communication, 1980). A somewhat higher concentration may exist in the immediate vicinity of the cell wall (possibly bound to DHFR).

Pediococcus cerevisiae (formerly called *Leuconostoc citrovorum*) is of particular interest because its specific requirements led ultimately to an understanding of its fastidious nutritional needs and to recognition of the dual transport systems involved with aromatic and reduced folic acid and the analogs, aminopterin and methotrexate. *Pediococcus cerevisiae* was first noticed because it would grow only on a substance (citrovorum factor) that soon was recognized as a reduced form of folate. Its uptake system dealt only with tetrahydrofolates. It concentrates 5-methyl-FAH_4 (which it cannot metabolize) quite as well as 5-formyl-FAH_4, which supports growth. The reduced folates were concentrated 140- and 80-fold respectively, by a system dependent on glucose. Folate did not compete, nor was aminopterin inhibitory (MANDELBAUM-SLAVIT and GROSSOWICZ 1970). However, the organism can grow on very high concentrations of folic acid, and cultures grown this way, after repeated transfers, require less and less folate for growth. In other words, it is possible to select clones which are able to transport folates. At the same time, aminopterin became inhibitory (NICHOL 1968). These findings point to ample DHFR in the cells, later verified by direct studies of cell lines sensitive and resistant to methotrexate (MANDELBAUM-SLAVET and GROSSOWICZ 1974).

I. Selective Rescue

The main point of the foregoing discussion is to emphasize the major difference between these folate-using bacteria and the mainstream of pathogenic bacteria. Whereas eukaryotic cells possess complicated dual transport mechanisms (FRIED-KIN et al. 1973) and intracellular enzymes that can deal with all types of folates, the run-of-the-mill pathogenic bacterium lacks all these refinements and subtleties and so perforce must continue to synthesize dihydrofolate de novo. This renders it sensitive to the effects of sulfonamides, and unable to take advantage of preformed folates when available. The difference between host and parasite in the ability to use preformed FAH_4 was exploited when high dose pyrimethamine was used in the treatment of toxoplasmosis (FRENKEL and HITCHINGS 1957) and in long-term therapy with TMP/SMX (JEWKES et al. 1970). *The ability to "rescue" the host without interfering with the therapeutic effectiveness of the drug* adds another factor in the selectivity of this type of drug. It *should be used whenever folic acid deficiency is suspected or anticipated*. It has not been used as frequently as it should have been in connection with therapy with TMP/SMX.

F. Mechanism of Action of TMP/SMX

The mechanism of action of TMP/SMX is probably better understood than that of any other antimicrobial agent. By "mechanism of action" is meant the factors that contribute to the selectivity of the action of the drug combination. The salient features are shown diagrammatically in Fig. 6. One of the more fundamental is the inability of pathogenic bacteria to use preformed folates. This condemns them to synthesize (dihydro) folate de novo, a reaction in which sulfonamides effectively displace the precursor, p-aminobenzoic acid (pABA). It also prevents them from absorbing and utilizing tetrahydrofolate (FAH_4) which would bypass the inhibitory blocks imposed both by sulfonamides and by trimethoprim. The human organism, on the other hand, lacks the biosynthetic mechanism, and is able to use preformed folates at all levels of oxidation. In the sense of direct biochemical interference, therefore, sulfonamides have no toxicity – the toxicities they exhibit are side reactions irrelevant to their main site of action. The ability of human beings to use preformed FAH_4 combined with the pathogen's inability to do so, adds an ancillary advantage to the host.

DHFR activity is common to almost all living things, but the enzymes that catalzye the reduction of FAH_2 differ dramatically in structure from species to species. The first inklings of this came in the 1950s with observations on the selective actions of various 2,4-diaminopyrimidines, and have become more explicit step-

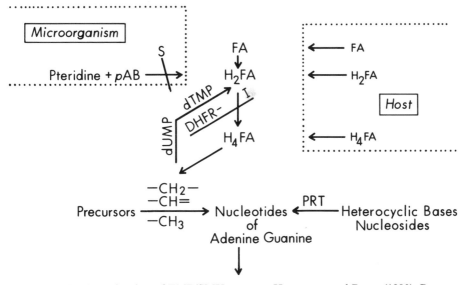

Fig. 6. Mechanism of action of TMP/SMX; see text. HITCHINGS and ROTH (1980). By permission of MacMillan Press Ltd., London

wise to current observations on amino acid sequences and X-ray-determined three-dimensional conformations (HITCHINGS and SMITH 1980). These later investigations deal with the how and why of inhibitor binding. By 1965, BURCHALL and HITCHINGS were able to show that there was an enormous difference in the binding of TMP to the DHFR from *E. coli* compared with the human liver enzyme.

Initially, the potentiation that occurs with combinations of sulfonamides and inhibitors of DHFR was regarded simply as a consequence of sequential blockade in an extended biochemical pathway (HITCHINGS 1962; BUSHBY and HITCHINGS 1968). Sequential blockade is a requisite, but not necessarily a sufficient condition for potentiation. The loop created by the oxidation of FAH_4 to FAH_2 during the biosynthesis of thymidylate is regarded by HARVEY (1978) as a conformation essential to potentiation. However, a rationalization for those not mathematically inclined would point out that blockade of DHFR by a competitive inhibitor such as TMP would be made more effective through the elimination of one of the two sources of FAH_2 – that produced by synthesis de novo which can be blocked by a sulfonamide.

The effects of the two inhibitors on growth are consistent with their modes of action. Sulfonamides alone stop the production of FAH_2 by competition with pABA (Chap. 6) and, through depletion and cell division, the cellular concentration of FAH_4 falls below the level at which normal activities can continue, and stasis ensues. The drug is bacteriostatic. Trimethoprim is capable of a much more rapid depletion of the cellular FAH_4. Each turnover of thymidylate synthetase traps one folate molecule in the FAH_2 (nonfunctional) state. Trimethoprim alone can be bactericidal, but its potency in this respect is enhanced in the presence of a sulfonamide (SEYDEL et al. 1972).

I. Thymineless Death

Cellular death morphologically resembles thymineless death (ANGEHRN and THEN 1973). The biochemical basis for this is reasonably well understood. Thymineless death results from unbalanced growth when a thymine deficiency occurs in the presence of adequate purine and amino acid concentrations (COHEN and BARNER 1956). A reductase inhibitor could bring this about if methylene-FAH_4 were depleted so rapidly that equilibrium between FAH_4 and the other cofactor forms could not be achieved. A thymineless state could also occur through depletion of FAH_4 in the presence of pools of purines and amino acids (but not thymine) adequate for growth.

The utilization of exogenous purine and amino acids is almost universal; that of thymine is irregular in bacteria, that of thymidine is more consistent, but still not completely universal. Nevertheless, media that contain thymidine are unsuitable for sensitivity testing and generally can be improved by the addition of thymidine phosphorylase which hydrolyzes thymidine to thymine plus ribose-1-phosphate (KOCH and BURCHALL 1971; FERONE et al. 1975; Chap. 4). The thymidine content of human serum fortunately is extremely low (NOTTEBROCK and THEN 1977). The purine content of plasma is relatively more adequate (e.g., HAJASHI and GILLING 1970). It is probably this relative imbalance that favors bactericidal action and thymineless death.

G. Summary

The mechanism of action of TMP/SMX has been described in terms of the biochemical events in which the drugs participate. Sulfonamides inhibit the biosynthesis of dihydrofolate, a biosynthetic reaction present in pathogenic microorganisms, but absent from human subjects. Trimethoprim is a highly selective inhibitor of the enzyme dihydrofolate reductase, very tightly bound to the enzyme from pathogenic bacteria and very weakly bound to that of the human. Tetrahydrofolate exists in the form of cofactors that participate in a number of important biosynthetic reactions. In one of them, thymidylate synthetase, the folate is oxidized to dihydrofolate. The reductase is necessary to restore tetrahydrofolate from the dihydrofolate formed in this way, as well as to reduce that formed de novo by microorganisms. The human, but not the microorganism, can utilize preformed folates.

References

Angehrn P, Then R (1973) Investigations on the mode of action of the combination sulfamethoxazole/trimethoprim. Chemotherapy 19:1–10

Blakley RL (1969) The biochemistry of folic acid and related pteridines. North Holland, Amsterdam London

Buchanan JM, Elford HL, Loughlin RE, McDougall BM, Rosenthal S (1964) The role of vitamin B_{12} in methyl transfer to homocysteine. Ann NY Acad Sci 112:756–773

Burchall JJ, Hitchings GH (1965) Inhibitor binding analysis of dihydrofolate reductases from various species. Mol Pharmacol 1:126–136

Bushby SRM, Hitchings GH (1968) Trimethoprim, a sulfonamide potentiator. Br J Pharmacol 33:72–90

Cleaver JE (1967) Thymidine metabolism and cell kinetics. American Elsevier, New York

Cohen L, MacKenzie RE (1978) Methylenetetrahydrofolate dehydrogenase-methenyltetra-hydrofolate cyclohydrolase-formyl tetrahydrofolate synthetase from porcine liver. Biochim Biophys Acta 522:311–317

Cohen SS, Barner HD (1956) Studies on the induction of thymine deficiency and on the effects of thymine and thymidine analogues in *Escherichia coli*. J Bacteriol 71:588–597

Dev IK, Harvey RJ (1978) A complex of N^5,N^{10}-methylenetetrahydrofolate dehydrogenase and N^5,N^{10}methenyltetrahydrofolate cyclohydrolase in *Escherichia coli*. J Biol Chem 253:4245–4253

Elstner EF, Suhadolnik RJ (1971) The biosynthesis of nucleoside antibiotics. IX Purification and properties of guanosine triphosphate 8-formyl hydrolase that catalyzes production of formic acid from the ureido carbon of guanosine triphosphate. J Biol Chem 246:6973–6981

Ferone R, Bushby SRM, Burchall JJ (1975) Identification of Harper-Causton factor as thymidine phosphorylase and removal from media of substances interfering with susceptibility testing to sulfonamides and diaminopyrimidines. Antimicrob Agents Chemother 7:91–98

Finkelstein JD (1979) Regulation of methionine metabolism in mammals. In: Usdin E, Borchardt RT, Creveling GR (eds) Transmethylation. Elsevier/North Holland, New York, pp 49–68

Frenkel JK, Hitchings GH (1957) Relative reversal by vitamins (para-aminobenzoic, folic and folinic acids) of the effects of sulfadiazine and pyrimethamine on toxoplasma, mouse and man. Antibiot Chemother 7:630–638

Friedkin M (1963) Enzymatic aspects of folic acid. Annu Rev Biochem 32:185–214

Friedkin M (1973) Thymidylate synthetase. Adv Enzymol 38:235–292

Hartman SC, Buchanan JM (1959) Biosynthesis of the purines. XXVI. The identification of the formyl donors of the transformylation reactions. J Biol Chem 234:1812–1816

Harvey RJ (1978) Interaction of two inhibitors which act on different enzymes of a metabolic pathway. J Theor Biol 74:411–437

Hajashi TT, Gilling B (1970) A method for determining plasma levels of oxypurines. Anal Biochem 36:343–351

Hiatt HH, Goldstein M, Tabor H (1958) Urinary excretion of formiminoglutamic acid by human subjects after antifolic acid therapy. J Clin Invest 37:829–832

Hitchings GH (1962) The utilization of biochemical differences between host and parasite as a basis for chemotherapy. In: Goodwin LE, Nurimo-Smith RH (eds) Drugs, parasites, and hosts. Churchill, London, pp 196–210

Hitchings GH (1975) The Bertner Foundation Memorial Award Lecture – Salmon, butterflies and cancer chemotherapy. In: Pharmacological basis of cancer chemotherapy. Williams and Wilkins, Baltimore, pp 25–43

Hitchings GH (1978) The metabolism of plasmodia and the chemotherapy of malarial infections. In: Wood C (ed) Tropical medicine from romance to reality. Academic Press, London, pp 79–98

Hitchings GH, Roth B (1980) Dihydrofolate reductases as targets for selective inhibitors. In: Sandler M (ed) Enzyme inhibitors as drugs. Macmillan, London, pp 263–280

Hitchings GH, Smith SL (1980) Dihydrofolate reductases as targets for inhibitors. In: Weber G (ed) Adv Enzyme Regul. Pergamon, Oxford New York, pp 349–371

Hitchings GH, Elion GB, Falco EA, Russell PB, Sherwood MB, Vanderwerff H (1950) Antagonists of nucleic acid derivatives. I. The *Lactobacillus casei* model. J Biol Chem 183:1–9

Huennekens FM, Vitols VS, Henderson GB (1978) Transport of folate compounds in bacterial and mammalian cell. In: Weber G (ed) Adv Enzymol 47:313–346

Jewkes RF, Edwards MS, Grant BJB (1970) Hematological changes in a patient on long-term treatment with a trimethoprim-sulphonamide combination. Postgrad Med J 16:723–726

Koch AE, Burchall JJ (1971) Reversal of the antimicrobial activity of trimethoprim by thymidine in commercially prepared media. Appl Microbiol 22:812–817

Lampen JO, Roepke RR, Jones MJ (1946) The replacement of *p*. aminobenzoic acid in the growth of a mutant strain of *Escherichia coli*. J Biol Chem 164:789–790

Lascelles J, Woods DD (1952) The synthesis of "folic acid" by *Bacterium coli* and *Staphylococcus aureus* and its inhibition by sulfonamides. Br J Exp Pathol 33:288–303

MacKenzie RE, Baugh CM (1980) Tetrahydropteroylpolyglutamate derivatives as substrates of two multifunctional proteins with folate-dependent enzyme activities. Biochim Biophys Acta 611:187–195

Mailänder B, Bacher A (1976) Biosynthesis of riboflavin. J Biol Chem 251:3623–3628

Mandelbaum-Slavit F, Grossowicz N (1970) Transport of folinate and related compounds in *Pediococcus cerevisiae*. J Bacteriol 104:1–7

Mandelbaum-Slavit F, Grossowicz N (1974) Dihydrofolate reductase in *Pediococcus cerevisiae* strains susceptible and resistant to amethopterin. Antimicrob Agents Chemother 6:369–371

Matthews DA, Alden RA, Bolin JT, Filman DJ, Freer StT, Hamlin R, Hol WGJ, Kislink RL, Pastore EJ, Plante LT, Xuong N-H, Kraut J (1978) Dihydrofolate reductase from *Lactobacillus casei*. X-ray structure of the enzyme methotrexate NADPH complex. J Biol Chem 253:6946–6954

Mitsuda H, Hakajima K, Nadamoto T (1977) The immediate nucleotide precursor, guanosine triphosphate, in the riboflavin biosynthetic pathway. J Nutr Sci Vitaminol (Tokyo) 23(1):23–34

Nichol CA (1968) Studies on dihydrofolate reductase related to the drug sensitivity of microbial and neoplastic cells. In: Weber G (ed) Adv Enzyme Regul 6:305–322

Nottebrock H, Then R (1977) Thymidine concentrations in serum and urine of different animal species and man. Biochem Pharmacol 26:2175–2179

Paukert JL, Strauss LDA, Rabinowitz JC (1976) Formyl methenyl-methylene tetrahydrofolate-synthetase-(combined). An ovine protein with multiple catalytic activities. J Biol Chem 251:5104–5111

Peters JM, Greenberg DM (1957) Studies on the conversion of citrovorum factor to a serine aldolase cofactor. J Biol Chem 226:329–338

Pinedo HM, Zaharko DS, Bull JM, Chabner BA (1976) The reversal of methotrexate toxicity to mouse bone marrow cells by leucovorin and nucleotides. Cancer Res 36:4416–4424

Rabinowitz JC (1960) Folic acid. Enzyme 2:185–252

Rabinowitz JC, Himes RH (1960) Folic acid coenzymes. Fed Proc 19:963–970

Rader JI, Huennekens FM (1973) Folate-coenzyme-mediated transfer of one-carbon groups. In: Boyend PD (ed) The enzymes IX. Academic Press, New York, pp 197–223

Reynolds JJ, Brown GM (1964) The biosynthesis of folic acid. IV. Enzymatic synthesis of dihydrofolic acid from guanine and ribose compounds. J Biol Chem 239:317–325

Richey DP, Brown GM (1969) The biosynthesis of folic acid. IX. Purification and properties of the enzymes required for the formation of dihydropteroic acid. J Biol Chem 244:1582–1592

Roth B, Hultquist ME, Fahrenbach MJ, Cosulich DB, Broquist HP, Brockman JA, Smith JM, Parker RP, Stokstad ELR, Jukes TH (1952) Synthesis of leucovorin. J Am Chem Soc 74:3247–3252

Schirch LV (1970) Formyl-methenyl-methylenetetrahydrofolate synthetase from rabbit liver (combined). Evidence for a single site in the conversion of 5,10-methylenetetrahydrofolate to 10-formyltetrahydrofolate. Arch Biochem Biophys 189:283–290

Semon JH, Grindey GB (1978) Potentiation of the antitumor activity of methotrexate by concurrent infusion of thymidine. Cancer Res 38:2905–2911

Seydel JK, Wempe E, Miller GH, Miller L (1972) Kinetics and mechanisms of action of trimethoprim and sulfonamides, alone or in combination, upon *Escherichia coli*. Chemotherapy 17:217–258

Snell EE, Peterson WH (1940) Growth factors for bacteria. X. Additional factors required by certain lactic acid bacteria. J Bacteriol 39:273–285

Tabor H, Rabinowitz JC (1956) Intermediate steps in the formylation of tetrahydrofolic acid by formiminoglutamic acid in rabbit liver. J Am Chem Soc 78:5705–5706

Tabor H, Wyngaarden L (1959) The enzymatic formation of formiminotetrahydrofolic acid, 5,10-methenyltetrahydrofolic acid, and 10-formyltetrahydrofolic acid in the metabolism of formiminoglutamic acid. J Biol Chem 234:1830–1846

Tan LUL, MacKenzie RE (1979) Methylene tetrahydrofolate dehydrogenase-methanyl-tetrahydrofolate cyclohydrolase-formyltetrahydrofolate synthetase from porcine liver. Location of the activities in two domains of the multifunctional polypeptide. Can J Biochem 57:806–812

Tan LUL, Drury EJ, MacKenzie RE (1977) Methylenetetrahydrofolate dehydrogenase-methenyltetrahydrofolate cyclohydrolase-formyltetrahydrofolate synthetase. A multifunctional protein from porcine liver. J Biol Chem 252:1117–1122

Taylor RT, Weissbach H (1973) N^5Methyltetrahydrofolate-homocysteine methyl transferase. In: Boyer PD (ed) The enzymes IX. Academic Press, New York London, pp 121–165

Teller JH, Powers SG, Snell EE (1976) Ketopantoate hydroxymethylase. I. Purification and role in pantotherate biosynthesis. J Biol Chem 251:3780–3785

Turner AJ (1979) The role of folates in adenosyl methionine biosynthesis and metabolism. In: Usdin E, Borchardt RT, Creveling CR (eds) Transmethylation. Elsevier/North Holland, New York, pp 69–76

White RH, Rudolph FB (1979) Biosynthesis of the pyrimidine moiety of thiamin in *Escherichia coli*. Incorporation of stable isotope-labeled glycines. Biochemistry 18:2632–2636

Williams RD (1944) The comparative antisulfanilamide activity of p-aminobenzoyl-1(+) glutamic acid and p-aminobenzoic acid. J Biol Chem 156:85–89

Wood RC, Hitchings GH (1959) A study of the uptake and degradation of folic acid, citrovorum factor, aminopterin, and pyrimethamine by bacteria. J Biol Chem 234:2381–2385

Wood RC, Ferone R, Hitchings GH (1961) The relationship of cellular permeability to the degree of inhibition by amethiopterin and pyrimethamine in several species of bacteria. Biochem Pharmacol 6:113–124

CHAPTER 2

Sulfonamides: Structure-Activity Relationships and Mechanism of Action

N. ANAND

A. Introduction

The discovery of the antibacterial activity of prontosil (1) in the early 1930s (DOMAGK 1935, 1957), the first effective chemotherapeutic agent to be employed for the systemic treatment of bacterial infection in humans (FOERSTER 1933), was the beginning of the present era of chemotherapy. The history of the development of sulfonamides as a major class of chemotherapeutic agents is one of the most fascinating chapters in drug research, highlighting the roles of skilful planning and serendipity. The synthesis of prontosil (1) was a carry-over of the interest generated in dyes in general as possible antimicrobials as a result of EHRLICH's studies on the relationship between selective staining by dyes and their antiprotozoal activity, and in the sulfonamide group as contributory to fastness for acid wool dyes as a result of the work of HORLEIN, DRESSEL and KETHE of I.G. Farbenindustrie (see MIETZSCH 1938), which led MIETZSCH and KLARER (1935) to synthesize a group of azo dyes containing a sulfonamide group, which included prontosil. The lack of correlation between in vitro and in vivo antibacterial tests prompted DOMAGK (1935) to resort to in vivo testing, a very fortunate decision, since otherwise the fate of sulfonamides might have been different. In fact, similar dyes had been synthesized almost a decade earlier, such as p-sulfonamidobenzeneazodihydrocupreine (HEIDELBERGER and JACOBS 1919), but tested in vitro, and thus understandably showing rather poor activity.

DOMAGK (1935) observed that prontosil protected mice against streptococcal infections and rabbits against staphylococcal infections, but had no effect on pneumococcal infections and was without action in vitro on bacteria. FOERSTER (1933) reported the first clinical success with prontosil in a case of staphylococcal septicaemia.

These epoch-making results, published between 1933 and 1935, aroused worldwide interest, and further developments took place at a very fast rate. TREFOUËL et al. (1935), working at the Pasteur Institute in Paris, prepared a series of azo dyes by coupling diazotized sulfanilamide with phenols, with and without amino or alkyl groups. They observed that variations in the structure of the phenolic moiety had very little effect on in vitro antibacterial activity, whereas even small changes in the sulfanilamide component abolished the activity. These observations pointed to the sulfanilamide component as the active structural unit and led to the conclusion that prontosil was converted in animals to p-aminobenzenesulfonamide [sulfanilamide, (2)]. They tested sulfanilamide and found that it was as effective as the parent dye-stuff in protecting mice infected with streptococci. They also showed that sulfanilamide exerted a bacteriostatic effect in vitro on susceptible organisms. Soon after, COLEBROOK and KENNY (1936) observed that, although prontosil was inactive in vitro, the blood of patients treated with it had bacteriostatic activity. They also reported the dramatic cure of 64 cases of puerperal sepsis by prontosil, while BUTTLE et al. (1936) showed that sulfanilamide could cure streptococcal and meningococcal infections in mice. FULLER's (1937) demonstration of the presence of sulfanilamide in the blood and its isolation from urine of patients (and mice) under treatment with prontosil firmly established that prontosil is reduced in the body to form sulfanilamide (2), a compound synthesized as early as 1908 by GELMO. The era of modern chemotherapy had begun.

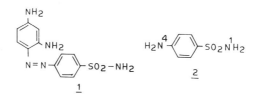

Some of the other developments resulting from this momentous discovery that had far-reaching effects on future progress, not only in the field of sulfonamides but on chemotherapy and drug research in general, may be mentioned. The standardization of a simple method for the assay of sulfonamides in body fluids and tissues (MARSHALL 1937; BRATTON and MARSHALL 1939) permitting precise determination of the absorption, distribution and excretion of these drugs, provided a rational basis for calculating the proper dosage requirements. Pharmacokinetic studies thus became an integral part of drug development programmes. WOODS' (1940) observation of the competitive reversal of the action of sulfanilamide by p-aminobenzoic acid (pABA) was the first definite demonstration of metabolite antagonism as a mechanism of drug action. The elucidation of this relationship provided the long sought-after mechanistic basis for a rational approach to chemotherapy, and led FILDES (1940) to propose his classical theory of antimetabolites, which has been the basis of numerous and intensive studies in chemotherapy and pharmacology. The development of dihydrofolate reductase inhibitors as antimicrobial agents was a direct result of this interest generated in antimetabolites (see HITCHINGS and BURCHALL 1965); their synergistic action with sulfonamides has added a new dimension to the clinical usefulness of sulfonamides.

B. Development of Sulfonamides and Sulfones

I. Sulfonamides

The demonstration that the antimicrobial activity of prontosil (1) was due to its metabolic reduction to sulfanilamide (2) was a most important event in this field. Sulfanilamide, being easy to prepare, cheap, and not covered by patents, became available for widespread use and brought a new hope for the treatment of microbial infections. Recognizing the potentiality of sulfonamides, almost all the major research organizations the world over initiated research programmes for the synthesis and study of analogues and derivatives of sulfanilamide, particularly with a view to: (i) enlarging the antimicrobial spectrum; (ii) improving the therapeutic index; (iii) increasing permeability and distribution in the body fluids and tissues; (iv) increasing half-life to reduce the frequency of administration; (v) increasing water solubility, both of the parent compound and its metabolites to reduce tendency to crystalluria and reduce toxicity; and (vi) delaying emergence of resistant forms and improving activity against resistant organisms. The analogues studied included position isomers, compounds having substituents on the functional groups, isosteres and ring annellates of the benzene ring. It was realized quite early that the p-aminobenzenesulfonyl unit is essential for maintaining the activity. Therefore, almost all the emphasis in later studies was laid on preparing N^1-substituted derivatives, many of which were found to possess vastly improved antimicrobial activity. The more important N^1-substituted derivatives of sulfonamides which were found useful clinically belonged to N^1-heterocycle and N^1-acyl class.

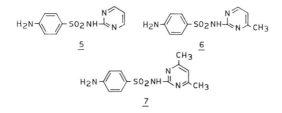

By varying the N^1-heterocyclic residue, it was possible to enlarge the usefulness of sulfonamides greatly. Sulfapyridine (3) reported in 1938, was one of the earliest new sulfonamides to be used in clinical practice for treatment of pneumonia, and remained the drug of choice till it was replaced by sulfathiazole (4), which possessed a higher therapeutic index. Sulfathiazole was in turn replaced by sulfadiazine (5), which has retained a prominent position among the sulfonamides ever since, because of its broad antibacterial spectrum, high in vivo activity, low toxicity and (subsequently discovered) relatively long duration of action. Two methylated derivatives of sulfadiazine, sulfamerazine (6), and sulfamethazine (7) were soon introduced in therapeutics. Sulfamerazine has greater solubility in water at pH 7.0,

is more quickly absorbed and more slowly excreted than sulfadiazine. Sulfamethazine is even more soluble than sulfamerazine at pH 5.5; though less active in vitro and in vivo than sulfadiazine and sulfamerazine, this property gives it a greater tolerance and some clinical advantage over the other two. Since these quantitative differences of the three sulfapyrimidines seemed to complement one another, they have been used in combination as a "triple sulfa," which made it possible to lower the dose of each individual component, thus reducing the toxicity of each and lowering significantly the tendency to crystalluria, improving the tolerance and activity and maintaining a higher total concentration in plasma and tissues over a longer period. The other clinically used N^1-heterocyclic sulfas of this period include sulfamethizole (8) and sulfisoxazole (9). Sulfamethizole has a relatively low minimum inhibitory concentration (MIC), high solubility, quick absorption and rapid excretion and finds use in kidney and urinary tract infections. Sulfisoxazole has significant activity against *Proteus vulgaris* and *Escherichia coli*. Though it is less active than sulfadiazine, in view of its high solubility and rapid excretion, it is also used in urinary tract infections.

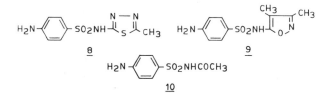

N^1-Acyl substitution leads to compounds which form highly soluble non-irritant neutral sodium salts, as opposed to highly basic salts formed by normal sulfonamides. The most important member of this group is sulfacetamide (10), which is quickly absorbed and rapidly excreted without danger of crystallization in the kidney. It is widely used in ophthalmic practice.

New sulfonamides were thus introduced in quick succession till about 1945 when, with the introduction of penicillin, interest gradually shifted to antibiotics. After about a decade, problems encountered with antibiotics, such as emergence of resistant strains, superinfection, and allergic reactions, brought a revival of interest in sulfonamides. Thus there are two distinct phases in the development of sulfonamides, the old (pre-1945) and the new (post-1955). The knowledge obtained during this period about the selectivity of action of sulfonamides on the parasite, the relationship between their solubility and toxicity, pharmacokinetics, and dose relationships, and that some sulfonamides were rapidly absorbed but slowly excreted, resulting in maintenance of adequate blood level for long periods, gave a new direction to further developments in this field; new sulfonamides with modified properties began to appear. Sulfamethoxypyridazine [(11), NICHOLS et al. 1956] was the first long-acting sulfonamide (half-life 37 h), to be introduced in clinical practice and needed to be administered once a day (WEINSTEIN et al. 1960). It was realized that some of the "older" sulfonamides such as sulfadiazine (5) and sulfamerazine (6) had a long half-life too (17 and 24 h respectively), and required much less frequent administration than was normally prescribed; it became obvi-

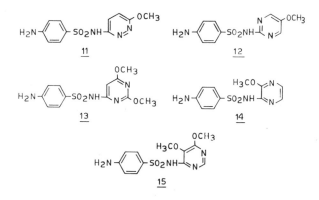

ous that the toxicity observed in earlier use with these drugs was often due to gross overdosage. Sulfamethoxydiazine [(12), half-life 35 h; HORSTMANN et al. 1961], sulfadimethoxine [(13), half-life 40 h; BRETSCHNEIDER et al. 1961; FUST and BÖHNI 1959; BÖHNI et al. 1969], sulfamethoxypyrazine [(14), half-life 65 h; CAMERINO and PALAMIDESSI 1960], and sulformethoxine [(15), half-life 150 h; HITZENBERGER and SPITZKY 1962; REBER et al. 1964] are amongst the other long-acting sulfonamides introduced during this period; sulformethoxine because of its ultra-long half-life needs to be administered only once a week and forms a very suitable combination with pyrimethamine in the treatment and prophylaxis of malaria (HITCHINGS and BURCHALL 1965).

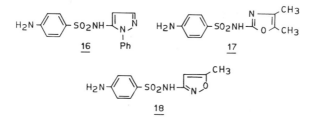

However, not all the sulfonamides discovered and introduced into clinical practice during this period have a long half-life; three such sulfonamides are sulfaphenazole [(16), TRIPOD et al. 1960], sulfamoxole [(17), DEININGER and GUTBROD 1960], and sulfamethoxazole [(18), FUST and BÖHNI 1962] having a half-life of 11 h. Sulfamethoxazole (18) is amongst the sulfonamides with the broadest antibacterial spectrum and the lowest MIC. On account of this fact and the matching half-life of sulfamethoxazole and trimethoprim, in clinical practice this is the most commonly used sulfa–dihydrofolate reductase inhibitor combination.

II. Sulfones

The demonstration that experimentally induced tuberculosis could be controlled by 4,4′-diaminodiphenylsulfone [dapsone, (19), RIST et al. 1940] and its N,N'-didextrose sulfonate (promin, FELDMAN et al. 1942) was a major advance in the chemotherapy of mycobacterial infections. Although dapsone and promin proved disappointing in the therapy of human tuberculosis, the interest aroused in the possibility of treatment of mycobacterial infections with sulfones led to the demonstration of the favourable effect of promin in rat leprosy (COWDRY and RUANGSIRI 1941). This was soon followed by the successful treatment of leprosy patients, first with promin and later with dapsone itself; dapsone has remained since then the drug of choice for the treatment of human leprosy (BROWNE 1969 a). An important advance in the use of sulfones took place with the demonstration that certain N,N'-diacyl derivatives and SCHIFF's bases of dapsone have a repository effect and re-

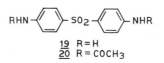

19 R = H
20 R = COCH₃

lease dapsone slowly. *N,N′*-Diacetamidodiphenylsulfone [acedapsone, (20)] is particularly useful as a repository form (ELSLAGER and WORTH 1965; ELSLAGER 1974); after a single intramuscular injection of 225 mg acedapsone, a therapeutic level of dapsone is maintained in the blood for as long as 68–80 days (SHEPARD et al. 1968).

III. Antimicrobial Spectrum

The antimicrobial activity of sulfonamides and sulfones extends to a number of microbial species having a folic acid pathway, which includes many gram-positive and gram-negative cocci and bacilli, mycobacteria, some large viruses, protozoa and fungi. In all cases their action is related to pABA antagonism. Their antibacterial spectrum is quite broad. Individual sulfonamides do differ in their antibacterial spectrum, but these differences are more quantitative than qualitative. The organisms most susceptible to sulfonamides include pneumococci, streptococci, meningococci, staphylococci, some coliform bacteria and shigellae, and lepra bacilli to sulfones. They have a weak activity against bacteria responsible for typhoid fever, diphtheria, and subacute bacterial endocarditis.

The antimalarial activity of sulfonamides and sulfones was noticed quite early (COGGESHALL 1938; COGGESHALL et al. 1941), but little notice was taken of it till the early 1960s when *Plasmodium falciparum* resistance to chloroquine took on a serious dimension. ARCHIBALD and ROSS (1960) investigating the cause of the lower prevalence of malaria in leprosy patients, showed that dapsone could clear the blood of trophozoites of both *P. falciparum* and *P. malariae*, though somewhat more slowly than chloroquine. It was soon found that dapsone potentiated the action of pyrimethamine, and a combination of the two drugs markedly delayed the development of resistance (RAMAKRISHNAN et al. 1962, 1963; BASU et al. 1964), and certain lines of *P. berghei*, *P. cynomolgi*, and *P. gallinaceum* made resistant to either of the drugs alone were still susceptible to the combination (BISHOP 1963; THOMPSON et al. 1965). Human malaria parasites vary greatly in their sensitivity to sulfones; *P. falciparum* is very sensitive, but *P. vivax* is rather weakly so. A number of long-acting sulfonamides such as sulfamethoxypyrazine (14) and sulformethoxine (15) have been shown to possess high antimalarial activity, and their effect is also potentiated by pyrimethamine (PETERS 1974). The action of sulfones and sulfonamides is against only the erythrocytic schizonts.

The observation of the activity of sulfonamides and sulfones against experimental toxoplasmosis (SABIN and WARREN 1941; BIOCCA 1943) and the synergization of this action by pyrimethamine (EYLES 1956; EYLES and COLEMAN 1955) has led to the wide use of this combination in human toxoplasmosis (APT 1970). Sulfonamides have been shown to be effective against *Eimeria* infection in chickens (LEVINE 1939, 1941; JOYNER et al. 1963), and are now commonly used, alone or preferably in combination with pyrimethamine, for the treatment of coccidiosis (KENDALL 1950; KENDALL and JOYNER 1958).

McCALLUM and FINDLAY (1938) showed that the "large virus" of *lymphogranuloma venereum* in mice was susceptible to sulfonamides. Later, other chlamydiae were also found to be inhibited by sulfonamides, which led to the successful clinical use of these drugs in the treatment of trachoma (TARIZZO 1972). Sulfonamides were also found to have marked activity in vitro against *Nocardia asteroides*

Table 1. Sensitivity of microorganisms to sulfonamides and sulfones

Gram-positive, acid fast	Gram-negative	Others
Highly sensitive		
Bacillus anthracis (some strains)	*Calymmatobacterium granulomatis*	*Chlamydia trachomatis*
Corynebacterium diphtheriae (some strains)	*Hemophilus ducreyi*	*Lymphogranuloma venereum* virus
Mycobacterium leprae	*Hemophilus influenzae*	Trachoma viruses
Staphylococcus aureus	*Neisseria gonorrhoeae*	*Plasmodium falciparum*
Streptococcus pneumoniae	*Neisseria meningitidis*	*Plasmodium berghei*
Streptococcus pyogenes (group A)	*Pasteurella pestis*	*Toxoplasma* spp.
	Proteus mirabilis	Coccidia
	Shigella flexneri	*Actinomyces bovis*
	Shigella sonnei	*Nocardia asteroides*
	Vibrio cholerae	
Weakly susceptible		
Clostridium welchii	*Aerobacter aerogenes*	*Plasmodium vivax*
Streptococcus viridans	*Brucella abortus*	*Plasmodium cynomolgi*
Mycobacterium tuberculosis	*Escherichia coli*	
	Klebsiella pneumoniae	
	Proteus vulgaris	
	Pseudomonas aeruginosa	
	Salmonella spp.	

and are largely used for the treatment of systemic nocardiosis (STRAUSS et al. 1951; CONNAR et al. 1951). Table 1 gives broadly the range of antimicrobial activity of sulfonamides and sulfones.

C. Structure and Biological Activity

Although the story of sulfonamides started with the discovery of their antimicrobial action, subsequent work has established their usefulness also as carbonic anhydrase inhibitors, diuretics, and antidiabetics. Compounds with each type of action possess certain specific structural features (ANAND 1979); modifications that do not alter these essential features only modulate the activity quantitatively. The present discussion is restricted only to the antimicrobial sulfonamides.

I. Structure-Activity Relationship

Antimicrobial sulfonamides (and sulfones) are characterized by their ability to interfere with the biosynthesis of folate coenzymes by competing with pABA for hydroxymethyldihydropterin (see Fig. 1) at the active site of dihydropteroate synthetase. As sulfanilamide (2) is a rather small molecule and there are not too many variations that can be carried out without changing the basic nucleus, the following generalizations regarding structure–activity relationships were arrived at quite early in the development of sulfonamides, which guided the subsequent work on molecular modification, and these generalizations still hold:

1. The amino and sulfonyl radicals on the benzene ring should be in 1,4 disposition for activity; the amino group should be unsubstituted or have a substituent that is removed readily in vivo.

2. Replacement of the benzene ring by other ring systems, or the introduction of additional substituents on it, decreases or abolishes the activity.

3. Exchange of the SO_2NH_2 by $SO_2C_6H_4$-p-NH_2 retains the activity, while exchange by $CONH_2$, COC_6H_4-p-NH_2 markedly reduces the activity.

4. N^1-Monosubstitution results in more active compounds with greatly modified pharmacokinetic properties; N^1-disubstitution in general leads to inactive compounds.

5. These generalizations also apply to sulfones, so that only N-monosubstituted dapsone derivatives retain the full activity.

The presence of a p-aminobenzenesulfonyl radical ($H_2N-\langle\,\rangle-SO_2$-) thus seems essential for maintaining good activity and practically all the subsequent attention was focused on N^1-substituents. These substituents seem to affect mainly the physicochemical, and in consequence the pharmacokinetic characteristics of the drugs. It has been suggested by MORIGUCHI and WADA (1968) that there are two binding sites on the enzyme, located about 6.7–7 Å apart, one being specific for the 4 − NH_2 group and the other non-specific where the acidic group of pABA or sulfonamide moiety binds.

II. Physicochemical Properties and Antimicrobial Activity

As it was realized quite early in the development of this field that any substitution in the benzene ring of sulfanilamide (1) led to lowering or loss of activity, in studies to find a correlation between structure, physicochemical properties and antimicrobial activity, attention was focused primarily on the amino and sulfonamido groups. Several groups of workers almost simultaneously in the early 1940s noted the relationship between bacteriostatic activity and degree of ionization of sulfonamides. The primary amino group in sulfonamides apparently plays a vital part in producing bacteriostasis, since any substituent on it causes complete loss of activity. SEYDEL et al. (1960) and SEYDEL and WEMPE (1964), from a study of the infrared (IR) spectrum and activity of a number of sulfonamides, concluded that the amount of negative charge on the aromatic amino group is significant for the activity. However, variation in activity within a series of compounds cannot be attributed to a change in ionic strength, since all the active sulfonamides (and sulfones) have a basic dissociation constant of about 2, which is close to that of pABA. FOERNZLER and MARTIN (1967) computed the electronic characteristics of 50 sulfonamides by the linear combination of atomic orbitals–molecular orbitals (LCAO–MO) method and found that the electronic charge on the 4-amino group did not vary with a change in the N^1-substituent. Thus, attention has been focused mainly on the acidic dissociation constant, which varies widely from about 3 to 11.

FOX and ROSE (1942) noted that sulfathiazole and sulfadiazine were about 600 times as active as sulfanilamide, against a variety of microorganisms, and that approximately 600 times as much pABA was required to antagonize their action as to antagonize the MIC of each drug. This suggested that the active species in both cases was similar. If only the ionized fraction at pH 7 was considered instead of the total concentration, the pABA:drug ratio was reduced to 1:1.6–6.4. They also observed that with a ten-fold increase in ionization of sulfanilamide on altering the pH from 6.8 to 7.8, there was an eight-fold increase in bacteriostatic activity. On the basis of these observations, Fox and Rose suggested that only the ionized fraction of the MIC is responsible for the antibacterial action. Schmelkes et al. (1942) also noted the effect of pH of the culture medium on the MIC of sulfonamides but suggested that the active agent in a sulfonamide solution is the anionic species.

Bell and Roblin (1942) in a comprehensive study of the relationship between the pK_a of a series of sulfonamides and their in vitro antibacterial activity against *E. coli*, found that the plot of log l/MIC against pK_a was a parabolic curve and that the highest points of this curve lay between pK_a 6 and 7.4; the maximal activity was thus observed in compounds whose pK_a approximated the physiological pH. Since the pK_a values are related to the nature of the N^1-substituent, the value of this relationship was emphasized for predicting the MIC of new sulfonamides. The pK_a of most of the active sulfonamides discovered since then, including the long-acting ones, falls in this range (see Table 2).

Cowles (1942) and Brueckner (1943) suggested that the sulfonamides penetrate the bacterial cell in the un-ionized form, but once inside the cell, the bacteriostatic action is due to the ionized form. Hence for maximum activity, the compound should have a pK_a that gives the proper balance between the intrinsic activity and penetration – the half-dissociated state appeared to present the best compromise between transport and activity. This was in consonance with the parabolic relationship observed by Bell and Roblin (1942) between pK_a and MIC.

Bell and Roblin (1942) laid emphasis on the polarizability of the SO_2 group and related the negative charge of this group to the MIC. Seydel et al. (1960), using IR spectroscopy, and Schnaare and Martin (1965) and Foernzler and Martin (1967), who calculated the electron density of the oxygen atom of the SO_2 group by the LCAO–MO method, could not find any evidence for this correlation. They have, therefore, attached greater importance to the electronic charge on the NH group at position 1. Foernzler and Martin (1967) found a correlation between pK_a, electron density, and MIC against *E. coli* of N^1-arylsulfonamides; this relationship was even more significant when the compounds were classified into smaller groups depending on the nature of the N^1-substituent.

Seydel (1966, 1968), Seydel et al. (1960), and Garrett et al. (1969) found an approximately linear relationship between bacteriostatic activity, Hammett sigma value, and electron density of the nitrogen atom at position 1 for a group of m- and p-substituted sulfanilides and emphasized the possibility of predicting the in vitro antibacterial activity of sulfanilamides by use of this relationship. Later, Seydel (1971 a, b) included in this study 3-sulfapyridines, carried out regression analysis of the data, and obtained a very acceptable correlation coefficient.

Yamazaki et al. (1970), in a study of the relationship between antibacterial activity and pK_a of 14 N^1-heterocyclic sulfanilamides, found that whereas the relationship between pK_a and activity is parabolic when total concentration is considered, it is linear for ionized and un-ionized states, giving two lines with opposite slopes and intersecting each other, the point of intersection corresponding to the pH of the culture medium. They found the pK_a for optimal activity to be between 6.61 and 7.4.

Miller et al. (1972) suggested that the observed parabolic dependence of the antibacterial activity to pK_a indicates that it is not the extracellular ionic concentration that governs the potency of the sulfonamides but rather the intracellular ionic concentration, which, in turn, is limited by the permeation of un-ionized compounds, thus supporting the postulates of Cowles (1942) and Brueckner (1943). They concluded that the lipophilic factors are not important in the cell-free system or for in vitro antibacterial activity when permeability is not limited by ionization.

The intensive work in this field over the last four decades has thus fully supported the conclusions of earlier studies which emphasized the functional relationship between acid dissociation and the antibacterial activity of sulfonamides. The pK_a is related to solubility, partition coefficient, permeability, tubular secretion and reabsorption in the kidneys. This, however, does not mean that the ions of different sulfonamides are equally active; other factors are also involved in explaining the differences in the activity of different sulfonamides such as hydrophobicity and affinity for the target enzyme.

In some recent studies on correlation of physicochemical properties with activity, therefore, additional parameters have been included, such as Hammett sigma values and hydrophobicity constant. Fujita and Hansch (1967), devised suitable equations for this correlation. In the case of sulfanilides they devised separate equations for the meta- and para-substituted compounds; the correlation for the para-substituted compounds was rather poor. The hydrophobicity of the compounds was also found to play a definite role in the activity.

The activities of sulfaguanidine and sulfones appear to be inconsistent with the ionization theory. This inconsistency is resolved by considering the availability of an electron pair as of critical importance. Sulfaguanidine has been shown by IR and nuclear magnetic resonance (NMR) spectroscopy to prefer the tautomeric structure $H_2NC_6H_4SO_2N=C(NH_2)_2$, represented as a resonance hybrid (Schwenker 1962; Rastelli et al. 1975). The activity of sulfones may be explained similarly when related to the resonance form having high electron availability at the position para to the amino group of the aminophenyl residue.

1. Water Solubility

The clinically used sulfonamides, being weak acids, are, in general, soluble in basic aqueous solutions. As the pH is lowered, the solubility of these N^1-substituted sulfonamides decreases, usually reaching a minimum in the pH range 3–5. This minimum corresponds to the solubility of the molecular species in water (Table 2). With a further decrease in pH, corresponding to that of a moderately strong acid, the sulfa drugs dissolve as cations.

The solubility of sulfonamides in the pH range of human urine (pH 5.5–6.5) is of clinical and toxicological significance because damage to kidneys is caused by crystallization of sulfonamides or their N^4-acetyl derivatives. One of the significant advances in the first phase of sulfonamide research was the development of compounds with greater water solubility, such as sulfisoxazole, which helped to overcome the problem of crystalluria noticed with earlier sulfonamides. However,

Table 2. Characteristics of commonly used sulfonamides and sulfones [a]

Generic name	Common proprietary names	In vitro activity[b] against Escherichia coli (μmol/l)	Water solubility[c] at 25 °C (mg/100 ml)	pK_a	Lipo-solubility (%)	Protein binding at 1.0 μmol/ml (% bound)	Plasma "half-life", human (h)
Sulfamethizole	Methisul, Lucosil	2.15	25 (pH 6.5)	5.5		22	2.5
Sulfisoxazole	Gantrisin, Urosulfin	1.7	35 (pH 6.0)	5.0	4.8	76.5	6.0
Sulfamethazine	Sulfadimidine, Diazil		150 (29 °C)	7.4	82.6	66	7
Sulfacetamide	Albucid	2.3	670	5.4	2.0	9.5	7
Sulfanilamide	Prontalbin	128	750	10.5	71	9	9
Sulfaphenazole	Orisul	1.0	150	6.09	69	87.5	10
Sulfamethoxazole	Gantanol	0.8	Sparingly soluble	6.9	20.5	60	11
Sulfadiazine	Debenal, Pyrimal	0.9	8	6.52	26.4	37.8	17
Sulfamerazine	Debenal M, Pyrimal M	0.95	16 (37 °C)	6.98	62.0	56.8	24
Sulfamethoxydiazine	Sulfameter, Durenat	2.0	Sparingly soluble	7.0	64.0	74.2	37
Sulfamethoxypyridazine	Lederkyn, Kynex	1.0	147 (37 °C, pH 6.5)	7.2	70.4	77	37
Sulfadimethoxine	Madribon	0.7	29.5 (37 °C, pH 6.7)	6.1	78.7	92.3	40
Sulfamethoxypyrazine	Sulfalene, Kelfizina	1.85	Sparingly soluble	6.1		65	65
Sulformethoxine	Sulfadoxine, Fanasil	0.8	Sparingly soluble	6.1	5	95	150
Diaminodiphenylsulfone	Dapsone, Avlosulphon	44	14	13 (pK_b)	13	50[d]	20
Diacetamidodiphenylsulfone	Acedapsone		0.3				43 days (i.m.)

[a] Unless otherwise stated, the data are from RIEDER (1963)
[b] From STRULLER (1968)
[c] From the Merck Index (1976), M. Windholz (ed.), Merck, Rahway, N. J.
[d] Martindale, the Extra Pharmacopoea, 26th edn., N. W. Blacow (ed.). Pharmaceutical Press, London, 1972

apart from the solubility of the parent compounds, the solubility of their N^4-acetyl derivatives, which are the main metabolic products, is of great importance because these are generally less soluble than the parent compounds. The solubility of sulfonamides and their principal metabolites in aqueous media, particularly in buffered solutions and body fluids, therefore, has been the subject of many studies aimed at enhancing our understanding of their behaviour in clinical situations (LEHR 1957; RIEDER 1963).

2. Lipid Solubility

An important factor for the chemotherapeutic activity of sulfonamides and their in vivo transport is the lipid solubility of the undissociated molecule. The partition coefficients measured in solvents of different dielectric constants (RIEDER 1963; GARRETT et al. 1969), and chromatographic R_m values in a number of thin layer chromatography systems (BIAGI et al. 1974) have been used to determine the lipid solubility and hydrophobicity constant. Lipid solubility of different sulfonamides (Table 2) varies over a considerable range. These differences unquestionably influence their pharmacokinetics and antibacterial activity. It has been noted by RIEDER (1963) and STRULLER (1968) that long-acting sulfonamides with a high tubular reabsorption are generally distinguished by a high degree of lipid solubility.

3. Protein Binding

Binding to proteins appears to have an important role in the action of sulfonamides. The unbound fraction of the drug in plasma seems to be significant for activity, toxicity, and metabolism, whereas protein binding appears to modulate the availability of the drug, its tissue distribution and half-life. The binding is reversible; thus the active free form is liberated gradually as its level in the blood is gradually lowered. The binding affinity of different sulfonamides varies widely with their structure and with the animal species (RIEDER 1963; SCHOLTAN 1963). In plasma the drug binds predominantly to the albumin fraction. The binding is weak (4–5 kcal/mol) and is easily reversible by dilution. It appears to be predominantly hydrophobic, with ionic binding playing a relatively less significant role (IRMSCHER et al. 1966; FUJITA 1972 a, b). Therefore, the structural features that favour binding are the same as those that increase lipophilicity, such as the presence of alkyl, alkoxy or aryl groups. N^4-Acetyl derivatives are more strongly bound than the parent drug. Introduction of hydroxyl or amino groups decreases protein binding, and glucuronidation almost abolishes it. SEYDEL (1971 b), in a study of the effect of the nature and position of substituents on protein binding and lipid solubility, has shown that among isomers, ortho-substituted compounds have the lowest protein binding. This would indicate that steric factors have a role in protein binding and that N-1 of the sulfonamide is involved. The binding seems to take place at the basic centres of arginine, lysine, and histidine in the proteins (RIEDER 1963). By high resolution NMR spectral studies the locus of binding of several sulfonamides to serum albumin has been shown to involve the benzene ring more than the heterocycle (JARDETZKY and WADE-JARDETZKY 1965).

There have been attempts to establish correlations between physicochemical properties of sulfonamides, their protein binding, and their biological activity.

MARTIN (1965) established a functional relationship between excretion and distribution and binding to albumin, and KRÜGER-THIEMER et al. (1965) have derived a mathematical relationship. MORIGUCHI et al. (1968) observed a parabolic relationship between protein binding and in vitro bacteriostatic activity in a series of sulfonamides, and suggested that too strong an affinity between sulfonamides and proteins would prevent them from reaching their site of action in bacteria. With too low an affinity, they would not be able to bind effectively with enzyme proteins to cause bacteriostasis, assuming that affinity for enzyme proteins is paralleled by affinity to bacterial proteins. In a multiparameter study of a series of N^1-heterocyclic sulfonamides, FUJITA and HANSCH (1967) developed suitable equations by regression analysis and showed that for a series of sulfonamides of closely related structures whose pK_a does not vary appreciably, the binding is governed mainly by the hydrophobicity of the N^1-substituent, which supports the earlier results of SCHOLTAN (1968).

The implications of protein binding for chemotherapeutic activity are not yet fully understood. The factors favouring protein binding are also those that would favour transport across membranes, tubular reabsorption, and increased binding to enzyme proteins. N^4-Acetyl derivatives are more strongly bound to proteins and yet are better excreted. No definite relationship has been found between half-life of sulfonamides and protein binding, although in general it appears that protein binding modulates bioavailability and prolongs the half-life of drugs.

III. Pharmacokinetics and Metabolism

1. Sulfonamides

The sulfonamides in clinical use vary widely in their pharmacokinetic properties (Table 2). Some of them, having additional acidic or basic groups, are not absorbed from the gastrointestinal tract after oral administration, leading to a high local concentration of the drug in that area; they are, therefore, used for enteric infections. A majority of the sulfonamides, however, are well absorbed, mainly from the small intestine, slightly from the large intestine and insignificantly from the stomach. Absorption occurs via the un-ionized form, in proportion to their lipid solubility. In rate and extent of absorption, most sulfonamides behave similarly within the pK_a range 4.5–10.5. After absorption they are fairly evenly distributed in all the body tissues. Those that are highly soluble do not, in general, attain a high tissue concentration, show no tendency to crystallize in the kidney, are more readily excreted, and are useful in treating genitourinary infections. The relatively less soluble ones build up high levels in blood, tissues and extravascular fluids and are useful for treating systemic infections. This wide range of solubilities and pharmacokinetic characteristics of sulfonamides permits their access to almost any site in the body, thus adding greatly to their usefulness as chemotherapeutic agents. The free, non-protein-bound drugs and their metabolic products are ultrafiltered in the glomeruli, then partly reabsorbed. Tubular secretion also plays an important role in the excretion of sulfonamides and their metabolites. The structural features of the compounds have a marked effect on these processes and determine the rate of excretion. The renal clearance rates of the metabolites are generally higher than those of the parent drugs.

Metabolism of sulfonamides takes place primarily in the liver and involves mainly N^4-acetylation, to a lesser extent N^1-glucuronidation and to a very small degree, C-hydroxylation of phenyl and heterocyclic rings and of alkyl substituents, and O- and ring N-dealkylation. N^1-Substituents markedly influence the metabolic fate of the sulfonamides (Table 2); the metabolism also differs markedly in different animal species (WILLIAMS and PARKE 1964; KOIZUMI et al. 1964; KAKEMI et al. 1965; NOGAMI et al. 1968; YAMAZAKI et al. 1968; ADAMSON et al. 1970). Some of the sulfonamides, such as sulfisomidine, are excreted almost unchanged; in most of them N^4-acetylation occurs to a substantial degree, but some of the newer sulfonamides, such as sulfadimethoxine and sulfaphenazole, are excreted mainly as the glucuronide (see also Chap. 7).

FUJITA (1972 b) has performed regression analysis on the rates of metabolism and renal excretion of sulfonamides in terms of their substituent constants. Equations showing the best correlation indicate that the most important factor governing the rate-determining step of the hepatic acetylation is the hydrophobicity of the drug and that pK_a does not play a significant role in this process. The excretion phenomenon seems to be more complex and it would be necessary to take into consideration additional parameters to obtain an acceptable correlation.

2. Sulfones

Dapsone is well absorbed after oral administration, and is evenly distributed in almost all the body tissues. It is excreted mainly through the kidneys. Less than 5% is excreted unchanged, very little N-acetylation takes place, and most of it is present as the mono-N-glucuronide (BUSHBY and WOIWOOD 1955, 1956; ELLARD 1966). Dapsone has a half-life of about 20 h. Acedapsone, following intramuscular injection, is very slowly absorbed and deacetylated. It has a half-life of about 42.6 days. It has been shown that there are marked species differences in the metabolism of dapsone; humans are relatively slow acetylators compared with rhesus monkeys (HUCKER 1970; GORDON et al. 1970). Similarly, mice deacetylate acedapsone efficiently, but rats do not (THOMPSON 1967).

IV. Half-Life

The half-life of sulfonamides is of great importance because the dosage regimen must be related to it. Dose schedule is a function of the inhibitory index and pharmacokinetic parameters. KRÜGER-THIEMER (1966) has developed a mathematical model for the relationship between these parameters and evolved a computer programme for calculating them.

The half-lives of the different clinically used sulfonamides vary widely, from 2.5 to 150 h (Table 2), and also show marked differences in different animal species. RIEDER (1963) correlated the pK_a, liposolubility, surface activity, and protein binding of a group of 21 sulfonamides with their half-life in humans. He found that long-acting sulfonamides were, in general, more lipid soluble than were the short-acting compounds, but no clear-cut relationship could be established; factors such as tubular secretion and tubular reabsorption seem to be involved. In 2-sulfapyrimidines, a 4-methyl group increases the half-life, 4,6-dimethyl reduces it to less than one-half, the corresponding methoxy derivatives have a much longer half-life, and both 5-methyl and 5-methoxy prolong the half-life to the same extent. Similarly, in 4-sulfapyrimidines, the 2,6-dimethyl derivative is short acting, 2,6-dimethoxy is long acting and the isomeric 5,6-dimethoxy is the most persistent sulfonamide known. Sulfamethoxypyridazine has a half-life about twice as long as that of sulfapyrazine. Thus, although no clear-cut pattern of relationship between structure and half-life is discernible, the methoxy group seems to prolong the half-life.

D. Mode of Antimicrobial Action

Sulfonamides are one of the few groups of drugs whose mechanism of action is now known at the molecular level. The discovery that sulfonamides act through inhibiting folic acid synthesis in microorganisms was a culmination of the efforts of many lines of investigation proceeding simultaneously, which included isolation and elucidation of the structure, function and biosynthesis of folic acid, and characterization of p-aminobenzoic acid (pABA) as the factor in yeast extract and other biological fluids responsible for antagonizing the action of sulfonamides.

I. Folic Acid Metabolism

Folic acid is a broadly distributed vitamin of the B-group, which was first detected in the course of studies in tropical macrocytic anaemia (tropical sprue), a disease cured by liver extracts. It was also called vitamin M by DAY et al. (1938) as it was a growth factor for monkeys, vit Bc by PFIFFNER et al. (1943, 1947) on account of its action on the anaemia of chicken, Sfr factor by MITCHELL et al. (1941) on account of its action on the growth of *Streptococcus faecalis (faecium)* R and LC factor (also termed "norite elution factor") on account of its action on the growth of *Lactobacillus casei* (SNELL and PETERSON 1940). The Sfr factor was named folic acid by MITCHELL et al. (1941) indicating its acidic nature and its abundance in green leaves (Latin: *folium* leaf). The vitamin was isolated in crystalline form from liver by PFIFFNER et al. (1943), and its structure established and confirmed by total chemical synthesis (ANGIER et al. 1946) as pteroylglutamic acid. It was soon shown that folic acid was also produced by fermentation in *Streptomyces* culture; the fermentation product was found to be pteroyltriglutamate, which on treatment with sodium hydroxide lost two residues of glutamic acid to form pteroylglutamate, identical with that obtained from liver.

Based on the observation that purines could be converted into pteridines in the presence of glyoxal, ALBERT (1954) suggested that in nature pteridines may be formed from purines. It was noticed both in insect systems and in bacterial cultures, that while radio activity from C-2-labelled purines was incorporated into pteridine moiety, that of C-8-labelled purines was lost, thus indicating imidazole ring opening (ZIEGLER-GUNDER et al. 1956; VIEIRA and SHAW 1961; REYNOLDS and BROWN 1964). The biochemical pathway for folate biosynthesis was worked out with extracts of *E. coli* (BROWN 1971; see Fig. 1); no inconsistencies with the scheme have appeared as other species have been investigated. It begins with the opening of the imidazole ring of guanosine triphosphate (GTP) and proceeds in a multistep sequence, to the formation of 2-amino-4-hydroxy-6-hydroxymethyldihydropteridine (Reynolds and Brown 1964), which condenses with pABA to form dihydropteroate (DHP). The enzymatic system catalyzing this synthesis was separated by Weisman and Brown (1964) in *E. coli* and by Ferone (1973) in *P. berghei* into its two components, dihydropterin pyrophosphokinase and dihydropteroate synthetase; Richey and Brown (1969) have purified the latter enzyme from *E. coli*, virtually free from pyrophosphokinase. In bacteria, an additional enzyme, dihydrofolate synthetase, that adds glutamate to dihydropteroate to form dihydrofolate (DHF), is widely distributed (Griffin and Brown 1964). DHP synthetase can also use p-aminobenzoylglutamate (pABG) as the substrate to form DHF directly. Plasmodia have been shown to possess DHP synthetase (Walter and Königk 1974; McCullough and Maren 1974), but DHF synthetase has not been reported, and plasmodial DHP synthetase will use pABG to produce DHF (Ferone 1973), but the binding of pABG is much poorer than with pABA, as is true with bacterial DHP synthetases (Brown 1971). It has been suggested that DHP synthetase is one single enzyme that can utilize either pABA or pABG (Shiota et al. 1969; Ortiz 1970); Shiota et al. (1969) have suggested that the enzyme may be allosteric. Toth-Martinez et al. (1975) have proposed a multiple enzyme complex for the biosynthesis of folates. They have suggested that the complex, among others, is composed of a glutamate pickup protein, reversibly attached to a pABA pickup protein, which in association with a dihydropteridine pickup protein functions as the enzyme dihydropteroate synthetase.

The enzyme synthesis of dihydropteroate and dihydrofolate was demonstrated in cell-free extracts by Shiota (1959), Shiota and Disraely (1961), and Shiota et al. (1964), using enzymes from *Lactobacillus plantarum* and *Veillonella* spp. and with an enzyme system from *E. coli* by Brown et al. (1961) and Weisman and Brown (1964). It has been noticed that almost all the folate compounds found in microorganisms occur as polyglutamates of pteroic acid. While the first glutamic acid is added to dihydropteroate, the other glutamic acid residues are added at the tetrahydro state of reduction (Robinowitz and Himes 1960). The exact significance of the presence of folates as polyglutamates is not fully understood; the polyglutamates can also serve as coenzymes.

Folic acid and dihydrofolate have no coenzyme activity. They are reduced to 5,6,7,8-tetrahydrofolate, the coenzyme form of folic acid. It has been shown that the cells convert folic acid to tetrahydrofolate in a two-stage reduction involving dihydrofolate as intermediate. Osborn and Huennekens (1958) were the first to isolate from acetone powder extracts of chicken liver, a partially purified NADPH-linked dihydrofolate reductase. Since then this enzyme has been shown to be widely present, both in microbial and mammalian systems.

Several substances related to folic acid have been recognized as formylating species in biological systems. Sauberlich and Baumann (1948) observed that *Leuconostoc citrovorum* required a growth factor (termed citrovorum factor, CF) present in liver and yeast. The CF was found to be more effective than folic acid in reversing the toxicity of aminopterin, and its structure was shown to be N^5-formyltetrahydrofolate (folinic acid, leucovorin). The enzymatic conversion of folinic acid to N^{10}-formyltetrahydrofolate was demonstrated by Greenberg (1954) in pigeon liver extracts; the participation of N^{10}-formyltetrahydrofolate as an intermediate in the enzymatic biosynthesis of folinic acid was shown by NICHOL et al. (1955) in microorganisms. Both groups presented evidence for the participation of N^5,N^{10}-methenyltetrahydrofolate (also called anhydroleucovorin, isoleucovorin) as an intermediate in purine biosynthesis. It thus appears that N^5,N^{10}-formyltetrahydrofolate, and N^5,N^{10}-methenyltetrahydrofolate are interconvertible. On reduction, the latter can form N^5,N^{10}-methylenetetrahydrofolate and N^5-methyltetrahydrofolate, which can also act as one-carbon donors. TABOR and WYNGAARDEN (1954) demonstrated that formyltetrahydrofolate are formed through formiminoamino acids such as formiminoglutamates, catalysed by formiminotransferases.

It is now well accepted that the introduction of one-carbon units in biosynthesis results from a transfer of one-carbon units fixed to folate cofactors onto one-carbon acceptors. As shown in Fig. 1, the pool of one-carbon donors consists of free formate and of their combinations with folate coenzymes at all levels of oxidation, such as methyl, methylene, hydroxymethyl, formyl or formimino groups (FRIEDKIN 1963; HITCHINGS and BURCHALL 1965). (See also Chap. 1.)

II. Action of Sulfonamides and Sulfones

The action of sulfonamides is characterized by a competitive antagonism of certain essential factors vital to the metabolism of microorganisms. Evidence for this antagonism started coming soon after the discovery of sulfonamides. It was found that substances antagonizing their action are present in peptones (LOCKWOOD et al. 1938), various body tissues and fluids, especially after autolysis or acid hydrolysis (MACLEOD 1940), pus (BOROFF et al. 1942), bacteria (STAMP 1939; GREEN 1940), and yeast extract (WOODS 1940; RATNER et al. 1944). WOODS (1940) obtained evidence that pABA is the probable antagonizing factor in yeast extract and showed that pABA could completely reverse the bateriostatic activity of sulfanilamide against various bacteria in vitro. SELBIE (1940) and FINDLAY (1940) soon after found that pABA could antagonize the action of sulfonamides in vivo as well. RUBBO and GILLESPIE (1940) isolated pABA as its benzoyl derivative, and KUHN and SCHWARTZ (1941) obtained it as the methyl ester from yeast extract. BLANCHARD (1941), RUBBO et al. (1941), and McILWAIN (1942) finally isolated pABA itself from these sources. WOODS (1940) suggested that pABA, because of its similarity of structure with sulfanilamide interfered with the utilization of pABA by the enzyme systems necessary for the growth of bacteria. Based on these observations, a more general and clear enunciation of the theory of metabolite antagonism to explain the action of chemotherapeutic agents was given by FILDES (1940) in his famous paper entitled *A Rational Approach to Research in Chemotherapy*.

Further studies showed that the inhibition of growth by sulfonamides in simple media can be reversed not only competitively by pABA, but also non-competitively by a number of compounds not structurally related to pABA, such as *l*-methionine, *l*-serine, glycine, adenine, guanine, and thymine (BLISS and LONG 1941; SNELL and MITCHELL 1943). The relationship of sulfonamides to purines was uncovered by the finding that sulfonamide-inhibited cultures accumulated 4-amino-5-imidazolecarboxamide ribotide (STETTEN and FOX 1945), a compound later shown by SHIVE et al. (1947) and GOTS (1953) to be a precursor of purine biosynthesis.

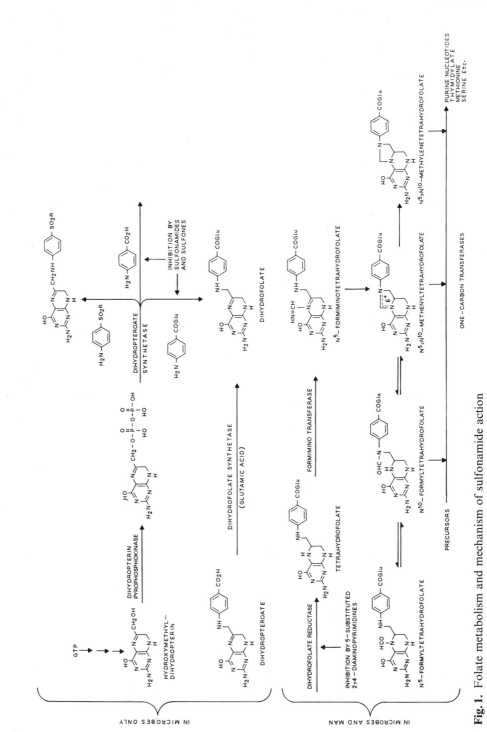

Fig. 1. Folate metabolism and mechanism of sulfonamide action

With the concurrent knowledge obtained on the structure and biosynthesis of folate coenzymes and the elucidation of their involvement (see Sect. D.I) where one-carbon units are added in biosynthesis, these isolated facts could be fitted into a pattern. It became obvious that amino acids, purines, and pyrimidines that were able to replace or spare pABA were precisely those whose formation requires one-carbon addition, catalyzed by folate coenzymes. Following the elucidation of the structure of folic acid, TSCHESCHE (1947) suggested that it is formed by the condensation of pABA or pABG with a pteridine, and that sulfonamides compete in this condensation.

Direct evidence of inhibition of folic acid synthesis by sulfonamides was soon obtained by studies on bacterial cultures. It was already known that a number of organisms could use pABA and folates as alternative essential growth factors (WOODS 1954). LAMPEN and JONES (1946, 1947) found that the growth of some strains of *Streptococcus faecalis*, *Lactobacillus arabinosus*, and *L. plantarum* in media containing pABA was inhibited competitively by sulfonamides, whereas folate caused a non-competitive type of reversal of this inhibition, suggestive of its being a product of the inhibited reaction. Inhibition of folate synthesis by sulfonamides was demonstrated by MILLER (1944) and MILLER et al. (1947) in growing cultures of *E. coli* and by LASCELLES and WOODS (1952) in cultures of *Staphylococcus aureus*, a pABA-requiring mutant of *E. coli* and its parent wild strain. NIMMO-SMITH et al. (1948) showed a similar inhibition of folate synthesis by sulfonamides and its competitive reversal by pABA in non-growing suspension of *L. plantarum*.

The success achieved in carrying out the synthesis of dihydropteroate and dihydrofolate in cell-free extracts, and isolation of enzymes involved therein provided the setting for studying the action of sulfonamides at the molecular level. BROWN (1962) working with enzymes from *E. coli* showed that the synthesis of dihydropteroate from pABA is sensitive to inhibition by a number of sulfonamides, and that in general the more potent inhibitors of folate biosynthesis were better growth inhibitors also. HOTCHKISS and EVANS (1960) have suggested that the differences in the response of various organisms to sulfonamides may be due to quantitative differences in the ability of individual enzymes to produce folic acid from pABA in the presence of sulfonamides. BROWN (1962) in the *E. coli* system and SHIOTA et al. (1964) in the *Veillonella* system found that the relation between a sulfonamide and pABA remained strictly competitive as long as the two compounds were added simultaneously or pABA was added first. If the enzyme and sulfonamide are preincubated with a low concentration of pteridine, the subsequent addition of pABA fails to reverse the inhibition. If, however, a high pteridine concentration is used, preincubation results in a much lesser degree of inhibition. BROWN (1962) showed that the enzyme was not irreversibly inactivated. These results were explained by assuming that the sulfonamide reacts enzymatically with the pteridine substrate during preincubation and were suggestive of its incorporation. Thus, when pABA is added after preincubation with sulfonamide at a low concentration of pteridine, very little pteridine remains, but at a high pteridine concentration there is very little inhibitor left. Using ^{35}S-labelled sulfanilic acid in this enzyme system, BROWN (1962) and WEISMAN and BROWN (1964) obtained evidence of incorporation. Though the nature of the resultant product was not elucidated, it was suggested that it may be a sulfanilic acid analogue of dihydropteroate or the fully aromatic form. BOCK et al. (1974) using ^{35}S-labelled sulfamethoxazole, have confirmed this incorporation by isolating the product formed using partially purified folate-synthesizing enzyme system and in growing cultures of *E. coli*, and identified the product as N^1-3-(5-methylisoxazolyl)-N^4-(7,8-dihydro-6-pterinylmethyl)sulfanilamide [(21), dihydropterinsulfonamide]. Metabolic incorporation of antimetabolites is not unknown.

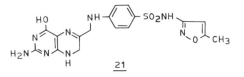

ROLAND et al. (1979) have in a recent study assessed the significance of this incorporation to the antimicrobial action of sulfonamides. The study has shown that inhibition by dihydropterinsulfonamides of dihydropteroate synthetase, or of the other folate enzymes tested, is not physiologically significant. The use of sulfonamides as alternative substrates by this enzyme contributes to growth inhibition only through preventing the accumulation of dihydropteropterine pyrophosphate, which would otherwise occur. Competition with pABA is thus the primary mode of action of sulfonamides. The consequent reduction in the rate of dihydropteroate synthesis decreases the concentration of tetrahydrofolate cofactors in the cell. This prevents or slows down the formation of a number of raw materials of protein, DNA, and RNA biosynthesis, thereby affecting a number of synthetic processes of the organism concurrently, thus reducing the cell growth rate. Sulfonamides inhibit only growing organisms, and the bacteriostasis of the latter is preceded by a lag phase. The lag phase can now be explained as being due to stored pABA and/or folates and its duration is dependent on the quantity stored.

The mechanism of action of dapsone (and other sulfones) is similar to that of sulfonamides, since the action is antagonized by pABA in mycobacteria (BROWNLEE et al. 1948; DONOVICK et al. 1952) as in other bacteria (LEVADITI 1941). The action of diaminodiphenylsulfoxide is similarly antagonized in vivo by pABA (LEVADITI 1941). The action of dapsone (19) against *P. gallinaceum*, like that of sulfonamides (MAIER and RILEY 1942; SEELER et al. 1943) against malarial parasites, is inhibited competitively by pABA and non-competitively by folic acid.

Similarly, in the case of chlamydia, it has been shown that the sulfonamide-sensitive members of this group, such as trachoma and inclusion conjunctivitis agents, have a folic acid metabolism similar to that of bacteria, and that the action of sulfonamides is competitively antagonized by pABA (MORGAN 1948; MOULDER 1962; KURNOSOVA and LENKEVICH 1964).

1. Selectivity of Action

The presence of the folate-synthesizing system has been demonstrated in a number of bacteria (BROWN 1962), protozoa (FERONE 1973; WALTER and KÖNIGK 1974; McCULLOUGH and MAREN 1974), yeasts (JAENICKE and CHAN 1960), and plants (MITSUDA and SUZUKI 1968; IWAI and OKINAKA 1968; OKINAKA and IWAI 1969), which explains the broad spectrum of action of sulfonamides. And since higher or-

ganisms (e.g., mammals) do not possess this biosystem and require pre-formed folate, they are unaffected by sulfonamides. This selectivity of action for the parasite
makes sulfonamides "ideal" chemotherapeutic agents.

III. Synergism with Dihydrofolate Reductase Inhibitors

In an attempt to synergize the action of sulfonamides and to avoid the development
of resistance to them, the most logical approach is to combine them with agents
that block the same metabolic pathway as that blocked by sulfonamides, but at different sites. The elucidation of the folic acid pathway and the demonstration of its
inhibition by both sulfonamides and "antifolates" provided this possibility
(HITCHINGS and BURCHALL 1965; Fig. 1).

GREENBERG (1949) and GREENBERG and RICHESON (1950, 1951) reported that
antifolate aryloxypyrimidines, and diaminopteridines (dihydrofolate reductase inhibitors) potentiate the action of sulfonamides in experimental *P. gallinaceum* infection. Since then, combinations of pyrimethamine (22) and sulfonamides have
been used for the treatment of plasmodial, toxoplasmal, and coccidial infections;
combinations of trimethoprim (23) and sulfonamides have been used for a number
of bacterial infections. This synergism is now recognized as being of general occurrence, and therapy with a combination of dihydrofolate reductase inhibitors and
sulfonamides has added a new dimension to treatment with these agents. This synergism is clearly a consequence of the sequential arrangement of the twin loci of
inhibition. Factors that contribute to the usefulness of such combinations include
several-fold increase in chemotherapeutic index, better tolerance of the drugs, ability to delay development of resistance and ability to produce cures where the curative effects of the individual drugs are minimal. The choice of drugs used in the
combination is based primarily on their half-life characteristics.

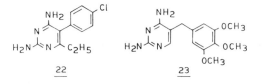

IV. Drug Resistance

Emergence of drug-resistant strains of parasites is one of the principal limitation
of sulfonamide therapy. The development of resistance is considered to arise owing
to one or more of a number of factors such as over-production of pABA (LANDY
et al. 1943; WHITE and WOODS 1965), altered permeability of the organisms to sulfonamides (AKIBA and YOKOTA 1962; PATO and BROWN 1963) and most important
of all to altered sensitivity of DHP synthetase to sulfonamides; the enzyme from
resistant cells has low affinity for sulfonamides and can bind pABA much more
tightly (PATO and BROWN 1963; WOLF and HOTCHKISS 1963; Ho et al. 1974; WISE
and ABOU-DONIA 1975) than the enzyme from the sensitive cells. Different sulfonamides show cross-resistance, but there is no cross-resistance to other antibacterials. Resistant strains develop by random mutation and selection (chromo-

somal) (PATO and BROWN 1963) or by transfer of resistance factors (R factor) by plasmids (extra-chromosomal) from resistant to susceptible strains by conjugation (WATANABE 1963). It has been observed that the frequency of conjugative plasmid encoding single sulfonamide resistance was very low from only sulfonamide-resistant strains, but the non-conjugative sulfonamide-resistant plasmid was demonstrated at a high frequency from strains of Shigella and E. coli carrying non-transferable sulfonamide resistance (MITSUHASHI et al. 1977); the physical properties of these plasmids are very different from those of conjugative multiple-resistance plasmids. It has been shown that there are two types of plasmid-mediated sulfonamide resistance, due to sulfonamide-resistant DHP synthetase making the strains diploid for this enzyme (SKÖLD 1976) and due to decreased permeation of the drug into cells; the latter is mediated only by conjugative plasmids encoding multiple resistance (NAGATE et al. 1978).

In plasmodia, in addition, resistance appears to be due to a bypass mechanism, i.e., ability to use pre-formed folic acid; BISHOP (1959, 1962) has described strains resistant to sulfonamides (and also to pyrimethamine) which can utilize the reduced forms of folic acid available in the host erythrocytes. In spite of the extensive use of sulfones in the mass treatment of leprosy for over 30 years, remarkably few cases of sulfone resistance have so far been reported (BROWNE 1969 b). Resistance may be developed in a stepwise manner (MORRISON 1968) and partial resistance may occur (PEARSON et al. 1968). The mechanism of resistance is not fully elucidated, but it is very likely due to altered sensitivity of the target enzyme.

E. Present Status in Therapeutics

Interest in sulfonamides has continued unabated since their discovery, and about twenty sulfonamides and one sulfone constitute the more largely used drugs of this group. They vary widely in their absorption, distribution, and excretion pattern (Table 2); this wide difference in their pharmacokinetic properties has greatly increased their scope for clinical use. This, coupled with their ease of administration, wide spectrum of antimicrobial action, non-interference with the host defence mechanism, and relative freedom from the problem of superinfection, is responsible for their extensive use in clinical practice, even after almost five decades since their discovery (WEINSTEIN et al. 1960). The demonstration of their synergism with dihydrofolate reductase inhibitors has considerably enlarged their use in therapeutics (GARROD et al. 1969). Sulfonamides are recommended for the prophylaxis of rheumatic fever, for meningococcal meningitis and for Hemophilus influenzae meningitis. They are largely used for the control of bacillary dysentery, particularly that caused by Shigella; their silver salts are used for treatment of burns. The sulfonamides, alone or in combination with trimethoprim, occupy an important place in the treatment of urinary tract infections; this combination has emerged as a useful treatment for salmonellosis and chronic bronchitis. Sulfonamides remain the drugs of choice in the treatment of chancroid, lymphogranuloma venereum, trachoma, inclusion conjunctivitis, and nocardiosis. Combined with pyrimethamine, they are recommended for treatment of toxoplasmosis, coccidiosis and chloroquine-resistant falciparum malaria. Dapsone remains the drug of choice for all forms of leprosy.

References

Adamson RH, Bridges JW, Kibby MR, Walker SR, Williams RT (1970) The fate of sulfa-dimethoxine in primates compared with other species. Biochem J 118:41–45

Akiba T, Yokota T (1962) Studies on the mechanism of transfer of drug resistance in bacteria 18. Incorporation of ^{35}S-sulfathiazole into cells of the multiple resistant strain and artificial sulfonamide resistant strain of *E. coli*. Med Biol 63:155–159

Albert A (1954) The transformation of purines into pteridines. Biochem J 57:X

Anand N (1979) Sulfonamides and sulfones. In: Wolff ME (ed) Burger's medicinal chemistry, 4th edn, Part II. Wiley and Sons, New York, p 1

Angier RB, Boothe JH, Hutchings BL, Mowat JH, Semb J, Stokstad ELR, SubbaRow Y, Waller CW, Cosulich DB, Fahrenbach MJ, Hultquist ME, Kuh E, Northey EH, Seeger DR, Sickels JP, Smith JM Jr (1946) Synthesis of a compound identical with the *L. casei* factor isolated from liver. Science 103:667–669

Apt W (1970) Tratamiento de la toxoplasmosis (in Spanish). Bol Chil Parasitol 25:65–68

Archibald HM, Ross CM (1960) Preliminary report on the effect of diaminodiphenylsulphone on malaria in Northern Nigeria. J Trop Med Hyg 63:25–27

Basu PC, Singh NN, Singh N (1964) Potentiation of activity of diphenylsulfone and pyrimethamine against *P. gallinaceum* and *P. cynomolgi bastianellii*. Bull WHO 31:699–703

Bell PH, Roblin RO Jr (1942) Studies in chemotherapy. VII. A theory of the relation of structure to activity of sulfanilamide type compounds. J Am Chem Soc 64:2905–2917

Biagi GL, Barbaro AM, Guerra MC, Forti GC, Fracasso ME (1974) Relationship between π and Rm values of sulfonamides. J Med Chem 17:28–33

Biocca E (1943) Quimioterapia sulfonica da toxoplasmose (in Portuguese). Arq Inst Biol (Sao Paulo) 27:7–10

Bishop A (1959) Drug resistance in protozoa. Biol Rev 34:445–500

Bishop A (1963) Some recent developments in the problem of drug resistance in malaria. Parasitology 53:10p

Blanchard KC (1941) The isolation of *p*-aminobenzoic acid from yeast. J Biol Chem 140:919–926

Bliss EA, Long PH (1941) Observations on the mode of action of sulfanilamide. The antibacteriostatic action of methionine. Bull Johns Hopkins Hosp 69:14–38

Bock L, Miller GH, Schaper KJ, Seydel JK (1974) Sulfonamide structure activity relationships in a cell-free system 2 Proof for the formation of a sulfonamide-containing folate analog. J Med Chem 17:23–28

Böhni E, Fust B, Reider J, Schaerer K, Havas L (1969) Comparative toxocological, chemotherapeutic, and pharmacokinetic studies with sulformethoxine and other sulfonamides in animals and man. Chemotherapy 14:195–226

Boroff DA, Cooper A, Bullowa JGM (1942) Inhibition of sulfapyridine in human serum, exudates, and transudates. J Immunol 43:341–348

Bratton AC, Marshall EK Jr (1939) A new coupling component for sulphanilamide determination. J Biol Chem 128:537–550

Bretschneider H, Klotzer W, Spiteller G (1961) Zweitsynthese des 6-sulfanilamido-2,4-dimethoxypyrimidins und Synthese des 6-sulfanilamide-2-methoxy-4,5-dimethylpyrimidins. Monatsh Chemie 92:128–134

Brown GM (1962) The biosynthesis of folic acid. Inhibition by sulfonamides. J Biol Chem 237:536–540

Brown GM (1971) The biosynthesis of pteridines. Adv Enzymol 35:35–77

Brown GM, Weisman RA, Molnar DA (1961) The biosynthesis of folic acid. I. Substrate and cofactor requirements for enzymatic synthesis by cell-free extracts of *E. coli*. J Biol Chem 236:2534–2543

Browne SG (1969a) The evaluation of present antileprosy compounds. Adv Pharmacol Chemother 7:211–246

Browne SG (1969b) Dapsone-resistant *M. leprae* in a patient receiving dapsone in low doses. Int J Lepr 37:296–301

Brownlee G, Green AF, Woodbine M (1948) Sulphetrone. A chemotherapeutic agent for tuberculosis. Pharmacology and chemotherapy. Br J Pharmacol 3:15–28

Brueckner AH (1943) The effect of pH on sulphonamide activity. Yale J Biol Med 15:813–821

Bushby SRM, Woiwood AJ (1955) Excretion products of 4:4′-diaminodiphenylsulfone. Am Rev Tuberc Pulm Dis 72:123–125

Bushby SRM, Woiwood AJ (1956) The identification of the major diazotizable metabolite of 4:4′-diaminodiphenylsulphone in rabbit urine. Biochem J 63:406–408

Buttle GAH, Grey WH, Stephenson D (1936) Protection of mice against streptococcal and other infections by p-aminobenzene sulfonamide and related substances. Lancet I:1286–1290

Camerino B, Palamidessi G (1960) Derivati della parazina II. Sulfonamdopir (in Italian). Gazz Chim Ital 90:1802–1815

Coggeshall LT (1938) The cure of P. knowlesi malaria in Rhesus monkeys with sulfanilamide and their susceptibility to reinfection. Am J Trop Med Hyg 18:715–721

Coggeshall LT, Maier J, Best CA (1941) The effectiveness of two new types of chemotherapeutic agents in malaria: sodium p,p′-diaminodiphenylsulphone-N,N′-di-dextrosesulfonate (Promin) and 2-sulfanilamidopyrimidine (sulfadiazine). JAMA 117:1077–1081

Colebrook L, Kenny M (1936) Treatment of human peripheral infections and of experimental infections in mice with prontosil. Lancet 1:1279–1286

Connar RG, Ferguson TB, Sealy WC, Conant NF (1951) Report of a single case with recovery. J Thorac Surg 22:424–426

Cowdry EV, Ruangsiri C (1941) Influence of promin, starch, and heptaldehyde in experimental leprosy in rats. Arch Pathol 32:632–640

Cowles PB (1942) Ionization and the bacteriostatic action of sulfonamides. Yale J Biol Med 14:599–604

Day PL, Langston WC, Darby WJ (1938) Failure of nicotinic acid to prevent nutritional cytopenia in the monkey. Proc Soc Exp Biol Med 38:860–863

Deininger R, Gutbrod H (1960) Die pharmakodynamische Wirkung des neun Sulfonamido, 2-(p-aminobenzol sulfonamido)-4,5-dimethyloxazole. Arzneim Forsch 10:612–619

Domagk G (1935) Ein Beitrag zur Chemotherapie der bakteriellen Infektionen. Dtsch Med Wochenschr 61:250–253

Domagk G (1957) Twentyfive years of sulfonamide therapy. Ann NY Acad Sci 69:380–384

Donovick R, Bayan A, Hamre D (1952) The reversal of the activity of antituberculous compounds in vitro. Am Rev Tuberc Pulm Dis 66:219–227

Ellard GA (1966) Absorption, metabolism and excretion of di-(p-aminophenyl)sulphone (Dapsone) and di(p-aminophenyl)-sulphoxide in man. Br J Pharmacol 26:212–217

Elslager EF (1974) New perspectives on the chemotherapy of malaria, filariasis and leprosy. Prog Drug Res 18:99–172

Elslager EF, Worth DF (1965) Repository antimalarial drugs: N,N′-diacetyl-4,4′-diaminodiphenylsulfone and related 4-acylaminodiphenylsulfones. Nature 206:630–631

Eyles DE (1956) Newer knowledge of the chemotherapy of toxoplasmosis. Ann NY Acad Sci 64:252–267

Eyles DE, Coleman N (1955) An evaluation of the curative effects of pyrimethamine and sulfadiazine, alone and in combination, on experimental mouse toxoplasmosis. Antibiot Chemother 5:529–539

Feldman WH, Hinshaw HC, Moses HE (1942) Promin in experimental tuberculosis. Am Rev Tuberc Pulm Dis 45:303–308

Ferone R (1973) The enzymic synthesis of dihydropteroate and dihydrofolate by Plasmodium berghei. J Protozool 20:459–464

Fildes P (1940) A rational approach to research in chemotherapy. Lancet I:955–957

Findlay GM (1940) The action of sulfanilamide on the virus of Lymphogranuloma venereum. Br J Exp Pathol 21:356–360

Foernzler EC, Martin AN (1967) Molecular orbital calculations on sulfonamide molecules. J Pharm Sci 56:608–615

Foerster R (1933) Sepsis im Anschluß an ausgehende Peritoritis. Heilung durch Streptozon. Zentral Haut Geschlechtskr 45:549–550

Fox CL Jr, Rose MM (1942) Ionisation of sulfonamides. Proc Soc Exp Biol Med 50:142–145

Friedkin M (1963) Enzymatic aspects of folic acid. Ann Rev Biochem 32:185–214

Fujita T (1972a) Hydrophobic bonding of sulfonamide drugs with serum albumin. J Med Chem 15:1049–1056

Fujita T (1972b) Substituent-effect analysis of the rates of metabolism and excretion of sulfonamide drugs. In: Gould RF (ed) Biological correlations – the Hansch approach. American Chemical Society, Washington DC, p 80

Fujita T, Hansch C (1967) Analysis of the structure-activity relationship of the sulfonamide drugs using substituent constants. J Med Chem 10:991–1000

Fuller AT (1937) Is p-aminobenzenesulfonamide an active agent in prontosil therapy? Lancet II:194–198

Fust B, Böhni E (1959) Tolerance and antibacterial properties of 2,4-dimethoxy-6-sulfanilamido-1,3-diazine (Madribon) and some other sulfonamides. Antiobiot Med 6(I):3–10

Fust B, Böhni E (1962) Vergleichende experimentelle Untersuchungen mit 5-Methyl-1,3-Sulfanilamido-Isoxazol, anderen Sulfanilamiden und Antibiotica. Schweiz Med Wochenschr 92:1599–1604

Garrett ER, Mielck JB, Seydel JK, Kessler HJ (1969) Kinetics and mechanisms of action of drugs on microorganisms. VIII. Quantification and prediction of the biological activities of m- and p-substituted N'-phenylsulfanilamides by microbial kinetics. J Med Chem 12:740–745

Garrod LP, James DG, Lewis AAG (1969) The synergy of trimethoprim and sulfonamides. Postgrad Med J [Suppl] 45:1–84

Geimo P (1908) Über Sulfamide der p-Amidobenzolsulphonsäure. J Prakt Chem 77:369–382

Gordon GR, Peters JH, Gelben R, Levy L (1970) Metabolic disposition of dapsone (4,4'-diaminodiphenylsulfone) in animals and man. Proc West Pharmacol Soc 13:17–24

Gots JS (1953) Occurrence of 4-amino-5-imidazolecarboxamide as a pentose derivative. Nature 172:256–257

Green HN (1940) The mode of action of sulfanilamide. Br J Exp Pathol 21:38–64

Greenberg GR (1954) A formylation cofactor. J Am Chem Soc 76:1458–1459

Greenberg J (1949) The antimalarial activity of 2,4-diamino-6,7-diphenylpterin: its potentiation by sulphadiazine and inhibition by pteroylglutamic acid. J Pharmacol Exp Ther 97:484–487

Greenberg J, Richeson EM (1950) Potentiation of the antimalarial activity of sulfadiazine by 2,4-diamino-5-aryloxypyrimidines. J Pharmacol Exp Ther 99:44–449

Greenberg J, Richeson EM (1951) Effect of 2,4-diamino-5-(p-chlorophenoxy)-6-methylpyrimidine and 2,4-diamino-6,7-diphenylpteridine on chlorguanide-resistant strain of Plasmodium gallinaceum. Proc Soc Exp Biol Med 77:174–176

Griffin MJ, Brown MJ (1964) The biosynthesis of folic acid. III. Enzymatic formation of dihydrofolic acid from dihydropteroic acid and of tetrahydropteroylpolyglutamic acid compound from tetrahydrofolic acid. J Biol Chem 239:310–316

Heidelberger M, Jacobs WA (1919) Synthesis in the Cinchona series. III. Azodyes derived from hydrocupreine and hydrocupreidine. J Am Chem Soc 41:2131–2147

Hitchings GH, Burchall JJ (1965) Inhibition of folate biosynthesis and function as a basis for chemotherapy. Adv Enzymol 27:417–468

Hitzenberger G, Spitzky KH (1962) Experimental studies of a new sulfonamide with depot character: sulfamethoxydiazine. Med Klin 57:310–313

Ho RI, Corman L, Morse SA, Artenstein MS (1974) Alterations in dihydropteroate synthetase in cell free extracts of sulfanilamide resistant Neisseria meningitidis and Neisseria gonorrhoeae. Antimicrob Agents Chemother 5:388–392

Horstmann H, Knott T, Scholtan W, Schraufstatter E, Walter A, Worffel U (1961) Beziehungen zwischen Struktur, Wirkung und protein-binding in der 2-Sulfanilamidopyrimidinreihe. Arzneim Forsch 11:682–684

Hotchkiss RD, Evans AH (1960) Fine structure of a genetically modified enzyme as revealed by relative affinities for modified substrate. Fed Proc 19:912–925

Hucker HB (1970) Species difference in drug metabolism. Am Rev Pharmacol 10:99–118

Irmscher K, Gabe D, Jahnke K, Scholtan W (1966) Untersuchungen zur Serumeiweißbildung und zur renalen Elimination von isomeren Sulfonamiden (5-Sulfanilamido-3-athyl-1,2,4-thiodiazol und 5-Sulfanilamido-2-athyl-1,3,4-thiodiazol. Arzneim Forsch 16:1019–1025

Iwai K, Okinaka O (1968) The biosynthesis of folic acid compounds in plants. I. Enzymatic formation of dihydropteroic acid, dihydrofolic acid from 2-amino-4-hydroxy-6-substituted pteridine by cell free extracts of pea seedlings. J Vitaminol (Kyoto) 14:160–169

Jaenicke L, Chan PC (1960) Die Biosynthese der Folsäure. Angew Chem [Engl] 72:752–753

Jardetzky O, Wade-Jardetzky NG (1965) The mechanism of the binding on sulfonamides to bovine serum albumin. Mol Pharmacol 1:214–230

Joyner LP, Davies SFM, Kendall SB (1963) Chemotherapy of coccidiosis. In: Schnitzer RJ, Hawking F (eds) Experimental chemotherapy. Academic Press, New York, p 445

Kakemi K, Arita T, Koizumi T (1965) Absorption and excretion of drugs. XXIII. Some pharmacokinetic aspects of absorption and excretion of sulfonamides 5. Acetylation of sulfonamides. Yakuzaigaku 25:22–25

Kendall SB (1950) A comparison of the efficacy of sulphamethazine and sulphaquinazoline in the control of experimentally induced caecal coccidiosis in chicks. Vet Record 62:381–382

Kendall SB, Joyner LP (1958) Potentiation of the coccidiostatic effects of sulphadimidine by five different folic acid antagonists. Vet Record 70:632–634

Koizumi T, Arita T, Kakemi K (1964) Absorption and excretion of drugs. XXI. Some pharmacokinetic aspects of absorption and excretion of sulfonamides. 3. Excretion from the kidney. Chem Pharm Bull (Tokyo) 12:428–432

Krüger-Thiemer E (1966) Die Lösung pharmakologischer Probleme durch Rechenautomaten. Arzneim Forsch 16:1431–1442

Krüger-Thiemer E, Wempe E, Töpfor M (1965) Die antibakterielle Wirkung des nicht eiweißgebundenen Anteils der Sulfanilamide im menschlichen Plasmawasser. Arzneim Forsch 15:1309–1317

Kuhn R, Schwartz K (1941) Isolation of the growth-promoting substance H from yeast. Chem Ber 74 B:1617–1624

Kurnosova LM, Lenkevich MM (1964) Mode of action of sulfonamides on trachoma virus. Acta Virol (Praha) 8:350–358

Lampen JO, Jones MJ (1946) The antagonism of sulfonamide inhibition of certain *lactobacilli* and *enterococci* by pteroylglutamic acid and related compounds. J Biol Chem 166:435–448

Lampen JO, Jones MJ (1947) The growth-promoting and antisulfonamide activity of *p*-aminobenzoic acid, pteroylglutamic acid, and related compounds for *L. arabinosus* and *Strept. plantarum*. J Biol Chem 170:133–146

Landy M, Larkum NW, Oswald EJ, Streightoff F (1943) Increased synthesis of *p*-aminobenzoic acid associated with the development of resistance in *Staph. aureus*. Science 97:265–267

Lascelles J, Woods DD (1952) The synthesis of folic acid by *Bacterium coli* and *Staphylococcus aureus* and its inhibition by sulphonamides. Br J Exp Pathol 33:288–303

Lehr D (1957) Clinical toxicity of sulfonamides. Ann NY Acad Sci 9:417–447

Levaditi C (1941) Woods phenomenon and N-containing sulfonamides, sulfoxides, and sulfones. C R Soc Biol 135:1109–1111

Levine PP (1939) The effect of sulfanilamide on the course of experimental avian coccidiosis. Cornell Vet 29:309–320

Levine PP (1941) The coccidiostatic effect of sulfaguanidine. Cornell Vet 31:107–112

Lockwood JS, Coburn AF, Stokinger HE (1938) Studies on the mechanism of the action of sulfanilamide. JAMA 111:2259–2264

Macleod CM (1940) The inhibition of the bacteriostatic action of sulfonamide drugs by substances of animal and bacterial origin. J Exp Med 72:217–232

Maier J, Riley E (1942) Inhibition of antimalarial action of sulfonamides by *p*-aminobenzoic acid. Proc Soc Exp Biol Med 50:152–154

Marshall EK Jr (1937) Determination of sulfanilamide in blood and urine. J Biol Chem 122:263–273

Martin BK (1965) Potential effects of the plasma proteins on drug distribution. Nature 207:274–276

McCallum FO, Findlay GM (1938) Chemotherapeutic experiments on the virus of *Lymphogranuloma inguinale* in the mouse. Lancet II:136–138

McCullough JL, Maren TH (1974) Dihydropteroate synthetase from *Plasmodium berghei*. Isolation, properties, and inhibition by dapsone and sulfadiazine. Mol Pharmacol 10:140–145

McIlwain H (1942) Correlation of drug action in vitro and in vivo through specific antagonists: Sulfanilamide and *p*-aminobenzoate. Br J Exp Pathol 23:265–271

Mietzsch F (1938) The chemotherapy of bacterial infections. Chem Ber 71 A:15–28

Mietzsch F, Klarer J (1935) Verfahren zur Herstellung von Azoverbindungen. Deutsches Reichspatent 607537

Miller AK (1944) Folic acid and biotin synthesis by sulphonamide-sensitive and sulphonamide-resistant strains of *E. coli*. Proc Soc Exp Biol Med 57:151–153

Miller AK, Bruno P, Berglund RM (1947) The effect of sulfathiazole on the in vitro synthesis of certain vitamins by *E. coli*. J Bacteriol 54:9

Miller GH, Doukas PH, Seydel JK (1972) Sulfonamide structure-activity relationship in a cell-free system. Correlation of inhibition of folate synthesis with antibacterial activity and physicochemical parameters. J Med Chem 15:700–706

Mitchell HK, Snell EE, Williams RJ (1941) The concentration of folic acid. J Am Chem Soc 63:2284

Mitsuda H, Suzuki Y (1968) Pteridines in plants. III. Biogenesis of folic acid in green leaves; inhibitors acting on the biosynthetic pathway for the formation of dihydropteroic acid from guanylic acid. J Vitaminol (Kyoto) 14:106–120

Mitsuhashi S, Inoue K, Inoue M (1977) Nonconjugative plasmids encoding sulfanilamide resistance. Antimicrob Agents Chemother 12:418–422

Morgan HR (1948) Studies on the relationship of pteroylglutamic acid to the growth of *Psittacosis* virus (strain 6 BC). J Exp Med 88:285–294

Moriguchi I, Wada S (1968) Protein bindings. IV. Relations of an index for electronic structure to binding constant with serum albumin and bacteriostatic activities of sulfonamides. Chem Pharm Bull (Tokyo) 16:734–738

Moriguchi I, Wada S, Nishizawa T (1968) Protein bindings. III. Binding of sulfonamides to bovine serum albumin. Chem Pharm Bull (Tokyo) 16:601–605

Morrison NE (1968) Sulfone resistant states (Abstr 199). Int J Lepr 36:652

Moulder JW (1962) The biochemistry of intracellular parasitism. University of Chicago Press, Chicago, p 105

Nagate N, Matsuhisa I, Inoue K, Mitsuhashi S (1978) Plasmid-mediated sulfanilamide resistance. Microbiol Immunol 22:367–375

Nichol CA, Anton AH, Zakrzewski SF (1955) A labile precursor of citrovorum factor. Science 121:275–279

Nichols RL, Jones WF Jr, Finland M (1956) Sulfamethoxypyridazine: preliminary observations on absorption and excretion of a new long-acting antibacterial sulfonamide. Proc Soc Exp Biol Med 92:637–640

Nimmo-Smith RH, Lascelles J, Woods DD (1948) Synthesis of folic acid by *Streptobacterium plantarum* and its inhibition by sulfonamides. Br J Exp Pathol 29:264–281

Nogami H, Hasegawa A, Hanano M, Imaoka K (1968) Absorption and excretion of drugs. XII. Pharmacokinetic studies on urinary excretion of sulfonamides. Yakugaku Zashi 88:893–899

Okinaka O, Iwai K (1969) Radioassay for dihydropteroate synthesizing enzyme activity. Anal Biochem 31:174–182

Ortiz PJ (1970) Dihydrofolate and dihydropteroate synthesis by partially purified enzymes from wild-type and sulfonamide-resistant pneumococci. Biochemistry 9:355–361

Osborn MJ, Huennekens FM (1958) Enzymatic reduction of dihydrofolic acid. J Biol Chem 233:969–974

Pato ML, Brown GM (1963) Mechanisms of resistance of *E. coli* to sulfonamides. Arch Biochem Biophys 103:443–448

Pearson JMH, Petit JMS, Rees RJW (1968) Studies on sulfone resistance in leprosy. 3. A case of partial resistance. Int J Lepr 36:171–178

Peters W (1974) Recent advances in antimalarial chemotherapy and drug resistance. Adv Parasitol 12:69–114

Pfiffner JJ, Binkley SB, Bloom ES, Brown RA, Bird OD, Emmett AD, Hogan AG, O'Dell BL (1943) Isolation of the antianemia factor (vit Bc) in crystalline form from liver. Science 97:404–405

Pfiffner JJ, Binkley SB, Bloom ES, O'Dell BL (1947) Isolation and characterisation of vit Bc from liver and yeast. Occurrence of an acid-labile chick antianaemia factor in liver. J Am Chem Soc 69:1476–1487

Ramakrishnan SP, Basu PC, Singh H, Singh N (1962) Studies on the toxicity and action of diaminodiphenylsulfone (DDS) in avian and simian malaria. Bull WHO 27:213–221

Ramakrishnan SP, Basu PC, Singh N, Wattal BL (1963) A study on the joint action of diaminodiphenylsulfone (DDS) and pyrimethamine in the sporogony cycle of *plasmodium gallinaceum*. Potentiation of the sporontocidal activity of pyrimethamine by DDS. Indian J Malariol 17:141–148

Rastelli A, De Beneditti PG, Battistuzzi GA, Albasini A (1975) The role of anionic, imidic and amidic forms in structure-activity relationships. Correlation of electronic indices and bacteriostatic activity in sulfonamides. J Med Chem 18:963–967

Ratner S, Blanchard M, Coburn AF, Green DE (1944) Isolation of a peptide of *p*-aminobenzoic acid from yeast. J Biol Chem 155:689–690

Reber H, Rutishauser G, Tholen H (1964) Untersuchungen am Menschen mit Sulfamethoxazol und Sulforthodimothoxin. In: Kuemmerle HP, Preziosi (eds) Third Int Congr Chemother Stuttgart 1963, vol 1. Thieme, Stuttgart, p 648

Reynolds JJ, Brown GM (1964) The biosynthesis of folic acid. IV. Enzymatic synthesis of dihydrofolic acid from guanine and ribose compounds. J Biol Chem 239:317–325

Richey DP, Brown GM (1969) The biosynthesis of folic acid IX Purification and properties of the enzymes required for the formation of dihydropteroic acid. J Biol Chem 244:1582–1592

Rieder J (1963) Physikalisch-chemische und biologische Untersuchungen an Sulfonamiden. Arzneim Forsch 13:81–88, 89–95, 95–103

Rist N, Bloch F, Hamon V (1940) Inhibiting action of sulfonamide and of a sulfone on the multiplication in vitro and in vivo of tubercle bacillus. Ann Inst Pasteur 64:203–237

Robinowitz JC, Himes RH (1960) Folic acid coenzymes. Fed Proc 19:963–970

Roland S, Ferone R, Harvey RJ, Styles YL, Morrison RW (1979) The characteristics and significance of sulfonamides as substrates for *E. coli* dihydropteroate synthase. J Biol Chem 254:10337–10345

Rubbo SD, Gillepsie JM (1940) *p*-Aminobenzoic acid as a bacterial growth factor. Nature 146:838–839

Rubbo SD, Maxwell M, Fairbridge RA, Gillespie JM (1941) The bacteriology, growth factor requirements and fermentation reactions of *Clostridium acctobutylicum* Weizman. Aust J Exp Biol Med Sci 19:185–198

Sabin AB, Warren J (1941) Therapeutic effect of the sulfonamides on infection by an intracellular protozoan (Toxoplasma). J Bacteriol 41:80

Sauberlich HE, Baumann CA (1948) A factor required for the growth of *Leuconostoc citrovorum*. J Biol Chem 176:165–173

Schmelkes FC, Wyss O, Marks HC, Ludwig BJ, Stranskov FB (1942) Mechanism of sulfonamide action. I. Acidic dissociation and antibacterial effect. Proc Soc Ex Biol Med 50:145–148

Schnaare RS, Martin AN (1965) Quantum chemistry in drug design. J Pharm Sci 54:1707–1713

Scholtan W (1963) The protein binding of long acting sulfonamides. Chemotherapia 6:180–189

Scholtan W (1968) Die hydrophobe Bindung der Pharmaka an Human-Albumin und Ribonucleinsäure. Arzneim Forsch 18:505–517

Schwenker G (1962) Infrared and nuclear magnetic resonance spectrophotometric study of the structure of sulfanil-guanidine. Arch Pharm (Weinheim) 295:753–758

Seeler AO, Graessle O, Dusenbery ED (1943) The effect of pAB on the chemotherapeutic activity of sulfonamides in *Lymphogranuloma venereum* and in duck malaria. J Bacteriol 45:205–209

Selbie FR (1940) The inhibition of the action of sulfanilamide in mice by *p*-aminobenzoic acid. Br J Exp Pathol 21:90–93

Seydel JK (1966) Prediction of in vitro activity of sulfonamides, using Hammett constants or spectrophotometric data of the basic amines for calculation. Mol Pharmacol 2:259–265

Seydel JK (1968) Molecular basis for the action of chemotherapeutic drugs: structure-activity studies on sulfonamides. In: Ariens EJ (ed) Physico-chemical aspects of drug action. Pergamon, New York, p 169

Seydel JK (1971 a) Prediction of the in vitro activity of sulfonamides synthesised from simple amines by use of electronic data obtained from simple amines. J Med Chem 14:724–729

Seydel JK (1971 b) Physicochemical approaches to the rational development of new drugs. In: Ariens EJ (ed) Drug design. Academic Press, New York, p 343

Seydel JK, Wempe E (1964) Physikalisch-chemische und bakteriologische Untersuchungen an N^1-acylierten Sulfamiden. Arzneim Forsch 14:705–708

Seydel JK, Krüger-Thiemer E, Wempe E (1960) Relation between antibacterial activity and IR of sulfanilamide. Z Naturforsch [C] 15 B:628–641

Shepard CC, Tolentino JG, McRae DN (1968) The therapeutic effect of 4,4′-diacetyldi-aminodiphenylsulfone (DADDS) in leprosy. Am J Trop Med Hyg 17:192–201

Shiota T (1959) Enzymic synthesis of folic acid-like compounds by cell-free extracts of Lactobacillus arabinosus. Arch Biochem Biophys 80:155–161

Shiota T, Disraely MN (1961) The enzymic synthesis of dihydrofolate from 2-amino-4-hy-droxy-6-hydroxymethyldihydropteridine and p-aminobenzoylglutamate by extracts of Lactobacillus plantarum. Biochim Biophys Acta 52:467–473

Shiota T, Disraely MN, McCann MP (1964) The enzymatic synthesis of folate-like compounds from hydroxymethyldihydropteridine pyrophosphate. J Biol Chem 239:2259–2266

Shiota T, Baugh CM, Jackson R, Dillard R (1969) The enzymatic synthesis of hydroxy-methyl-dihydrofolate. Biochemistry 8:5022–5028

Shive W, Ackerman WC, Gordon M, Getzendaner ME, Eakin RE (1947) 5(4)-Amino-4(5)-imidazolecarboxamide, a precursor of purines. J Am Chem Soc 69:725–726

Sköld O (1976) R-Factor-mediated resistance to sulfonamides by a plasmid-borne drug re-sistance dihydropteroate synthase. Antimicrob Agents Chemother 9:49–54

Snell EE, Mitchell HK (1943) Some sulfonamide antagonists as growth factors for lactic acid bacteria. Arch Biochem 1:93–101

Snell EE, Peterson WH (1940) Growth factors for bacteria. X. Additional factors required by certain lactic acid bacteria. J Bact 39:273–284

Stamp TC (1939) Bacteriostatic action of sulphanilamide in vitro. Lancet II:10–17

Stetten MR, Fox CL (1945) An amine formed by bacteria during sulphonamide bacterio-stasis. J Biol Chem 161:333–349

Strauss AM, Kliggman AM, Pillsbury DM (1951) The chemotherapy of actinomycosis and nocardiosis. Am Rev Tuberc Pulm Dis 63:441–448

Struller T (1968) Progress in sulfonamide research. Prog Drug Res 12:389–457

Tabor H, Wyngaarden L (1954) The enzymatic formation of formimino-tetrahydrofolic acid, 5,10-methylenetetrahydrofolic acid and 10-formyltetrahydrofolic acid in the me-tabolism of formimino-glutamic acid. J Biol Chem 234:1830–1846

Tarizzo ML (1972) Chemotherapy of trachoma. WHO Chronicle 26:99–101

Thompson PE (1967) Antimalarial studies on 4,4′-diaminodiphenyl sulfone (DDS) and re-pository sulfones in experimental animals. Int J Lepr 35:605–615

Thompson PE, Olszewski B, Waitz JA (1965) Laboratory studies on the repository antimalarial activity of 4,4′-diacetyl-aminodiphenylsulfone, alone and mixed with cycloguanil pamoate (CI-501). Am J Trop Med Hyg 14:343–353

Toth-Martinez RJ, Papp S, Dinya Z, Hernadi FJ (1975) New vistas for p-aminobenzoate participation in the biosynthesis of dihydrofolate: a tentative model of the tetrahydro-folate multienzyme complex. Biosystems 7:172–182

Trefouël J, Trefouël MMe J, Nitti F, Bovet D (1935) Activite du p-aminophenylsulfamide sur les infections streptococciques experimentales de la souris et du lapin. C R Soc Biol 120:756–758

Tripod J, Neipp L, Padowtz W, Sackmann W (1960) Relations experimentales entre l'action curative et les taux sanguins de sulfamides, en particulier du sulfaphenazol. Antibiot Chemotherapia 8:17–31

Tschesche R (1947) A new explanation of the mode of action of the sulfonamides. Z Natur-
  forsch [C] 2b:10–11
Vieira E, Shaw E (1961) The utilisation of purines in the biosynthesis of folic acid. J Biol
  Chem 236:2507–2510
Walter RD, Königk E (1974) Biosynthesis of folic acid compounds in plasmodia; purification and properties of 7,8-dihydropteroate synthesising enzyme from *Plasmodium cha-
  baudi*. Hoppe Seylers Z Physiol Chem 355:431–437
Watanabe T (1963) Infective heredity of multiple drug resistance in bacteria. Bacteriol Rev
  27:87–115
Weinstein L, Madoff MA, Samet CM (1960) The sulfonamides. Engl J Med 263:793–800,
  842–849, 900–907
Weisman RA, Brown GM (1964) The biosynthesis of folic acid. V. Characteristics of the
  enzyme system that catalyses the synthesis of dihydropteroic acid. J Biol Chem 239:326–
  331
White PJ, Woods DD (1965) The synthesis of *p*-aminobenzoic acid and folic acid by staphy-
  lococci sensitive and resistant to sulphonamides. J Gen Microbiol 40:243–253
Williams RT, Parke DV (1964) Metabolic fate of drugs. Ann Rev Pharmacol 4:85–114
Wise EM Jr, Abou-Donia MM (1975) Sulfonamide resistance mechanism in *E. coli*: R plasmids can determine sulfonamide-resistant dihydropteroate syntheses. Proc Natl Acad
  Sci USA 72:2621–2625
Wolf B, Hotchkiss RD (1963) Genetically modified folic acid synthesising enzymes of pneu-
  mococcus. Biochemistry 2:145–150
Woods DD (1940) Relation of *p*-aminobenzoic acid to mechanism of action of sulphanil-
  amide. Br J Exp Pathol 21:74–90
Woods DD (1954) Metabolic relations between *p*-aminobenzoic and folic acids in microor-
  ganisms. In: Chemistry and biology of pteridines, CIBA Foundation Symposium. Little
  Brown, Boston, Mass, p 220
Yamazaki M, Aoki M, Kamada A (1968) Biological activities of drugs. III. Physicochemical
  factors affecting the excretion of sulfonamides in rabbits. Chem Pharm Bull (Tokyo)
  16:707–714
Yamazaki M, Kakeya N, Morishita T, Kamada A, Aoki A (1970) Biological activity of
  drugs. X. Relation of structure to the bacteriostatic activity of sulfonamides (1). Chem
  Pharm Bull (Tokyo) 18:702–707
Ziegler-Gunder I, Simon H, Wacker A (1956) Metabolism of guanine-2-^{14}C and hypoxan-
  thine-8-^{14}C in amphibians. Zentral Naturforsch IIb:82–85

CHAPTER 3

Dihydrofolate Reductase

J.J. Burchall

A. Introduction

The discovery of the antibacterial activity of the sulfonamides had two important consequences. First, a new agent of unprecedented efficacy became available for the treatment of infectious diseases. Less obvious was the support it gave to the concept that biochemical differences between humans and their parasites could serve as the basis for a rational approach to the design of chemotherapeutic agents. Knowledge of the mechanism of action of the sulfonamides (Woods 1940) suggested that chemotherapeutic effort be directed toward essential enzymes and pathways present in prokaryotic parasites, but lacking in their mammalian host. That such an approach would be fruitful was not obvious. At least superficially, it appeared to run counter to the increasingly well-documented concept of "the unity of biochemistry" which emphasized the commonality of pathways employed by both prokaryotes and eukaryotes for their growth and reproduction (Florkin 1974).

In the years following the introduction of the sulfonamides, numerous attempts were made to apply the antimetabolite strategy to the synthesis of antimicrobial and anticancer agents (Wooley 1952). In spite of some success, no major breakthrough was forthcoming and enthusiasm for the approach gradually diminished. It was argued that selective toxicity could be achieved more readily by exploiting differences in rates of cell growth or drug metabolism between the parasite and host rather than by the identification of unique biochemical loci.

In spite of this outlook, interest in folic acid metabolism and its inhibition remained high. The synthesis of x-methylfolate (Franklin et al. 1947) and amethopterin (Seeger et al. 1947) provided the first compounds capable of inducing folate deficiency in animals. Knowledge of the folate pathway was extended greatly by the observation of Broquist et al. (1950) that citrovorum factor, a reduced form of folate, antagonized aminopterin toxicity, and the discovery by Nichol and Welch (1950) that folate conversion of citrovorum factor was blocked by aminopterin. These findings were explained at the molecular level by the experiments of Osborn and Huennekens (1958) who demonstrated that methotrexate (MTX) inhibits dihydrofolate reductase (DHFR), the enzyme which converts dihydrofolate (FAH$_2$) to its active cofactor form, tetrahydrofolate.

As an inhibitor of DHFR, methotrexate was notable, both for its inhibition constant ($\leq 1 \times 10^{-10}$ M) and its lack of selectivity (Blakeley 1969). The discovery by Hitchings et al. (1948) that certain diaminopyrimidines also were acting as antifols radically altered the outlook for the design and synthesis of truly selective enzyme inhibitors. Unlike methotrexate, these compounds showed potent antibacterial and antiprotozoal activity which could be separated from mammalian toxicity, although the enzymatic basis of their selectivity was not clear.

When viewed against this background, the development of successful chemotherapeutic agents based on the selective inhibition of DHFR takes on special importance. To this day, drugs such as trimethoprim and pyrimethamine provide convincing arguments for the concept that drugs may be discovered by a rational approach which attempts to exploit chemotherapeutic differences in the submolecular structure of enzymes and receptors of parasites and hosts (BURCHALL 1979). In this chapter, our current knowledge of DHFR is reviewed with particular emphasis on research which has contributed to our understanding of the comparative biochemistry of this enzyme and its importance for the design of selective antimicrobial agents.

B. Assay and Kinetic Studies

Dihydrofolate reductase (5,6,7,8-tetrahydrofolate: oxidoreductase, EC 1.5.1.3) catalyzes the reaction shown in Eq. (1).

$$FAH_2 + NADPH + H^+ \rightarrow FAH_4 + NADP^+. \tag{1}$$

The central role of this enzyme in cellular metabolism is discussed elsewhere in this volume (Chap. 1). As noted there, the role of DHFR is to supply tetrahydrofolate, the carrier of a one-carbon unit, required for the biosynthesis of purines, pyrimidines, and amino acids. Normally tetrahydrofolate is regenerated intact after serving as a one-carbon carrier in these reactions. The sustained demand for DHFR arises as a consequence of the oxidation of the cofactor methylenetetrahydrofolate to dihydrofolate during the synthesis of thymidylate. Cells capable of using preformed thymidylate tolerate higher levels of reductase inhibitors after losing thymidylate synthetase activity through mutation. Thus, under normal circumstances, DHFR is essential to the growth and survival of bacterial and mammalian cells.

The enzyme is most commonly assayed by following spectrophotometrically the decrease in absorbance at 340 nm which accompanies the reduction. Numerous versions of the procedure are in use. The method of BACCANARI et al. (1975) has been used for many of the studies involving reductase inhibitors such as trimethoprim. The convenience and rapidity of the 340 nm assay makes it the method of choice for most enzymes, but more sensitive methods are occasionally needed to allow collection of accurate kinetic data when concentrations of substrates are low relative to their Michaelis constant K_m values and when crude extracts are used. Fluorescent methods have been proposed to follow activity by measuring the production of NADP (BERTINO et al. 1964) and tetrahydrofolate (LINDQUIST et al. 1977). Radiometric assays employing labeled substrate have been devised and readers may wish to consult the recent papers of HAYMAN (1980) and ROTHENBERG et al. (1980) for illustrative examples. HUENNEKENS et al. (1976) provide a good introduction to methods and procedures commonly used in DHFR research.

Dihydrofolate and NADPH are the preferred substances for bacterial DHFRs but alternatively folate can be used, albeit less efficiently. For example, *Escherichia coli* DHFR can use folate as a substrate, but the pH must be as low as 4.5 for optimal rate of reduction. Even at this pH, the K_m for folate is 16 μM and the V_{max} is 1/1,000 of the rate obtained with dihydrofolate. NADH can be oxidized in place of NADPH but the K_m value of the former is 268 μM as contrasted to 3.2 μM for the natural substrate (BACCANARI et al. 1975). Folate and its oxidized pteroyloligo-γ-L-glutamates are substrates for mammalian DHFRs, although they are used less well than dihydrofolate. COWARD et al. (1974) have determined the K_m and V_{max} values of folate and several of its polyglutamates forms for DHFR from L 1210/ MTX, erythrocyte, AML and ALL cells. Among the oxidized pteroyl-γ-L-glutamates, there is no clear preference for any particular number of glutamate residues. All of the dihydropteroyloligo-γ-L-glutamates are more active than their oxidized congeners.

C. Mechanism of Action

The mechanism of action of DHFR has been examined using enzymes from bacterial and mammalian sources. Studies of the enzyme isolated from L 1210 (McCULLOUGH et al. 1971), *E. coli* (BURCHALL 1970), and porcine liver (S. SMITH et al. 1979 a) demonstrate a rapid equilibrium random Bi–Bi mechanism, although differences exist in the number of dead-end complexes observed. An ordered sequential mechanism has been reported for reductase *Streptococcus faecium (faecalis)* A. (BLAKLEY et al. 1971).

The reviews of BENKOVIC (1980) and GREADY (1980) provide an excellent overview of current knowledge of the mechanism of action of folate-requiring enzymes. Several other observations that have been made in the course of mechanism studies have been helpful in understanding the nature of inhibitor binding. First, it appears that the hydrogen of NADPH is transferred from the A side of the pyridine ring based on studies with bacterial (BLAKLEY et al. 1963), mammalian, and avian enzymes (PASTORE and FRIEDKIN 1962). This observation, as we shall see later, has proved useful in determining whether reductases bind dihydrofolate and amethopterin in the same manner. Second, there is considerable evidence that dihydrofolate and its analogs may bind in a cooperative manner with the pyridine nucleotide. Studies of *E. coli* reductase show that the binding of either substrate is enhanced if the other substrate is already bound to the enzyme (BURCHALL 1970). PERKINS and BERTINO (1966) observed a similar situation with respect to the folate analog, triampterene (2,4,7-triamino-6-phenylpteridine). More recently, PATTISHALL et al. (1976), using equilibrium dialysis, have presented evidence which suggests that some reductase inhibitors, such as trimethoprim, bind more tightly in the ternary than the binary complex, whereas others such as pyrimethamine do not show this behavior, at least when studied with *E. coli* DHFR.

Many of the apparently unrelated data, obtained from these various kinetic and mechanism studies, have become clearer as new information from nuclear magnetic resonance (NMR), X-ray crystallography, and amino acid sequencing techniques has allowed the rationalization of these data in terms of direct interactions between ligands and specific amino acid residues. Some conclusions of this type of analysis will be presented later in this chapter.

Table 1. Kinetic parameters of several dihydrofolate reductases

Source	$K_m (\mu M)$		Optimal pH	Reference
	FAH$_2$	NADPH		
Escherichia coli	8.9	6.4	4, 7	BACCANARI et al. (1975, 1977)
L1210 lymphoma	0.4	5.0	4, 7.5	HUENNEKENS et al. (1976)
Porcine liver	0.74	3.2	5, 7.5	MCCULLOUGH et al. (1971)
				s. SMITH et al. (1979a)

D. Basis of Selectivity

I. Kinetic Studies

At first glance, dihydrofolate reductase is perhaps an unlikely target for antibacterial or antiprotozoal chemotherapy. The enzyme has been found in almost every organism and tissue that has been examined for its presence, and no biochemical pathway has been found which could perform a similar role in purine, pyrimidine, and amino acid synthesis. For these reasons, rationalization of the selective effects of reductase inhibitors must rest on the documentation of species-dependent differences in the primary structures of the enzymes.

The data presented in Table 1 describing the basic kinetic parameters of reductase from several phylogenetically separated species, provide little encouragement for the hypothesis that such differences exist. The K_m values of FAH$_2$ and NADPH for most bacterial and mammalian enzymes are in the μM range (HITCHINGS and SMITH 1980). K_m values for NADPH appear relatively constant (about 5 μM) for most species of reductase examined. There does appear to be a consistent trend toward lower K_m values for FAH$_2$ in the mammalian reductase group, but it should be noted that the 340 nm absorbance assay used for most of these determinations lacks sensitivity and reproducibility below μM levels of substrate. Optimal pH values tend to be bimodal for mammalian and bacterial reductases (BACCANARI et al. 1975), but further differentiation on this basis is not possible.

Measurements of molecular weight and turnover number have been made on most reductases studied. Mammalian reductases in general are slightly larger ($\sim 21,000$ daltons) than bacterial enzymes ($\sim 18,000$ daltons) and each consists of a single chain of amino acids. Protozoal DHFRs have molecular weights in the range of 100,000–240,000 daltons as measured by gel filtration. FERONE et al. (1969) first observed that *Plasmodium berghei* DHFR had a molecular weight 9- to 10-fold higher than that reported for most other DHFRs. Similar observations were made in studies of the DHFRs from trypanosomes and crithidia (GUTTERIDGE et al. 1969) and coccidia (WANG et al. 1975). Recently, FERONE and ROLAND (1980) have shown that purified enzyme (107,000 daltons) is composed of two polypeptides, each of which possesses DHFR and thymidylate synthetase activity. This arrangement presumably increases the efficiency of carbon and hydrogen transfer and may be widespread in the protozoa. R plasmid dihydrofolate reductase which has a molecular weight of 33,780 daltons, consists of four identical

Table 2. Biologic effects of 5-benzylpyrimidines

Substituents			Plasmodium gallinaceum MED$_{50}$ (mg/kg)[a]	Staphylococcus aureus MIC (μg/ml)[b]	Mouse LD$_{50}$ (mg/kg)[c]
R$_1$	R$_2$	R$_3$			
H	H	H	100	32	40
CH$_3$	H	H	5	128	60
H	H	Cl	100	8	80
CH$_3$	H	Cl	1.5	64	30
H	OCH$_3$	OCH$_3$	100	< 1	> 500
CH$_3$	OCH$_3$	OCH$_3$	10	30	> 100

[a] Minimum effective dose
[b] Minimal inhibitory concentration
[c] Median lethal dose

subunits (S. SMITH et al. 1979 b). Calculated turnover numbers defy rationalization with variations of over ten-fold within the group of bacterial and the group of mammalian enzymes (HITCHINGS and SMITH 1980).

II. Inhibitor Binding Analysis

The inadequacy of the kinetic approach for the demonstration of interspecific variations in dihydrofolate turned attention to compounds known to interfere with folate metabolism. Table 2 lists some of the biologic effects observed in a series of closely related 5-benzylpyrimidines. The effects of each substituent on the spectrum of activity of the compounds is striking. On the pyrimidine ring, substitution in position R$_1$ with hydrogen favors antibacterial activity while methyl substitution clearly enhances antimalarial *(Plasmodium gallinaceum)* effects. The effect of substituents on the benzyl ring depends largely on the electron-donating or electron-withdrawing properties of the group involved. For example, electron-withdrawing groups such as Cl increased the activity of the compound against all three species listed whereas electron-donating groups such as methoxy enhance antibacterial activity while at the same time lowering activity against *P. gallinaceum* and decreasing rodent toxicity by over eight-fold. (See also Chap. 5.)

It was inferred from these data that the selectivity of these compounds might result from their differential binding to DHFRs from the various species tested, although selective effects due to pharmacokinetic parameters could not be ruled out. When a related set of compounds was tested on several different reductases obtained from bacterial and mammalian sources, the data shown in Table 3 were obtained. These data show clearly that the potency and selectivity of the diaminoheterocyclic inhibitors can be explained satisfactorily, mainly by measurement of their relative binding to reductases from various species. For example, the highly potent and toxic compound, methotrexate binds very tightly to all reductases tested and is lethal to any cell it can enter. On the other hand, trimethoprim shows

Table 3. Comparative binding of inhibitors to dihydrofolate reductases from various species

Compound	IC_{50} ($\times 10^{-8}$ M)		
	Escherichia coli	Staphylococcus aureus	Rat liver
MTX	0.01	0.02	0.02
PYR	250	300	180
TMP	0.7	1.5	35,000
DHT	65,000	50,000	24

MTX: 2,4-diamino-N^{10}-methylpteroylglutamate (methotrexate)
PYR: 2,4-diamino-5-p-chlorophenyl-6-ethylpyrimidine (pyrimethamine)
TMP: 2,4-diamino-5-(3',4',5'trimethoxybenzyl)pyrimidine (trimethoprim)
DHT: 1-(p-butylphenyl)-1,2-dihydro-2,2-dimethyl-4,6-diamino-5-triazine

a remarkable ability to distinguish between bacterial and mammalian reductases (BURCHALL and HITCHINGS 1965). This important relative difference in binding serves as the basis of the high chemotherapeutic index of the compound. The data obtained with the dihydrotriazine compound illustrates the extent to which subtle variations in enzyme structure (see Sect. D.V) may be illustrated by inhibition studies with the appropriate compounds. In this case, the reverse of that seen with trimethoprim, the rat liver DHFR is powerfully inhibited whereas the activity of the bacterial enzymes is only weakly effected.

For a very large number of compounds, measurements of enzyme binding are predictive of the activity of the compounds on the growth rate of *E. coli* and other organisms. Where correlations cannot be made, the usual observation is that the compound does not inhibit the growing bacteria as well as predicted by the enzyme data. Because these compounds usually contain bulky, lipophilic groups, it is widely assumed that their relative inactivity reflects diminished uptake into the bacterial cell. However, the biochemical literature contains no record that this hypothesis has been directly tested using radiolabeled compounds. There is indirect evidence that the resistance of *Pseudomonas aeruginosa* to DHFR inhibitors may be due to lack of uptake. HITCHINGS et al. (1968) have shown that the several diaminopyridopyrimidines exhibit increased activity against *Pseudomonas aeruginosa* when incubated with the organisms in the presence of detergents. They concluded that, at least with that organism, uptake of this type of inhibitor appears to be slow and meager.

Of the compounds listed in Table 3, trimethoprim shows the largest difference in its binding between bacterial and mammalian reductases. This specificity can be dissected in greater detail by the examination of a number of compounds closely related to trimethoprim. Table 4 lists the activity of some analogs of this type against DHFR from *E. coli* and rat liver. The compound with the unsubstituted benzyl ring shows weak activity against both enzymes. Substitution in the para position with methyl, or better still methoxy groups enhances the ability of the compound to bind selectively to the bacterial reductase. Increasing the number of methoxy groups to three simultaneously improves bacterial enzyme binding while making the compounds less potent inhibitors of the mammalian enzyme.

Table 4. Binding of diaminobenzylpyrimidines to bacterial and mammalian dihydrofolate reductases

Substitutions			IC_{50} ($\times 10^{-8}$ M)		
R_1	R_2	R_3	Escherichia coli	Rat	E. coli/rat
H	H	H	406	15,000	37
H	CH_3	H	230	10,000	43
H	OCH_3	H	110	17,000	155
OCH_3	H	H	49	18,900	386
OCH_3	OCH_3	H	5	7,000	1,400
OCH_3	OCH_3	OCH_3	0.7	35,000	50,000

Table 5. Binding of trimethoprim to reductases from various species

	IC_{50} ($\times 10^{-6}$ M) Average
Mammals (4)[a]	235
Lower vertebrates (3)[b]	94
Invertebrates (2)[c]	18
Bacterial (3)[d]	0.008
Protozoa (1)[e]	0.17

[a] Human, rat, guinea pig, rabbit liver
[b] Turtle, frog, carp
[c] Tapeworm, lobster
[d] *Escherichia coli, Staphylococcus aureus, Proteus vulgaris*
[e] *Plasmodium berghei*

The examples given show that there are clear differences between bacterial and mammalian reductases and that these differences are of sufficient magnitude to be exploited chemotherapeutically. Even more surprising is the finding that such species differences exist among reductases over the entire phylogenetic scale. The data in Table 5 show that the study of even a single compound, in this case trimethoprim, is often sufficient to detect these differences. For example, the average median inhibitory concentration (IC_{50}) of trimethoprim for four well-studied mammalian reductases is 235 μM. The corresponding values for the lower vertebrates are less than half this value while the invertebrates bind TMP over ten-fold as well. At the other end of the phylogenetic spectrum, typical bacteria DHFRs have IC_{50} values about 30,000-fold lower than that seen with mammalian reductases.

Protozoal DHFRs are more difficult to characterize by "inhibitor binding profiles" since they, like yeast and tapeworm reductases, do not show great differences in their affinity for inhibitors of varying chemical type (J. BURCHALL, unpublished work 1972). This group of enzymes shows some characteristics of both the mammalian and bacterial DHFRs. For example, they bind trimethoprim only at concentrations greater than those needed to inhibit bacterial reductases, but 100-fold less than the IC_{50} for the invertebrate reductases.

III. Enzyme Conformation and Cooperativity

The analysis of enzyme inhibition becomes more complicated when one considers that inhibitors may bind to either the enzyme alone (binary complex) or to an enzyme–NADPH complex (ternary complex). As mentioned previously, PERKINS and BERTINO (1966) suggested that inhibitors may bind more tightly in the ternary complex than to the enzyme alone. The dissociation constants of methotrexate and triampterene were determined by fluorescence quenching techniques. In the binary complex, triampterene was characterized by a dissociation constant of 3.4×10^{-7} M, while in the ternary complex with NADPH, the binding increased 25- to 60-fold.

It is incorrect to conclude from these data that the analysis of enzyme inhibition is without difficulty. As BACCANARI and JOYNER (1981) have pointed out, the binding of ligands to DHFR is a complex process involving a variety of protein conformations. As mentioned previously, the limit of sensitivity of the assay is below the reported K_m value of some mammalian enzymes. Also, the substrates are unstable and their degradation products are not all known.

In addition to these problems, the measurement of enzyme inhibition may be complicated by time dependence. J. WILLIAMS et al. (1980) have shown that inhibition by many compounds proceeds in two stages: an initial rapid formation of an enzyme–NADPH–inhibitor complex and the subsequent slow isomerization of the ternary complex. BACCANARI and JOYNER (1981) have pointed out that *E. coli* DHFR exhibits hysteretic behavior which must be considered in a study of enzyme inhibition. For example, pyrimethamine eliminated hysteresis when dihydrofolate was used to start the reaction, whereas trimethoprim increased the hysteresis when either enzyme or NADPH was used to start the reaction. These authors have proposed a method to avoid hysteresis and allow the calculation of reliable inhibition constants.

M. WILLIAMS et al. (1973a), using NMR techniques and *E. coli* dihydrofolate reductase, showed that cooperativity was also important in the binding of methotrexate. The dissociation constants observed were 0.36 nM (binary) and <0.01 nM (ternary). Interpretation of these data were complicated by the further observation of these authors (M. WILLIAMS et al. 1973b) that *E. coli* DHFR may possess more than one NADPH binding. Ultrafiltration experiments suggests two NADPH binding sites; however, fluorometric analysis shows only a single binding site.

POE et al. (1974) reported that *E. coli* DHFR possesses two NADPH binding sites, as measured by UV difference spectroscopy. In addition, the ternary complex showed a ratio of 1 enzyme: 1 methotrexate: 2 NADPH. Regardless of the number of NADPH binding sites, the cooperative nature of cofactor binding seems well established. Studies of methotrexate binding to *Lactobacillus casei* DHFR by PASTORE et al. (1974), using proton magnetic resonance spectroscopy also support the view that the conformation of the enzyme–MTX complex differs from the enzyme–MTX–NADPH complex. When both enzyme–NADPH and enzyme–MTX are converted to ternary complexes by the addition of MTX or NADPH, similar NMR spectra are observed. These results also support the suggestion (see Sect. C) that the enzyme adds substrates in a random rather than ordered sequence.

BIRDSALL et al. (1978) have explored the problem of cooperativity further by examining the binding of diaminopyrimidine (DAP) and p-aminobenzoyl-L-glutamate which may be considered as "fragments" of methotrexate. A number of important findings have come from these NMR studies. DAP and pABG were shown to bind with about 54-fold cooperativity to *L. casei* DHFR. NADPH was shown to increase the binding of both compounds without altering the cooperativity between them. These findings were given further weight by other studies (BIRDSALL et al. 1980a) in which coenzyme analogs were shown also to enhance "fragment" binding with cooperativity ranging from 1.8- to 428-fold. DUNN and KING (1980) using stop-flow fluorescence have studied further the nature of the very tightly binding enzyme–MTX–NADPH complex. They have shown that the main effect of NADPH is to decrease the off rate of MTX from the enzyme–MTX–NADPH complex. In agreement with the findings of BIRDSALL et al. (1978), they conclude that these results are best explained by postulating the existence of more than one interconvertible form of the free enzyme, in contrast to the binary complex which can exist in only one form.

The suggestion that free DHFR can exist in more than one form recalls the observations of PATTISHALL et al. (1976) on the binding of trimethoprim and pyrimethamine to *E. coli* DHFR. In this study it was concluded that two species of free DHFR were present in about equal proportions. However, BACCANARI et al. (1977) showed that *E. coli* DHFR preparations normally contain two isozymes and it is possible that reductases from other species also are composed of two similar but not identical isozymes. For this reason, final judgment on experiments demonstrating multiple binding sites for substrates, cofactors, and inhibitors must be reserved until the molecular homogeneity of these preparations is confirmed beyond doubt.

IV. Amino Acid Sequences

At present about 13 DHFRs have been completely or partially sequenced from bacterial, mammalian, or avian sources. It is likely that amino acid sequences deduced from DNA sequencing experiments will shortly be available, particularly those reductases coded by resistance-determining sequences of plasmid DNA. Table 6 gives the enzyme sequences that have been published.

While careful statistical analysis and correlation with X-ray data will no doubt reveal increasingly subtle aspects of substructure, certain features of comparative enzyme structure can be discerned after even crude realignment of the residues to produce an approximate fit. Some of these conclusions are listed.

1. General. Bacterial reductases contain about 160 residues whereas mammalian and avian forms have about 186 residues which are linked in a single chain. The R plasmid R 67-coded reductase which confers resistance to trimethoprim, in contrast, consists of four identical subunits each with a molecular weight of 8,444 daltons.

2. Mammalian reductases show greater similarity to each other than other groups of reductase. About 125 of 186 amino acids of the enzymes sequenced are identical. There is strong antigenic cross-reactivity among these enzymes.

Table 6. Published sequences of dihydrofolate reductases

Source	Reference
Bacterial	
Escherichia coli, forms 1 and 2	BACCANARI et al. (1981)
Escherichia coli MB148	BENNETT et al. (1978)
Escherichia coli K12	D. SMITH and CALVO (1980)
Escherichia coli Rplasmid (R67)	STONE and SMITH (1979)
Escherichia coli Rplasmid (R388)	ZOLG and HÄNGGI (1981)
Streptococcus faecium I	FREISHEIM et al. (1977)
Streptococcus faecium II	GLEISNER et al. (1974)
Lactobacillus casei	BITAR et al. (1977), FREISHEIM et al. (1978)
Mammalian	
L1210 lymphoma	STONE and PHILLIPS (1977), STONE et al. (1979)
Sarcoma 180	RODKEY and BENNETT (1976)
Pig liver	S. SMITH et al. (1979a)
Bovine liver	BAUMANN and WILSON (1975), LAI et al. (1979)
Avian	
Chicken liver	FREISHEIM et al. (1979)

3. Bacterial reductases are not as homogeneous as mammalian enzymes. However, there is evidence for common ancestry since about 30 of approximately 160 residues are identical. There is antigenic cross-reactivity in this group, but not as complete as that seen in studies of mammalian reductases.

4. A small number of residues is shared by both bacterial and mammalian enzymes, and are probably important to the mechanism of action of all reductases. HITCHINGS and ROTH (1980) count 16 such residues, but if identity to the R plasmid reductase is ignored, 20 conserved amino acids can be identified. These amino acids form a starting point for analysis of the essential components of the DHFR active site by X-ray crystallography.

5. R plasmid R 67 DHFRs show no homology to any reductase studied thus far. No antigenic relationship has been observed either.

6. DHFRs, regardless of their source, show greater homology towards their amino terminal rather than carboxy terminal residues. The tendency is more pronounced in the bacterial enzymes. In most cases, the carboxy terminal region of the enzymes has the highest proportion of hydrophobic amino acids.

Comparative studies of amino acid sequence among DHFRs have yielded information of both immediate and longer-term value. Specifically, it provided one test of the usefulness of inhibition analysis as a means of characterizing DHFRs as well as providing an essential element in the solution of the three-dimensional structure of these enzymes by X-ray crystallography. For example, initial studies of several bacterial and mammalian DHFRs suggested that although the bacterial enzymes showed certain common affinities, they could be distinguished from each other (especially between gram-negative and gram-positive bacteria) by proper selection of inhibitors. On the other hand, mammalian enzymes appeared to be a homogeneous group which responded almost identically to each of the inhibitors chosen. All of these inferences are supported by the homologies observed in the sequence studies. The inability of reductase inhibitors to attack tumor tissue selectively can also be rationalized simply by the observations that L 1210 lymphoma and sarcoma 180 DHFRs are almost identical to other fully sequenced mammalian reductases. Inhibition analysis also predicts that protozoal reductases differ substantially from bacterial and mammalian reductases, but to date no sequence data are available to support or disprove the inference.

V. Three-Dimensional Structures of DHFR

Using the then unpublished *E. coli* sequence data of BENNETT et al. (1978), MATTHEWS et al. (1977) provided the first three-dimensional view of a DHFR. The structure proposed is remarkable, both for its ability to explain numerous important observations made previously and for certain wholly unexpected insights. The *E. coli* reductase can be viewed as a clamshell–like structure consisting of two main lobes connected by a short peptide bridge. More accurately, it is a central eight-stranded, β-pleated sheet. The inhibitor, methotrexate, sits in the 15 Å deep cavity with the pteridine moiety in a hydrophobic pocket. At least 13 amino acids are involved in the binding of methotrexate. The aspartate at position 27 is of particular interest. This amino acid is conserved in all bacterial sequences examined thus far and is replaced in mammalian reductases by its close congener, glutamic acid. Located near the N-1 of methotrexate, the carboxyl group may share a proton with this most basic atom in the pteridine ring.

This observation may help to explain the extremely tight binding of methotrexate to all reductases. Methotrexate differs from the much weaker binding folic acid (by over four orders of magnitude) in the presence of an amino rather than a hydroxyl group at position C-4 and less importantly by the presence of a methyl group at position N-10. The 4-amino group acts to increase indirectly the basicity of the pteridine ring by 3 pK units and strongly promotes protonation at the N-1 position. The authors conclude that the hydrogen bonding of the 4-amino substituent itself would not enhance the binding of MTX relative to folate or dihydrofolate.

Isozymes of DHFR differing in only a few amino acids are useful in allowing a precise evaluation of the role of individual amino acids in inhibitor binding. For example, BACCANARI et al. (1981) have purified to homogeneity two *E. coli* DHFR isozymes designated forms 1 and 2. They differ in a single amino acid: arginine occurs at residue 28 in form 2 and leucine in form 1. The isozymes are important since it has been proposed that Asp-27 is a key factor in inhibitor binding and catalysis (MATTHEWS et al. 1977). BACCANARI et al. (1981) have demonstrated that the behavior of both isozymes with respect to trimethoprim binding, pH activity profile, sensitivity to $BaCl_2$, and turnover numbers can all be explained on the basis of the presence or absence of charge interactions between Asp-27 and the amino acid present at residue 28.

Of equal interest with the study of binding of folate-like antagonists is the contribution of these studies to our knowledge of the NADPH binding site. Previous kinetic studies showed that NADPH is preferred as a reductant by many bacterial and mammalian reductases. T. WILLIAMS et al. (1977), for example, demonstrated that a standardized *L. casei* DHFR preparation had a specific activity of 23.5 U/ mg with NADPH, while NADH, thio-NADPH, and acetylpyridine-NADPH all give values of less than 5 U/mg. Interestingly, deamino-NADPH raised the specific activity to 33.5 U/mg.

The tighter binding of NADP compared with NAD may come in large part from the involvement of 2'-phosphate group. BIRDSALL et al. (1977), using ^{31}P NMR, showed that NADP ($K_i = 1.8$ µM) binds more tightly than NAD ($K_i = 50$ µM) and noted that the ΔG^0 of 2'-AMP is -4.6 kcal/mol whereas the binding of 5'-AMP was too weak to determine a ΔG^0 value. HYDE et al. (1980) showed that the binding of thionicotinamide and acetylpyridine analogs of NADPH may differ because of the different environments of the nicotinamide rings on the *L. casei* DHFR. The authors also note that although the addition of methotrexate or folate has little effect on the environment of the NADP$^+$ nicotinamide ring, trimethoprim produces large changes in this region.

BIRDSALL et al. (1980 b) have attempted to correlate the findings of their NMR studies with the three-dimensional structure of the *L. casei*–MTX–NADPH ternary complex (MATTHEWS et al. 1978). As observed with other dehydrogenases, the reduced pyridine nucleotide is bound much more tightly than is the oxidized congener. DANNENBERG et al. (1978) suggested that phenyladenine dinucleotide, which is planar and lacks a charge, behaves like NADH since both compounds show a parallel increase in K_d values as pH is raised. They conclude that NAD and NADP$^+$ differ in binding owing to charge and not stereochemical orientation of the reduced nicotinamide ring. BIRDSALL et al. (1980 b) suggest that the explanation is more complicated and involves changes in the environment of the cofactor, perhaps owing to conformational changes.

Studies of the ternary complexes of methotrexate and trimethoprim with reduced cofactors show major increases in binding of the inhibitors or cofactors compared with the binary complexes. The increased binding energy does not come exclusively from direct interaction between the substrate and cofactor since the nicotinamide ring of NADPH and the pteridine ring of MTX show only partial overlap and are not parallel, but more likely from protein conformational changes.

Although the NADPH binding site of DHFR had not been studied previously by crystallographic methods, it is possible to infer something of its nature, even from the methotrexate binary complex. The spatial arrangement of the pyridine nucleotide binding site is the same in DHFR and lactic dehydrogenase (ROSSMAN et al. 1975), but, in DHFR, helices do not connect adjacent β-pleated sheets, but rather those separated by intervening strands. Inspection of the proposed binding site suggests that there is sufficient room for substrate to bind and not restrict movement of the other molecule; an observation which is consistent with a random Bi–Bi kinetic mechanism.

More detailed information on the NADPH and the methotrexate ternary complex appeared in three subsequent studies of the *L. casei* DHFR (MATTHEWS et al. 1978, 1979; MATTHEWS 1979). X-ray studies at the 2.5 Å level of resolution showed that NADPH binds in an extended conformation with adenine in a nonspecific hydrophobic cleft and nicotinamide in another cavity, one wall of which is the pyrazine ring of MTX. In view of the kinetic inhibition studies which suggest that

NADPH and methotrexate bind cooperatively in the ternary complex, it is interesting to note that the binding of NADPH causes shifts of up to 3 Å in the enzyme backbone in the flexible loop regions of residues 12–21 and 125–128. There was no homology seen between the NADPH binding site of *L. casei* DHFR and four other dehydrogenases, but as with other dehydrogenases binding occurs at the carboxyl end of the parallel β-pleated sheet flanked by a pair of α-helices.

In their paper, MATTHEWS et al. (1979) make the important point that the pteridine ring may be rotated 180° along the C-6–C-9 axis and still fit well into its hydrophobic cleft. This observation allows the further speculation that perhaps folate and dihydrofolate are bound in one conformation while methotrexate is bound in another. This hypothesis is important since it explains how the substrates, which are most basic at position N-5 (POE 1977), can align this atom in sufficient proximity to the nicotinamide ring of NADPH to allow hydride ion transfer. A number of other studies support this suggestion. CHARLTON et al. (1979) have shown that the reduction of folate involves the transfer of the 4-pro-R-hydrogen of NADPH to the si-face of folate. Taken together with the observation of FONTICELLA-CAMPS et al. (1979) who determined the absolute configuration of the C-6–C-9 bond of 5,10-methylenetetrahydrofolate, it was possible to conclude that reduction at C-6 and C-7 involve the same face of NADPH and the same face of folate, and that this orientation is substantially different from that determined for the orientation of methotrexate in the ternary complex of *L. casei* DHFR (see HITCHINGS and ROTH 1980; HITCHINGS and SMITH 1980). POE (1980) reached similar conclusions in his study of the stereochemistry of reduction of folic acid by chicken liver DHFR.

Much less is known about the binding of trimethoprim to DHFR. Of the greatest importance is an explanation at the molecular level for the great specificity of this compound for bacterial rather than mammalian reductases (see Sect. D.II). CAYLEY et al. (1979), have studied by NMR techniques the binding of trimethoprim to reductases of *L. casei* and *E. coli*. Assuming that the pyrimidine ring of trimethoprim binds in the same way as the corresponding part of the methotrexate molecule, it is possible to infer a probable configuration of the trimethoprim–enzyme complex on the basis of the three-dimensional structure of the *E. coli* reductase and ring current effects of each of the rings of trimethoprim. In addition, a rapid flipping of the bound trimethoprim molecule around the C-7–C-1′ bond was observed. Verification of this suggestion by X-ray crystallography is awaited with interest.

BAKER et al. (1981) have provided the first information on the crystal structure of the trimethoprim–*E. coli*–DHFR complex. The conformation of trimethoprim is compatible with that deduced by solution NMR studies and with the crystal structure of trimethoprim hydrobromide. The diaminopyrimidine ring is surrounded by Asp-27, Phe-31, Ile-94, and Thr-113 while the trimethoxy moiety is enclosed by Phe-31, Ile-50, and Leu-28. There are small dissimilarities in the difference Fourier electron density between the trimethoprim and methotrexate complexes. FEENEY et al. (1980) have attempted to study the effect of various ligands, including NADPH and trimethoprim, on the surface accessibility of several aromatic residues in dihydrofolate reductase. Changes in the availability of at least three amino acids are seen.

E. Plasmid-Coded Reductases

In 1972, 4 years after the commercial introduction of trimethoprim, FLEMING et al. (1972) reported the existence of R plasmids containing strains of *E. coli* which were highly resistant to trimethoprim. AMYES and SMITH (1974) and SKÖLD and WIDH (1974) showed this resistance to be due to a novel DHFR with greatly diminished affinity for all diaminoheterocycles, including methotrexate. A different plasmid-coded reductase (R 67) having almost total resistance to trimethoprim was reported by PATTISHALL et al. (1977). Amino acid sequence analysis confirmed that these enzymes constitute a new type of reductase bearing no obvious relationships to reductases isolated previously from bacterial, mammalian, avian, protozoan, or other sources (STONE and SMITH 1979).

The R 67 R plasmid DHFR reported by PATTISHALL et al. (1977) has been studied in greater detail by S. SMITH et al. (1979 b). In these studies, strains of *E. coli* prepared by FLING et al. (1978) with amplified levels of the resistant DHFR were employed. A hybrid plasma, pIE 028 was constructed from EcoR1 restricted DNA from *E. coli* R 67 and the cloning vehicle pBR 313. After transformation and selection with trimethoprim, organisms were isolated which contained a minimum of 28 plasmid copies for each genome equivalent. This strain (*E. coli* C 600 pIE 028) had about 25 times more enzyme than the parent strain.

Purification and characterization of this amplified enzyme was reported by S. SMITH et al. (1979 a). Unlike any other DHFR studied to date, the resistant enzyme was shown to consist of four identical subunits, each with a molecular weight of 8,444 daltons. The amino acid sequence showed no homology with any other known dihydrofolate reductase. Further studies by S. SMITH and BURCHALL (1980) demonstrated that 4 mol folate and 1 mol NADPH are bound to each 34,000 daltons tetramer in the binary complexes. The binding of folate shows strong positive cooperativity, but this type of interaction has not been demonstrated with NADPH. There was no suggestion that units smaller than the tetramer were active.

The differences observed between the amino acid sequence of the R 67 plasmid DHFR and all other DHFRs previously sequenced is in agreement with immunologic studies in which antibodies prepared against the trimethoprim-sensitive chromosomal reductases of *E. coli* and L 1210 cells failed to inactivate R 67 reductase. Interestingly, antibody prepared against the R 67 enzyme did react with the trimethoprim-resistant reductase coded by plasmid R 388 (S. SMITH and BURCHALL 1980). The relationship is confirmed by the finding of ZOLG and HÄNGGI (1981) that the nucleotide sequence of the R 388 enzyme codes for a protein which differs in amino acid sequence from the R 67 enzyme by only 17 residues. Previously, D. SMITH and CALVO (1980) determined the nucleotide sequence of the chromosomal DHFR of *E. coli* K 12 and showed that the amino acid sequence it predicted was very close to that determined for *E. coli* B by STONE et al. (1977).

The origin of plasmid-coded DHFRs remains obscure. There are indications that the enzymes in this group may not be closely related (S. SMITH and BURCHALL 1980). AMYES and SMITH (1976) suggested that the DHFR coded by plasmid R 388 may have its source in a bacteriophage. However, MOSHER et al. (1977) showed important differences between the DHFR of bacteriophage T 4 and the R 483 plasmid-coded DHFR in several criteria. As we have suggested elsewhere (S. SMITH et al. 1979 b) the plasmid-coded DHFR may be a rather different type of oxidoreductase which has lost some degree of substrate specificity, but which as a result has acquired the ability to reduce dihydrofolate. Thus, trimethoprim resistance would arise as a consequence of a "preadaptive" evolutionary sequence which optimized a different function and by chance became the instrument of the organisms' survival in the presence of trimethoprim.

F. Genetics of DHFR

The control of DHFR in bacterial and mammalian cells has received increased attention, particularly as recombinant DNA techniques have made its investigation more feasible. The study of control is complicated by the fact that certain DHFR inhibitors appear to stabilize the enzyme against proteolytic degradation (BURCHALL 1968; HAKALA and SUOLINNA 1966). Evidence for genuine hyperproduction of dihydrofolate reductase in *Diplococcus pneumoniae* has been reported by McCUEN and SIROTNAK (1974). The hyperproduction is associated with a mutation in the structural gene for dihydrofolate reductase. These findings have been confirmed and extended to fol-regulatory mutants of *E. coli* K 12 by SHELDON (1977). BREEZE et al. (1975) and D. SMITH and CALVO (1979) have studied strains of *E. coli* resistant to trimethoprim. In the latter case, it was concluded that resistance was due to a mutation in a regulatory region of the genome which resulted in an increase in DHFR mRNA.

Analogous increases in the levels of dihydrofolate reductase in mammalian cells exposed to methotrexate have been reported. HILLCOAT et al. (1967) reported that human lymphoblast-like cells showed a 12-fold increase in total DHFR when grown in the presence of methotrexate. The time-dependent effects suggested that this increase was due to decreased degradation of the enzyme when complexed with methotrexate. However, not all increases in DHFR levels are due to enzyme stabilization. SCHIMKE et al. (1978) have shown in experiments with cultured murine cells that increased DHFR levels which accompany methotrexate can be due to amplification of the genes coding for this enzyme. Some resistant cell lines are stable in the absence of methotrexate while others rapidly lose gene copies and resistance to the drug. This mechanism of drug selection for gene amplification undoubtedly accounts for other types of resistance observed in nature. It remains to be seen whether this mechanism is important in resistance to methotrexate observed during cancer chemotherapy.

Recombinant DNA appears to provide an important tool for answering some of the most important remaining questions about DHFR. CHANG et al. (1978) have reported the construction of bacterial plasmids which phenotypically express mouse dihydrofolate reductase in *E. coli*. The selection procedure used takes advantage of the resistance to trimethoprim conferred on *E. coli* by the presence of mammalian DHFR, a type of DHFR known to be relatively insensitive to this antimicrobial. Detailed analysis of this mouse dihydrofolate reductase gene has been reported by NUNBERG et al. (1980). These studies have shown that this gene has a 42,000 base DNA sequence which is interrupted by at least five intervening sequence (interons). In no other gene analyzed to date have intervening sequences comprised such a high fraction of the total genome. Based on a molecular weight of 21,500 daltons for the L 1210 DHFR gene (STONE and PHILLIPS 1977) the genome can be calculated to contain over 50 times the minimum number of base pairs needed to code for this enzyme. Identical results were obtained from methotrexate-sensitive and methotrexate-resistant cells. The significance of this surprising finding remains unclear.

Dihydrofolate reductase continues to fascinate scientists and clinicians for whom it provides a target for antibacterial and anticancer chemotherapy, a model for the rational design of chemotherapeutic agents and a basic genetic tool for the study of microevolution. Recent studies which have revealed new and unexpected complexities in its catalytic function, structural organization, and biosynthetic control suggest that more surprises of consequence lie ahead.

References

Amyes SGB, Smith JT (1974) R-factor trimethoprim resistance mechanism: an insusceptible target site. Biochem Biophys Res Commun 58:412–418

Amyes SGB, Smith JT (1976) The purification and properties of the trimethoprim resistant dihydrofolate reductase mediated by the R-factor, R 388. Eur J Biochem 61:597–603

Baccanari DP, Joyner SS (1981) Dihydrofolate reductase hysteresis and its effect on inhibitor binding analyses. Biochemistry 20:1710–1716

Baccanari D, Phillips AW, Smith S, Sinski D, Burchall J (1975) Purification and properties of *Escherichia coli* dihydrofolate reductase. Biochemistry 14:5267–5273

Baccanari D, Averett D, Briggs C, Burchall J (1977) *Escherichia coli* dihydrofolate reductase: Isolation and characterization of two isozymes. Biochemistry 16:3566–3572

Baccanari D, Stone D, Kuyper L (1981) Effect of a single amino acid substitution on *Escherichia coli* dihydrofolate reductase. J Biol Chem 256:1738–1747

Baker DJ, Beddell CR, Champness JN, Goodford PJ, Norrington FEA, Smith DR, Stammers DK (1981) The binding of trimethoprim to bacterial dihydrofolate reductase. FEBS Lett 126:49–52

Bauman H, Wilson KJ (1975) Dihydrofolate reductase from bovine liver. Eur J Biochem 60:9–15

Benkovic SJ (1980) On the mechanism of action of folate- and biopterin-requiring enzymes. Annu Rev Biochem 49:227–251

Bennett CS, Rodkey JA, Sondey JM, Hirschman R (1978) Dihydrofolate reductase: the amino acid sequence of the enzyme from a methotrexate-resistant mutant of *Escherichia coli*. Biochemistry 17:1328–1337

Bertino JR, Booth BA, Bieber AL, Cashmore A, Sartorelli AC (1964) Studies on the inhibition of dihydrofolate reductase by the folate antagonists. J Biol Chem 239:479–485

Birdsall B, Roberts GCK, Feeney J, Burgen ASV (1977) ^{31}PNMR studies of the binding of adenosine-2'-phosphate to *Lactobacillus casei* dihydrofolate reductase. FEBS Lett 80:313–316

Birdsall B, Burgen ASV, deMiranda JR, Roberts GCK (1978) Cooperativity in ligand binding to dihydrofolate reductase. Biochemistry 17:2102–2110

Birdsall B, Burgen ASV, Roberts GCK (1980a) Effects of coenzyme analogues on the binding of p-aminobenzoyl-L-glutamate and 2,4-diaminopyrimidine to *Lactobacillus casei* dihydrofolate reductase. Biochemistry 19:3732–3737

Birdsall B, Burgen ASV, Roberts GCK (1980b) Binding of coenzyme analogues to *Lactobacillus casei* dihydrofolate reductase: binary and ternary complexes. Biochemistry 19:3723–3731

Bitar KG, Blankenship DT, Walsh KA, Dunlap RB, Reddy AV, Freisheim JH (1977) Amino acid sequence of dihydrofolate reductase from an amethopterin resistant strain of *Lactobacillus casei*. FEBS Lett 80:119–122

Blakley RL (1969) The biochemistry of folic acid and related pteridines. John Wiley and Sons, New York

Blakley RL, Ramasastri BU, McDougall BM (1963) The biosynthesis of thymidylic acid. V. Hydrogen isotope studies with dihydrofolate reductase and thymidylate synthetase. J Biol Chem 238:3075–3079

Blakley RL, Schrock M, Sommer K, Nixon PF (1971) Kinetic studies of the reaction mechanism of dihydrofolate reductase. Ann NY Acad Sci 186:119–130

Breeze AS, Sims P, Stacey KA (1975) Trimethoprim resistant mutants of E. coli K 12: preliminary genetic mapping. Genet Res 25:207–214

Broquist HP, Stockstad ELR, Jukes TH (1950) Some biological and chemical properties of the citrovorum factor. J Biol Chem 185:399–409

Burchall JJ (1968) Protection of microbial dihydrofolate reductase against inactivation by pronase. Mol Pharmacol 4:238–248

Burchall JJ (1970) Purification and properties of dihydrofolate reductase from Escherichia coli. In: Iwai K, Akino M, Goto M, Iwanami Y (eds) Chemistry and biology of pteridines. Int Acad Printing Co, Tokyo, Japan, pp 351–355

Burchall JJ (1979) The development of the diaminopyrimidines. J Antimicrob Chemother [Suppl B] 5:3–14

Burchall JJ, Hitchings GH (1965) Inhibitor binding analysis of dihydrofolate reductases from various species. Mol Pharmacol 1:126–136

Cayley PJ, Albrand JP, Feeney J, Roberts GCK, Piper EA, Burgen ASV (1979) Nuclear magnetic resonance studies of the binding of trimethoprim to dihydrofolate reductase. Biochemistry 18:3886–3894

Chang ACY, Nunberg JH, Kaufman RJ, Erlich HA, Schimke RT, Cohen SN (1978) Phenotypic expression in E. coli of a DNA sequence coding for mouse dihydrofolate reductase. Nature 275:617–624

Charlton PA, Young DW, Birdsall B, Feeney J, Roberts GCK (1979) Stereochemistry of reduction of folic acid using dihydrofolate reductase. J Chem Soc Chem Commun 20:922–924

Coward JK, Parameswaran KN, Cashmore AR, Bertino JR (1974) 7,8-dihydropteroyloligo-γ-L-glutamates: synthesis and kinetic studies with purified dihydrofolate reductase from mammalian sources. Biochemistry 13:3899–3903

Dannenberg PV, Dannenberg KD, Cleland WW (1978) The interaction of liver alcohol dehydrogenase with phenyl adenine dinucleotide, a novel analog of pyridine nucleotide coenzymes. J Biol Chem 253:5886–5887

Dunn SMJ, King RW (1980) Kinetics of ternary complex formation between dihydrofolate reductase coenzyme and inhibitors. Biochemistry 19:766–773

Feeney J, Roberts GCK, Kapstein R, Birdsall B, Gronenborn A, Burgen ASV (1980) Photo-CIDNP studies of the influence of ligand binding on the surface accessibility of aromatic residues in dihydrofolate reductase. Biochemistry 19:2466–2472

Ferone R, Roland S (1980) Dihydrofolate reductase: thymidylate synthetase, a functional polypeptide from Crithidia fasciculata. Proc Natl Acad Sci USA 77:5802–5806

Ferone R, Burchall J, Hitchings G (1969) Plasmodium berghei dihydrofolate reductases. Isolation, properties and inhibition by antifolates. Mol Pharmacol 5:49–59

Fleming MP, Datta N, Gruneberg RN (1972) Trimethoprim resistance determined by R-factors. Br Med J 1:726–728

Fling M, Elwell LP, Inamine JH (1978) Cloning and amplification of DNA sequence encoding a trimethoprim-resistant dihydrofolate reductase gene. In: Boyer HW, Nicosia S (eds) Genetic engineering. Elsevier/North Holland, Amsterdam, pp 173–180

Florkin M (1974) Concepts of molecular biosemiotics and of molecular evolution. In: Florkin M, Stotz EH (eds) Comprehensive biochemistry, vol 29 A. Elsevier, Amsterdam, pp 1–124

Fontecilla-Camps JC, Bugg CE, Temple C, Rose JD, Montgomery JA, Kisliuk RL (1979) X-ray crystallographic studies of the structure of 5,10-methylenetetrahydrofolic acid. In: Kisliuk RL, Brown GM (eds) Chemistry and biology of pteridines. Elsevier/North Holland, New York, pp 235–240

Franklin AL, Stockstad ELR, Belt M, Jukes TH (1947) Biochemical experiments with a synthetic preparation having an action antagonistic to that of pteroylglutamic acid. J Biol Chem 169:427–435

Freisheim JH, Ericsson CH, Bitar KG, Dunlap RB, Reddy AV (1977) An active center tryptophan residue in dihydrofolate reductase: chemical modification, sequence surrounding the critical residue, and structure homology consideration. Arch Biochem Biophys 180:310–317

Freisheim JH, Bitar KG, Reddy AV, Blankenship DT (1978) Dihydrofolate reductase from amethopterin-resistant *Lactobacillus casei*. J Biol Chem 253:6437–6444

Freisheim JH, Kumar AA, Blankenship DT, Kaufman BT (1979) Structure-function relationships of dihydrofolate reductase: sequence homology considerations and active center residues. In: Kisliuk RL, Brown GM (eds) Chemistry and biology of pteridines. Elsevier/North Holland, New York, pp 419–424

Gleisner JM, Peterson DL, Blakley RL (1974) Amino acid sequence of dihydrofolate reductase from a methotrexate-resistant mutant of *Streptococcus faecium* and identification of methionine residue at the inhibitor binding site. Proc Natl Acad Sci USA 71:3001–3005

Gready JE (1980) Dihydrofolate reductase: binding of substrates and inhibitors and catalytic mechanism. Adv Pharmacol Chemother 17:37–102

Gutteridge WE, Jaffe JJ, McCormack JJ (1969) The gel-filtration behaviour of dihydrofolate reductases from culture forms of trypanosomatids. Biochim Biophys Acta 191:753–755

Hakala MT, Suolinna EM (1966) Specific protection of folate reductase against chemical and proteolytic inactivation. Mol Pharmacol 2:465–480

Hayman R, McGready R, Van der Weyden MB (1980) A rapid radiometric assay for dihydrofolate reductase. Anal Biochem 87:460–465

Hillcoat BL, Swett V, Bertino JR (1967) Increase of dihydrofolate reductase activity in cultured mammalian cells after exposure to methotrexate. Proc Natl Acad Sci USA 58:1632–1637

Hitchings GH, Roth B (1980) Dihydrofolate reductase as targets for selective inhibitors. In: Sandler M (ed) Enzyme inhibitors as drugs. Macmillan, London Basingstoke, pp 263–280

Hitchings GH, Smith SL (1980) Dihydrofolate reductases as targets for inhibitors. In: Weber G (ed) Adv Enzyme Regul, pp 349–370

Hitchings GH, Elion GB, Vanderwerff H, Falco EA (1948) Pyrimidine derivatives as antagonists of pteroylglutamic acid. J Biol Chem 174:765–766

Hitchings GH, Burchall JJ, Ferone R (1968) The comparative enzymology of dihydrofolate reductase and the design of chemotherapeutic agents. In: Welch AD (ed) Proc 3rd Int Pharmacol Meeting. The control of growth processes by chemical agents, vol 5. Pergamon, New York, pp 3–18

Huennekens FM, Vitols KS, Whiteley JM, Neef VG (1976) Dihydrofolate reductase. Methods Cancer Res 13:199–225

Hyde EI, Birdsall B, Roberts GCK, Feeney J, Burgen ASV (1980) Proton nuclear magnetic resonance saturation transfer studies of coenzyme binding to *Lactobacillus casei* dihydrofolate reductase. Biochemistry 19:3738–3746

Lai PH, Pan YC, Gleisner JM, Peterson DL, Blakeley RL (1979) Primary sequence of bovine liver dihydrofolate reductase. In: Kisliuk RL, Brown GM (eds) Chemistry and biology of pteridines. Elsevier/North Holland, New York, pp 437–440

Lindquist CA, Cadman EC, Bertino JR (1977) A fluorometric assay for dihydrofolate reductase. Anal Biochem 83:20–25

Matthews DA, Alden RA, Bolin JT, Freer ST, Hamlin R, Xuong N, Kraut J, Poe M, Williams M, Hoogsteen K (1977) Dihydrofolate reductase: X-ray structure of the binary complex with methotrexate. Science 197:452–455

Matthews DA (1979) Interpretation of nuclear magnetic resonance spectra for *Lactobacillus casei* dihydrofolate reductase based on the x-ray structure of the enzyme-methotrexate-NADPH complex. Biochemistry 18:1602–1610

Matthews DA, Alden RA, Bolin JT, Filman DJ, Freer ST, Hamlin R, Hol WGJ, Kisliuk RL, Pastore EJ, Plante LT, Xuong N, Kraut J (1978) Dihydrofolate reductase from *Lactobacillus casei* x-ray structure of the enzyme-methotrexate-NADPH complex. J Biol Chem 253:6946–6954

Matthews DA, Alden RA, Freer ST, Xuong N, Kraut J (1979) Dihydrofolate reductase from *Lactobacillus casei*/Stereochemistry of NADPH binding. J Biol Chem 254:4144–4151

McCuen RW, Sirotnak FM (1974) Hyperproduction of dihydrofolate reductase in *Diplococcus pneumonia* by mutation in the structure gene. Biochim Biophys Acta 338:540–544

McCullough JL, Nixon PF, Bertino JR (1971) Kinetic investigations of the reaction mechanisms of dihydrofolate reductase from L 1210 cells. Ann NY Acad Sci 186:131–142

Mosher RA, DiKenzo AB, Mathews CK (1977) Bacteriophage T_4 virion dihydrofolate reductase; approaches to quantitation and assessment of function. J Virol 23:645–658

Nichol CA, Welch AD (1950) Synthesis of citrovorum factor from folic acid by liver slices; augmentation by ascorbic acid. Proc Soc Exp Biol Med 74:52–55

Nunberg JH, Kaufman RJ, Chang ACY, Cohen SN, Schimke RT (1980) Structure and genomic organization of the mouse dihydrofolate reductase gene. Cell 19:355–364

Osborn MJ, Huennekens FM (1958) Inhibition of dihydrofolate reductase by aminopterin and amethopterin. Proc Soc Exp Biol Med 97:429

Pastore EJ, Friedkin M (1962) The enzymatic synthesis of thymidylate. II. Transfer of tritium from tetrahydrofolate to the methyl group of thymidylate. J Biol Chem 237:3802–3810

Pastore EJ, Kisliuk RL, Plante LT, Wright JM, Kaplan NO (1974) Conformational changes induced in dihydrofolate reductase by folates, pyridine nucleotides coenzymes and methotrexate. Prox Natl Acad Sci USA 71:3849–3853

Pattishall KH, Burchall JJ, Harvey RJ (1976) Interconvertible forms of *Escherichia coli* dihydrofolate reductase with different affinities for analogs of dihydrofolate. J Biol Chem 251:7011–7020

Pattishall KH, Acar J, Burchall JJ, Goldstein FW, Harvey RJ (1977) Two distinct types of TMP-resistant dihydrofolate reductases specified by R-plasmids of different compatibility groups. J Biol Chem 252:2319–2323

Perkins JP, Bertino JR (1966) Dihydrofolate reductase from L 1210 murine lymphoma. Fluorometric measurements of the interactions of the enzyme with coenzymes, substrates and inhibitors. Biochemistry 5:1005-1012

Poe M (1977) Acidic dissociation constants of folic acid, dihydrofolic acid and methotrexate. J Biol Chem 252:3724–3728

Poe M (1980) Stereochemistry of reduction of folic acid by chicken liver dihydrofolate reductase. Fed Proc 39:1856

Poe M, Greenfield NJ, Williams MN (1974) Dihydrofolate reductase from a methotrexate-resistant *Escherichia coli*. J Biol Chem 249:2710–2716

Rodkey JA, Bennett CD (1976) Micro-Edman degradation: the use of high pressure liquid chromatography and gas chromatography in the amino terminal sequence determination of 8 nanomoles of dihydrofolate reductase from a mouse sarcoma. Biochem Biophys Res Commun 72:1407–1413

Rossman MG, Liljos A, Bränden GI, Banoszak LJ (1975) Evolutionary and structural relationships among dehydrogenases. In: Boyer PD (ed) The enzymes, 3rd edn, vol 11. Academic Press, New York, pp 61–102

Rothenberg SP, Perivair-Igbal M, DaCosta M (1980) An amplified radioenzymatic assay using [^{3}H]dihydrofolate. Anal Biochem 103:152–156

Schimke RT, Kaufman RJ, Alt FW, Kellems RF (1978) Gene amplification and drug resistance in cultured murine cells. Science 202:1051–1055

Seeger DR, Smith JM, Hultquist ME (1947) Antagonists for pteroylglutamic acid. J Am Chem Soc 69:2567

Sheldon R (1977) Altered dihydrofolate reductase in *fol* regulatory mutants of *Escherichia coli* K 12. Molec Gen Genet 151:215–219

Sköld O, Widh A (1974) A new dihydrofolate reductase with low trimethoprim sensitivity induced by an R-factor mediating high resistance to trimethoprim. J Biol Chem 249:4324–4325

Smith DR, Calvo JM (1979) Regulation of dihydrofolate reductase in *Escherichia coli.* Molec Gen Genet 175:31–38

Smith DR, Calvo JM (1980) Nucleotide sequence of the *E. coli* gene coding for dihydrofolate reductase. Nucleic Acids Res 8:2255–2273

Smith SL, Burchall JJ (1980) Studies of *E. coli* R plasmid dihydrofolate reductase. Fed Proc 39:1771

Smith SL, Patrick P, Stone D, Phillips AW, Burchall JJ (1979 a) Porcine liver dihydrofolate reductase: purification, properties, and amino acid sequence. J Biol Chem 254:11475–11484

Smith SL, Stone D, Novak P, Baccanari D, Burchall J (1979 b) R-plasmid dihydrofolate reductase with subunit structure. J Biol Chem 254:6222–6225

Stone D, Phillips AW (1977) The amino acid sequence of dihydrofolate reductase from L 1210 cells. FEBS Lett 74:85–87

Stone D, Smith SL (1979) The amino acid sequence of a trimethoprim-resistant dihydrofolate reductase specified in *E. coli* by R-plasmid R 67. J Biol Chem 254:10857–10861

Stone D, Phillips AW, Burchall JJ (1977) The amino acid sequence of dihydrofolate reductase of a trimethoprim-resistant strain of *Escherichia coli.* Eur J Biochem 72:613–624

Stone D, Paterson SJ, Raper JH, Phillips AW (1979) The amino acid sequence of dihydrofolate reductase from the mouse lymphoma L 1210. J Biol Chem 254:480–488

Wang CC, Stotish RL, Poe M (1975) Dihydrofolate reductase from *Eimeria tenella:* rationalization of chemotherapeutic efficacy of pyrimethamine. J Protozool 22:564–568

Williams JW, Duggleby RG, Cutler R, Morrison JR (1980) The inhibition of dihydrofolate reductase by folate analogs: structural requirements for slow- and tight-binding inhibition. Biochem Pharmacol 29:589–595

Williams MN, Poe M, Greenfield NJ, Hirschfield JM, Hoogsteen W (1973 a) Methotrexate binding to dihydrofolate reductase from a methotrexate resistant strain of *Escherichia coli.* J Biol Chem 248:6375–6379

Williams MN, Greenfield NJ, Hoogsteen K (1973 b) Evidence for two reduced triphospho-pyridine nucleotide binding sites on dihydrofolate reductase from a methotrexate-resistant strain of *Escherichia coli.* JBC 248:6380–6386

Williams TJ, Kee TK, Dunlap RB (1977) Dihydrofolate reductase from amethopterin-resistant *Lactobacillus casei.* Arch Biochem Biophys 181:569–579

Woods DD (1940) The relation of *p*-aminobenzoic acid to the mechanism of action of sulphonilamide. Br J Exp Pathol 21:74–90

Wooley DW (1952) A study of antimetabolites. Wiley, New York

Zolg JW, Hänggi UJ (1981) Characterization of a R-plasmid associated, trimethoprim-resistant dihydrofolate reductase and determination of the nucleotide sequence of the reductase gene. Nucleic Acids Res 9:697–709

CHAPTER 4

Antibacterial Activity

S.R.M. BUSHBY

A. Introduction

From the results of an extensive study of substituted pyrimidines, HITCHINGS et al. (1948) concluded that as a class the 2,4-diaminopyrimidines are antifolates. Further studies revealed that within the series considerable selectivities for various biologic systems were exhibited (HITCHINGS et al. 1952 b). Thus the 5-phenyl derivatives yielded the antimalarial, pyrimethamine, whereas the 5-alkoxybenzyl derivatives were recognized as having interesting antibacterial activities (HITCHINGS et al. 1952 a) and these were soon seriously considered as chemotherapeutic antibacterial agents. After exploratory experiments with selected members of the series, trimethoprim (TMP) was chosen in 1959 from among close analogs for more extensive prior to clinical trials (ROTH et al. 1962).

The locus of action of the class was defined in 1952 as "interference with the conversion of folic to folinic acid" (HITCHINGS et al. 1952 a) but it took some years to resolve all the apparent discrepancies suggested by reversal experiments. The significance of the synergy between sulfonamides and 2,4-diaminopyrimidines, first observed by GREENBERG and RICHESON (1950), was not overlooked (HITCHINGS et al. 1952 b) and soon became the basis for studies of potentiation which were applied to a wide spectrum of bacterial pathogens, both in vitro and in vivo (HITCHINGS and BUSHBY 1961). The site of action of TMP in the biosynthesis of the folate coenzymes and its relation to that of the sulfonamides are discussed in Chaps. 1 and 2.

Several sulfonamides and two pyrimidines, TMP and its close analog tetroxoprim (2,4-diamino-5-[3,5-dimethoxy-4-(2-methoxyethoxy)benzyl]pyrimidine) have been used in combinations for treating bacterial infections. The combination of TMP and sulfamethoxazole (SMX) in the ratio of 1:5, generically co-trimoxazole, has had much the most extensive use.

B. In Vitro Activity

I. Effects of Medium and Size of Inoculum

The antibacterial activity of the sulfonamides was first detected in mice infected with streptococci and only subsequently demonstrated in vitro. The in vitro activity varied greatly, depending on the organism and on the constituents of the medium, but media giving unsatisfactory results could be greatly improved by adding lysed horse blood (HARPER and CAWSTON 1945). In contrast to that of the sulfonamides, the antibacterial activity of the 2,4-diaminobenzylpyrimidines was first detected in vitro in media that were suitable for sulfonamides and, as with the sulfonamides, unsuitable media could be improved by adding lysed horse blood (S. Bushby 1973). The cross-unsuitability of media for these two classes of antibacterials indicated the factor responsible to be probably an end product of folate metabolism, produced beyond the metabolic blocks imposed by either the sulfonamide or the 2,4-diaminobenzylpyrimidine. This indication was confirmed by Koch and Burchall (1971), who showed that activity varied inversely with the concentration of thymidine in the medium, and by Ferone et al. (1975), who showed that the improvement was due to thymidine phosphorylase.

Among the commonly available animal species, the presence of thymidine phosphorylase in the red cells appears to be unique to the horse (Ferone et al. 1975); certainly Harper and Cawston (1945) found that, of lysed blood from several species, only that from the horse improved media. The action of the enzyme is to convert the thymidine to thymine which is used 30–100 times less effectively by the pathogens that can utilize thymidine (M. Bushby et al. 1978). The improvement is therefore limited by the concentration of thymidine present and is minimal when the concentration is greater than 1 µg/ml but, according to Amyes and Smith (1978), the addition of uridine to the medium will prevent the antagonism by thymine through, paradoxically, competitively inhibiting intracellular thymidine phosphorylase.

Not all bacterial species, e.g., *Neisseria gonorrhoeae*, are capable of using thymidine as a growth factor and therefore their susceptibilities to these antifolate drugs are not affected by the medium. Even with species that can use it, the ability to use it as an antagonist varies. The concentration that begins to affect the suitability of the medium is about 0.01 µg/ml (S. Bushby 1973; Then 1977) and although at this concentration the inhibition is only partial, it may be sufficient to abolish killing. In bacteriostatic measurements, using the serial dilution method, partial inhibition causes long-trailing end points and, using the diffusion method, it causes graded growth within the main zone of inhibition. Unless the concentration in a test medium is known to be below the critical level (0.01 µg/ml), thymidine phosphorylase, either as the actual enzyme or as lysed horse blood, should be added when measuring the antibacterial activities. The addition is particularly necessary when endeavoring to measure bactericidal activity (see Sect. B.III). For example, Table 1 shows the effects of 2% lysed horse blood on the number of viable cells of *Escherichia coli* when exposed to varying concentrations of TMP during 24 h at 37 °C in a nutrient broth, this medium was highly satisfactory for bacteriostatic sensitivity testing, and yet there is little evidence of killing except when the enzyme was present.

Because sulfonamides act by competing with p-aminobenzoic acid and, because this metabolite antagonizes the action of sulfonamides in vitro, it has often been assumed to be the sulfonamide antagonist in media. However, this can rarely be the case, seeing that lysed horse blood usually prevents the antagonism.

As with the sulfonamides, the minimum inhibitory concentration (MIC) of TMP varies with number of organisms present. Table 2 shows the increases in the MIC for one strain each of *E. coli*, *Staphylococcus aureus*, and *Proteus vulgaris* when the inocula were increased from 5 to 5×10^5 organisms; the maximum in-

Table 1. Effect of lysed horse blood on bactericidal activity[a] of trimethoprim

TMP (μg/ml)	Presence of 2% lysed horse blood	Reduction of inoculum with time (%)		
		3 h	6 h	24 h
0.1	−	0	0	0
	+	88	93	30
0.3	−	0	0	0
	+	90	98.9	99
1.0	−	0	0	3
	+	98	99.7	> 99.9

[a] Reduction in the number of *E. coli* present in Oxoid Sensitivity Test Broth, with and without 2% lysed horse blood, during incubation at 37 °C for 24 h. The reduction is expressed as a percentage of those present at 0

Table 2. Effect of inoculum size on MIC[a] of TMP

Inoculum	MIC of TMP (μg/ml)		
	Escherichia coli	*Staphylococcus aureus*	*Proteus vulgaris*
10^0	> 50	> 50	> 50
10^{-1}	5	50	50
10^{-2}	0.5	0.5	15
10^{-3}	0.5	0.5	5
10^{-4}	0.5	0.15	5
10^{-5}	0.15		1.5

[a] Titration showing increase in MIC of trimethoprim with increase in the size of inoculum; 10^0 inoculum contains approximately 5×10^5 organisms streaked over 1 cm. The medium was Wellcotest Sensitivity Test Agar which is basically a soya digest agar with a low thymidine content. The MIC was read as 90% inhibition of macroscopic growth

crease in MIC is greater than 300-fold. In the diffusion method, the size of the zone of inhibition varies inversely with that of the inoculum and, with excessively large inocula, the zone may be completely abolished.

II. Bacteriostatic Activity

On a weight basis, the antibacterial in vitro activity of TMP is to date broader and higher than that reported for any other member of the 2,4-diaminobenzyl-pyrimidines. Its MICs compared with those of sulfamethoxazole (SMX) for 29 rep-

Table 3. Activities[a] of TMP and SMX   **b**

Organism	MIC (μg/ml)	
	TMP	SMX
Streptococcus pyogenes	0.5	95
Streptococcus pneumoniae type II	1.5	28.5
Viridans streptococci	0.15	9.5
Streptococcus faecalis	0.5	95
Streptococcus agalactiae	5.0	28.5
Staphylococcus aureus	0.15	2.85
Erysipelothrix rhusiopathiae	5.0	> 95
Corynebacterium pyogenes	0.5	> 95
Corynebacterium diphtheriae	0.5	> 95
Clostridium perfringens	50	28.5
Mycobactericum tuberculosis	150	>950
Nocardia asteroides	15	2.85
Escherichia coli	0.15	9.5
Citrobacter freundii	0.15	2.85
Klebsiella pneumoniae	0.5	28.5
Enterobacter aerogenes	5.0	> 95
Salmonella typhi	0.5	2.85
Shigella sp.	0.5	2.85
Vibrio cholerae	1.5	28.5
Pasteurella septica	0.15	9.5
Haemophilus influenzae	0.5	9.5
Moraxella lacunata	5.0	9.5
Proteus sp.	1.5	28.5
Providencia rettgeri	1.5	28.5
Pseudomonas aeruginosa	150	28.5
Neisseria gonorrhoeae	15	0.95
Neisseria meningitidis	5.0	0.285
Brucella abortus	15	2.85

[a] The MIC's of TMP and SMX were compared in Wellcotest Sensitivity Test Agar containing 7.5% lysed horse blood. For *H. influenzae*, *N. gonorrhoeae*, and *N. meningitidis*, the medium was heated at 80 °C for 5 min, and in the case of *M. tuberculosis*, Peizer–Schector medium was used. One-third dilutions were used

resentative strains of various bacterial species, measured in a medium of low thymidine content, are shown in Table 3, and the range of MICs reported by BACH et al. (1973) for 11–36 strains of 18 species are shown in Table 4. These results show that, although, in general TMP and SMX have similar spectra of activities, the MIC of TMP is usually some ten-times lower than that of the sulfonamide. Species which are, in general, relatively insensitive to TMP are *Pseudomonas aeruginosa*, *Neisseria* spp., *Brucella* spp., *Nocardia* spp., *Bacterioides* spp., *Clostridium* spp., and *Mycobacterium tuberculosis*.

The activity of tetroxoprim compared with that of TMP is shown in Table 5 ·and, according to HÖXER (1980), who compared the MICs of tetroxoprim with those of TMP for 404 strains of 15 bacterial species, tetroxoprim is 2–8 times less

Table 4. Susceptibility of strains of various bacteria to TMP and SMX. (Adapted from BACH et al. 1973)

Organism (no. of strains)	MIC (µg/ml)			
	TMP		SMX	
	Range	Median	Range	Median
Streptococcus pyogenes (35)	0.02–0.8	0.1	3.1–1,000	12.5
Enterococcus (25)	0.02–0.2	0.1	all >1,000	>1,000
Streptococcus pneumoniae (33)	0.04–0.8	0.4	6.3–>1,000	50
Staphylococcus aureus (36)	0.4 –1.6	0.8	25 –>100	50
S. epidermidis (35)	0.2 –6.3	0.4	12.5–>1,000	100
Neisseria gonorrhoeae (35)	0.2 –3.1	0.8	6.3–1,000	50
Neisseria meningitidis (11)	3.1 –25	6.3	0.4–>100	1.6
Haemophilus influenzae (35)	0.2 –0.4	0.4	100 –>1,000	1,000
Escherichia coli (36)	0.2 –0.8	0.4	25 –1,000	100
Klebsiella pneumoniae (33)	all 3.1	3.1	50 –>1,000	1,000
Enterobacter spp. (35)	0.2 –1.6	0.8	12.5–>1,000	50
Serratia marcescens (27)	0.4 –3.1	0.8	1,000 –>1,000	>1,000
Proteus spp. (35)	0.4 –6.3	3.1	3.1–>1,000	100
Providencia spp. (35)	0.8 –6.3	1.6	3.1–>1,000	100
Pseudomonas aeruginosa (35)	50 –1,000	1,000	50 –>1,000	1,000
Salmonella spp. (34)	0.1 –0.2	0.1	12.5–>1,000	1,000
Shigella spp. (31)	0.1 –0.8	0.4	12.5–>1,000	>1,000
Acinetobacter calcoaceticus (16)	3.1 –12.5	6.3	3.1–12.5	6.3

The medium was MUELLER–HINTON agar except for *H. Influenzae* when trypticase soy agar with 5% lysed horse blood was used

Table 5. In vitro activity of tetroxoprim (TET) compared with that of trimethoprim on MUELLER–HINTON agar

Organisms		MIC (µg/ml)	
		TET	TMP
Streptococcus pyogenes	CN10	5.0	0.5
Streptococcus pyogenes	S3640	0.5	0.1
Streptococcus faecalis	CN478	0.5	0.1
Staphylococcus aureus	CN491	1.0	0.1
Vibrio cholerae	ATCC14035	5.0	1.0
Pasteurella multocida	ATCC6587	5.0	0.1
Candida albicans	CN1863	>50	>50
Mycobacterium smegmatis	S3254	1.0	0.5
Salmonella typhimurium (LT-2)	S8587	1.0	0.1
Salmonella typhosa	CN512	1.0	0.05
Shigella flexneri	CN6007	5.0	0.1
Escherichia coli	CN314	1.0	0.1
Serratia marcescens	CN2398	>50	5.0
Serratia marcescens	UNC18	10	0.5
Klebsiella pneumoniae	CN3632	5.0	0.5
Enterobacter aerogenes	2200/86	5.0	0.5
Citrobacter freundii	2200/77	5.0	0.5
Pseudomonas aeruginosa	CN200	>50	50
Proteus vulgaris	CN329	50	1.0
Proteus mirabilis	S2409	>50	5.0

active than is trimethoprim; BYWATER et al. (1979) conducted a similar study and found the difference to be in general 8–16 times.

By determining the number of viable units present in a culture of *E. coli*, in logarithmic growth phase, before and after the addition of inhibitory concentrations of SMX, SEYDEL et al. (1973) confirmed that there is a lag phase of about five generations before the sulfonamide exerts significant inhibition, whereas there is little or no lag phase with trimethoprim. These differences are attributable to the sulfonamide interfering with the de novo synthesis of folates and not affecting their recycling, whereas TMP interferes with the formation of tetrahydrofolate from both sources.

III. Bactericidal Activity

Both TMP and sulfonamides are bactericidal, but apparently only under conditions in which their inhibition of protein synthesis is circumvented by the presence of methionine, glycine, and a purine, and in which their inhibition of DNA synthesis is not antagonized (ANGEHRN and THEN 1973; AMYES and SMITH 1974). Under these conditions, the bacteria enlarge without dividing and die; this is the so-called thymineless death. If the inhibition of protein synthesis is not circumvented, then the effects of the antibacterials are merely bacteriostatic. The two amino acids and the necessary purine are present in most bacteriologic media, but in many there is also thymidine which antagonizes the effect on the synthesis of DNA. Traces of thymidine (0.01 µg/ml) will convert the bactericidal activity to bacteriostasis and higher concentrations will interfere with the bacteriostasis. Whether or not the drugs are bactericidal in vivo is not known, but in vitro the conditions in normal blood and urine are, according to THEN and ANGEHRN (1974), suitable for killing and they can be rendered unsuitable by adding thymine or, more effectively, thymidine.

IV. Demonstration of Synergy

The synergy between the benzylpyrimidines and the sulfonamides can be demonstrated in vitro by:
1. A reduction in the MIC of each drug
2. An increase in the size of the zone of inhibition in the diffusion method
3. A reduction in the minimum bactericidal concentrations.

The reduction in the MIC varies with the ratio of the drugs present. Therefore, maximum protentiation can only be determined by measuring activity with the drugs present in multiple ratios as in a two-dimensional, serial dilution procedure (S. BUSHBY and HITCHINGS 1968). In order to simplify the comparison of results obtained with strains of bacteria of different sensitivities to the single drugs, the MIC of each drug in the various ratios may be expressed as a decimal fraction of the MIC of the respective drug when acting alone. This fraction was termed the fractional inhibitory concentration (FIC) by ELION et al. (1954). When the sum of the FICs for each of the drugs at any particular ratio is less than unity, synergy is indicated and the lowest sum, i.e., maximum synergy, is termed the FIC index; so, the lower this index, the greater is the synergy (Table 6). The result can also be pre-

Table 6. Potentiation[a] in combinations of TMP and sulfadiazine (SDZ)

Ratio TMP:SDZ	TMP MIC µg/ml	FIC	SDZ MIC µg/ml	FIC	Sum of FICs[b]
1: 0	0.1	1.00	0.00	–	–
1: 1.24	0.05	0.50	0.062	0.03	0.53
1: 5	0.025	0.25	0.125	0.06	0.31
1: 20	0.012	0.12	0.25	0.13	0.25[c]
1: 83	0.006	0.06	0.5	0.25	0.31
1:333	0.003	0.03	1.0	0.5	0.53
0: 1	0.000	–	2.0	1.00	–

[a] The MICs of the drugs, singly and in various combination for *Proteus vulgaris* (CN 329), determined in Wellcome Nutrient Agar plus 2% lysed horse blood

[b] FIC = (MIC of drug alone/MIC of drug in combination)
[c] FIC index

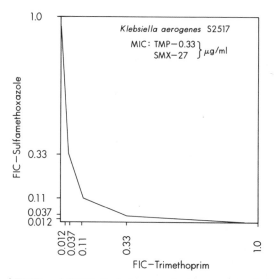

Fig. 1. Synergy of TMP and SMX. Isobologram showing synergy between trimethoprim and sulfamethoxazole constructed from two-dimensional titration of bacteriostatic activity. FIC = Fractional inhibitory concentration, i.e. (MIC of drug in combination/MIC of drug acting alone). Organism is *Klebsiella aerogenes* S 2517; MICs 033, and 27 µg/ml for TMP and SMX, respectively

sented graphically as an isobologram, in which plots falling below the diagonal indicate synergy. An example is shown in Fig. 1.

The results of examining many strains of different species have shown that the isobolograms of TMP and SMX are symmetrical. This observation is important for it indicates that the optimum ratio, as measured by maximum reduction in the

Table 7. Effect on MIC of combining 1 part TMP with 20 parts SMX

Organism	MIC (μg/ml)			
	SMX		TMP	
	Alone	Mixture	Alone	Mixture
Streptococcus pyogenes	>100	1	1	0.05
Streptococcus pneumoniae	30	2	2	0.1
Staphylococcus aureus	3	0.3	1	0.015
Haemophilus influenzae	10	0.3	1	0.015
Bordetella pertussis	50	4	3	0.2
Klebsiella pneumoniae	>100	4	1	0.2
Klebsiella aerogenes	>100	4	1	0.2
Escherichia coli	3	1	0.3	0.05
Salmonella typhimurium	10	1	0.3	0.05
Shigella sonnei	10	1	0.3	0.05
Proteus vulgaris	30	3	3	0.15

MICs of both drugs, is that in which the drugs are present in proportions corresponding to their respective MICs when acting singly. For example, if the MIC for TMP is 0.5 μg/ml and that for SMX is 10 μg/ml, the optimum ratio is 1:20. It should be emphasized, however, that potentiation occurs over a wide range of ratios; at other ratios, the MIC of one of the components will be above and that of the other will be below those of the optimum ratio. The optimum ratio is therefore "optimum" only in terms of economy of drug (see Sect. G). From the results of growth rate studies, SEYDEL et al. (1973) reached similar conclusions; their studies showed that, although maximal effects occurred with the drugs present in equipotent concentrations, they still occurred with ratios ranging from 1:19 to 19:1 of the maximum.

Because of the wide variation in sensitivities of organisms to TMP and sulfonamides, the optimum ratio is very variable but, in general, the MIC of TMP is usually 20–100 times less than that if SMX and therefore, when examining strains for enhanced susceptibility to the combination, investigators have generally preferred to use a single fixed ratio, near the model optimal, i.e., 1:20, rather than the multiratio, time-consuming two-dimensional technique. Examples of the increase in activity using the 1:20 ratio are shown in Table 7.

The degree of bacteriostatic synergy varies with the medium and, according to THEN (1973); it is maximum when the medium contains the complete set of antagonists, i.e., a purine, methionine, glycine, and thymine. With these antagonists present, however, the concentrations of drugs necessary to produce the inhibition are increased and THEN interprets these findings as showing that the basic mechanism of the synergy is depletion of the tetrahydrofolate pool which, in the presence of all the one-carbon metabolites, selectively inhibits the formylation of Met-tRNA.

By the diffusion method, synergy can be detected by using three discs, two of which contain TMP and SMX, singly, and a third containing the drugs together in the same quantities as they are in the single discs. Because the two drugs diffuse

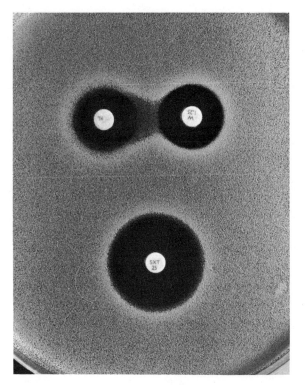

Fig. 2. Demonstration of synergy by the disc diffusion method. The upper discs contain 23.75 SMX (*left*) and 1.25 TMP (*right*), respectively, and the lower one contains these same quantities in combination. Synergy is shown by the bridging of the zones of inhibition by the single discs and by the zone of the combination disc being larger than that of either of the single discs

at the same rate (GRACE et al. 1975), an increase in the size of the zone produced by the combination disc, compared with those produced by the single discs, is indicative of enhanced susceptibility. An alternative method is to place the two single discs at a distance apart that is 5 mm or so greater than the sum of the widths of the expected zones of inhibition, measured from the edge of the disc. With this arrangement there will be a gap between the zones, which will be undistorted when there is not synergy, but when there is synergy there will be local enlargement of the zones between the discs, possibly with bridging of the zones (Fig. 2).

In media, in which TMP and the SMX induce "thymineless death" of susceptible bacteria, i.e., in media that are virtually thymidine free and contain a purine, methionine, and glycine (Sect. B.III), synergy reduces the minimum bactericidal concentrations, and two-dimensional titrations show that the optimum ratio, in terms of economy of drug (Sect. F), is similar to that for bacteriostatic activity (Fig. 3). These titrations, and the studies by SEYDEL and WEMPE (1978, 1979), show that the rate of killing is not appreciably affected by raising the concentration above the minimum; in fact, there is evidence which indicates that high concentrations, especially of the sulfonamide, reduce the bactericidal activity (Sect. H).

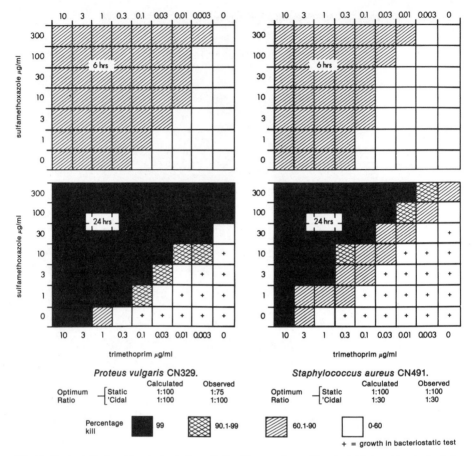

Fig. 3. Bactericidal and bacteriostatic activity. Comparison of bactericidal and bacteriostatic activities, each measured by a two-dimensional titration in Oxoid Sensitivity Test Broth + 2% lysed horse blood. The "calculated" optimum ratio is the ratio of the MIC of each drug when acting singly and the "observed" optimum ratio is that of the combination showing the lowest FIC value

In clinical situations, the advantages of the combinations over those of the single components are not readily demonstrated because, when the concentration of one of the components at the infection site is sufficient for that component to be effective, the presence of the second drug is of no advantage. Therefore, to demonstrate synergy in vivo, the dose must be carefully adjusted according to the susceptibility of the causal organism. These conditions are easily satisfied in experimental mouse infections, employing a large number of animals, and synergy between TMP and a sulfonamide has been convincingly documented (S. BUSHBY and HITCHINGS 1968; GRUNBERG 1973; BÖHNI 1969a); an example of such an experiment is shown in Table 8. Statistical evidence of synergy has also been demonstrated in dogs under experimental conditions by POWERS et al. (1980) using relatively few animals. In this experiment, groups of six dogs were injected intrave-

Table 8. Synergistic effects in vivo of TMP and SDZ against *Proteus vulgaris*

Drugs		Experiment 1		Experiment 2	
TMP (mg)	SDZ (mg)	Survival (%)	Average survival time (days)	Survival (%)	Average survival time (days)
5.0		67	4.7	50	3.2
2.0		0	<1.0	0	<1.0
2.0	2.0	100	7.0	100	7.0
1.0	1.0	83	6.0	100	7.0
0.5	2.0	100	7.0	100	7.0
0.5	1.0	83	6.0	83.3	6.0
0.2	1.0	67	5.0	33.3	3.0
	2.0	0	<1.0	16.6	1.5
		0	<1.0	0	<1.0

The organism, *P. vulgaris* (CN329), was grown in O'Meara broth for 6 h, and 0.5 ml 1:10 dilution was injected intraperitoneally into groups of six mice. The drugs were administered orally immediately after infection and 6 h and 24 h later. The experiment was terminated on day 7

Table 9. Average scores of clinical signs of infection in groups of six dogs, infected with *Streptococcus zooepidemicus*, measured on day 0 and day 4 of treatment with trimethoprim and sulfadiazine, singly and in concentration

TMP (mg/kg)	SDZ (mg/kg)	Average total score on treatment day		Adjusted score [a] on day 4
		0	4	
		18.0	12.2	17.9
5		9.3	11.0	9.6
2.5		12.0	13.1	11.4
	25	8.5	16.0	6.7
	12.5	8.7	14.2	7.6
5	25	2.6	12.3	2.4
2.5	12.5	3.4	13.0	2.8
1.25	6.25	1.5	7.7	3.3

[a] Adjusted for differences in the scores between groups on day 0
See text for criteria of scores

nously with *Streptococcus zooepidemicus*, which consistently produced joint lameness, and the effects of treatment were clinically assessed by a system of scoring (lameness 0–15, lymphadenitis 0–8, color of mucus membrane 0–5, alertness 0–4, hair coat 0–4, and dehydration 0–4: maximum total 40). According to this scoring, maximum effects in the untreated control dogs occurred on day 4 and the score of each group on this day is shown in Table 9. Those results, along with other data which consisted of leukocyte counts, blood cultures, and bacteriologic culturing of tissues, taken at necropsy on the day 7, showed the combination of TMP and sulfadiazine to be statistically superior to the individual components at each dose level ($P \leq 0.05$), with synergy being conclusively demonstrated according to the model developed by Piserchia and Shah (1975).

C. Synergy and Sulfonamide-Resistant Strains

The basis for the use of the combinations is that the reduction by the sulfonamide of the synthesis of dihydrofolate lowers the concentration of the benzylpyrimidine needed to inhibit growth through blocking the conversion of the folate to its active forms. Justification for using the combination therefore depends upon the causal organism's being sensitive to the sulfonamide; "sensitive" under these circumstances, however, must be distinguished from "sensitive" when the sulfonamide is tested alone.

When examined by conventional susceptibility methods, an organism is regarded as resistant when its macroscopic growth is not affected by the sulfonamide, but being resistant by this definition does not necessarily mean that the sulfonamide has not reduced the de novo folate biosynthesis of the organism. Although there are no recorded comparative estimations of the amount of dihydrofolate in cells of sulfonamide-resistant bacteria grown in the presence and absence of a sulfonamide, these organisms are known to contain altered dihydropteroate synthetases. Pato and Brown (1963) showed that these enzymes of *E. coli*, made resistant to sulfonamides by serial passage, combined less effectively with the sulfonamide than did those of the parent strain. Also, Wise and Abou-Donia (1975) showed that strains carrying sulfonamide-resistant plasmids contain two similar synthetases, one of which was the normal enzyme of sensitive strains and was inactive in the presence of the sulfonamide, whilst the other was active in its presence; together these enzymes produced activities that varied quantitatively. Thus, the TMP sensitivity of sulfonamide-resistant strains will be variably increased in the presence of a sulfonamide, because the amount of substrate against which TMP competes will be variably reduced.

Reports concerning the detection of synergy by conventional susceptibility testing methods with sulfonamide-resistant strains are conflicting but, in some instances failure to demonstrate potentiation may be due to the presence of antagonistic substances in the medium or to the use of an inappropriate ratio of the drugs. The results of tests specifically designed to detect the interaction indicate that many sulfonamide-resistant strains are more susceptible to the action of the combination than to TMP alone, although with the more highly resistant strains, the degree of the potentiation may not be of clinical importance (Grüneberg et al. 1975; Grey et al. 1979 a).

The enhanced susceptibility of these strains has been demonstrated in vivo; it was reported by Grunberg (1973) and by Böhni (1974) in mice infected with sulfonamide-resistant strains. Also, Sourander et al. (1972) reported that of 55 patients with long-lasting urinary infections due to sulfonamide-resistant bacterial strains, 21 out of 24 treated daily with 1.92 g co-trimoxazole were cured, which compared with 8 out of 19 cured when treated with 320 mg TMP and 1 out of 12 cured when treated daily with 1.6 g SMX. The question of whether potentiation occurs with strains that are sulfonamide sensitive but TMP resistant is of less clinical importance, for these strains are less common.

D. Reversal of Activity of TMP

Sulfonamide interfere with the synthesis of dihydrofolic acid and TMP prevents its conversion to tetrahydrofolic acid. Therefore, the presence of an exogenous source of the latter folate should, theoretically, diminish or even abolish the antibacterial activity of trimethoprim and/or a sulfonamide in the host. In vitro folinic acid affects the sensitivities of only the enterococci, which are the only common pathogens known to utilize exogenous folates (S. BUSHBY and HITCHINGS 1968) and, when administered subcutaneously to mice infected with either *Streptococcus pneumoniae*, *Streptococcus pyogenes*, *E. coli*, *P. vulgaris*, *Salmonella schottmuelleri*, or *Salmonella typhimurium*, folinic acid did not affect the ability of trimethoprim to potentiate the protection afforded by sulfamethoxazole (BÖHNI 1969 b; *Grunberg* et al. 1970).

The in vitro interference with the action of TMP and the sulfonamides by thymidine also raises the question of whether its presence could affect in vivo activity. According to THEN and ANGEHRN (1974, 1975), the concentration of thymidine in the blood and urine of normal humans is below that which interferes with the in vitro bactericidal activity of TMP (Sect. B.IV). The concentration during bacterial infections is unknown, but, the half-life of tritiated thymidine, injected intravenously is very short, being about 1 min (RUBINI et al. 1960) and, although NOTTEBROCK and THEN (1977) found that the concentration of thymidine in the blood and urine of infected mice seemed to be increased, S. BUSHBY (1973) did not find that the intraperitoneal injection of thymidine, before and during a proteus infection of mice, interfered with the chemotherapeutic activity of TMP/SMX (Table 10).

E. Development of Resistance

Resistance to the benzylpyrimidines can occur by mutation and can be transferred by plasmids (R factors). The mutation in vitro was first reported by DARRELL et al. (1968), who showed that if large inocula of various species were exposed to increasing concentrations of TMP, the MIC increased during five passages from 32- to 124-fold. When the organisms were sulfonamide sensitive and a sulfonamide was present, the increase was delayed, but when the organisms were sulfonamide resistant, the sulfonamide did not have this delaying effect. S. BUSHBY (1972) showed, however, that the delaying effect depended on the degree of resistance to the sulfonamide and that the clinical importance of these mutants is doubtful. He showed that most of these mutants grew very slowly, and, in the case of typeable *E. coli*, as more than 99% of the mutants were untypeable and "rough," he concluded that they were, on the whole, avirulent.

A further mechanism by which organisms can become resistant to an antibacterial is by alteration in metabolism, so that the biochemical step at which the anti-

Table 10. Effect of thymidine in vivo

Drug dose (mg)		Average survival time (days)		Survival (%)	
TMP	SMX	Without thymidine	With thymidine	Without thymidine	With thymidine
2.0		3.7	6.0	50	83.3
1.0		<0.17	<0.17	0	0
0.5		<0.17	1.2	0	16.7
	2.0	1.2	1.3	16.7	16.7
	1.0	<0.17	1.5	0	16.7
1.0	2.0	6.0	7.0	83.3	100
0.5	2.0	4.2	7.0	50	100
0.25	2.0	2.3	7.0	16.7	100
0.12	2.0	1.2	4.8	0	66.7
1.0	1.0	7.0	6.2	100	83.3
0.5	1.0	4.3	7.0	50	100
0.25	1.0	2.0	6.0	0	83.3
0.12	1.0	3.0	5.0	33.3	66.7
		<0.17	<0.17	0	0

Groups of six mice were infected intraperitoneally with 0.05 ml 6-h culture of *Proteus vulgaris* CN329 in O'Meara broth and the drugs were administration orally, at 0, 6, and 24 h after infection. Thymidine at doses of 10 mg was administered intraperitoneally at 18 h before infection and at 0, 6, and 24 h after infection. The experiment was terminated on the day 8

bacterial acts is no longer involved. TMP has been used as a tool by biochemists since 1965 for selecting mutants which are deficient in thymidylate synthetase (Stacey and Simson 1965). This enzyme, in association with the specific folate coenzyme, converts uridylate to thymidylate, and mutants overcome this deficiency by using exogenous thymidine or thymine. These organisms are therefore resistant to TMP and similar mutants have been isolated occasionally from patients undergoing therapy with co-trimoxazole (Barker et al. 1972; Okubadejo and Maskell 1973, 1974; Tanner and Bullin 1974; Tapsall et al. 1974; Hayek and Netherway 1976; Sparham et al. 1978; Haltiner et al. 1980) and from food animals treated with trimethoprim/sulphadiazine (Devriese and Hommez 1974).

In practice, these thymine-dependent mutants are recognized by their ability to grow in the primary isolation medium which contains adequate amounts of thymidine, but not in media suitable for susceptibility testing to benzylpyrimidine/sulfonamide because of their low thymidine content. Barker et al. (1972) suggested that the occurrence of these mutants may be more common than is generally supposed because they are often not recognized and, although Okubadejo and Maskell (1974) reported that they had isolated three thymine-dependent strains in 1971–1972 and during 1973–1974, despite a very careful watch, only one further strain from over 75,000 specimens, they (Maskell et al. 1977) later reported clinical details of 16 patients from whom they had isolated thymine-dependent strains.

Since these mutants readily occur in vitro, the thymidine content in tissues, etc., would appear to be usually too low to support their growth and this conclusion is supported by the indirect measurements of Then and Angehrn (1975), who concluded that the concentrations are normally less than 0.05 µg/ml. MASKELL et al. (1977), however, detected thymine-like substances in the urine of the six patients from whom these mutants had been isolated. An alternative explanation for the apparent rarity of their occurrence is that these mutants have decreased infectivity and are, in consequence, readily eliminated by the host; this suggestion is supported by the observation of WILLIAMS SMITH and TUCKER (1976) who found thymine-dependent salmonellae to be less invasive. However, whatever the explanation, they can in practice rarely be a problem, for otherwise the benzylpyrimidines would be poor therapeutic agents. In each of the instances in which these mutants have been isolated from patients, the treatment was with co-trimoxazole, and so the presence of the sulfonamide has not affected the survival of the mutant; this would be expected, for the presence of thymidine also reverses the activity of the sulfonamide. These mutants have emerged from species of the genera *Escherichia, Klebsiella, Serratia, Proteus, Salmonella, Enterobacter, Haemophilus*, and *Staphylococcus*, and from enterococci.

For several years after the introduction of TMP, it seemed that the transfer of resistance to TMP by plasmids must be a rare event. The first published report of episomal transfer was by LEBEK (1972) but, as the resistance was of a low order and subsequent reports have shown episomal resistance to be usually of a high order ($> 1,000$ µg/ml), there is some doubt of the authenticity of this claim. Although the first published claim may be that of FLEMING et al. (1972), according to GRÜNEBERG et al. (1975) the first, but unpublished, detection occurred in 1971. When first detected, this form of resistance was expected to spread rapidly and limit the usefulness of TMP but 8 years later there was no convincing evidence that, at least in Great Britain, where, in combination with SMX, TMP has been in use for 10 years, it had become widespread (HAMILTON-MILLER 1979). During this period the frequency may have increased somewhat in some other European countries and there are now suggestions that it is occurring in Britain, where according to WILLIAMS SMITH (1980) the incidence is high in the fecal flora of pigs; he suggests this is due to the wide use of the TMP/sulfadiazine combination in veterinary medicine. The resistance is usually associated with multiple drug resistance, including that to sulfonamides and it is fully discussed in Chap. 11.

Resistance to TMP is also encoded by transposons, which are segments of DNA which transfer from plasmids to chromosome or to plasmids. The first reported transfer of TMP resistance by this mechanism (BARTH et al. 1976) was from the plasmid R 483, which originally was first detected in a strain of *E. coli* isolated from a calf in Britain (HEDGES et al. 1972), and TMP resistance though this mechanism appears to be increasing (TOWNER et al. 1980; WILLIAMS SMITH 1980; BRUMFITT et al. 1980).

Cross-resistance, not plasmid encoded, between TMP, chloramphenicol, and nalidixic acid was reported by WILLIAMS SMITH (1976) and TRAUB and KLEBER (1977). WILLIAMS SMITH showed that with the species, *Klebsiella pneumoniae*, one-step chromosomal mutation occurred during exposure to TMP, chloramphenicol, or nalidixic acid, and that the MICs of these antibacterials for these mutants were 25–50 times greater than those for the parent strain. Morphologically, the colonies of the mutants were similar to those of the parents and the capsular antigens of the five strains examined were unchanged; virulence for mice of one strain examined was also unchanged. Like their parents, the mutants were prototropic. These mutants could also be isolated from cloaca of chicks, infected orally when 1 day old with klebsiellae and treated with trimethoprim. TRAUB and KLEBER (1977) isolated similarly cross-resistant mutants from strains of *Serratia marcescens*. That this cross-resistance may be of clinical importance is suggested by the finding of RONALD et al. (1978), which showed that of 74 nalidixic acid-resistant enterobacteria from urinary infections, 23 were resistant to trimethoprim. Before the introduction of trimethoprim, *K.pneumoniae* had a moderately high proportion of strains that were resistant to TMP (HAMILTON-MILLER and GREY 1975); so this cross-resistance may be partly responsible.

F. Spectrum of Activity of TMP/SMX

The wide and high activity of TMP alone and with SMX as originally reported by S. BUSHBY and BARNETT (1967), has been fully confirmed by several groups of workers using the serial dilution method (S. BUSHBY and HITCHINGS 1968; DARRELL et al. 1968; BÖHNI 1969 a; BARNETT and BUSHBY 1970; JARVIS and SCRIMGEOUR 1970; SNG and LAM 1970, 1971; BACH et al. 1973). The range of activities of the combination is similar to that of TMP alone, but the activity is higher, especially with species of the genera *Brucella*, *Nocardia*, and *Neisseria*, because of their higher susceptibility to sulfonamides.

Although all investigators agree that bacteroides are relatively insensitive to TMP, there is disagreement over their sensitivity to the combination. According to ROSENBLATT and STEWART (1974), the majority of strains are too insensitive to the combination for co-trimoxazole to be clinically useful; in contrast, several groups of investigators (OKUBADEJO 1974; PHILLIPS and WARREN 1976; PERCIVAL and CUMBERLAND 1978; WÜST and KAYSER 1980; THEN and ANGEHRN 1979) consider that there is sufficient synergy with strains that are sensitive to 32 µg/ml SMX or less to justify conducting clinical trials with co-trimoxazole in infections by bacteroides, especially as strains with this degree of sensitivity represent the majority. The synergy is most marked with the 1:1 ratio which would probably be close to the ratio in most sites of these infections during treatment with co-trimoxazole. With respect to this controversy, it is of interest that bacteroides, along with lactobacilli, represent the major component of the flora of the gut and, according to NÄFF (1971), treatment with 960 mg co-trimoxazole twice a day for 10 days does not affect them, whereas it eliminates the enterobacteria, e.g., *E. coli*, from the feces; similar effects were also reported by KNOTHE (1973). This differential effect could be due to the higher sensitivity of the enterobacteria to TMP, along with an insufficient concentration of SMX to produce the necessary synergy to affect bacteroides but, alternatively, it could merely reflect low activity of the combination for these organisms, thus supporting the claim by ROSENBLATT and STEWART (1974). Incidentally, the failure to affect the major components of the gut flora probably accounts for the rarity of intestinal upsets during therapy with TMP or co-trimoxazole.

Table 11 shows the incidence of susceptible strains among approximately 73,000 strains of 33 species detected by the disc diffusion method using the stan-

Table 11. Susceptibility of organisms to TMP/SMX

Species	Strains	
	No. examined	Susceptibility (%)
Alcaligenes sp.	67	74
Bacteroides fragilis	9	55
Citrobacter freundii	1,031	91
Clostridium perfringens	4	50
Enterobacter aerogenes	1,521	95
Enterobacter agglomerans	419	90
Enterobacter cloacae	3,049	96
Enterococcus (*Streptococcus faecalis*)	5,561	63
Escherichia coli	33,937	96
Flavobacterium sp.	38	63
Haemophilus influenzae	787	79
Hafnia alvei	99	95
Klebsiella pneumoniae	10,052	89
Lactobacillus sp.	28	50
Moraxella sp.	67	89
Morganella morganii	932	90
Neisseria gonorrhoeae	28	75
Neisseria meningitidis	40	77
Peptostreptococcus sp.	15	20
Proteus mirabilis	8,209	95
Proteus vulgaris	613	85
Providencia rettgeri	216	55
Providencia stuartii	869	46
Pseudomonas aeruginosa	8,773	9
Salmonella sp.	410	97
Serratia liquefaciens	295	88
Serratia marcescens	1,814	80
Shigella flexneri	34	94
Shigella sonnei	154	95
Staphylococcus aureus	4,157	94
Staphylococcus epidermidis	4,804	82
Streptococcus pyogenes (A)	250	47
Streptococcus agalactiae (B)	682	24
Streptococcus pneumoniae	249	91

Data collected by Professional Marketing Research Inc. during June 1980–August 1980 from 216 acute-care hospitals in the United states

dard sensitivity disc containing 1.25 µg TMP and 23.75 µg SMX and regarding zones of 16 mm or more as indicative of susceptibility. The results are based on data from 216 acute-care hospitals of 100 beds or more in the United States during December 1978 to February 1979. Because the accuracy of the disc method depends on the medium being virtually thymidine free, the results tend to overestimate the incidence of resistance. Among the gram-negative organisms, *Pseudomonas aeruginosa* is a notable exception, for only 9% of strains are reported as susceptible. The relatively low incidence of susceptible strains of streptococci is probably an underestimate, particularly with those of *Streptococcus faecalis (fae-*

Table 12. Species, others than those of Table 10, which are reported to be sensitive to TMP/SMX

Achromobacter xylosoxidans	HOLMES et al. (1977); TOMIOKA et al. (1978)
Aeromonas hydrophila	NORD et al. (1974)
Brucella abortus	S. BUSHBY (1973)
Corynebacterium pyogenes	S. BUSHBY (1973)
Flavobacterium sp.	ABER et al. (1978); ALTMANN and BOGOKOVISKY (1971)
Legionella pneumophilia	THORNSBERRY et al. (1978); POHLOD et al. (1980)
Listeria monocytogenes	PACHECO and SIMONI DA SILVA (1973), LARSSON et al. (1978), WINSLOW and PANKEY (1980)
Mycobacterium fortuitum	LASZLO and EIDUS (1979), SWENSON et al. (1980b)
Mycobacterium marinum	BARROW and HEWITT (1971), BLACK and EYKYN (1977)
Nocardia sp.	BEAUMONT (1970), S. BUSHBY (1973)
Pseudomonas cepacia	MOODY and YOUNG (1975), TOMIOKA et al. (1978)
Pseudomonas fluorescens	NORD et al. (1974)
Pseudomonas maltophilia	MOODY and YOUNG (1975), FELEGIE et al. (1979), TOMIOKA et al. (1978)
Pseudomonas pseudomallei	EVERETT and KISHIMOTO (1973), BEAUMONT (1970), BASSETT (1971), TANPHAICHITRA et al. (1980)
Pseudomonas putrefaciens	THONG (1976), NORD et al. (1974)
Pseudomonas thomasii	PHILLIPS et al. (1972)
Vibrio cholerae	NORTHRUP et al. (1972), DUTTA et al. (1978), COLAERT et al. (1979)
Pasteurella haemolytica	S. BUSHBY (1973)
Propiobacterium acnes	HOEFFLER et al. (1976)
Yersinia enterocolitica	HAMMERBERG et al. (1977), GUTMAN et al. (1973)
Yersinia pestis	NGUYEN-VAN-AI et al. (1972, 1973), BUTLER et al. (1974)

cium) because its susceptibility is reversed by very low concentrations of thymidine or thymine, but the same is probably true, although to a lesser extent, for the susceptibilities of *S. pyogenes* and group B streptococci. The activity against *E. coli*, includes the entertoxigenic strains (DUPONT et al. 1978).

Organisms, other than those listed in Table 11 and which have been reported to be sensitive to the combination, are listed in Table 12. The incidence of resistance among the strains of *K. pneumoniae* is very variable but is higher among those from hospital inpatients, e.g., McGILL (1978) found that 32% of 142 strains from inpatients, compared with only 6% of 58 from general practice or outpatients, were resistant. Other species which have been reported to be resistant to the combination are *Campylobacter fetus* (WALDER 1979; VANHOOF et al. 1980), *Clostridium difficile* (BURDON et al. 1979; FEKETY et al. 1979), *Clostridium botulinum* (SWENSON et al. 1980a), and *Gardnerella (Haemophilus) vaginalis* (McCARTHY et al. 1979); according to LEVINSON et al. (1979), however, the latter organism is usually sensitive to 1.6 µg/ml TMP and this concentration is present in the vagina during treatment with standard doses of co-trimoxazole.

G. Choice of Sulfonamide

SMX was the first sulfonamide to be marketed in a combination with TMP. The combination was developed jointly by the Wellcome Foundation and by Hoffmann La Roche. This sulfonamide was chosen because its half-life in human blood is similar to that of TMP and, in the ratio of 5 parts to 1 part trimethoprim, it produces in the blood a ratio of around 20:1 which is close to the modal mean of the optimum ratio for most pathogens. However, contrary to the widely held view, the ratio is seldom important and the frequent reference in the literature to the "optimum ratio" is primarily responsible for the misunderstanding. "Optimum" is based on the results of in vitro studies and its use has led to the impression that at this ratio the drugs are most active. In fact, this ratio is "optimum" only in terms of economy of drugs because, except for the possible effects of a marked excess of the sulfonamide on the bactericidal activity of TMP (Sect. H), identical effects on the bacteria occur over a wide range of ratios. At the optimum ratio, the minimum effective concentrations are lowest for each of the drugs and, although at other ratios, the minimum effective concentration of one of the components will be higher than that at the optimum, that of the other will be less (see Sect. B.IV). Also, even if it were considered preferable in the clinical situation to expose organisms to the combination at its optimum ratio, this would be difficult in practice because the optimum ratio, which corresponds to that of the MIC of the components when acting singly (Sect. B.IV), varies greatly for the various pathogens. Another complicating factor is the difference in the pharmacokinetic distribution of the components. In contrast to the sulfonamide, TMP rapidly passes from the blood, where its ratio is around 1:20, into the tissues, where it tends to concentrate. The ratios of the drugs in the tissues therefore differ from those in the blood and these differ from those in the urine, each of which differs from that in the pharmaceutical preparation. A circumstance in which it might be necessary to attain the optimum ratio occurs when there is a problem of reaching adequate concentrations of both components at the infection site but, usually, an excess of one component will compensate for a deficiency of the other and, even under the exceptional circumstance when this does not occur, the problem could theoretically be solved by merely increasing the dose of the combination. A frequently raised objection to overcoming this problem by simply increasing the dose of the combination is that in the case of infections due to the organisms which are more sensitive to SMX than to TMP it would be more rational to increase the dose of TMP so that the ratio of the drugs at the infection site would be nearer to the optimum. This procedure has been advocated for the treatment of gonorrhea and nocardiosis, and it does have the merit of avoiding the theoretical effects of excess sulfonamide on bactericidal activity (Sect. H).

With most strains, the ratio of the MIC of TMP to that of SMX for gonococci is about 1:5 (PHILLIPS et al. 1977; STOLZ et al. 1977), but, as the difference between this ratio and most other bacterial species is due to lower sensitivity of the gonococcus to TMP, adjustment of the ratio of the drugs given to the patient should theoretically be by increasing the dose of TMP and not reducing that of SMX. The ratio of SMX to TMP at the site of gonococcal infections of patients treated with the standard dose of co-trimoxazole (160 mg TMP and 800 SMX twice a day) is not known, but it is probably close to 1:1 and, if this is true, then to increase it to 1:5 would require raising the dose of TMP to 800 mg. However, in opposition to this suggestion is the observation that patients with gonorrhea who fail to respond to treatment with co-trimoxazole tend to be those with the more sulfonamide-resistant strains (AUSTIN and HOLMES 1975; ELLIOTT et al. 1977).

Recently, other TMP/sulfonamide fixed-ratio combinations have been introduced or are being investigated as marketable products. The sulfonamides in these combinations are sulfadiazine, sulfamoxole, sulfalene, and sulfametral and, with TMP now available in several major countries as a single agent, members of the medical profession in those countries are now able to use trimethoprim with the sulfonamide and at the ratio of their choice. Theoretically, synergy with TMP occurs with all sulfonamides and this has been documented with some ten or so. Justification for using a different sulfonamide from SMX could be more favorable pharmacokinetics, pK_a, or higher antibacterial activity, but based on the problems associated with defining and reaching the most active synergic concentrations of the TMP/SMX combination, superiority in practice of any other combination will be difficult to substantiate, except perhaps with respect to side effects, e.g., crystalluria. Presently, tetroxoprim is available with sulfadiazine in the ratio of 1:4.

H. 2,4-Diaminopyrimidines as Single Agents

Unlike the sulfonamides, both TMP and tetroxoprim were first introduced in combination with a sulfonamide, and this was in spite of their activities being, in general, 20 times greater than those of the sulfonamides. The reasons for this unusual procedure were two-fold; first, to take advantage of the synergy, and second, and more importantly, because experimental evidence indicated that resistance would develop rapidly if the benzylpyrimidines were used without a sulfonamide.

The synergy is undoubtedly advantageous in the treatment of infections in which the concentrations of either of the components given singly would be near or below their effective concentration at the site of infection. However, under circumstances, in which the concentrations are consistently above the minimum effective concentration, no therapeutic advantage can be expected from using the combination; in fact, there is evidence that indicates that marked excess of a sulfonamide interferes with killing (THEN and ANGEHRN 1973; SEYDEL and WEMPE 1978, 1979), possibly through inhibition of syntheses other than that of thymidylate. These circumstance occur, possibly uniquely, in urine where the concentration of both components are many fold greater than the in vitro minimum effective concentration.

The expectancy of rapid emergence of resistance (see Sect. E) was based on the in vitro observations of DARRELL et al. (1968), and were later confirmed by SMITH et al. (1972) and by GRUNBERG and BESKID (1977). The observations suggested that the clinical use of TMP alone would quickly lead to the emergence of TMP-resistant strains but, in the case of sulfonamide-sensitive but not of sulfonamide-resistant strains, the emergence would be delayed if it were used in combination with a sulfonamide. However, the results of several years of clinical experience with the combination indicate that the expectancy that resistance would rapidly emerge if TMP were used alone was unfounded. In spite of the incidence of sulfonamide resistance ranging from 25%–50%, especially among strains of enterobacteria of the intestinal flora and of those causing urinary infection (BALL and WALLACE 1974; KAYSER and SANTANAM 1974; HAMILTON-MILLER 1979; GRÜNEBERG 1980), reports published 4–8 years after its introduction in Europe showed there was, in general, little or no increase in frequency of resistance to TMP (BRUMFITT and PURSELL 1972; LACEY et al. 1972; LEWIS and LACEY 1973; BALL and WALLACE 1974; FRUENS-GÅARD and KORNER 1974; WÜST and KAYSER 1980; GREY et al. 1979 b; GRÜNEBERG 1980), except transitionally in closed communities, as in hospitals (GRÜNEBERG et al. 1975). Also, if the development of resistance to TMP were the problem, as indicated by the experiments of DARRELL et al. (1968), then, during prolonged administration of trimethoprim, resistance should develop among the myriads of enterobacteria present in the gut. This would be especially so when the dose of TMP is adjusted to reduce the numbers of these organisms without completely eliminating them, and, because TMP would be constantly present, the resistant mutants should become the dominant enterobacterium for as long as the drug was being administered.

In a study, conducted by the writer, profound falls in the number of enterobacteria occurred in the eight subjects taking 50 mg TMP daily for 3 months, and lesser falls in five subjects who took 10 mg doses for the same period, but in no subject did TMP-resistant enterobacteria become established and the dominant member of this family. By using a medium containing TMP as a selective medium, TMP-resistant enterobacteria were isolated intermittently and in very low numbers from eight of the thirteen TMP-treated subjects, but similarly TMP-resistant enterobacteria were isolated from two of the subjects before the commencement of treatment and from two of the five control subjects who took SMX without TMP. Similar findings, but using a less highly selective method of isolation, were reported by BRUMFITT and PURSELL (1972), TOIVANEN et al. (1976), and SIETZEN and KNOTHE (1978). Negative findings were also reported by SPELLER and BRUTEN (1972), MOORHOUSE and FARRELL (1973), and LACEY et al. (1980) for patients who received TMP or co-trimoxazole, but positive results were reported by GRÜNEBERG and his colleagues in a series of papers (GRÜNEBERG et al. 1975, 1976; SMELLIE et al. 1976). These latter investigators examined 2,010 strains of coliform bacilli from 545 rectal swabs taken from 130 children during prophylactic treatment for recurrent urinary infections with doses of 12 mg kg^{-1} day^{-1} co-trimoxazole and found 426 to be TMP resistant. These resistant strains, which came from 55 swabs from 37 of the children, were intermittently present and, although their presence would seem to be a direct consequence of the treatment with TMP/SMX, their frequency according to the GRÜNEBERG and colleagues was less than that which occurs with sulfonamides alone or with ampicillin, and they quickly disappeared after cessation of treatment. Apart from these clinical data not supporting the expectancy of rapid development of resistance, S. BUSHBY (1972) had shown that although these in vitro delaying effects of the sulfonamide were quantitatively related to the degree of sulfonamide resistance, the majority of the TMP-resistant mutants showed changes, strongly suggesting decreased infectivity.

Therefore, in vitro and in vivo data do not support the original expectancy that resistance to TMP would develop rapidly if it were used without a sulfonamide; in fact, resistance appears to be no more likely to emerge with TMP than with most other antibacterials in current use. Consequently, there is little justification for using TMP with a sulfonamide under circumstances in which synergy cannot occur because the concentration of TMP at the infection site is far above its minimum effective concentration. Uncomplicated urinary infections, are probably the only certain example in which these circumstances occur and in these conditions the presence of a sulfonamide contributes little or nothing to the antibacterial effects of TMP, as is supported by the results obtained in the bladder model of GREEN-WOOD and O'GRADY (1978) and GREENWOOD (1979). In this model, the continuous ureteric infusion of urine, with the periodic emptying of the bladder, is mimicked and the growth of bacteria is continuously monitored photometrically. In it, the response to sulfamethoxazole was shown to be slow and the response to TMP was not enhanced by the presence of the sulfonamide. Concentrations of 0.25 µg/ml TMP were very effective and raising them to 10 µg/ml did not increase the effect.

In Sect. E, reference is made to possible recent increases in the incidence of transferable resistance to TMP among strains of *E. coli* in Britain. The increase antedates the introduction of TMP as a single agent, but as the majority of the strains are highly resistant to sulfonamides, the increase would not be appreciably affected by the concomitant use of sulfonamides. The clinical use of TMP as a single agent is discussed in Chap. 12.

J. Susceptibility Testing

Although serial dilution methods, especially the microautomated ones in the United States, are becoming widely used for routine susceptibility testing, the most commonly used method is probably the disc diffusion method. Other methods based on the effects of the antibacterials on growth rates are also being used. Each of these methods is suitable for the benzylpyrimidines and the sulfonamides, provided a standard inoculum is used and the growth medium does not contain antagonists. In practice, thymidine is the usual antagonist and it is present in many media (Sect. A); its effects, except on the testing of the enterococci, can be largely overcome by adding thymidine phosphorylase to the medium, either as the pure enzyme (M. BUSHBY et al. 1978) or as lysed horse blood (see the discussion at the end of this section).

The problems associated with the disc diffusion method, in general, were fully discussed by ERICSSON and SHERRIS (1971) and, although the same basic method is used worldwide, it varies greatly in detail, even within the same country. The principle variations are in the size of the disc, the concentrations of the antibacterials in the disc, the constituents of the medium, the depth of medium, and the size of the inoculum. In the United States, the procedures described by BAUER et al. (1966) are officially recommended by the BUREAU of FOOD and DRUG ADMINISTRATION (1972). The medium is Mueller-Hinton but, depending on its source, the thymidine content can vary greatly (THEN 1977).

There is little disagreement regarding the determination of susceptibilities to the sulfonamides and the benzylpyrimidines as individual drugs, but there is with respect to that of their combinations. A combination disc containing 1.25 µg TMP and 23.75 µg SMX is widely used and if the zone of inhibition is of a certain size (16 mm or more in the United States), then the organism is regarded as fully sensitive. The use of this disc is critized on the grounds that the results do not indicate whether or not there is synergy and that the inhibition may be due solely to one of the drugs. However, in view of the virtual impossibility of deciding whether, in any particular case, synergy will occur in vivo, in spite of its being demonstrated in vitro (Sect. F), some investigators consider it essential to show that the organism is sensitive to trimethoprim before deciding whether the combination is indicated; others will only accept that the combination is indicated when the organism is sensitive to both components. In either case, it entails testing with the individual drugs.

If synergy is to be demonstrated by the diffusion method, then discs containing the individual drugs may be placed at the appropriate distance apart to give distorted zones as depicted in Fig. 2. Alternatively, the combination disc, and discs containing the single components in the same quantities as in the combination disc, may be used; synergy is assumed when the combination disc produces a larger zone of inhibition than either of the single discs.

The 1:19 ratio was chosen for the combination disc because, for most organisms, it is close to their optimum ratio (Sect. B.IV) and because it is also the ratio of the concentrations of the TMP and SMX present in the blood of patients treated with the standard dose of co-trimoxazole. However, the ratio is inappropriate for bacteria that are more sensitive to the sulfonamide than to TMP. The ratio also differs from that of the concentrations in the urine and in tissues, which are nearer 1:1 and 1:5, respectively.

For testing susceptibility prior to treatment with trimethoprim as a single agent, a disc containing 5 μg TMP is used in the United States. This quantity, like those in the combination disc, is relatively low as compared with those present in other sensitivity discs but, if larger quantities were used in either, the zones of inhibition would frequently interfere with those of adjacent discs of other drugs in multiple disc susceptibility testing. Organisms with zones 16 mm or greater are regarded as fully sensitive; if the infection is confined to the urine, those producing a 10 mm zone are also considered sensitive because of the high concentrations of TMP in the urine. The regression lines relating zone sizes with MICs for both the 5 μg TMP disc and the 1.25 μg/23.75 μg SxT combination disc, using the diffusion method recommended in the United States, and from which the interpretative standards were selected are shown in Fig. 4.

Both TMP and SMX are relatively insoluble in water, but suitable aqueous solutions for use in the serial dilution methods can be prepared by dissolving TMP in lactic acid or hydrochloric acid and SMX in sodium hydroxide. A convenient stock solution of TMP containing 1 mg/ml can be prepared by dissolving 100 mg TMP in 10 ml 0.05 M lactic acid or hydrochloric acid followed by increasing the volume to 100 ml with distilled water. Dissolution may be aided by gentle heating prior to the addition of the distilled water. Similarly, a stock solution of SMX containing 19 mg/ml can be prepared by dissolving 1.9 g SMX in 100 ml 0.1 M sodium hydroxide. Depending on anticipated needs, lesser volumes of these stock solutions can be conveniently prepared by using proportionally small quantities. At these concentrations, TMP and SMX may precipitate if mixed together; consequently, stock solutions should not be mixed together but added separately to the test medium.

In the solid state, TMP and SMX are stable for indefinite periods and in these solutions kept at 2°–4 °C they are stable for 6 months. The solutions should be discarded if a precipitate forms and persists on warming to room temperature (15°–30 °C), or if the solutions darken in color. The drugs are heat stable and can be sterilized by autoclaving at 121 °C. The sterilizing procedure can be performed ei-

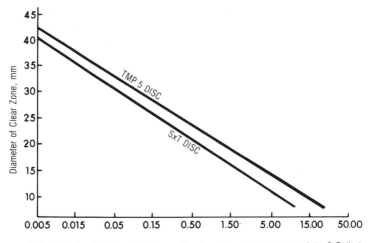

MIC of trimethoprim, in µg/ml (plus × 19 sulfamethoxazole in the case of the SxT disc)

Fig. 4. Relationship between zone sizes of the SxT and of the TMP 5 µg diffusion discs and MICs. The regression line for the TMP 5 µg disc was based on data from 359 urinary pathogens and that for the SxT 25 µg disc on data from 612 pathogens of 22 species, including *Memophilus influenzae*. The zone sizes were determined by the standard diffusion method of the United States and the MICs were those that produced $\geqq 90\%$ inhibition. For TMP 5 µg disc: zone diameter $= 42.31 - 9.45 \log x$; for SxT disc: zone diameter $= 40.65 - 10.09 \log x$; $x = \mathrm{MIC}/0.005$

ther before or after addition to the medium. Stored at 2°–4 °C, the drugs are stable in the medium for periods of at least 1 month.

The inoculum used in the serial dilution method should be smaller than that usually used with other antibacterials. On solid media, where a multiple inoculator is used, the inoculum should contain approximately 500 organisms. This approximate number can usually be achieved by using a 10^{-3} dilution of an overnight broth culture. When using a fluid medium, the concentration of organisms in the final test should be approximately 1,000/ml. When reading the results, the minimum inhibitory concentration should be read as the smallest concentration of the drugs which inhibits 90% or more of growth, as judged by eye when compared with that of the control tube or plate containing no drug.

When thymidine phosphorylase is added to the medium to convert the thymidine to thymine, it should be added to give a final concentration of 0.025–0.1 international units (IU)/ml. The medium can be pretreated with the enzyme or the enzyme can be added at the time of use. The enzyme is heat labile, so when it is added to molten agar media, the medium must be precooled to 48°–50 °C before its addition and then immediately poured into plates. The enzyme can also be used on prepoured plates by swabbing the surface with a cotton applicator (throat swab) dipped into a solution containing about 30 IU/ml enzyme. The plate should be allowed to dry before inoculating with the test organism. When the enzyme is added as 2%–5% lysed horse blood, the cells can be hemolyzed by freezing and thawing the blood twice or by adding 5% of a 10% solution of saponin.

References

Aber RC, Wennersten C, Moellering R (1978) Antimicrobial susceptibility of flavobacteria. Antimicrob Agents Chemother 14:483–487

Altmann G, Bogokovsky B (1971) In-vitro sensitivity of *Flavobacterium meningosepticum* to antimicrobial agents. J Med Microbiol 4/2:296–299

Amyes SGB, Smith JT (1974) Trimethoprim action and its analogy with thymine starvation. Antimicrob Agents Chemother 5:169–178

Amyes SGB, Smith JT (1978) Trimethoprim antagonists: effect of uridine on thymine and thymidine uptake in mineral salts medium. J Antimicrob Chemother 4:415–419

Angehrn P, Then P (1973) Nature of trimethoprim-induced death in *Escherichia coli*. Arzneim Forsch 23:447–451

Austin TW, Holmes KK (1975) The use of trimethoprim sulfamethoxazole in gonococcal infections. Can Med Assoc J 112:375–395

Bach MC, Maxwell F, Gold O, Wilcox C (1973) Susceptibility of recently isolated pathogenic bacteria to trimethoprim and sulfamethoxazole separately and combined (suppl). J Infect Dis [Suppl] 128:5508–5533

Ball AP, Wallace ET (1974) A ten-year study of the sensitivities of urinary pathogens in a pyelonephritis unit. J Int Med Res 2:18–22

Barker J, Healing D, Hutchison JGP (1972) Characteristics of some co-trimoxazole-resistant Enterobacteriaceae from infected patients. J Clin Pathol 25:1086–1088

Barnett M, Bushby SRM (1970) Trimethoprim and the sulphonamides. Vet Rec 87:43–51

Barrow GI, Hewitt M (1971) Skin infection with *Mycobacterium marinum* from a tropical fish tank. Br Med J 2:505–506

Barth PT, Datta N, Hedges RW, Grinter NJ (1976) Transposition of a deoxyribonucleic acid sequence encoding trimethoprim and streptomycin resistances from R 483 to other replicons. J Bacteriol 125:800–810

Bassett DCJ (1971) The sensitivity of *Pseudomonas pseudomallei* to trimethoprim and sulphamethoxazole *in vitro*. J Clin Pathol 24:798–800

Bauer AW, Kirby WMM, Sherris JC, Turck M (1966) Antibiotic susceptibility testing by a standardized single disk method. Am J Clin Pathol 45:493–496

Beaumont RJ (1970) Trimethoprim as a possible therapy for nocardiosis and melioidosis. Med J Aust 2:1123–1127

Black MM, Eykyn SJ (1977) The successful treatment of tropical fish tank granuloma *(Mycobacterium marinum)* with co-trimoxazole. Br J Dermatol 97:689–692

Böhni E (1969 a) Comparative bacteriologic investigations with the combination trimethoprim/sulfamethoxazole in vitro and in vivo (in German). Chemotherapy [Suppl] 14:1–21

Böhni E (1969 b) Chemotherapeutic activity of the combination of trimethoprim and sulphamethoxazole in infections of mice. Postgrad Med J [Suppl] 45:18–21

Böhni E (1974) Co-trimoxazole in sulfonamide resistant infections. In: Daikos GK (ed) Progress in chemotherapy. Proc 8 th Int Congr Chemother. 2:204–210. Hellinic Society of Chemotherapy, Athens

Brumfitt W, Pursell R (1972) Double-blind trial to compare ampicillin, cephalexin, co-trimoxazole, and trimethoprim in treatment of urinary infection. Br Med J 2:673–676

Brumfitt W, Hamilton-Miller JM, Gooding A (1980) Resistance to trimethoprim. Lancet 1/8183:1409–1410

Burdon DW, Brown JD, Youngs DJ et al. (1979) Antibiotic susceptibility of *Clostridium difficile*. J Antimicrob Chemother 5:307–310

Bureau of Food and Drug Administration (1972) Federal Register 37:20527–29

Bushby MB, Bushby SRM, Krenitsky TA (1978) Thymidine phosphorylase: improving media for testing susceptibility to sulfonamides and trimethoprim. In: Siegethaler W, Luthy R (eds) Current chemoterapy. Proc 10 th Int Congr Chemother, Zurich, Switzerland, vol I. The American Society of Microbiology, Washington, DC, pp 469–471

Bushby SRM (1972) Effects of sulphonamides on the emergence of trimethoprim-resistant variants. In: Hejzlar M, Semonsky M, Masak S (eds) Advances in antimicrobial and antineoplastic chemotherapy. Proc 7 th Int Congr Chemother, vol VI/2. Urban and Schwarzenberg, Munich, pp 847–848

Bushby SRM (1973) Trimethoprim/sulfamethoxazole in vitro: microbiological aspects. J Infect Dis [Suppl] 128:S442–S462

Bushby SRM, Barnett M (1967) Trimethoprim-sulphonamides – in vitro sensitivity of 384 strains of bacteria. In: Spitzy KH (ed) Proc 5th Intern Congr Chemother, Vienna, Austria, vol VI/2. Verlag Wien Med Acad, Vienna, pp 753–757

Bushby SRM, Hitchings GH (1968) Trimethoprim, a sulphonamide potentiator. Br J Pharmacol 33:72–90

Butler T, Bell WR, Linh NN, Tiep ND, Arnold K (1974) *Yersina pestis* infection in Vietnam. I. Clinical and hematologic aspects. J Infect Dis [Suppl] 129:S78–S84

Bywater MJ, Holt HA, Reeves DS (1979) Activity in vitro tetroxoprim-sulphadiazine. J Antimicrob Chemother [Suppl B] 5:51–60

Colaert J, Van Dyck E, Ursi JP, Piot P (1979) Antimicrobial susceptibility of *Vibrio cholerae* from Zaire and Rwanda. Lancet 2:849

Darrell JH, Garrod LP, Waterworth PM (1968) Trimethoprim: laboratory and clinical studies. J Clin Pathol 21:202–209

Devriese LA, Hommez J (1974) Thymine-requiring *Escherichia coli* mutants isolated from animals. An unusual type of resistance to trimethoprim. Zentralbl Veterinaermed [B] 21:211–215

Dupont HL, West H, Evans DG et al. (1978) Antimicrobial susceptibility of enterotoxigenic *Escherichia coli*. J Antimicrob Chemother 4:100–102

Dutta JK, Santhanam S, Misra BS, Ray SN (1978) Effect of trimethoprim-sulphamethoxazole on vibrio clearance in cholera (El Tor): a comparative study. Trans R Soc Trop Med Hyg 72:40–42

Elion GB, Singer S, Hitchings GH (1954) Antagonists of nucleic acid derivatives. VIII. Synergism in combinations of biochemically related antimetabolites. J Biol Chem 208:477

Elliott WC, Reynolds G, Thornsberry C et al. (1977) Treatment of gonorrhea with trimethoprim-sulfamethoxazole. J Infect Dis 135:939–943

Ericsson HM, Sherris JC (1971) Antibiotic sensitivity testing. Report of an international collaborative study. Acta Pathol Microbiol Scand [A] [Suppl] 217:1–90

Everett ED, Kishimoto RA (1973) In vitro sensitivity of 33 strains of *Pseudomonas pseudomallei* to trimethoprim and sulfamethoxazole. J Infect Dis [Suppl] 128:S539–S542

Fekety R, Silva J, Toshniwal R et al. (1979) Antibiotic-associated colitis: effects of antibiotics on *Clostridium difficile* and the disease in hamsters. Rev Infect Dis 1:386–396

Felegie TP, Yu VL, Rumans LW, Yee RB (1979) Susceptibility of *Pseudomonas maltophilia* to antimicrobial agents, singly and in combination. Antimicrob Agents Chemother 16:833–837

Ferone R, Bushby SRM, Burchall JJ, Moore WD, Smith D (1975) Identification of Harper-Cawston factor as thymidine phosphorylase and removal from media of substances interfering with susceptibility testing to sulfonamides and diaminopyrimidines. Antimicrob Agents Chemother 7:9–98

Fleming MP, Datta N, Grüneberg RN (1972) Trimethoprim resistance determined by R factors. Br Med J 1:726–728

Fruensgaard K, Korner B (1974) Alterations in the sensitivity pattern after use of trimethoprim/sulfamethoxazole for two years in the treatment of urinary tract infections. Chemotherapy 20:97–101

Grace ME, Bushby SRM, Sigel CW (1975) Diffusion of trimethoprim and sulfamethoxazole from susceptibility disks into agar medium. Antimicrob Agents Chemother 8:45–49

Greenberg J, Richeson EM (1950) Potentiation of the antimalarial activity of sulfadiazine by 2,4-diamino-5-aryloxypyrimidines. J Pharmacol Exp Ther 99:444–449

Greenwood D (1979) Relevance of in vitro synergy to therapy: does synergy between diaminopyrimidines and sulphonamides operate at concentrations achievable in urine? J Antimicrob Chemother [Suppl B] 5:85–89

Greenwood D, O'Grady F (1978) An in vitro model of the urinary bladder. J Antimicrob Chemother 4:113–120

Grey D, Hamilton-Miller JMT, Brumfitt W (1979a) Combined action of sulphamethoxazole and trimethoprim against clinically-isolated sulphonamide-resistant bacteria. Chemotherapy 25:296–302

Grey D, Hamilton-Miller JMT, Brumfitt W (1979b) Incidence of mechanisms of resistance to trimethoprim in clinically isolated gram-negative bacteria. Chemotherapy 25:147–156

Grüneberg RN (1980) Antibiotic sensitivities of urinary pathogens, 1971–8. J Clin Pathol 33:853–856

Grüneberg RN, Leakey A, Bendall MJ, Smellie JM (1975) Bowel flora in urinary tract infection: effect of chemotherapy with special reference to cotrimoxazole. Kidney Int [Suppl] 8:S122–S129

Grüneberg RN, Smellie JM, Leakey A, Atkin WS (1976) Long-term low-dose co-trimoxazole in prophylaxis of childhood urinary tract infection: bacteriological aspects. Br Med J 2:206–208

Grunberg E (1973) The effect of trimethoprim on the activity of sulfonamides and antibiotics in experimental infections. J Infect Dis [Suppl] 128:S478–S485

Grunberg E, Beskid G (1977) Studies on the in vitro development of drug resistance of proteae to sulfonamides, trimethoprim, and combinations of a sulfonamide and trimethoprim. Chemotherapy 23:309–313

Grunberg E, Prince HN, De Lorenzo WF (1970) The in vivo effect of folinic acid (Citrovorum Factor) on the potentiation of the antibacterial activity of sulfisoxazole by trimethoprim. J Clin Pharmacol 10:231–234

Gutman LT, Wilfert CM, Quan T (1973) Susceptibility of *Yersina enterocolitica* to trimethoprim-sulfamethoxazole. J Infect Dis [Suppl] 128:S538

Haltiner RC, Migneault PC, Robertson RG (1980) Incidence of thymidine-dependent enterococci detected on Mueller-Hinton agar and low thymidine content. Antimicrob Agents Chemother 18:365–368

Hamilton-Miller JMT (1979) Mechanisms and distribution of bacterial resistance to diaminopyrimidines and sulphonamides. J Antimicrob Chemother [Suppl B] 5:61–73

Hamilton-Miller JMT, Grey D (1975) Resistance to trimethoprim in klebsiellae isolated before its introduction. J Antimicrob Chemother 1:213–218

Hammerberg S, Sorger S, Marks MI (1977) Antimicrobial susceptibilities of *Yersinia enterocolitica* biotype 4, serotype 0:3. Antimicrob Agents Chemother 11:566–568

Harper GJ, Cawston WC (1945) The in vitro determination of the sulphonamide sensitivity of bacteria. J Pathol 47:59–66

Hayek LJ, Netherway J (1976) Thymine-requiring bacteria (Letter). Lancet 1:1080

Hedges RW, Datta N, Fleming MP (1972) R factors conferring resistance to trimethoprim but not sulphonamides. J Gen Microbiol 73:573–575

Hitchings GH, Bushby SRM (1961) 5-Benzyl-2,4-diaminopyrimidines, a new class of systemic antibacterial agents. Abstr Vth Int Congr Biochem, vol 9, biochemical antibiotics. Pergamon, Oxford, Abstr p 223

Hitchings GH, Elion GB, VanderWerff H, Falco EA (1948) Pyrimidine derivatives as antagonists of pteroylglutamic acid. J Biol Chem 174:765–766

Hitchings GH, Rollo IM, Goodwin LG et al. (1952a) Daraprim as an antagonist of folic and folinic acids. Trans R Soc Trop Med Hyg 46:467–497

Hitchings GH, Falco EA, VanderWerff H, Russell PB, Elion GB (1952b) Antagonists of nucleic acid derivatives. VII. 2,4-diaminopyrimidines. J Biol Chem 199:43–56

Hoeffler U, Ko HL, Pulverer G (1976) Antimicrobial susceptibility of *Propionibacterium acnes* and related microbial species. Antimicrob Agents Chemother 10/3:387–394

Höxer K (1980) Activity of the new compound tetroxoprim against gram-positive and gram-negative microorganisms. In: Nelson JD, Grassi C (eds) Current chemotherapy and infectious disease. Proc 11th Int Congr Chemother and 19th Intersci Conf Antimicrob Agents Chemother, Boston USA, vol I. The American Society for Microbiology, Washington, DC, pp 420–421

Holmes B, Snell JJS, Lapage SP (1977) Strains of *Achromobacter xylosoxidans* from clinical material. J Clin Pathol 30:595–601

Jarvis KJ, Scrimgeour G (1970) In vitro sensitivity of *Shigella sonnei* to trimethoprim and sulphamethoxazole. J Med Microbiol 3:554–557

Kayser FH, Santanam P (1974) Sulfamethoxazol-trimethoprim: bakteriologische Erfahrungen nach 5 Jahren Anwendung. Schweiz Med Wochenschr 104:1950–1954

Knothe H (1973) The effect of a combined preparation of trimethoprim and sulphamethox-azole following short-term and long-term administration on the flora of the human gut. Chemotherapy 18:285–296

Koch AE, Burchall JJ (1971) Reversal of the antimicrobial activity of trimethoprim by thymidine in commercially prepared media. Appl Microbiol 22:812–817

Lacey RW, Bruten DM, Gillespie WA, Lewis EL (1972) Trimethoprim-resistant coliforms. Lancet 1:409–410

Lacey RW, Gunasekera HKW, Lord VL, Leiberman PJ, Luxton DEA (1980) Comparison of trimethoprim alone with trimethoprim sulphamethoxazole in the treatment of respiratory and urinary infections with particular reference to selection of trimethoprim resistance. Lancet 2:1270–1273

Larsson S, Cronberg S, Winblad S (1978) Clinical aspects on 64 cases of juvenile and adult listeriosis in Sweden. Acta Med Scand 204:503–508

Laszlo A, Eidus L (1979) Differentiation of rapidly growing mycobacteria with trimethoprim (TMP). Can J Microbiol 25:991–994

Lebek G (1972) Extrachromosomal, transmissible antibiotic resistance in human pathogens. Hippokrates 43:45–60

Levison ME, Trestman I, Quach R et al. (1979) Quantitative bacteriology of the vaginal flora in vaginitis. Am J Obstet Gynecol 133:139–144

Lewis EL, Lacey RW (1973) Present significance of resistance to trimethoprim and sulphonamides in coliforms, *Staphylococcus aureus*, and *Streptococcus faecalis*. J Clin Pathol 26:175–180

Maskell R, Okubadejo OA, Payne RH, Pead L (1977) Human infections with thymine-requiring bacteria. J Med Microbiol 11:33–45

McCarthy LR, Mickelsen PA, Smith EG (1979) Antibiotic susceptibility of *Haemophilus vaginalis (Corynebacterium vaginale)* to 21 antibiotics. Antimicrob Agents Chemother 16:186–189

McGill RET (1978) Trimethoprim-resistant *Klebsiella aerogenes*. Lancet 2:156

Moody MR, Young VM (1975) In vitro susceptibility of *Pseudomonas cepacia* and *Pseudomonas maltophilia* to trimethoprim and trimethoprim-sulfamethoxazole. Anticrob Agents Chemother 7:836–839

Moorhouse EC, Farrell W (1973) Effect of co-trimoxazole on faecal enterobacteria: no emergence of resistant strains. J Med Microbiol 6:249–252

Näff H (1971) Über die Veränderungen der normalen Darmflora des Menschen durch Bactrim. (On the changes in the intestinal flora induced in man by Bacterim.) Pathol Microbiol 37:1–22

Nguyen-Van-Ai, Nguyen-Duc-Hanh (1972) Successful treatment of bubonic plague and septicaemia with trimethoprim-sulphamethoxazole (preliminary note). Bull Soc Pathol Exot Filiales 65:770–780

Nguyen-Van-Ai, Nguyen-Duc-Hanh, Pham-Van-Dien, Nguyen-Van-Le (1973) Co-trimoxazole in bubonic plague (Letter). Br Med J 4:108–109

Nord CE, Waldstrom T, Wretlind B (1974) Sensitivity of different Pseudomonas species and *Aeromonas hydrophilia* to trimethoprim and sulfamethoxozole separately and in combination. Med Microbiol Immunol 160:1–7

Northrup RS, Doyle MA, Feeley JC (1972) In vitro susceptibility of El Tor and classical *Vibrio cholerae* strains to trimethoprim and sulfamethoxazole. Antimicrob Agents Chemother 1:310–314

Nottebrock H, Then R (1977) Thymidine concentrations in serum and urine of different animal species and man. Biochem Pharmacol 26:2175–2179

Okubadejo OA (1974) Susceptibility of *Bacteroides fragilis* to co-trimoxazole. Lancet 1:1061

Okubadejo OA, Maskell RM (1973) Thymine-requiring mutants of *Proteus mirabilis* selected by co-trimoxazole *in vivo*. J Gen Microbiol 77:533–535

Okubadejo OA, Maskell RM (1974) Co-trimoxazole resistance (Letter). Br Med J 1:227

Pacheco G, Simoni da Silva D (1973) Sensibilide da *Listeria monocytogenes* „in vitro": a differentes antibiotics a quimioterapicos. (In vitro sensitivity of *Listeria monocytogenes* to various antibiotic and chemical agents.) Rev Bras Med 30:561–563

Pato ML, Brown GM (1963) Mechanisms of resistance of *Escherichia coli* to sulfonamides. Arch Biochem Biophys 103:443–448

Percival A, Cumberland N (1978) Antimicrobial susceptibilities of gram-negative anaerobes. J Antimicrob Chemother [Suppl] 4:3–13

Phillips I, Warren C (1976) Activity of sulfamethoxazole and trimethoprim against *Bacteroides fragilis*. Antimicrob Agents Chemother 9:736–740

Phillips I, Eykyn S, Laker M (1972) Outbreak of hospital infection caused by contaminated autoclaved fluids. Lancet 1:1258–1260

Phillips I, Watts BA, Tayler E (1977) Activity of trimethoprim and sulphamethoxazole against *Neisseria gonorrhoeae*. In: Skinner FA, Walker PD, Smith H (eds) Gonorrhoea: epidemiology and pathogenesis. Academic Press, London, pp 231–241

Piserchia PV, Shah BV (1975) A design for the detection of synergy in drug mixtures. In: Proc 21st Conf on Design of Experiments. US Army Research Office, Research Triangle Park, NC, pp 323–335

Pohlod D, Saravolatz L, Quinn E, Somerville M (1980) Susceptibility of *Legionella pneumophila* to 17 antimicrobial agents. In: Nelson JD, Grassie C (eds) Current chemotherapy and infectious disease. Proc 11th Int Congr Chemother and 19th Intersci Conf Antimicrob Agents Chemother, Boston USA, vol II. The American Society for Microbiology, Washington, DC, pp 997–998

Powers TE, Powers JD, Garg RC, Scialli VT, Hajian GH (1980) Trimethoprim and sulfadiazine: experimental infection of beagles. Am J Vet Res 41:1117–1122

Ronald AR, Cates C, Hoban S et al. (1978) The epidemiology of nalidixic acid (NA) and/or trimethoprim (TMP) resistant Enterobacteriaceae. Abstr Annu Meet Am Soc Microbiol. The American Society for Microbiology, Washington, DC, p 285

Rosenblatt JE, Stewart PR (1974) Lack of activity of sulfamethoxazole and trimethoprim against anaerobic bacteria. Antimicrob Agents Chemother 6:93–97

Roth B, Falco EA, Hitchings GH, Bushby SRM (1962) 5-Benzyl-2,4-diaminopyrimidines as antibacterial agents. I. Synthesis and antibacterial activity in vitro. J Med Pharm Chem 5:1103–1123

Rubini JR, Cronkite EP, Bond VP, Fliedner TM (1960) The metabolism and fate of tritiated thymidine in man. J Clin Invest 39:909–918

Seydel JK, Wempe E (1978) Potentiation of trimethoprim action with various sulfonamides: a comparison using bacterial growth kinetic techniques *(Escherichia coli)*. In: Siegenthaler W, Lüthy R (eds) Current chemotherapy. Proc 10th Int Congr Chemother, Zurich Switzerland. I. The American Society for Microbiology, Washington, DC, pp 658–660

Seydel JK, Wempe E (1979) Synergistic antibacterial activity in vitro of trimethoprim and sulphonamides and the importance of pharmacokinetic properties for optimal therapy. Infection [Suppl] 7:S313–S320

Seydel JK, Wempe E, Miller GH, Miller L (1973) Quantification of the antibacterial action of trimethoprim alone and in combination with sulfonamides by bacterial growth kinetics. J Infect Dis [Suppl] 128:S463–S469

Sietzen W, Knothe H (1978) Effect of trimethoprim, trimethoprim-sulfamethoxazole, and sulfamethoxazole on the occurence of drug-resistant *Enterobacteriaceae* in the human bowel flora. In: Siegenthaler W, Lüthy R (eds) Current chemotherapy. Proc 10th Int Congr Chemother, Zurich Switzerland, I. The American Society for Microbiology, Washington, DC, pp 660–662

Smellie JM, Grüneberg RN, Leakey A, Atkin WS (1976) Long-term low-dose co-trimoxazole in prophylaxis of childhood urinary tract infection: clinical aspects. Br Med J 2:203–206

Smith DD, Bell SM, Levey JM, Loy YT (1972) The action of trimethoprim-sulphamethoxazole against urinary pathogens. Med J Aust 1:263–265

Sng EH, Lam S (1970) The susceptibility of 44 strains of shigellae to eleven antimicrobial agents. Singapore Med J 11:162–165

Sng EH, Lam S (1971) The susceptibility of 168 strains of salmonellae to eleven antimicrobial agents. Singapore Med J 12:8–12

Sourander L, Saarimaa H, Arvilommi H (1972) Treatment of sulfonamide-resistant urinary tract infections with a combination of sulfonamide and trimethoprim. Acta Med Scand 191:1–3

Sparham PD, Lobban DI, Speller DC (1978) Thymidine-requiring *Staphylococcus aureus* (Letter). Lancet 1:104–105

Speller DCE, Bruten DM (1972) Faecal flora after prolonged co-trimoxazole treatment (Letter). Br Med J 3:416

Stacey KA, Simson E (1965) Improved method for the isolation of thymine-requiring mutants of *Escherichia coli*. J Bacteriol 90:554–555

Stolz E, Michel MF, Zwart HGF (1977) Potentiation of sulphamethoxazole by trimethoprim in *Neisseria gonorrhoeae* strains. Chemotherapy 23:65–72

Swenson JM, Thornsberry C, McCroskey LM, Hatheway CL, Dowell VR Jr (1980a) Susceptibility of *Clostridium botulinum* to thirteen antimicrobial agents. Antimicrob Agents Chemother 18:13–19

Swenson JM, Thornsberry C, Silcox V (1980b) Susceptibility of rapidly growing mycobacteria to 34 antimicrobial agents. In: Nelson JD, Grassi C (eds) Current chemotherapy and infectious disease. Proc 11th Int Congr Chemother and 19th Intersci Conf Antimicrob Agents Chemother, Boston USA, vol II. The American Society for Microbiology, Washington, DC, pp 1077–1079

Tanner EI, Bullin CH (1974) Thymidine-dependent *Escherichia coli* infection and some associated laboratory problems. J Clin Pathol 27:565–568

Tanphaichitra D, Stahel R, Shaw R (1980) Melioidosis: current therapy and cellular immunity. In: Nelson JD, Grassi C (eds) Current chemotherapy and infectious disease. Proc 11th Int Congr Chemother and 19th Intersci Conf Antimicrob Agents Chemother, Boston USA, vol II. The American Society for Microbiology, Washington, DC, pp 1016–1018

Tapsall JW, Wilson E, Harper J (1974) Thymine dependent strains of *Escherichia coli* selected by trimethoprim-sulphamethoxazole therapy. Pathology 6:161–167

Then R (1973) Influence of sulfonamide antagonists on the synergism of sulfamethoxazole/trimethoprim in *Escherichia coli*. Zentralbl Bakteriol Hyg I Abt [Orig A] 225:34–41

Then R (1977) Thymidine content in commercially prepared media. Zentralbl Bakteriol [Orig A] 237:372–377

Then R, Angehrn P (1973) Sulphonamide-induced "thymineless death" in *Escherichia coli*. J Gen Microbiol 76:255–263

Then R, Angehrn P (1975) The biochemical basis of the antimicrobial action of sulfonamides and trimethoprim in vivo. II. Experiments on the limited thymine and thymidine and urine. Biochem Pharmacol 23:2977–2982

Then R, Angehrn P (1975) The biochemical basis of the antimicrobial action of sulfonamides and trimethoprim in vivo. II. Experiments on the limited thymine and thymidine availability in blood and urine. Biochem Pharmacol 24:1003–1006

Then RL, Angehrn P (1979) Low trimethoprim susceptibility of anaerobic bacteria due to insensitive dihydrofolate reductases. Antimicrob Agents Chemother 15:1–6

Thong ML (1976) *Pseudomonas putrefaciens* from clinical material. Southeast Asian J Trop Med Public Health 7:363–366

Thornsberry C, Baker CN, Kirven LA (1978) In vitro activity of antimicrobial agents on Legionnaires disease bacterium. Antimicrob Agents Chemother 13:78–80

Toivanen A, Kasanen A, Sundquist H, Toivanen P (1976) Effect of trimethoprim on the occurrence of drug-resistant coliform bacteria in the faecal flora. Chemotherapy 22:97–103

Tomioka S, Kobayashi Y, Uchida H (1978) Susceptibilities of glucose-nonfermentative gram-negative rods to 20 antimicrobial agents. In: Siegenthaler W, Lüthy R (eds) Current chemotherapy. Proc 10th Int Congr Chemother, Zurich, Switzerland, vol I. The American Society for Microbiology, Washington, DC, pp 440–442

Towner KJ, Pearson NJ, Pinn PA, O'Grady F (1980) Increasing importance of plasmid-mediated trimethoprim resistance in enterobacteria: two six-month clinical surveys. Br Med J 280:517–519

Traub WH, Kleber I (1977) Selected and spontaneous variants of *Serratia marcescens* with combined resistance against chloramphenicol, nalidixic acid, and trimethoprim. Chemotherapy 23/6:436–451

Vanhoof R, Gordts B, Dierickx R, Coignau H, Butzler JP (1980) Bacteriostatic and bactericidal activities of 24 antimicrobial agents against *Campylobacter fetus* subsp. *jejuni.* Antimicrob Agents Chemother 18:118–121

Walder M (1979) Susceptibility of *Campylobacter fetus* subsp. *jejuni* to twenty antimicrobial agents. Antimicrob Agents Chemother 16:37–39

Williams Smith H (1976) Mutants of *Klebsiella pneumoniae* resistant to several antibiotics. Nature 259:307–308

Williams Smith H (1980) Antibiotic-resistant *Escherichia coli* in market pigs in 1956–1979: the emergence of organisms with plasmid-borne trimethoprim resistance. J Hyg (Camb) 84:467–477

Williams Smith H, Tucker JF (1976) The Virulence of trimethoprim-resistant thymine-requiring strains of *Salmonella.* J Hyg (Camb) 76:97–108

Winslow DL, Pankey GA (1980) In vitro activity of trimethoprim-sulfamethazole (TMP/SMX) against *Listeria monocytogenes.* Abstr 20th Intersci Conf Antimicrob Agents Chemother, New Orleans, Abstr 618. Am Soc Microbiol Washington, DC

Wise DM Jr, Abou-Donia MM (1975) Sulfonamide resistance mechanism in *Escherichia coli:* R plasmids can determine sulfonamide-resistant dihydropteroate synthases. Proc Natl Acad Sci USA 7:2621–2625

Wüst J, Kayser FH (1980) Activity of sulfamethoxazole/trimethoprim against aerobic and anaerobic bacteria. In: Nelson JD, Grassi C (eds) Current chemotherapy and infectious disease. Proc 11th Int Congr Chemother and 19th Interscience Conf Antimicrob Agents Chemother, Boston, USA, vol I. The American Society for Microbiology, Washington, DC, pp 501–502

CHAPTER 5

Selective Inhibitors
of Bacterial Dihydrofolate Reductase:
Structure-Activity Relationships*

B. ROTH

A. Introduction

Although trimethoprim (TMP); (1) has been in the public domain since 1959
(HITCHINGS and ROTH 1959) and available to the public since 1968 in combination
with sulfamethoxazole as a broad spectrum antibacterial agent, it still stands almost alone in this field as a species-specific dihydrofolate reductase (DHFR) inhibitor. It was preceded by its close relative diaveridine (2) (FALCO et al. 1951a;
HITCHINGS 1955), which found its utility as an anticoccidial agent, and was followed by ormetoprim (3) (HOFFER et al 1971), which again found its use in the latter
category. Very recently another very close relative, tetroxoprim (4) (HEUMANN
1974; ASCHOFF and VERGIN 1979) has been introduced in combination with sulfadiazine as an antibacterial competitor of TMP/SMX, with the claim of higher water solubility. Other competitors have masked trimethoprim (TMP) in the form of
various prodrugs, or in the form of various soluble or insoluble salts, in an effort
to modify its pharmacokinetic properties. This type of modification will not be discussed in this chapter, because of the difficulty of evaluating proprietary claims.

The fact that so few antibacterial DHFR inhibitors have reached the public
does not mean that the chemist and biologist have been idle in this area for the past

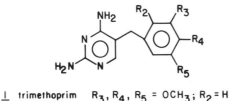

<u>1</u>	trimethoprim	$R_3, R_4, R_5 = OCH_3; R_2 = H$
<u>2</u>	diaveridine	$R_3, R_4 = OCH_3; R_2, R_5 = H$
<u>3</u>	ormetoprim	$R_2 = CH_3; R_4, R_5 = OCH_3; R_3 = H$
<u>4</u>	tetroxoprim	$R_3, R_5 = OCH_3; R_2 = H;$
		$R_4 = OCH_2CH_2OCH_3$

---

* *Editorial Note.* The following chapter by BARBARA ROTH represents some revisions and
condensations of the chapter as originally written. In particular the full text deals extensively with quantitative structure–activity relationships. This full text is being published
separately and will be made available to interested medicinal chemists on application to
the author. Some of the numberings of the figures of the longer text have been retained
in the present version in order to avoid possible confusion. The editor wishes to express
his appreciation to Dr. Roth for her cooperation in adapting her text to the current volume

20 years, however. It is the purpose of this chapter to highlight the most interesting among the hundreds of diaminopyrimidines and other substituted nitrogen-containing heterocycles which have been synthesized and evaluated as antibacterials or as bacterial DHFR inhibitors in the intervening years, and to try to place them in perspective, insofar as this is possible with the available published information.

To place a relative evaluation upon the known antibacterial DHFR inhibitors from various laboratories is a difficult task at best. Perhaps the most cogent reason is that a large proportion of the derivatives which one might expect to be among those most active (for example, trisubstituted benzylpyrimidines) lie buried in the patent literature, and it has only been in very recent years that patents have included useful biologic data. One then proceeds by inference, from the scope of claims made, variety of syntheses recorded, or frequency of occurrence of a given compound – as well as from one's own previous experience.

As is always true, data from different sources are difficult to compare, and can only be compared when the same standards have been used. In many cases there are insufficient data presented to draw any meaningful conclusions, as for example when high antibacterial activity is claimed and *Streptococcus faecium (faecalis)* is the only organism documented. In many cases, the only bacterial data recorded involve synergistic combinations with sulfonamides. Such data will not be compared here. SEYDEL and WEMPE (1980) have discussed the problems of such comparisons. Our structure–activity discussion will be restricted to the DHFR inhibitors alone (see Chap. 6).

Another type of problem concerns the crude enzymes and crude assay procedures which were used in the earlier days. It has been a common procedure in most laboratories to record enzyme inhibitory data by use of I_{50} values and to compare data from different enzyme sources using this figure rather than the kinetic rate constant K_i. Since the Michaelis constants K_M for the substrate dihydrofolate differ from enzyme to enzyme (a figure used in the calculation of K_i), and since for multisubstrate reactions the relation between I_{50} and K_i for dissociation of the inhibitor from an enzyme–inhibitor complex is dependent both on the type of inhibition and the concentrations of fixed substrates, an inaccurate picture of relative inhibitory potencies can result (BLAKLEY and MORRISON 1970; CHENG and PRUSOFF 1973). However, it would seem satisfactory to use I_{50} values to compare a given series in a relative manner, provided that the inhibition is competitive in all cases.

Some of the pitfalls of determining the inhibition of DHFR by folate analogs have recently been pointed out (M. WILLIAMS et al. 1973; J. WILLIAMS et al. 1980). Many compounds have been found to bind to DHFR and other enzymes in a time-dependent manner. In such cases, the inhibition observed will depend on the order of adding the components to the assay, as well as the times of measurement. Thus, the reaction rate may increase or decrease with time, depending on which component is added last in order to start the reaction. I_{50} values then can be rather misleading, even meaningless, unless these problems are recognized. It is rather sobering to find it necessary to report at the beginning of this chapter that trimethoprim is one of the compounds which behaves in this manner. Some comparative K_i values for TMP and analogs (WILLIAMS et al. 1980; BACCANARI and JOYNER 1981) conducted under conditions which recognize these facts are presented in the appropriate sections which follow.

The publication of the X-ray structures of *Escherichia coli* DHFR crystals in binary complex with methotrexate (MTX) and *Lactobacillus casei* DHFR in ternary complex with MTX plus NADPH (MATTHEWS et al. 1977, 1978; for details see Sect. E and Chap. 3) marks the leap to a new plane of endeavor in the study of inhibitor binding to this enzyme. A report has just appeared on the X-ray structure of TMP–*E. coli* DHFR binary complex (BAKER et al. 1981). Soon we may learn how vertebrate DHFR enzymes differ in architecture from those of bacteria. The days of the routine I_{50} assay will soon be replaced by more sophisticated techniques, which are now in use or under serious evaluation, so that a better quantitative picture may be obtained of relative inhibitor binding. To attempt to understand specificity will require a knowledge of energetics of binding as well as the total hydrogen bonding picture with the various small molecule–DHFR complexes. To assess the relative importance of these interactions is a difficult challenge (ROBERTS 1978). The nature of quantitative structure–activity relationship studies on this enzyme is already reaching a new plane which is keeping pace with the new age of computer graphics, as inhibitors are fitted to the enzyme which is seen three-dimensionally, sometimes in color, on a two-dimensional screen, and which can be rotated to view all angles (LANGRIDGE et al. 1981; FELDMANN et al. 1978; GUND et al. 1980). It may be predicted that a structure–activity discussion will utilize a new language 5 years from now. In the meantime, we offer no apology for using the less precise language of the age of "enlightened empiricism" (a term introduced by G. H. HITCHINGS), which in itself elevated us to a new plane a generation ago.

B. Historical Perspective

In 1947, two laboratories independently announced their discoveries that 2,4-diaminopteridines were powerful inhibitors of the activity of folic acid (5). The 4-amino derivative of folic acid itself, aminopterin, (6a) provided what was apparently the closest possible analogy to the parent vitamin. The announcement of the potent inhibitory effects of (6a) against growth of *Streptococcus faecium* (SEE-

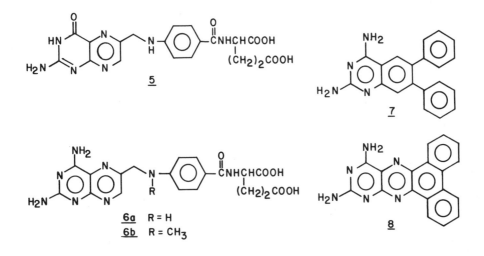

GER et al. 1947, 1949) as well as its growth inhibitory properties in mammalian systems paved the way to the development of methotrexate (6 b) (SEEGER et al. 1947, 1949 and references therein), one of the most widely used antitumor drugs available today. The drug was later found to owe its activity largely to its competitive inhibitory action against the enzyme DHFR (ZAKRZEWSKI and NICHOL 1958; WERKHEISER 1960).

The second series of announcements of 1947 (DANIEL and NORRIS 1947; MALLETTE et al. 1947; DANIEL et al. 1947) concerned 2,4-diaminopteridines which lacked the p-aminobenzoylglutamic acid moiety. Several such compounds [(7) and (8), for example] were reported to inhibit the growth, not only of the folate-requiring bacteria, S. faecium and L. casei, but also of Lactobacillus arabinosus, E. coli, and Staphylococcus aureus, which synthesized their own needs of folic acid (FA). Furthermore, a synergistic effect was observed on adding a sulfonamide to the medium (DANIEL et al. 1947). The authors stated that "synergism between the pterins and sulfonamides is to be expected, since they are competing with two different parts of the FA molecule ... The results ... point to the possibility of using the inhibitory pterins in conjunction with sulfonamides in therapy, thereby decreasing the amount of sulfonamides required." This early insight into synergism can be ascribed to the teachings of WOODS (1940) and of LAMPEN and JONES (1946), concerning the mechanism of action of sulfonamides. DANIEL reasoned that pterins related to the pteridine portion of FA might well behave similarly. Although this lead did not produce a useful antibacterial agent, and despite the fact that no specificity of action against bacteria was demonstrated, these findings (even if imperfect in concept) nevertheless stand as a landmark which helped to pave the way to combination chemotherapy with a diaminopyrimidine and sulfa drug.

The specific critical clue that was to lead to TMP and pyrimethamine was announced by 1948 (HITCHINGS et al.). This was the discovery that simple 2,4-diaminopyrimidines, such as the 5,6-dimethyl derivative (9 a) or the diamino analog of thymine (9 b) originally synthesized as possible antagonists to the nucleic acid bases, actually inhibited the growth of L. casei owing to interference with the utilization of FA, rather than thymine or purines. This was rapidly followed by publications on the potent antimalarial activities of 5-aryloxy-2,4-diaminopyrimidines (10 a), (FALCO et al. 1951 a), 5-benzyl- (10 b) (FALCO et al. 1951 c), and 5-aryl-2,4-diamino analogs (10 c) (RUSSELL and HITCHINGS 1951), and then by the discovery that some of these compounds (notably benzylpyrimidines lacking 6-substituents on the pyrimidine ring) were more active against bacteria than plasmodia (FALCO et al. 1951 b; HITCHINGS 1955; ELION et al. 1960; BUSHBY and HITCHINGS 1968; HITCHINGS and BUSHBY 1961). The effort to optimize these results led

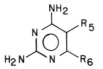

<u>9a</u> R_5, R_6 = CH_3
<u>9b</u> R_5 = CH_3, R_6 = H

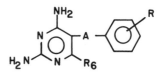

<u>10a</u> A = O, R_6 = H, alkyl
<u>10b</u> A = CH_2, R_6 = H, alkyl
<u>10c</u> A = —, R_6 = H, alkyl

eventually to TMP (HITCHINGS and ROTH 1959; HITCHINGS and BUSHBY 1961; ROTH et al. 1962). However, what put TMP into perspective as a candidate antibacterial agent was the announcement (BURCHALL and HITCHINGS 1965) of the tremendous specificity of TMP for bacterial DHFR, coupled with equally astonishing specificity of a dihydrotriazine for mammalian enzymes, and of pyrimethamine for plasmodial enzymes, despite ubiquitous DHFR activity for MTX. Here indeed then had been found a "magic bullet," and a most unusual enzyme, with many possibilities for exploitation.

C. Some General Requirements for DHFR Inhibition and Antibacterial Activity

Although many close analogs of folic acid, such as methotrexate (MTX), are powerful inhibitors of the growth of folate-requiring bacteria, such as *S. faecium* and *L. casei*, they do not inhibit the growth of the great majority of bacteria, which synthesize their own dihydrofolate. Such bacteria do not have a transport mechanism for the incorporation of folate and its analogs. In any event, most folate analogs show no selectivity for bacterial DHFR.

Most antibacterial DHFR inhibitors are incorporated into bacteria by passive diffusion. Very large molecules (of the size of folic acid and greater) seldom diffuse easily into bacterial cells, and a negative charge (as with folate) normally blocks cell entry by passive means. The ease of penetration into various bacterial cells depends in part on the lipophilicity of the inhibitor, which should be neither too great nor too small, so that it may pass through a lipid membrane layer without being trapped. Many DHFR inhibitors do not have a broad spectrum because of such problems.

D. Inhibitors of Specific DHFRs

I. The 5-Phenyl Derivatives and Related Compounds

A discussion of specific antimalarial DHFR inhibitors is beyond the scope of this review. Literally hundreds of such compounds have been prepared in the search for a successor to the clinically important pyrimethamine, developed by HITCHINGS and his colleagues in the early 1950s. A symposium on this drug (HITCHINGS et al. 1952) contains much useful structure–activity information from that period. The following statement by HITCHINGS (1952) shows that the concept of specificity had been recognized even though the target enzyme was as yet uncharacterized.

Where an antimetabolite differs from the metabolite by a single structural change, it may be expected to produce a deficiency of the metabolite in a variety of biological species, for it must possess nearly all of the structural features which determine the affinity of the metabolite for the cell receptors. An antimetabolite which differs more widely from the metabolite in chemical structure may be expected to show much greater variations from species to species. Daraprim may be regarded as a structural analogue of folinic acid of a rather remote sort, but well adapted to the displacement of this metabolite from its apoenzyme in plasmodia.

However, the mechanism of action was viewed as "preventing the conversion of folic to folinic acid in the organism."

One final historical note must be added. The antimalarial, proguanil [iso-PrNHC(=NH)NHC(=NH)NHC$_6$H$_4$Cl-4], a biguanide developed by CURD et al. (1945) under entirely different lines of research, was found to owe its activity in vivo to a cyclic metabolite which proved to be a diaminodihydrotriazine (cycloguanil, see formula *CG*; CARRINGTON et al. 1951). The similarity in structure of this metabolite to pyrimethamine (formula *PYR*) was recognized by HITCHINGS et al. (1956), and the formal analogy of chlorproguanil to pyrimethamine by FALCO et al. (1951 b). Both compounds were indeed found later to act on the same target enzyme DHFR. Thus began the many-faceted search down the diamino trail, which goes on with new emphasis today. For a discussion of the antimalarial activities of pyrimethamine see Chap. 13.

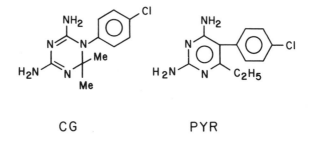

CG   PYR

II. 5-Benzyl-2,4-Diaminopyrimidines and Close Relatives

1. The 6-Unsubstituted Derivatives
a) Activity and Specificity Among Mono-, Di-,
and Trisubstituted Benzyl Analogs

This class of compounds, which embraces trimethoprim, includes the single most important category of selective antibacterial DHFR inhibitors known to date. During the last three decades, the skills of the medicinal chemist have been applied to every feature of the benzylpyrimidine molecule. Many compounds in this class do *not* have species specificity for bacterial reductases, however. Furthermore, many of them do not have broad spectrum inhibitory activity against all bacterial DHFR enzymes. In addition, many of them are not able to get into bacterial cells, or into some types of cells, such as the gram-negative bacteria. The reasons for these differences are not fully understood. Much current work is being undertaken in an attempt to understand these phenomena at the molecular level.

Literally hundreds of 5-(substituted benzyl)-2,4-diaminopyrimidines have been synthesized as potential antibacterial agents since the original report of their activity (FALCO et al. 1951 a, b). The main features of selective antibacterial structures were soon apparent. It became clear at a very early date that 3′,4′,5′-trisubstituted derivatives were in general more active and selective than disubstituted, which were in turn more active than monosubstituted analogs; and alkoxy groups showed promise of being desirable. Lipophilic substituents in general aided gram-positive bacterial activity, but were deleterious for the gram-negative bacteria. These points are exemplified by the data of Table 1, which also demonstrate the relatively feeble binding of these compounds to a mammalian DHFR.

Table 1. Comparative antibacterial activity and DHFR inhibition of selected benzyl-pyrimidines

No.	Benzene substituents				In vitro antibacterial activity MIC (µg/ml)[a]			I_{50} vs DHFR ($\times 10^{-8}$ M)[b]	
	R_2	R_3	R_4	R_5	Proteus vulgaris	Staphylococcus aureus	Streptococcus pyogenes	E. coli	Rat liver
(27)					50	25	4	340	15,000
(28)			OMe		320	20	<2	110	17,000
(29)			Me		50	12	2	230	10,000
(30)			Cl		50	12	4	210	9,000
(31)			OH					180	16,000
(32)			NMe$_2$		50	25	4		
(33)		OMe			25	6	2	49	4,300
(34)		Cl	Cl		100	2	0.5		
(2)		OMe	OMe		4	1	2	10	7,000
(35)	NO$_2$		OMe	OMe	12	0.3	4		
(36)		OMe		OMe	16	2	4		
(37)	OMe	OMe			250	16	<2		
(38)		OMe	OMe	Cl	32	0.5	0.25	4	10,000
(39)		OMe	OMe	Br	16	1	1	2	8,000
(1)		OMe	OMe	OMe	1	0.5	0.25	0.5	26,000
(40)		OMe	OH	OMe				1.1[c]	11,000[c]
(41)	Br		OPr-n	OMe	250	0.12	0.5		
(42)	Br	OMe	OMe	OMe	32	0.06	1		

[a] Roth et al. (1962)
[b] Hitchings et al. (1966)
[c] Roth et al. (1980a)

Inhibitory activities against partially purified DHFRs were first reported by Baker (1964) and by Burchall and Hitchings (1965). These data documented the highly selective actions of compounds of this type. A second report comparing the E. coli and rat liver DHFR inhibition of ten benzylpyrimidines appeared a year later (Hitchings et al. 1966; see Table 1). Although no direct comparisons with in vitro results are possible with these data, it is apparent that the better DHFR inhibitors are also in general better in vitro antibacterial agents, particularly with the gram-positive bacteria. In other words, the antibacterial activity is a function of DHFR inhibition, as has been amply shown in a host of additional experiments, too numerous to document here. The few trimethoprim analogs which have found commercial distribution to date are shown in formulae (2–4) in Sect. A.

b) The 3'4',5'-Trisubstituted Benzylpyrimidines:
Activity and Specificity

α) *Variations in the 4'-Substituent.* A large number of 3',5'-dialkoxy-4'-substituted analogs of TMP have been reported. It is among this class of compounds that the highest specificities and activities have been found. Among the compounds prepared by Kompis et al. (1980) was the 4'-isopropenyl derivative (59), which shows the greatest selectivity of any compound reported to date against bacterial DHFR,

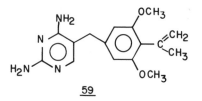

59

and also a somewhat increased inhibitory activity against *E. coli* DHFR over that of TMP. It also has high antibacterial activity in the species reported.

ROTH et al. (1980a) suggested that one factor involved with TMP selectivity might be the out-of-plane 4'-methoxy group. The 4'-hydroxy analog, for example, was slightly less inhibitory toward *E. coli* DHFR, but more inhibitory against rat liver DHFR; I_{50} against DHFR $= 1.1 \times 10^{-8}$ *M (E. coli)*; 9,200 (rat liver). A second paper (ROTH et al. 1981) pointed out that the highly selective Kompis compounds all have 4'-substituents which are presumed to be out-of-plane in *both* directions from the benzene ring. This has recently been confirmed by X-ray crystallography (CODY and DEJARNETTE 1981). Interference at one face of the benzene ring may decrease binding to the mammalian enzyme.

A series of thirty-eight 3',5'-dimethoxy-4'-OR substituted TMP analogs and two 4'-alkyl derivatives was reported by ROTH et al. (1981); see also ROTH and STRELITZ (1972). It was suggested that one important function of any 4'-substituent (other than H) may be to force the two meta-methoxy groups to bend away from it, in plane with the ring, (69) and thus favor meta-space interactions with the enzyme.

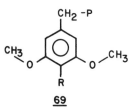

69

A number of 4-amino-3,5-disubstituted TMP analogs have been claimed to have high antibacterial activity (KOMPIS et al. 1975, 1981; PERUN et al. 1975, 1978). The 4-amino-3,5-dimethoxy derivative was later found to be a diuretic agent, however (DAUM et al. 1980). The 4-methylthio-3,5-dimethoxy derivative has recently received considerable attention (FRITSCHE et al. 1979; KOMPIS and WICK 1979; KOMPIS et al. 1981).

β) Variations in the 3'- and 5'-Substituents. ROTH et al. (1972; see also ROTH 1973, 1974; ROTH et al. 1974, 1980b; also unpublished work) made a systematic study of the meta-space requirements of substituted benzylpyrimidines for optimal binding to bacterial DHFR, by varying alkyl substituents in both positions. Optimal *E. coli* DHFR activity was found with the 3',5'-diethyl and ethyl-*n*-propyl derivatives, which inhibit the enzyme to approximately the same extent as TMP, and which can also presumably occupy similar space on the enzyme. This finding strongly suggests that it is the *shape* of the meta-substituents, rather than the lipophilicity or polarity, which is important for *E. coli* DHFR binding. Greater binding to rat liver DHFR occurs with slightly greater bulk, and the I_{50} values show dependence on the nature of the 4'-substituent.

All of the 3',5'-dialkyl derivatives to date have considerably less selectivity for bacterial DHFR than does TMP. The 3',5'-ether oxygens then play a role in this phenomenon, which could relate to ring conjugation and planarity of such substituents or to hydrogen bonding possibilities. KOMPIS et al. (1981) have called attention to the fact that in a number of instances where comparable 3',5'-dimethoxy-4'-R- and 3',4'-dimethoxy-5'-R-derivatives were available, the former had both greater bacterial DHFR inhibitory activity and greater selectivity.

The 3'-hydroxymethyl-4',5'-dimethoxy-TMP derivative has been prepared (S. DALUGE and R. FERONE, unpublished work 1980) and found to be 24-fold less inhibitory to *E. coli* DHFR than TMP ($I_{50} = 12 \times 10^{-8}$ M). The 4'-isomer (KOMPIS et al. 1980) is slightly less active than TMP ($I_{50} = 2 \times 10^{-8}$ M). One can infer that the meta-methyl groups of TMP have hydrophobic interaction with the enzyme, since these isomeric hydroxymethyl substituents, presumably hydrogen bonded at their terminal hydroxyl groups, are contraindicated. A large number of 3',5'-dialkylamino- and monoalkylamino-4'-substituted benzylpyrimidines have been explored (KOMPIS et al. 1976).

c) Polyfunctional Benzylpyrimidines
Other than 3',4',5'-Trisubstituted Derivatives

These studies have all pointed toward fine tuning the vicinal substituents in the 3',4',5'-positions for optimal activity and selectivity. Brief mention should be made of other substituent patterns that have been studied, such as 2',4',5'- or 2',3',4'-substituted benzylpyrimidines.

Ormetoprim (3), the 2'-methyl-4',5'-dimethoxyl derivative, was found to be much less active than TMP as an antibacterial when tested in vivo in mice (HOFFER et al. 1971) although it gave good potentiation with sulfa drugs. It is also less active as an *E. coli* DHFR inhibitor ($I_{50} = 5 \times 10^{-8}$ M; R. FERONE, unpublished work 1970). This compound, as well as diaveridine (2), are effective coccidiostats, however. Ortho-substituents other than methyl are revealed in related patents (HOFFER 1967, 1969; ROSEN 1977).

The 2',3',4'-trimethoxybenzyl TMP analog has been prepared in several laboratories (HOFFER 1967; TOKUYAMA 1974; R. BALTZLY and R. FERONE, unpublished work 1967). It is very much less active than is TMP (I_{50} against DHFR = 92×10^{-8} M *(E. coli)*, 5,800 (rat liver), from BALTZLY and FERONE, unpublished work 1967). The 2',3',4',5'- and 2',3',5',6'-tetramethoxy analogs are also disclosed in the ormetoprim patents without data.

2. 6-Substituted Derivatives

A series of diverse 6-substituted TMP analogs was prepared by ROTH et al. (1980 b). All had considerably lower activity than TMP, both as enzyme inhibitors and as antibacterial agents. The authors postulated that if TMP interacted with the enzyme in the known conformation of its hydrobromide salt, a conformation in which the H-6 of the pyrimidine ring points toward the center of the benzene ring, such a conformation would be hindered owing to crowding by the 6-substituent. With the publication of the conformation of TMP in interaction with *E. coli* DHFR (BAKER et al. 1981) the postulate has been shown to be correct for the binary complex. A second reason for low activity is that the inductive effect of the 6-substituent will in most cases (except alkyl) lower the pK_a of the pyrimidine (ROTH and STRELITZ 1969) and thus decrease the ionic attraction of the protonated N-1 atom to Asp-27 of *E. coli* DHFR. A 6-chloro substituent, for example, will lower the dissociation constant by about 4 units, to give a pK_a value of about 3. This compound is then virtually un-ionized at physiologic pH.

3. Substitution of a Heterocyclic Ring for the Benzene Moiety

KOMPIS et al. (1977) synthesized a series of TMP analogs in which the benzene ring was replaced by pyridine, with the nitrogen in the 2',3', or 4'-position. The compounds are all relatively weak inhibitors of DHFR.

4. Variations in the Bridge Between the Pyrimidine and Benzene Rings

Among direct analogs of TMP, a number of modifications have been made in the methylene bridge between the two rings. One of the metabolites of TMP in humans and animals is the inactive hydroxymethylene derivative (SCHWARTZ et al. 1970; BROSSI et al. 1971). In vivo it was inactive at 1,000 mg/kg against most bacteria. With the current knowledge that the methylene bridge of TMP lies buried in a hydrophobic cleft (BAKER et al. 1981), it is not surprising that the alcohol is inactive. The hydrophilic substituent may also change the torsional angles between the two rings. The corresponding ketone was likewise inactive (ROTH and YEOWELL 1971; BROSSI et al. 1971). These comments would also apply to the ketone, but in addition, the electron-withdrawing substituent in the pyrimidine-5-position results in the very low pK_a value of approximately 4.5 (ROTH and STRELITZ 1969).

REY-BELLET et al. (1975) prepared eleven additional bridge variations. All of these compounds had very low DHFR and antibacterial activity. Either there is a lack of space tolerance for even a methyl group, or the torsional angles are changed thereby. STOGRYN (1972) varied the bridge to give X = O, N = N, CONH, NHCO, COO, CH = N, CH_2NH, NHCONH, and NHCSNH. The activity was very low in all cases.

A number of 5-arylthiopyrimidines (X = S) have been reported, all of which have low antibacterial activity (FALCO et al. 1961). Such compounds have pK_a values below 6 (ROTH and STRELITZ 1969) as well as the bulkier bridge. 5-Anilinopyrimidines have likewise been reported to have very low activity (GERNS et al. 1966).

The methylene bridge has also been eliminated to give the 3',4',5'-trimethoxyphenyl analog of TMP (ROTH and STRELITZ 1969). This molecule of necessity has an entirely different conformation from that of TMP, and has very low inhibitory activity against *E. coli* DHFR ($I_{50} = 26,000 \times 10^{-8}$ *M*) (R. FERONE, unpublished work 1981). The antimalarial, pyrimethamine (the 4'-chlorophenyl-6-ethyl analog), has an intermediate degree of *E. coli* DHFR activity. The two aromatic rings of pyrimethamine have been found to be nearly perpendicular to each other, along a common axis, in the crystal state (PHILLIPS and BRYAN 1969).

III. The 1,2-Dihydro-1,3,5-Triazines

The 1965 report by BURCHALL and HITCHINGS on the striking species specificity of DHFR from various sources was exemplified in part by two extremes in activity; that of trimethoprim on the one hand, with its tremendous affinity for bacterial DHFR, and of a dihydrotriazine (132) (ROTH and BURCHALL 1971) on the other, which was reported to have an I_{50} for human DHFR of 55×10^{-8} M, as opposed to $65,000 \times 10^{-8}$ M for $E.\,coli$ DHFR. (More recent assays with purified enzymes (R. FERONE and J. J. BURCHALL, unpublished work 1980) give values of 24×10^{-8} and $3,200 \times 10^{-8}$ M, respectively.)

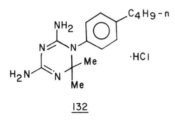

132

ROTH et al. (1960, 1963) prepared a series of 1-aryldihydrotriazines which either contained ortho-substituents in the benzene ring or bulky groups in the triazine 2-position, with putative selective DHFR activity against parasitic organisms. Such compounds were found to have excellent anthelmintic activity against intestinal parasites (*Syphacia obvelata* and *Aspiculuris tetraptera*) in mice, and very low toxicity. They were active against immature, as well as mature, forms of the parasite. Compound (134) was submitted to extensive anthelmintic and pharmacologic investigation. It was tested clinically, and found active against the pinworm of humans, *Enterobius vermicularis*. The mechanism of action of (134) is not known, but the possibility must be strongly considered that the compound is species specific for the parasitic DHFR. This series shows no appreciable inhibition for *E. coli* or mammalian DHFR. It was this report that triggered the synthesis of a barrage of dihydrotriazines by B. R. BAKER and his colleagues, with cancer as their target (BAKER et al. 1960; BAKER 1964, 1967).

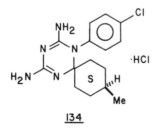

134

IV. Bicyclic Analogs of the Diaminopyrimidines

A very large number of bicyclic and some tricyclic DHFR inhibitors have been prepared, including direct analogs of folic acid and methotrexate, as well as simpler compounds without the *p*-aminobenzoylglutamate side chain of folic acid. The main classes of simple bicyclic compounds studied include the pteridines (137), the pyrido[2,3-d]pyrimidines (138), and the quinazolines (139). These compounds differ chiefly in their pK_a values (ROTH and STRELITZ 1969), solubilities, and lipophilicities, with the basicity and lipophilicity increasing as electron-withdrawing nitrogen atoms are removed from a ring. All are protonated on the N-1 nitrogen of the pyrimidine ring, and it is not unlikely that they are bound to DHFR in the manner described by MATTHEWS et al. (1977, 1978) for methotrexate.

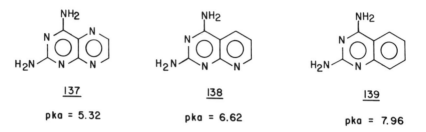

137	138	139
pka = 5.32	pka = 6.62	pka = 7.96

A very early study by HITCHINGS et al. (1954) compared several such bicyclic systems for their ability to inhibit growth of *S. faecium* and *L. casei*. It is of interest that although no direct isosteres were tested, the quinazoline was more active than the pyridopyrimidine, which was in turn more active than the pteridine, a result which might be predicted from comparative pK_a values alone. HITCHINGS and LEDIG (1960) found that 2,4-diaminopyrido[2,3-d]pyrimidines containing alkyl or alkylene groups at the 5- and 6-positions were very active against pathogenic bacteria.

HURLBERT et al. (1968) prepared a large series of 5- and 6-substituted pyrido[2,3-d]pyrimidines, some of which are very potent antibacterial agents. The striking effect on the inhibitory activity of adding alkyl substituents is evident, but the effect on the mammalian enzyme parallels that on *E. coli* DHFR. In vitro, the activity of the 5-methyl-6-*sec*-butyl derivative against *Pseudomonas aeruginosa* is noteworthy. In vivo, the effect of the compounds was potentiated by sulfadiazine in mice, and complete cures were effected in *Staphylococcus aureus* and *Proteus vulgaris* infections. Such compounds might be useable were it not for the availability of combinations with better chemotherapeutic indices.

HITCHINGS et al. (1960) prepared a series of 2,4-diaminoquinazolines analogous to the pyrido[2,3-d]pyrimidines described by HITCHINGS and LEDIG (1960). The 5-methyl and 6-methyl derivatives were particularly active in a bacterial plating test, with a spectrum showing activity against such troublesome organisms as *Proteus vulgaris* and *Pseudomonas aeruginosa*. In a review of quinazolines and related compounds as antimalarial agents, ELSLAGER and DAVOLL (1974) cited the 6-aryloxyquinazolines (ELSLAGER et al. 1972) as having potent broad spectrum activity in vitro against pathogenic bacteria, with MIC values of <0.25–20 μg/ml. The corresponding 6-arylthioquinazoline analogs were tested by HYNES et al. (1974) as inhibitors of *S. faecium* and rat liver DHFR, and found to be nonselective.

E. Discussion

A number of new developments have brought new insight to the action of old inhibitors and promise new approaches to the design of new agents. Some modifi-

Table 2. Comparison of inhibitory rate constants, dissociation constants, and cell growth rates for benzylpyramidines with DHFR enzymes and with *Escherichia coli* cells

No.	Benzene substituents			I_{50} (μM), growth[a] *E. coli* ML-30 whole cells	Inhibitory rate constants and dissociation constants with DHFR (nM)			
					E. coli form 1[b]		*E. coli* form 2[b]	
	R_3	R_4	R_5		K_i	Binary K_D	K_i	Binary K_D
(1)	OMe	OMe	OMe	0.3	1.3	15	106	864
(35)	OMe	OMe		1.9	8.3	9	494	296
(36)	OMe		OMe	1.2	8.6	18	426	101
(33)	OMe			10.6	73	18.5	2,102	158
(28)		OMe		11.8	78	24.5	2,530	264
(27)				120	671	54	10,370	215

[a] Glucose minimal medium
[b] BACCANARI et al. (1981b). Forms 1 and 2 are two isoenzymes from a TMP-resistant strain of *E. coli* (RT500) which differ in a single amino acid

cations of reported Michaelis constants seem required in response to new findings. Recent reports have discussed the problem of curvature in rate plots with tight-binding inhibitors of DHFR, and on the methodology developed (in their laboratories) to avoid these problems (DIETRICH et al. 1980; WILLIAMS et al. 1980; BACCANARI and JOYNER 1981). In all cases, carefully purified enzymes were used.

A recent study of TMP, its parent benzylpyrimidine and the monomethoxy and dimethoxy analogs in interaction with DHFR from *E. coli* and mouse lymphoma, and with *E. coli* cells (BACCANARI et al. 1981a) gives insight as to selectivity and to cooperativity in binding to the ternary, rather than binary, complexes of DHFR (Table 2). The *E. coli* DHFR K_i values parallel the whole cell antibacterial activity. It will be noted that the monomethoxy derivatives are about ten-fold more active than the unsubstituted benzylpyrimidine, the dimethoxy analogs another ten-fold more active, and TMP roughly six-fold more active again. The binary dissociation constants of the pyrimidine–enzyme complexes, studied by equilibrium dialysis of ^{14}C derivatives, are remarkably similar to each other, however. The authors conclude that cooperativity in binding with the ternary complex is largely responsible for the high affinity of TMP for *E. coli* DHFR, and that this increases with methoxy substitution.

There is poor cooperativity with the mammalian enzyme, a factor which may also be important in the selectivity of TMP. To understand the nature of the cooperativity will require knowledge of the X-ray structure of the ternary *E. coli* DHFR complex with TMP and NADPH. In diametric opposition to TMP as a selective DHFR enzyme inhibitor, lies MTX. Despite the lack of utility of MTX as an antibacterial agent, it nevertheless is a very potent inhibitor of bacterial, as well as mammalian, DHFRs (*S. faecium*, $K_i = 58 \times 10^{-12}$ M; WILLIAMS et al. 1979); *E. coli*, $K_i = 21 \times 10^{-12}$ M; BACCANARI and JOYNER 1981; L1210 cells, $K_i = 5.3 \times 10^{-12}$ M; L578Y cells, $K_i = 3.1 \times 10^{-12}$ M; JACKSON et al. 1976; human lymphoblastic W1-L2 cells, $K_i = 6.9 \times 10^{-12}$ M; JACKSON and NIETHAMMER 1977).

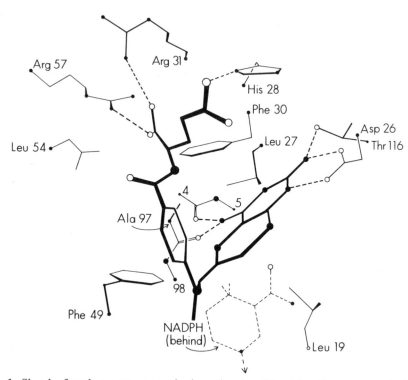

Fig. 1. Sketch of methotrexate as seen in the active site of *Lactobacillus casei* dihydrofolate reductase, with neighboring amino acid side chains, and nicotinamide ring of NADPH. Hitchings and Roth (1980)

Many studies have been carried out with MTX as a stoichiometric binder to DHFR, in an effort to learn more about the enzyme.

Beginning about 1975, DHFRs from various sources in approximately pure form began to accumulate, mainly as a result of improved methods of purification (Hitchings and Roth 1980; Hitchings and Smith 1980). The availability of pure enzymes permitted the determination of amino acid sequences, and by 1980 eight or ten of these had been reported. These amply verified the diversity among the enzymes that the inhibitor studies had detected. The differences were even more profound than had been suspected, and the homologies even more limited. Thus, among those available in 1980, there were only 16 apparently identical residues among the sequences then available. It is perhaps significant that all of these have been identified as probable participants in active site binding, as discussed in the following paragraphs (Hitchings and Smith 1980).

A quantum leap in understanding the interactions of the inhibitors with the enzymes came with the reports of the X-ray diffraction patterns of crystalline enzyme complexes. The first to be reported was that of the *E. coli* DHFR–MTX complex (Matthews et al. 1977) followed shortly by that of the ternary complex formed with the *L. casei* enzyme, MTX, and NADPH (Matthews et al. 1978). The principal interactions of enzyme residue with features of the inhibitor are depicted in Fig. 1.

MTX resides in a large cleft of DHFR in which the only conserved ionized residues that interact with the inhibitor are Asp-27 and Arg-57 (*E. coli* numbering for the amino acid sequence; MATTHEWS et al. 1977). The former residue interacts through its carboxy group with N-1, the most basic nitrogen of the pteridine ring of MTX. The latter forms hydrogen bonds with the α-carboxy group of the glutamate moiety of the inhibitor. The 2-amino group of the pteridine is situated so that it can form a hydrogen bond with Thr-113. The 4-amino group donates a hydrogen bond to the carbonyl backbone of Ile-5; also, the plane of the Ala-6–Ala-7 peptide bond is approximately parallel with, and 3.5 Å from, the plane of the pyrimidine ring, suggesting π–π interactions with N-1, C-2, 2-NH$_2$, and N-3. Side chains of Ile-5, Ala-7, Leu-28, Phe-31, and Ile-94 form a hydrophobic pocket surrounding the pteridine ring, and Leu-28, Ile-50, Leu-54, and Ile-94 similarly surround the benzene ring. Thus, the hydrophobic cavity so often referred to by BAKER and other workers in the field (see for example, BAKER 1967) is described.

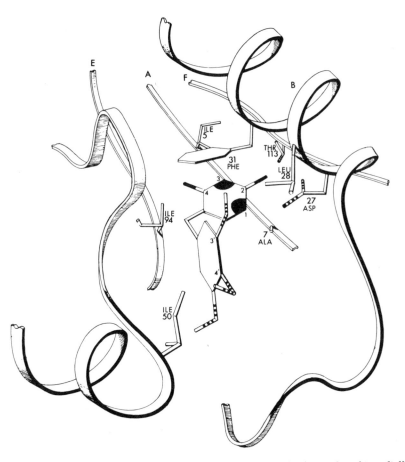

Fig. 2. Schematic illustration of the binding site for trimethoprim in *Escherichia coli* dihydrofolate reductase. Nitrogen atoms are shown black, oxygen striped. Only those side chains which might interact with trimethoprim are shown. BAKER et al. (1981)

It has been assumed the diaminopyrimidines and their bicyclic analogs are bound to DHFR in the manner of MTX, with the N-1 nitrogen (the most basic site) attracted to Asp-27. CAYLEY et al. (1979) have used this assumption in deriving two possible conformations for TMP in the active site of DHFR, based on NMR spectroscopy. It has now been confirmed that in its binary complex TMP is indeed bound to *E. coli* DHFR with its N-1 nitrogen in ionic interaction with Asp-27 (BAKER et al. 1981; see Fig. 2). There may be slight differences in the tilt of the pyrimidine rings in the MTX and TMP complexes, but this will require more highly resolved X-ray structures to determine. The benzene ring of TMP is directed outwards from the cleft with its ring plane roughly aligned with the cleft, and at a somewhat different locus from the benzene ring of MTX. It is only partially enclosed by Phe-31, Ile-50, and Leu-28; crystallographic studies of the ternary complex with NADPH will be required to explain the greater than 100-fold increase in binding upon adding the coenzyme (BACCANARI et al. 1981 b).

The publication of the MTX–DHFR crystal structure immediately raised doubts that dihydrofolate is bound in the same manner, since its more basic nitrogen is at N-5 (POE 1977; GUND et al. 1977), and since Asp-27 provides the most ready site for proton transfer to N-5 during the catalytic reduction across the 5,6 double bond (MATTHEWS et al. 1978; HITCHINGS and ROTH 1980). Verification that the pteridine ring of DHFR must indeed be inverted came from several interdependent sources (FONTECILLA-CAMPS et al. 1979; CHARLTON et al. 1979; BLAKLEY et al. 1963; PASTORE and FRIEDKIN 1962). It will be of considerable interest to obtain information on the hydrogen bonding patterns of folate and dihydrofolate in interaction with DHFR. Both substrates have been shown to be reduced at the same face by the enzyme (CHARLTON et al. 1979). We also await information on the crystal structure of a vertebrate DHFR.

F. Conclusion

Among the many hundreds of diaminopyrimidines and condensed pyrimidines and analogs which have been made over the past 30 years, many have shown potent inhibitory activity for DHFR, but to date there is only one series of compounds which has shown any useful degree of specificity for bacterial DHFR. That series is the 2,4-diamino-5-(substituted benzyl) pyrimidines – trimethoprim and its close analogs. High specificity furthermore is limited, as far as is known, to derivatives with 3',4',5'-tri-substitution in the benzene ring, and this class is further restricted to compounds containing substituents with appropriate shape and polarity. The nature of the binding of trimethoprim to *E. coli* DHFR is now known for the binary complex. Hopefully, information will soon be forthcoming on the nature of the ternary complex with the coenzyme NADPH, and of the corresponding binary and ternary vertebrate complexes. At such a point we may hope to begin to understand the nature of this specificity, and, hopefully, gain insight which will lead to new series of improved antibacterial agents.

References

Aschoff HS, Vergin H (1979) Tetroxoprim – a new inhibitor of bacterial dihydrofolate reductase. J Antimicrob Chemother [Suppl B] 5:19–25

Baccanari DP, Joyner SS (1981) Dihydrofolate reductase hysteresis and its effect on inhibitor binding analyses. Biochemistry 20:1710–1716

Baccanari DP, Daluge S, King R (1981 a) Inhibition of dihydrofolate reductase: effect of NADPH on the selectivity and affinity of diaminopyrimidines. Fed Proc 40:1748

Baccanari DP, Stone D, Kuyper L (1981 b) Effect of a single amino acid substitution on *Escherichia coli* dihydrofolate reductase catalysis and ligand binding. J Biol Chem 256:1738–1747

Baker BR (1964) Differential inhibition of dihydrofolate reductase from different species. J Pharm Sci 53:1137–1138

Baker BR (1967) Design of active-site-directed irreversible inhibitors. John Wiley, New York Chichester

Baker BR, Lee WW, Skinner WA, Martinez AP, Tong E (1960) Potential anticancer agents. L. Non-classical metabolites. II. Some factors in the design of exo-alkylating enzyme inhibitors, particularly of lactic dehydrogenase. J Med Pharm Chem 2:633–657

Baker DJ, Beddell CR, Champness JN, Goodford PJ, Norrington FEA, Smith DR, Stammers DK (1981) The binding of trimethoprim to bacterial dihydrofolate reductase. FEBS Lett 126:49–52

Blakley RL, Morrison JF (1970) The determination of inhibition effects of folate analogues on dihydrofolate reductase. In: Chemistry and biology of pteridines. Proceedings of the Fourth International Symposium on Pteridines. International Academic Press, Tokyo, pp 315–327

Blakley RL, Ramasastri BV, McDougall BM (1963) The biosynthesis of thymidylic acid. D. Hydrogen isotope studies with dihydrofolate reductase and thymidylate synthetase. J Biol Chem 238:3075–3079

Brossi A, Grunberg E, Hoffer M, Teitel S (1971) Synthesis and chemotherapeutic activity of two metabolites of trimethoprim. J Med Chem 14:58–59

Burchall JJ, Hitchings GH (1965) Inhibitor binding analysis of dihydrofolate reductases from various species. Mol Pharmacol 1:126–136

Bushby SRM, Hitchings GH (1968) Trimethoprim, a sulfonamide potentiator. Br J Pharmacol Chemother 33:72–90

Carrington HC, Crowther AF, Davey DG, Levi AA, Rose FL (1951) A metabolite of "paludrine" with high antimalarial activity. Nature 168:1080

Cayley PJ, Albrand JP, Feeney J, Roberts GCK, Piper EA, Burgen ASV (1979) Nuclear magnetic resonance studies of the binding of trimethoprim to dihydrofolate reductase. Biochemistry 18:3886–3894

Charlton PA, Young DW, Birdsall B, Feeney J, Roberts GCK (1979) Stereochemistry of reduction of folic acid using dihydrofolate reductase. J Chem Soc Chem Commun 922–924

Cheng YC, Prusoff WH (1973) Relationship between the inhibition constant (K_i) and the concentration of inhibitor which causes 50% inhibition (I_{50}) of an enzymatic reaction. Biochem Pharmacol 22:3099–3108

Cody V, DeJarnette E (1981) Structural comparisons of 2,4-diamino-5-(3,5-dimethoxy-4-(2-propene)benzyl)pyrimidine with trimethoprim as an inhibitor of dihydrofolate reductase. Fed Proc 40:1797

Curd FHS, Davey DG, Rose FL (1945) Studies on synthetic antimalarial drugs. X. Some biguanide derivatives as new types of antimalarial substances with both therapeutic and causal prophylactic activity. Ann Trop Med Parasitol 39:208–216

Daniel LJ, Norris LC (1947) Growth inhibition of bacteria by synthetic pterins. II. Studies with *Escherichia coli*, *Staphylococcus aureus*, and *Lactobacillus arabinosus* showing synergism between pterin and sulfonamide. J Biol Chem 170:747–756

Daniel LJ, Norris LC, Scott ML, Heuser GF (1947) Growth inhibition of bacteria by synthetic pterins. I. Studies with *Streptococcus faecalis*, *Lactobacillus casei*, and *Lactobacillus arabinosus*. J Biol Chem 169:689–697

Daum A, Fernex M, Wick AE (1980) Diuretic compositions containing potassium retaining agents – comprising 2,4-diamino-5-aminobenzyl-pyrimidine derivatives. German Patent 2,936,244

Dietrich SW, Blaney JM, Reynolds MA, Jow PYC, Hansch C (1980) Quantitative structure-selectivity relationships. Comparison of the inhibition of *Escherichia coli* and bovine liver dihydrofolate reductase by 5-(substituted-benzyl)-2,4-diaminopyrimidines. J Med Chem 23:1205–1212

Elion GB, Singer S, Hitchings GH (1960) Potentiation in combinations of three biochemically related antimetabolites. Antibiot Chemother 10:556–564

Elslager EF, Davoll J (1974) Synthesis of fused pyrimidines as folate antagonists. In: Castle RN, Townsend LB (eds) Lectures in heterocyclic chemistry, vol II. Hetero, Oren, Utah, pp s 97–s 133

Elslager EF, Clarke J, Johnson J, Werbel LM, Davoll J (1972) Folate antagonists. 5. Antimalarial and antibacterial effects of 2,4-diamino-6-(aryloxy and aralkoxy) quinazoline antimetabolites. J Heterocycl Chem 9:759–773

Falco EA, Russell PB, Hitchings GH (1951 a) 2,4-Diaminopyrimidines as antimalarials. I. 5-Aryloxyl and 5-alkoxy derivatives. J Am Chem Soc 73:3753–3758

Falco EA, Goodwin LG, Hitchings GH, Rollo IM, Russell PB (1951 b) 2,4-Diaminopyrimidines – a new series of antimalarials. Br J Pharmacol 6:185–200

Falco EA, DuBreuil S, Hitchings GH (1951 c) 2,4-Diaminopyrimidines as antimalarials. II. 5-Benzyl derivatives. J Am Chem Soc 73:3758–3762

Falco EA, Roth B, Hitchings GH (1961) 5-Arylthiopyrimidines. I. 2,4-Diamino derivatives. J Org Chem 26:1143–1146

Feldman RL, Bing DH, Furie BC, Furie D (1978) Interactive computer surface graphics approach to study of the active site of bovine trypsin. Proc Natl Acad Sci USA 75:5409–5412

Fontecilla-Camps JC, Bugg CE, Temple C, Rose JD, Montgomery JA, Kisliuk RL (1979) X-Ray crystallography studies of the structure of 5,10-methenyltetrahydrofolic acid. In: Kisliuk RL, Brown GM (eds) Chemistry and biology of pteridines. Elsevier North Holland, New York, pp 235–240

Fritsche E, Liebenow W, Prikryl J (1979) 2,4-Diamino-5-(4'-methylthio)benzylpyrimidines, compounds, compositions, and methods of use. U.S. Patent 4,180,578

Gerns FR, Perrotta A, Hitchings GH (1966) 5-Arylaminopyrimidines. J Med Chem 9:108–115

Gund P, Poe M, Hoogsteen KH (1977) Calculations by complete neglect of differential overlap (CNDO/2) on dihydrofolic acid: role of N(5) in reduction of dihydrofolate reductase. Mol Pharmacol 13:1111–1115

Gund P, Andose JD, Rhodes JB, Smith GM (1980) Three-dimensional molecular modeling and drug design. Science 208:1425–1431

Heumann L Co GmbH (1974) 4'-Alkyl dioxyalkylene-5-benzylpyrimidines, the preparation thereof and compositions containing them. Belgian Patent 812,375

Hitchings GH (1952) Daraprim as an antagonist of folic and folinic acids. Trans R Soc Trop Med Hyg 46:467–473

Hitchings GH (1955) Purine and pyrimidine antagonists. Am J Clin Nutr 3:321–327

Hitchings GH, Bushby SRM (1961) 5-Benzyl-2,4-diaminopyrimidines, a new class of systemic antibacterial agents. In: Sissakian NM (ed) V th International Congress of Biochemistry, Moscow, pp 165–171

Hitchings GH, Ledig KW (1960) 2,4-Diamino-5,6-dialkylpyrido(2,3-d)pyrimidines. U.S. Patent 2,937,284

Hitchings GH, Roth B (1959) Trialkoxybenzylpyrimidines and method. U.S. Patent 2,909,522

Hitchings GH, Roth B (1980) Dihydrofolate reductases as targets for selective inhibitors. In: Sandler M (ed) Enzyme inhibitors as drugs. MacMillan, London, pp 263–280

Hitchings GH, Smith SL (1980) Dihydrofolate reductases as targets for inhibitors. In: Weber G (ed) Advances in enzyme regulation, vol 18. Pergamon, Oxford New York

Hitchings GH, Elion GB, Vanderwerff H, Falco EA (1948) Pyrimidine derivatives, as antagonists of pteroylglutamic acid. J Biol Chem 174:765–766

Hitchings GH, Rollo IM, Goodwin LG, Coatney GR (1952) Symposium on daraprim. Trans R Soc Trop Med Hyg 46:467–497

Hitchings GH, Elion GB, Singer S (1954) Derivatives of condensed pyrimidines as antimetabolites. In: Wolstenholme (ed) Chemistry and biology of pteridines. Churchill Livingstone, London Edinburgh, pp 290–303

Hitchings GH, Russell PB, Whittaker N (1956) Some 2:6-diamino and 2-amino-6-hydroxy derivatives of 5-aryl-4:5-dihydropyrimidines. A new syntheses of 4-alkyl-5-aryl-pyrimidines. J Chem Soc 1019–1028

Hitchings GH, Falco EA, Ledig KW (1960) Diaminoquinazolines and method of making. U.S. Patent 2,945,859

Hitchings GH, Burchall JJ, Ferone R (1966) Comparative enzymology of dihydrofolate reductases as a basis for chemotherapy. Proc Int Pharmacol Meet, 3 rd 5:3–18

Hoffer M (1967) Processes and intermediates for pyrimidine derivatives. U.S. Patent 3,341,541

Hoffer M (1969) 2,4-Diamino-5-(2′,4′,5′-substituted benzyl)pyrimidines, intermediates and processes. U.S. Patent 3,485,840

Hoffer M, Grunberg E, Mitrovic M, Brossi A (1971) An improved synthesis of diaveridine, trimethoprim, and closely related 2,4-diaminopyrimidines. J Med Chem 14:462–463

Hurlbert BS, Ferone R, Herrmann TA, Hitchings GH, Barnett M, Bushby SRM (1968) Studies on condensed pyrimidine systems. XXV. 2,4-Diaminopyrido[2,3-d]-pyrimidines. Biological data. J Med Chem 11:711–717

Hynes TB, Ashton WT, Bryansmith D, Freisheim JH (1974) Quinazolines as inhibitors of dihydrofolate reductase. 2. J Med Chem 17:1023–1025

Jackson RC, Niethammer D (1977) Acquired methotrexate resistance in lymphoblasts resulting from altered kinetic properties of dihydrofolate reductase. Eur J Cancer 13:567–575

Jackson RC, Hart LI, Harrap KR (1976) Intrinsic resistance to methotrexate of cultured mammalian cells in relation to the inhibition kinetics of their dihydrofolate reductases. Cancer Res 36:1991–1997

Kompis I, Wick AE (1979) 2,4-Diamino-5-benzylpyrimidine und Verfahren zu deren Herstellung. German Patent 2,847,825

Kompis I, Rey-Bellet G, Zanetti G (1975) Neue Benzylpyrimidine. German Patent 2,443,682

Kompis I, Rey-Bellet G, Zanetti G (1976) Benzylpyrimidines. German Patent 2,558,150

Kompis I, Mueller W, Boehni E, Then R, Montavon M (1977) 2,4-Diamino-5-(pyridyl-methyl)-pyrimidine als potentielle Chemotherapeutica. Eur J Med Chem 12:531–536

Kompis I, Then R, Boehni E, Rey-Bellet G, Zanetti G, Montavon M (1980) Synthesis and antimicrobial activity of C(4′)-substituted analogs of trimethoprim. Eur J Med Chem 15:17–22

Kompis I, Then R, Wick A, Montavon M (1981) 2,4-Diamino-5-benzylpyrimidines as inhibitors of dihydrofolate reductase. In: Brodbeck U (ed) Enzyme inhibitors. Verlag Chemie, Weinheim, pp 178–189

Lampen JO, Jones MJ (1946) The antagonism of sulfonamide inhibition of certain lactobacilli and enterococci by pteroylglutamic acid and related compounds. J Biol Chem 166:435–448

Langridge R, Ferrin TE, Kuntz ID, Connolly ML (1981) Real-time color graphics in studies of molecular interactions. Science 211:661–666

Mallette MF, Cain CK, Taylor EC Jr (1947) Pyrimido[4,5-b]pyrazines. II. 2,4-Diamino-pyrimido[4,5-b]pyrazine and derivatives. J Am Chem Soc 69:1814–1816

Matthews DA, Alden RA, Bolin JT et al. (1977) Dihydrofolate reductase: X-ray structure of the binary complex with methotrexate. Science 197:452–455

Matthews DA, Alden RA, Bolin JT et al. (1978) Dihydrofolate reductase from *Lactobacillus casei*. X-Ray structure of the enzyme-methotrexate NADPH complex. J Biol Chem 253:6946–6954

Pastore EJ, Friedkin M (1962) The enzymatic synthesis of thymidylate. II. Transfer of tritium from tetrahydrofolate to the methyl group of thymidylate. J Biol Chem 237:3802–3810

Perun TJ, Rasmussen RR, Horrom BW (1975) Pharmaceutical 2,4-diamino-5-benzyl-pyrimidines. U.S. Patent 4,008,236

Perun TJ, Rasmussen RR, Horrom BW (1978) 2,4-Diamino-5-benzylpyrimidines. U.S. Patent 4,087,528

Phillips T, Bryan RF (1969) The crystal structure of the antimalarial agents daraprim and trimethoprim. Acta Crystallogr Sect A 25:S 200

Poe M (1977) Acidic dissociation constants of folic acid, dihydrofolic acid and methotrexate. J Biol Chem 252:3724–3728

Rey-Bellet G, Bohni E, Kompis I, Montavon M, Then R, Zanetti G (1975) 2,4-Diamino-5-benzylpyrimidine als potentielle Chemotherapeutica. Eur J Med Chem 10:7–9

Roberts GCK (1978) Origins of specificity in the binding of small molecules to dihydrofolate reductase. Ciba Found Symp 60:89–104

Rosen P (1977) 2,4-Diaminopyrimidine derivatives and processes. U.S. Patent 4,033,962

Roth B (1973) Alkyl substituted benzyl pyrimidines. U.S. Patent 3,772,289

Roth B (1974) 2,4-Diamino-5-benzylpyrimidines. U.S. Patent 3,822,264

Roth B, Burchall JJ (1971) Small molecule inhibitors of dihydrofolate reductase. Methods Enzymol 18 B:779–786

Roth B, Strelitz JZ (1969) The protonation of 2,4-diaminopyrimidines. I. Dissociation constants and substituent effects. J Org Chem 34:821–836

Roth B, Strelitz JZ (1972) Substituted 2,4-diamino-5-benzylpyrimidines. U.S. Patent 3,692,787

Roth B, Burrows RB, Hitchings GH (1960) Abstracts 137th Meeting, American Chemical Society, Cleveland, 31 N

Roth B, Falco EA, Hitchings GH, Bushby SRM (1962) 5-Benzyl-2,4-diaminopyrimidines as antibacterial agents. I. Synthesis and antibacterial activity in vitro. J Med Pharm Chem 5:1103–1123

Roth B, Burrows RB, Hitchings GH (1963) Anthelmintic agents. 1,2-Dihydro-s-triazines. J Med Chem 6:370–378

Roth B, Yeowell DA (1971) The synthesis of 5-benzoylpyrimidines. [Abstr] Third International Congress of Heterocyclic Chemistry, Sendai, Japan, pp 358–361

Roth B, Aig E, Lane K, Ferone R, Bushby SRM (1972) An analysis of trimethoprim geometry from analog studies. Abstracts 164th American Chemical Society National Meeting, New York MEDI 23

Roth B, Stuart A, Paterson T (1974) 2,4-Diamino-5-benzylpyrimidines and processes for their production. British Patent 1,375,162

Roth B, Strelitz JZ, Rauckman BS (1980a) 2,4-Diamino-5-benzylpyrimidines and analogues as antibacterial agents. 2. C-Alkylation of pyrimidines with Mannich bases and application to the synthesis of trimethoprim and analogues. J Med Chem 23:379–384

Roth B, Aig E, Lane K, Rauckman BS (1980b) 2,4-Diamino-5-benzylpyrimidines as antibacterial agents. 4. 6-Substituted trimethoprim derivatives from phenolic Mannich intermediates. Application to the synthesis of trimethoprim and 3,5'-dialkylbenzyl analogues. J Med Chem 23:535–541

Roth B, Aig E, Rauckman BS et al. (1981) 2,4-Diamino-5-benzylpyrimidines and analogues as antibacterial agents. 5. 3',5'-Dimethoxy-4'-substituted benzyl analogues of trimethoprim. J Med Chem 24:933–941

Russell PB, Hitchings GH (1951) 2,4-Diaminopyrimidines as antimalarials. IV. 5-Aryl derivatives. J Am Chem Soc 73:3763–3770

Schwartz DE, Vetter W, Englert G (1970) Trimethoprim metabolites in rat, dog and man: Qualitative and quantitative studies. Arzneim Forsch 20:1867–1871

Seeger DR, Smith JM Jr, Hultquist ME (1947) Antagonist for pteroylglutamic acid. J Am Chem Soc 69:2567

Seeger DR, Cosulich DB, Smith JM Jr, Hultquist ME (1949) Analogs of pteroylglutamic acid. III. 4-Amino derivatives. J Am Chem Soc 71:1753–1758

Seydel JK, Wempe E (1980) Bacterial growth kinetics of E. coli in the presence of various trimethoprim derivatives alone and in combination with sulfonamides. Chemotherapy 26:361–371

Stogryn EL (1972) Synthesis of trimethoprim variations. Replacement of CH_2 by polar groupings. J Med Chem 15:200–201

Tokuyama K (1974) 2,4-Diamino-5-benzylpyrimidine derivatives. Japan Patent 69,679

Werkheiser WC (1960) Specific binding of 4-amino folic acid analogues by folic acid reductase. J Biol Chem 236:888–893

Williams JW, Morrison JF, Duggleby RG (1979) Methotrexate, a high-affinity pseudosubstrate of dihydrofolate reductase. Biochemistry 18:2567–2573

Williams JW, Duggleby RG, Cutler R, Morrison JF (1980) The inhibition of dihydrofolate reductase by folate analogues: structural requirements for slow and tight-binding inhibition. Biochem Pharmacol 29:589–595

Williams MN, Poe M, Greenfield NJ, Hirshfield JM, Hoogsteen K (1973) Methotrexate binding to dihydrofolate reductase from a methotrexate resistant strain of *Escherichia coli*. J Biol Chem 248:6375–6379

Woods DD (1940) The relation of p-aminobenzoic acid to the mechanism of the action of sulphanilamide. Br J Exp Pathol 21:74–90

Zakrzewski SF, Nichol CA (1958) On the enzymatic reduction of folic acid by a purified hydrogenase. Biochim Biophys Acta 27:425–426

CHAPTER 6

Kinetics of Antibacterial Effects

J.K. SEYDEL

A. Introduction: Bacterial Growth Kinetics in the Presence of Folate Inhibitors

Several bacteriologic and biochemical investigations have been done to evaluate the effectiveness and mode of action of the drug combination, Septrin, Eusaprim, and Bactrim, consisting of trimethoprim, 2,4-diamino-5-(3′,4′,5′-trimethoxybenzyl)pyrimidine (TMP) and a sulfonamide, sulfamethoxazole (SMX). Many of these studies have been concerned with the mode of action, sensitivity testing procedures, or the development of resistance (HITCHINGS and BURCHALL 1965; BUSHBY and BARNETT 1967; BÖHNI 1969; TIESLER 1970). A potentiating effect of TMP on sulfonamides (or vice versa) has been stated to occur (BUSHBY and HITCHINGS 1968; FOWLE 1970; BUSHBY 1970; THEN and ANGEHRN 1973; THEN 1977). This has been said to be the consequence of the fact that the sites of action of the inhibitors are two different steps in the same biosynthetic pathway (HITCHINGS and BURCHALL 1965). In addition, decrease in the rate of development of resistance has been claimed when the bacterial strain is initially sensitive to both antibacterials (BUSHBY and BARNETT 1967). A review article has summarized these studies as well as the pharmacologic and clinical investigations of the antibacterial combination (GARROD 1971).

Studies which have demonstrated synergism between the components of the combination have been done, using serial dilution techniques (BUSHBY 1970; KNOTHE 1975), disc sensitivity tests (TIESLER 1970; DORNBUSCH 1971; BÖHNI 1976), turbidimetric measurements (GREENWOOD and O'GRADY 1976), or experimental animal infections (BUSHBY and HITCHINGS 1968). In addition to the differences between the definitions of synergism and additivity of drug action among various authors, these methods do not seem suitable for the quantification of the effects of chemotherapeutic agents for theoretical reasons. This has already been pointed out by JAWETZ and GUNNISON (1953) and JAWETZ et al. (1952). A linear relationship between inhibition and inhibitor concentration cannot be presumed and would not be expected to exist. Also the summation of the "kill" of numbers of bacteria is not necessarily synonymous with a summation of rate constants for bacterial death. Diffusion of the two drugs in agar plate tests may not be independent of each other, resulting in a false presumption of synergy of antibacterial action. Whole animal experiments, while perhaps best related to the clinical effects of the combination, may show synergy as a result of pharmacologic or pharmacokinetic interaction rather than antibacterial effects. For these reasons, it is important to

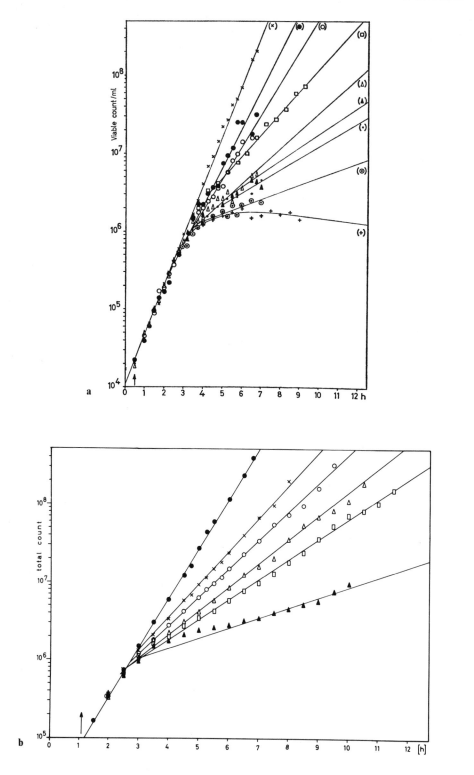

study the antibacterial actions of the combination in an experimental situation not subject to these limitations (BOCK et al. 1974; SEYDEL 1975; SEYDEL et al. 1972, 1973; SEYDEL and MILLER 1973; SEYDEL and WEMPE 1975, 1977, 1978, 1979, 1980; SEYDEL and SCHAPER 1978, 1980; KUHNE et al. 1976).

GARRETT (1958, 1971) has described mathematical models for the differentiation of drug synergism, antagonism, and additivity. Experimental methods have been developed which use the kinetics of bacterial growth to study the effects of antibiotic combinations. In these experiments, the activity of the drug is defined in terms of decrease in growth rate caused by the drug, as a function of the drug concentration. Viable and total count techniques have been used to quantify the decrease in the generation rates of *Escherichia coli* as a result of different antibiotic concentrations, and to discriminate between inhibition, uninhibited growth simultaneous with kill, and inhibition simultaneous with or followed by kill (GARRETT 1966; GARRETT and BROWN 1963; GARRETT and MILLER 1965).

This general approach has been used to determine whether the combined action of TMP and sulfonamides is additive or more than additive, i.e., synergistic (SEYDEL et al. 1972, 1973; SEYDEL and MILLER 1973; SEYDEL and WEMPE 1975, 1977, 1978, 1980; THEN and ANGEHRN 1973; THEN 1977; NOLTE 1973). Before these experiments were performed it was necessary to quantify the relative potencies of the single drugs by these same methods and in particular to determine if they were acting by pure inhibition or inhibition with kill. The growth dependence of *E. coli* cultures in the presence of the individual drugs was therefore evaluated.

B. Sulfonamides (Synthetase Inhibitors)

I. Effect of Sulfonamides on Generation Rates of E. coli

To *E. coli* cultures in the logarithmic growth phase, various sulfonamides, especially SMX, were added. Samples were taken at appropriate time intervals, and the number of viable cells (plate count) and/or the total number of cells (Coulter counter measurement) was counted. Typical examples are given in Fig. 1. As already reported by KOHN and HARRIS (1941), HIRSCH (1943), and GARRETT and WRIGHT (1967), a lag phase of about five generations exists before there is any significant effect of drug concentration on the growth of *E. coli* at 37 °C. This lag phase appears to be independent of the specific activities of different sulfonamides. Subsequently, the viable count and total count techniques showed a diminishing rate of increase in the numbers of *E. coli*. Apparent first-order generation rate con-

---

◄ **Fig. 1a, b.** Typical generation rate curves of *Escherichia coli* (mutaflor) at 37 °C in the presence of various concentrations of SMX. **a** viable count method. Curves (concentrations in μmol/l) are as follows: *crosses* control; *full circles* 0.5; *open circles* 1.0; *squares* 2.0; *open triangles* 3.0; *full triangles* 4.0; *dots* 5.0; *circled dots* 10.0; *plus signs* 400.0. *Arrows* indicate addition of drug; **b** total count method. Curves (concentrations in μmol/l) are as follows: *full circles* 0.0; *crosses* 0.6; *open circles* 1.2; *open triangles* 2.1; *squares* 3.3; *full triangles* 7.5. (SEYDEL et al. 1972)

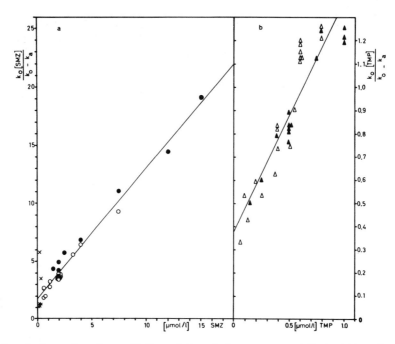

Fig. 2, a, b. Examples of quantitative relations between apparent *Escherichia coli* growth rate constants k_{app}. Curves are plotted in accordance with the expression $k_0 \cdot C/k_0 - k_{app} = K_a + K_b C$. **a** SMX. *Crosses* and *open circles* total count method; *full circles* viable count method; **b** TMP. *Open triangles* total count method; *full triangles* viable count method. (Seydel et al. 1972)

stants, k_{app}, have been obtained from the slopes of these new growth curves in accordance with the general rate expression:

$$\log N = \frac{k_{app} t}{2.303} + \text{constant},\tag{1}$$

where N is the number of cells generated in time t.

The coincidence between total and viable count experiments supports the contention that sulfonamides are bacteriostatic and not bactericidal. Even at very high sulfonamide concentrations, the rate constants were positive and no decrease in viable cells could be observed. It should be emphasized that there does not exist a linear relationship between either the generation rate constant, k_{app}, and the sulfonamide concentration, C, or the logarithms of these two parameters. A linear relationship is however obtained with a Lineweaver–Burk plot (Garrett and Wright 1967) according to the equation:

$$\frac{1}{k_0 - k_{app}} = \frac{K_a}{C} + K_b,\tag{2}$$

where k_0 is the generation rate constant in the absence of sulfonamide, k_{app} is the apparent rate constant in the presence of certain sulfonamide concentrations and K_a and K_b are constants. K_a is a measure of the molar activity of the particular sulfonamide tested and C is its concentration. An example is given in Fig. 2a. In this plot, Eq. (2) has been multiplied by the inhibitor concentration C [Eq. (3)] and normalized for the rate constant k_0 of the controls in the various experiments.

$$\frac{k_0 [\text{SMX}]}{k_0 - k_a} = K_a + K_b \times C . \tag{3}$$

In this case, the specific inhibitory activity constant K_a for the sulfonamide is obtained as intercept. The value for SMX is 4.25×10^{-3} mol l^{-1} s^{-1}. K_a values for other sulfonamides studied are listed in Table 1.

C. Trimethoprim (TMP): Dihydrofolate Reductase Inhibitor

I. Effect of TMP on Generation Rates of E. coli

Similar experiments were done in the presence of graded concentrations of TMP alone. Compared with the results of sulfonamide inhibition several important differences have been observed. In contrast to sulfonamides, only a very short lag phase is observed before onset of inhibition. Depending upon culture conditions and TMP concentration, the onset of inhibition may be seen almost immediately (Fig. 3). This difference in lag phase is consistent with the suggested sites of action of the two inhibitors. Cellular division seems to be required before sulfonamide activity is observed. There are approximately five cellular divisions before onset of sulfonamide inhibition and the stored folate in the cells, dihydrofolic acid, may be depleted while de novo synthesis is inhibited by sulfonamides. Only after the stored folate is depleted does the inhibition of folate synthesis become critical for cell division. On the other hand, TMP presumably blocks the synthesis of tetrahydrofolate directly at the level of dihydrofolic acid (HITCHINGS and BURCHALL 1965; BAKER and BENG-THONG 1964). As TMP seems to block a stage beyond the site of folate storage, one would expect to observe a relatively rapid onset of action. After the short lag phase, cells grow in the presence of low TMP concentrations at a reduced logarithmic rate. The same relationship between the concentration of the antibacterial and the rate constants for bacterial growth is observed as for sulfonamides (Fig. 2b). It can be seen from Fig. 2 that, under the experimental conditions of this study, the ratio of activities, as expressed by the intercept of the lines, SMX:TMP is about 1:5. This ratio is similar to the ratio of minimum inhibitory concentration (MIC) values for the two drugs obtained in similar experiments with the same E. coli strain (TMP 0.175 µmol/l, SMX 0.8 µmol/l; see also Table 1). Since the activity of neither drug alone is linearly related to drug concentration, estimates of the potency of combinations, based on linear relationships between potency and concentration, are subject to error. For example, SMX at 2 µmol/l produces a 50% inhibition of growth rate in our system. Half the concentration at 1 µmol/l does not produce a 25% inhibition, but rather a 33% inhibition.

Table 1. Structure, name, specific inhibition constant K'_A and K''_A and MIC values of trimethoprim, some of its derivatives and of sulfonamides used in the combination. (Seydel and Wempe 1980)

No.	Structure	R_3	Name	K'_A (mol l^{-1} s^{-1} × 10^{-3})	K''_A (mol l^{-1} s^{-1} × 10^{-3})	MIC (*Escherichia coli*) (μmol/l)
	R_1	R_2				
I	OCH$_3$	OCH$_3$	OCH$_3$	Trimethoprim (TMP)	0.78	0.41	0.17
II	OCH$_3$	H	OCH$_3$	Diaveridine	4.22		5.6
III	OCH$_3$	OCH$_2$CH$_2$OCH$_3$	OCH$_3$	Tetroxoprim	1.84		2.8–5.6
IV	Br	NH$_2$	Br	A-47077	2.3	1.3	3.5
V	Cl	NHC$_2$H$_5$	Cl	A-44733	8.8	5.9	22.5
VI				Pyrimethamin (PMA)	226	43.3	45–64
VII				Sulfamethylisoxazole Sulfamethoxazole (SMX)	4.25		0.8
VIII				Sulfamoxazole Sulfadimethyloxazole (SDMO)	20.36		3.5
IX				Sulfadiazine (SDZ) Sulfapyrimidine	6.0		1
				N^1-Phenylsulfanilamide	55		16

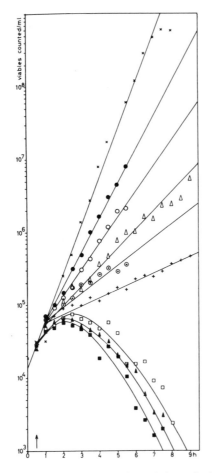

Fig. 3. Typical generation rate curves of *Escherichia coli* (mutaflor) at 37 °C in the presence of various concentrations of TMP. Curves (concentrations in µmol/l) are as follows: *Crosses* 0.0; *full circles* 0.125; *open circles* 0.25; *open triangles* 0.5; *circled dots* 0.75; *plus signs* 1.0; *open squares* 2.0; *full triangles* 3.0; *full squares* 4.0. (SEYDEL et al. 1972)

II. Influence of TMP Concentration and Inoculum Size on the "Bactericidal" Effect of TMP

The second major difference between the effects of TMP (Fig. 3) and SMX is that negative rate constants are obtained from experiments with viable counts at concentrations of 2 µmol/l. At the TMP concentration of Fig. 4a, the total and viable counts determined simultaneously are not the same; a kill is caused by TMP, whereas at lower TMP concentrations viable and total counts are the same and there is no kill (Fig. 4b).

This means that TMP is bacteriostatic at low concentrations, but at higher concentrations a kill is observed together with inhibition. The threshold concentration seems to lie between 1 and 2 µmol/l under the conditions used. It is important to

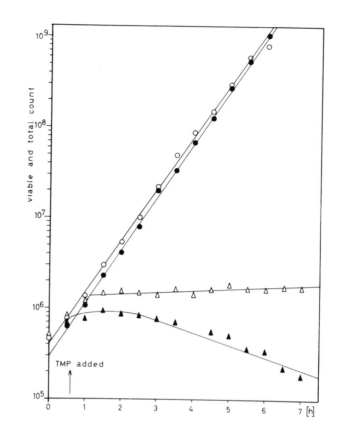

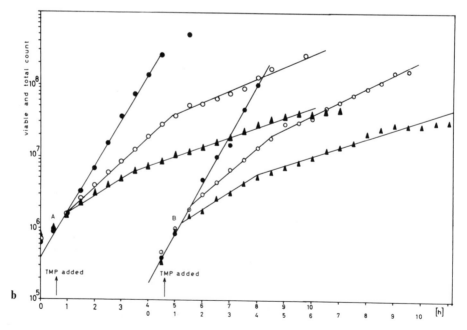

Table 2. Apparent first-order generation rate constants k_{app} for the kill rate of *Escherichia coli* in the presence of various concentrations of TMP at different inoculum sizes of *E. coli* at 37 °C, using viable count method. (SEYDEL et al. 1972)

TMP (μmol/l)	Inoculum size of *E. coli* (ml^{-1})	$k_0 (s^{-1}) \times 10^{-4}$	$k_{app} (s^{-1}) \times 10^{-4}$
2	10^4	4.39 ± 0.083	-1.70 ± 0.071
2	10^4	4.04 ± 0.124	-1.65 ± 0.240
3	10^4	4.04 ± 0.124	-2.23 ± 0.210
4	10^4	4.04 ± 0.124	-2.13 ± 0.460
2	10^6	3.72 ± 0.133	-0.82 ± 0.025
4	10^6	3.72 ± 0.133	-0.88 ± 0.036
6	10^6	3.80	-0.86 ± 0.080
10	10^6	3.72 ± 0.133	-0.87 ± 0.071

note that the kill rate becomes independent of the TMP concentration after a certain threshold concentration has been passed (see Fig. 3 and Table 2). Although the rate constants are independent of the TMP concentration, they are dependent upon the number of microorganisms (Table 2).

III. Reversibility of TMP Action

The bacteriostatic effects of sulfonamides have been shown to be easily reversed by dilution into antibacterial-free media (GARRETT and WRIGHT 1967) or as classically performed by the addition of *p*-aminobenzoic acid (THEN 1973). Since equilibration of TMP between medium and biophase is fast, as expressed by a relatively rapid onset of action, reversibility of the action of TMP in subbactericidal concentrations may be expected.

It was therefore of interest to see if the effects of TMP could be reversed at concentrations where a kill rate can be observed. The results of such an experiment are shown in Fig. 5. It is clearly demonstrated that an immediate increase in generation rate occurs after dilution of the antibacterial concentration. Thus, dilution with fresh broth is sufficient to reverse the effects of TMP at "bactericidal" concentrations. The kill rate observed at higher TMP concentrations is not identical with the bactericidal effect known with other antibiotics like penicillin, where an inhibition of cell wall synthesis occurs. In the case of higher TMP concentrations (1 mmol/l), the bacterial cells starve, as a result of total folate metabolism blockade. This type of statistical kill which becomes independent of inhibitor concentration has been classified as thymineless death.

◄ **Fig. 4. a** Generation rate curves of *Escherichia coli* (mutaflor) in the presence of 6 μmol/l TMP, showing no coincidence of total (*open triangles*) and viable count (*full triangles*). **b** Coincidence of positive generation curves for *E. coli* (mutaflor) at 37 °C, obtained by A total and B viable count in the presence of low concentrations (μmol/l) of TMP as follows: *full circles* 0.0; *open circles* 0.395; *triangles* 0.79. (SEYDEL et al. 1972)

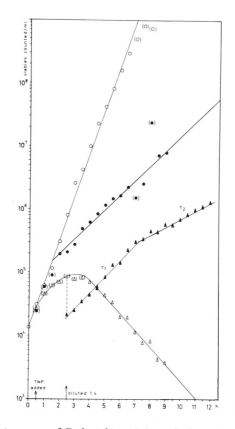

Fig. 5. Generation rate curves of *Escherichia coli* (mutaflor) at 37 °C on addition of TMP, and after dilution of the culture. Viable count method; curves are as follows:

	Final concentration (µmol/l)	Generation rate constant $k_{app}(s^{-1})$	r
Open circles	0	4.39×10^{-4}	0.998
Full circles	0.5	1.49×10^{-4}	0.991
Full triangles c_1	0.5	1.62×10^{-4}	0.996
Full triangles c_2	0.5	0.86×10^{-4}	0.994
Open triangles	2.0	-1.7×10^{-4}	0.992

SEYDEL et al. (1972)

IV. Influence of Culture Broth Constituents on Biphasic Inhibition

The third major difference between the effects of sulfonamides and TMP is also dependent upon the number of organisms present. When experiments such as that described in Fig. 3 are performed with a higher number of *E. coli*, an additional growth phase is obtained. After addition of drug and a short lag phase, the cultures are inhibited to an extent similar to that seen in Fig. 3 at low TMP concentrations, however, after a period of growth, a new, more inhibited growth phase is observed (Figs. 4b and 5). Both viable and total count methods show this effect. The occurrence of this second, more strongly inhibited growth phase seems to be related to

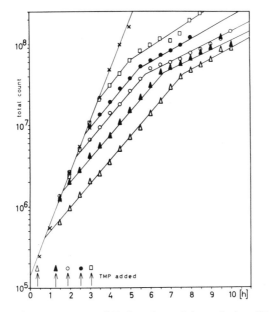

Fig. 6. Typical generation rate curves of *Escherichia coli* (mutaflor) at 37 °C in the presence of a constant concentration of TMP, 0.6 µmol/l, showing the onset of new TMP-affected steady state phase, phase II independent of the time of addition, but at a constant number of organisms (total count). (SEYDEL et al. 1972)
In all figures numbers of viable and total counts are given per ml

the number of cells present. Figure 6 shows an experiment in which a single concentration of TMP was addedt to cultures containing different numbers of log phase cells. This was achieved by adding the TMP to replicate cultures at different times. The onset of the second phase of inhibition occurs at a nearly constant number of cells, regardless of the growth time required to attain this particular cell number. That is, the number of generation times required for transition from the initial inhibited state (phase I) to the second, more inhibited, state (phase II) is not a constant, but increases as the number of the cells present at the time of TMP addition decreases. A mechanism which postulates depletion of a stored metabolite after addition of antibacterial can, therefore, not be assumed. Such a mechanism would imply a constant number of cell divisions after addition of antibacterial until exhaustion of the stored metabolite, as is found in the case of the onset of action of sulfonamides.

The experiments are, however, consistent with the idea that the culture medium contains a drug antagonist which is utilized by both inhibited and uninhibited cells and which is present in a concentration proportional to the initial organism concentration. In Fig. 6, the initial organism concentration was the same in all cultures. Experiments in which a different initial organism concentration was used showed different transition points for the shift from phase I to phase II. In this model, the total number of cell divisions prior to onset of phase II, including both uninhibited and phase I inhibited growth, would be expected to be approximately constant.

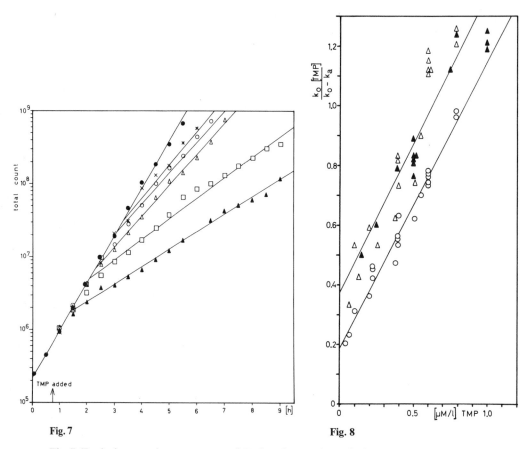

Fig. 7   **Fig. 8**

Fig. 7. Typical generation rate curves of *Escherichia coli* (mutaflor) at 37 °C, performed with saline-washed inocula. The appearance of phase I is not observed. Rates coincide with phase II using unwashed inocula. (SEYDEL et al. 1972)

Fig. 8. Examples of quantitative relations between apparent *Escherichia coli* growth rate constants k_{app} and TMP concentrations using unwashed inocula (*open triangles* viable count method; *full triangles* total count method) and saline-washed inocula (*open circles* total count method). (SEYDEL et al. 1972)

Thus, in an experiment such as Fig. 6, the transition point would occur at a constant number of cells. Since phase I inhibited cells might be expected to use more of the drug antagonist for growth than uninhibited cells, some small variation in the number of cell division might be expected. Other experiments (see, e.g., Fig. 4b) have shown that the total number of cell divisions before onset of phase II varies slightly with the TMP concentration or the degree of inhibition in phase I.

The source of the postulated drug antagonist in these experiments might be expected to arise from either of two sources: (1) present in the casamino acids–dextrose salts broth; or (2) introduced into the medium as a "contaminant" in the *E. coli* used to inoculate the broth. Preliminary experiments, described below in the discussion of reversibility of TMP inhibition Sect. C.III), suggested that the antag-

Table 3. Apparent first-order generation rate constants, k_{app} for the growth of *Escherichia coli* in the presence of various concentrations of either TMP or SMX at 37 °C. These experiments were performed with saline-washed inocula using the total count method. (SEYDEL et al. 1972)

TMP (μmol/l)	k_0 (s^{-1})× 10^{-4}	k_{app} (s^{-1})× 10^{-4}	SMX (μmol/l)	k_0 (s^{-1})× 10^{-4}	k_{app} (s^{-1})× 10^{-4}
0.040	4.15	3.30	0.2	4.05	3.91
0.060	4.15	3.08	0.3	4.05	3.70
0.100	4.15	2.79	0.6	4.05	3.16
0.200	4.15	1.82	1.2	4.05	2.55
0.400	4.15	1.52	4.0	4.05	1.52
0.219	4.05	2.10	2.0	4.05	1.66
0.224	4.22	1.97	2.0	4.22	1.94
0.224[a]	4.23[a]	2.11[a]	2.0[a]	4.23[a]	1.89[a]

[a] Generation rate constants obtained by the viable count method simultaneously with the rate constants obtained by the total count method, see same concentration, directly above

onist was not present in the culture medium. In order to test the hypothesis that an antagonist was present in the *E. coli* used to inoculate the culture, experiments were performed in which the inoculum was washed with saline solution prior to its use in the experimental cultures. The experimental details of this procedure are described elsewhere (SEYDEL et al. 1972). In principle, the usual culture used for inoculation was filtered onto a sterile membrane filter (0.22 μm) and washed with warm saline. The filter paper was suspended in fresh broth and, after logarithmic growth had been established, a portion of this culture was used as an inoculum for the experimental cultures. Figure 7 shows the effect of TMP upon cultures prepared in this manner. After an initial short lag phase, an inhibited state is produced which is maintained throughout the entire growth of the culture. The degree of inhibition of these cultures is much greater than that seen in phase I and is characteristic of phase II. Apparent generation rate constants obtained from these cultures are listed in Table 3.

Figure 8 shows a Lineweaver–Burk plot of these rate constants and also the rate constants obtained previously using unwashed *E. coli* inocula. As mentioned previously, the intercept of such plots is a measure of the degree of inhibition caused by the antibacterial. When saline-washed inocula are used TMP is seen to be about twice as effective as when normal cells are used for culture inoculation. This difference is similar to that seen between phase I and phase II, and suggests that the biphasic growth curves obtained previously were caused by the presence of a drug antagonist in the *E. coli* inocula. Similar experiments have been performed using SMX in place of TMP. No difference in sulfonamide activity could be observed between experiments performed using washed or unwashed *E. coli* inocula. Apparent generation rate constants for this experiment are listed in Table 3. Since only one phase of inhibited growth had been observed in the sulfonamide experiments, it seems natural that washing the inocula should have little or no effect on sulfonamide. However, this seems to imply that the drug antagonist removed by washing is specific for TMP. It is hard to imagine an antagonist of TMP which is not also an antagonist of sulfonamide if the mechanism of action of TMP is sol-

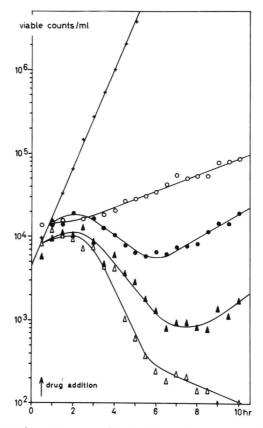

Fig. 9. Typical generation rate curves of *Escherichia coli* (mutaflor) at 37 °C in the presence of various concentrations of tetroxoprim (III) and TMP derivative V (viable count method). Tetroxoprim concentrations (µmol/l) are as follows: *crosses* control; *full triangles* 5.0; *open triangles* 10.0. TMP derivative V concentrations (µmol/l) are as follows; *crosses* control; *open circles* 10.0; *full circles* 20.0. (SEYDEL and WEMPE 1980)

ely an inhibition of dihydrofolate reductase. These findings suggest that TMP may have an additional mode of action. It is interesting to note that some TMP derivatives (see Sect. D.III and Table 1) do not show a biphasic inhibition. The influence of culture broth constituents on the inhibitory effect of TMP has also been studied by THEN (1973).

V. Development of Resistance Against Dihydrofolic Acid Reductase Inhibitors

An interesting observation is the steady decrease of the negative rate constant in experiments with "bactericidal" inhibitor concentrations (SEYDEL and WEMPE 1980). The generation rate finally becomes positive again. This is especially observed for TMP derivatives with smaller inhibitory activity, but can also be ob-

Table 4. Apparent first-order generation rate constants k_{app} for the growth or *Escherichia coli* in the presence of various concentrations of tetroxoprim, and inhibition at 37 °C. (SEYDEL and WEMPE 1980)

Tetroxoprim (μmol/l)	Normal conditions		Treated culture[a]	
	k_{app} $(s^{-1}) \times 10^{-4}$	Inhibition (%)	k_{app} $(s^{-1}) \times 10^{-4}$	Inhibition (%)
0	3.45		3.32	
0.2	3.02	12.46	3.26	1.81
0.4	2.50	27.54	3.05	8.13
0.6	2.08	39.71	2.67	19.58
0.8	1.88	45.51	2.24	32.53
1.0	1.72	50.14	1.94	41.57

[a] Culture treated with 5 μmol/l tetroxoprim for 22 h, after this the inhibitor was removed and bacteria were recultured in fresh medium in the presence of the stated concentrations

served for more active derivatives. Examples are given in Fig. 9 for *E. coli* cultures in the presence of high concentrations of tetroxoprim (5 and 10 μmol/l) and TMP derivative A-44733 (10 and 20 μmol/l; compound V in Table 1). It was shown that the decrease in inhibitory power is a consequence of the selection of more resistant bacteria. Cultures were treated with tetroxoprim or other TMP derivatives for 22 h, the bacteria were harvested and washed to remove the inhibitor and recultured in fresh medium in the absence (control) and presence of graded concentrations of inhibitors. Generation rates of *E. coli* for fresh cultures and cultures pretreated with a certain inhibitor concentration in the presence of inhibitor are given in Table 4. It is obvious that the pretreated cultures are affected to a smaller degree by the inhibitor. This supports the assumption that there is indeed a selection of less sensitive bacteria which is responsible for a change from negative to positive generation rates in the presence of "bactericidal" concentrations of TMP or its derivatives alone (SEYDEL and WEMPE 1980). In case of TMP/sulfonamide combinations, such a selection of less sensitive bacteria has not been observed (SEYDEL and WEMPE 1977; SEYDEL et al. 1972).

D. Combined Action of Sulfonamides and Trimethoprim (Folate Inhibitors)

I. Effect of TMP/SMX on Generation Rates of E. coli

A typical example of the effects on the growth of *E. coli* of a combination of TMP and SMX is given in Fig. 10. Because of the lag time in sulfonamide, the drugs were given to the cultures at different times of the logarithmic growth phase. SMX was added first, and after 1.5 h TMP was added. The graph shows the effects of the drugs on the growth rates of the cultures inhibited with either SMX (2 μmol/l) or TMP (0.5 and 1.0 μmol/l) alone and also in combination of these concentrations. It can be seen that the effects of the combinations are significantly greater than when either drug is used alone. If the effects of the two drugs are independently

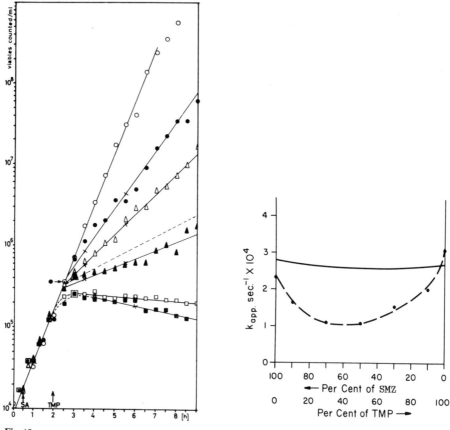

Fig. 10   **Fig. 11**

Fig. 10. Typical generation rate curves of *Escherichia coli* (mutaflor) at 37 °C in the presence of SMX alone and in combination with various concentrations of TMP. TMP was added five generations later (1.5 h) when SMX-affected steady state was obtained. *Dotted line* is the calculated generation rate curve for the combination of 2.0 μmol/l SMX and 0.5 μmol/l TMP using Eq. 4; calculated value of $k_{app} = 0.83 \times 10^{-4}$. Curves are as follows:

	SMX (μmol/l)	TMP (μmol/l)	k_{app} (s^{-1})
Open circles	0.0	0.0	4.03×10^{-4}
Full circles	2.0	0.0	2.11×10^{-4}
Open triangles	0.0	0.5	1.60×10^{-4}
Full triangles	0.0	1.0	0.64×10^{-4}
Open squares	2.0	0.5	-0.11×10^{-4}
Full squares	2.0	1.0	-0.93×10^{-4}

SEYDEL et al. (1972)

Fig. 11. Generation rate constants k_{obs} obtained by the total count method are plotted as a function of the percentages of initial concentrations of 1 μmol/l. SMX and 0.105 μmol/l TMP, present in the culture. These concentrations are equivalent in activity. The *solid line* was calculated from Eq. 4, assuming additivity of the combination. The difference between the *solid line* and the *dashed line* connecting the experimental points indicates the synergy observed at any given ratio of TMP to SMX. (SEYDEL et al. 1973)

additive, one may predict the effects of the combination by combining the two expressions [Eq. (2)] that were shown to hold for each drug alone, to obtain:

$$k_{\text{app}} = k_0 \left(1 - \frac{K_1 [\text{SMX}]}{1 + K_1 [\text{SMX}]}\right)\left(1 - \frac{K_2 [\text{TMP}]}{1 - K_2 [\text{TMP}]}\right) \tag{4}$$

$$\text{where } K_1 = \frac{1}{K_{\text{SMX}} k_0} \quad \text{and} \quad K_2 = \frac{1}{K_{\text{TMP}} k_0}.$$

Figure 10 shows as a dotted line the calculated value on the generation rate constants obtained in this way. It can be clearly seen that the combination effects are much greater than those predicted by simple additivity, i.e., the inhibitory effect of the combination is more than additive.

The synergism was further demonstrated by the method of continuous variations (Fig. 11) to prove whether or not the inhibitory effect of the combination is more than equivalent. In this experiment, generation rates were evaluated for a series of five cultures inhibited by mixtures of TMP and SMX as well as for each drug alone. The mixtures were chosen so that the concentration of each drug was a fraction of its concentration in its single drug culture, and so that the sum of the two drug fractions was always 1. Equation (4) has been used to calculate a curve showing the generation rates expected if the combinations were acting in an additive manner. The experimentally obtained generation rates are considerably lower than those predicted by this curve. Maximal synergy is observed when equipotent combinations of TMP and SMX are used, but appreciable potentiation is observed, even when the potency ratio of TMP to SMX is as low as 1:9 or as high as 9:1 (Fig. 11). Therefore, differences in concentrations of the two inhibitors obtained in various body tissues during therapy should not have a large effect on the maximum antibacterial effect (SEYDEL et al. 1973). As the combined action has been shown to be more than additive and more than equivalent, the inhibitory effect of the combination is synergistic, i.e., more than additive (for definition see GARRETT 1958).

II. Influence of Inhibitory Power and Concentration of Sulfonamides or Sulfones on the Degree of Synergism

During the last decade, new combinations with TMP and other sulfonamides have been evaluated and marketed (Supristol, Triglobe, Lidaprim). It was therefore of interest to evaluate which sulfonamide concentrations at a constant TMP concentration and which TMP concentration at a constant sulfonamide concentration result in an optimal antibacterial effect under the conditions of the experiment.

Do we need higher concentrations of a sulfonamide combination with TMP if we use a sulfonamide with lower intrinsic activity, i.e., having a higher MIC if tested alone? If this question has to be answered "yes," does this have any influence on the necessary dose recommended for clinical treatment?

For this reason, the influence on bacterial growth rate was tested under conditions where the TMP concentration was kept constant and the sulfonamide concentration was varied, and vice versa. The combined effect and the effects of the single drugs were evaluated. The results are given in Tables 5 and 6 (SEYDEL and WEMPE 1977, 1978). Two results are of major interest:

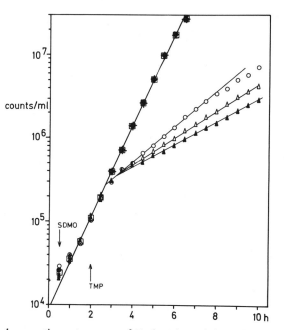

Fig. 12. Typical generation rate curves of *Escherichia coli* (mutaflor) at 37 °C in the presence of TMP and various concentrations of SDMO alone and in combination. The final drug concentrations (μmol/l) and observed steady state rate growth curves are as follows (total count method):

	SDMO	TMP
Plus signs	0.0	0.0
Open circles	0.0	0.5
Squares	0.05	0.0
Full circles	0.1	0.0
Open triangles	0.05	0.5
Full triangles	0.1	0.5

SEYDEL and WEMPE (1979)

1. Small concentrations of sulfonamide or TMP which are subinhibitory, i.e., which do not cause significant deviations from the growth rates of the control cultures, exert strong potentiating effects in combination with TMP or sulfonamide respectively (Fig. 12; SEYDEL and WEMPE 1977).

2. Even with relatively small sulfonamide concentration, a maximum effect (kill rate) is observed. For example, if SMX reduces the growth rate approximately 10% (0.055 μg/ml) then 0.1455 μg/ml TMP is sufficient to obtain the maximum potentiating effect, k_{pot}, which has been observed under the conditions of the experiment. This is independent of the sulfonamide used (Table 5). The potentiating effect, k_{pot}, is defined as:

$$k_{pot} = k_{obs(TMP+SA)} - k_{obs(TMP)} \tag{5}$$

and represents the difference of the rate constant observed in the presence of both inhibitors minus the rate constant observed in the presence of TMP alone.

Table 5. Antibacterial effect of TMP sulfonamide (SA) combinations at constant TMP concentrations: 0.145 µg/ml. (SEYDEL and WEMPE 1979)

SDMO (µg/ml)	Reduction in growth rate compared with control rate (%)	TMP (0.145 µg/ml) reduction compared with control (%)	$k_{pot} = k_{obs(TMP+SA)} - k_{obs(TMP)}$ $(s^{-1}) \times 10^{-4}$	0.145 µg/ml TMP + χ µg/ml SA. Reduction compared with control (%)
0.013	0	63	−0.289	71.51
0.027	0	67	−0.536	81.40
0.040	1.98	57	−0.71	76.6
0.054	2.83	57	−0.85	80.4
0.067	2.00	67	−0.97	92.1
0.133	4.90	71	−1.48	>100
0.267	7.50	67	−1.61	≫100
0.534	20.70	67	−1.68	≫100
1.068	33.7	66	−2.17	≫100
2.136	45.0	66	−2.19	≫100
4.005	84.6	>100 (0.52 µg/ml)	−0.91	≫100
SMX				
0.00076	0	66	−0.09	67.9
0.0076	0	60	−0.62	75.2
0.0056	0	67	−0.487	79.4
0.0025	0	60	−0.26	66.3
0.0011	0	67	−0.851	88.5
0.015	0	72	−0.890	92.9
0.022	0	72	−0.98	95.1
0.038	6.4	73	−1.38	>100
0.076	19.7	73	−1.34	≫100
0.506	47.64	60	−1.71	≫100
18.75	100	100 (1 µg/ml)	0	≫100
Sulfanilamide				
1.72	0	61	−1.46	100
3.44	0	61	−1.46	100

Table 6. Antibacterial effect of TMP/SMX combinations at constant SMX concentration: 0.25 µg/ml. (SEYDEL and WEMPE 1979)

TMP (µg/ml)	Reduction in growth rate compared with control rate (%)	SMX (0.25 µg/ml). Reduction compared with control (%)	$k_{pot} = k_{obs(TMP+SA)} - k_{obs(SA)}$ $(s^{-1}) \times 10^{-4}$	0.25 µg/ml SMX + χ µg/ml TMP. Reduction compared with control (%)
0.00072	0	44	−0.58	58
0.00116	0.5	47	−0.74	68
0.00145	0	44	−0.71	62
0.0022	5.6	51	−1.18	82
0.0029	5.3	51	−1.32	86
0.0072	8.25	47	−2.12	100

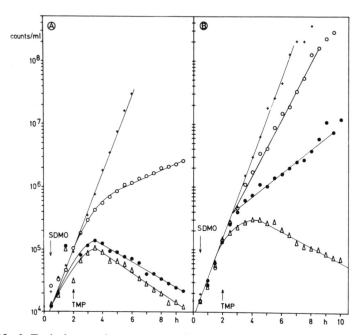

Fig. 13a, b. Typical generation rate curves of *Escherichia coli* (mutaflor) at 37 °C. **a** 15 µmol/l SDMO alone and in combination with 1.8 µmol/l TMP; curves are as follows (viable and total count method):

	SDMO (µmol/l)	TMP (µmol/l)	k_{obs} (s^{-1})
Plus signs	0.0	0.0	4.09×10^{-4}
Open circles	15.0	0.0	0.63×10^{-4}
Full circles	0.0	1.8	-0.89×10^{-4}
Triangles	15.0	1.8	-1.08×10^{-4}

b 4 µmol/l SDMO alone and in combination with 0.5 µmol/l TMP; curves are as follows:

	SDMO (µmol/l)	TMP (µmol/l)	k_{obs} (s^{-1})
Plus signs	0.0	0.0	4.16×10^{-4}
Open circles	4.0	0.0	2.76×10^{-4}
Aull circles	0.0	0.5	$1.4 \ \times 10^{-4}$
Triangles	4.0	0.5	-0.77×10^{-4}

Seydel and Wempe (1979)

The question can therefore be answered as follows. We do need higher concentration of a sulfonamide with lower intrinsic activity. For example five times more sulfadimethyloxazole (SDMO) is required to obtain the same effect as with SMX in the presence of a constant (0.145 µg/ml) TMP concentration. The important result is the observation that the maximum possible effect, a kill rate of

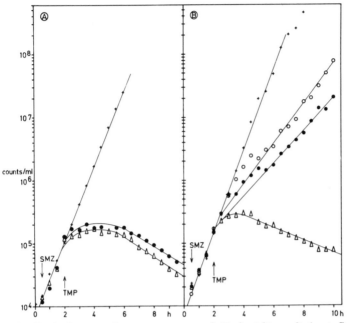

Fig. 14a, b. Typical generation rate curves of *Escherichia coli* (mutaflor) at 37 °C.
a 75 µmol/l SMX alone and in combination with 3.5 µmol/l TMP; curves are as follows
(viable and total count method):

	SMX (µmol/l)	TMP (µmol/l)	k_{obs} (s^{-1})
Plus signs	0.0	0.0	3.84×10^{-4}
Full circles	0.0	3.5	-0.95×10^{-4}
Triangles	75.0	3.5	-0.95×10^{-4}

b 3 µmol/l SMX alone and in combination with 0.5 µmol/l TMP; curves are as follows:

	SMX (µmol/l)	TMP (µmol/l)	k_{obs} (s^{-1})
Plus signs	0.0	0.0	4.25×10^{-4}
Open circles	3.0	0.0	1.85×10^{-4}
Full circles	0.0	0.5	1.52×10^{-4}
Triangles	3.0	0.5	-0.61×10^{-4}

SEYDEL and WEMPE (1979)

approximately $0.7 \times 10^{-4}\,\mathrm{s}^{-1}$ which corresponds to a half-life of 165 min, is
also obtained with a sulfonamide with lower antibacterial activity, far below the
minimum plasma water concentration achieved during therapy (Tables 5 and 6).
As already shown, very small amounts of various sulfonamides (Fig. 12) combined with TMP exert a strong and significant synergistic effect. On the contrary,

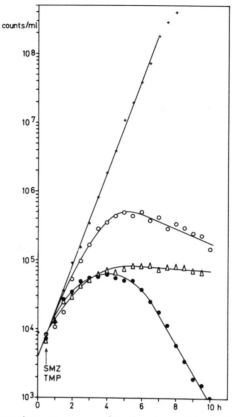

Fig. 15. Typical generation rate curves of *Escherichia coli* (mutaflor) at 37 °C. Final drug concentrations are as follows:

	SMX (µg/ml)	TMP (µg/ml)
Plus signs	0.0	0.0
Open circles	100.0	0.0
Full circles	0.0	0.58
Triangles	100.0	0.58

Seydel and Wempe (1979)

the relative potentiating effect decreases if TMP or sulfonamide is present in such high concentrations that the optimal possible effect is already achieved by the single drug. This is demonstrated in two examples. Figure 13 shows results with SDMO and TMP alone and in combination at concentrations obtained as minimum plasma water concentrations (Fig. 13 a; 4 µg/ml SDMO, 0.5 µg/ml TMP) and at much lower concentrations (Fig. 13 b; 1 µg/ml SDMO, 0.145 µg/ml TMP). There is no significant difference in the antibacterial action. Figure 14 represents similar experiments with TMP/SMX concentrations achieved as minimum plasma water concentrations during therapy (Fig. 14 a; 18.7 µg/ml SMX, 1 µg/ml TMP) and with much smaller concentrations (Fig. 14 b; 0.78 µg/ml SMX and 0.145 µg/ml TMP). It is obvious that in Figs. 13 a and 14 a no potentiating effect of SMX is obtained. The maximum effect is already obtained by TMP alone.

If one increases the sulfonamide concentration even further in the mixture (100 µg/ml SMX), an antagonistic effect of SMX on the action of TMP is observed (Fig. 15). The effect of TMP alone, which was bactericidal, is reduced to a merely bacteriostatic action in the combination. This indicates that for this type of combination, the usual assumption in the therapy of infectous diseases that "more is better" is at least doubtful with respect to the degree of synergism.

III. Influence of Inhibitory Power of TMP Derivatives on the Degree of Synergism and Maximal Possible Effect

It has been shown (SEYDEL and WEMPE 1975) that, despite the much lower antibacterial effect of pyrimethamine (PMA) compared with TMP (1: 290), the same maximal kill rate in *E. coli* cultures is observed for a PMA sulfonamide combination at a comparable sulfonamide concentration. The PMA concentration required for a maximal effect is only 20 times (not 290 times) higher than the necessary TMP concentration (Fig. 16). It is interesting to note that PMA alone, even at very large concentrations, has only a bacteriostatic effect (SEYDEL and WEMPE 1975).

Similar results have been obtained for a series of TMP derivatives, the single activities of which are summarized in Table 1. On combination with sulfonamide all derivatives show strong synergism and the maximal possible kill rate is obtained for all derivatives, despite significantly lower inhibitory activity of the single derivatives in some cases. A plasma water concentration to obtain the maximal kill rate under therapy conditions could always be achieved easily (Table 7). Small concentrations of sulfonamides which are subinhibitory, i.e., which do not cause significant deviations from the growth rates of the control cultures exert strong potentiating effects in combination with the TMP derivatives. The combinations not only show strong synergistic effects, but in addition no development of resistant bacteria under the condition of the experiments can be detected. In cultures inhibited to the same degree by TMP derivatives alone, however, development of *E. coli* bacteria with lower sensitivity against these inhibitors occurs.

IV. Selection Criteria for Combination of TMP and TMP Derivatives with Sulfonamides

The experimental results discussed provide support for combination of TMP or TMP derivatives with sulfonamides with regard to an optimal pharmacokinetic fit, optimal pharmacokinetic properties, and most convenient dosage regimen. A *small* decrease in antibacterial activity of the TMP or sulfonamide derivatives seems not to influence the inhibitory power of the combination significantly because of strong synergism. Selection criteria could be
1. Comparable biologic half-life and distribution pattern of the two drugs
2. Low protein binding, because of the decrease in dose needed
3. Low metabolic rate

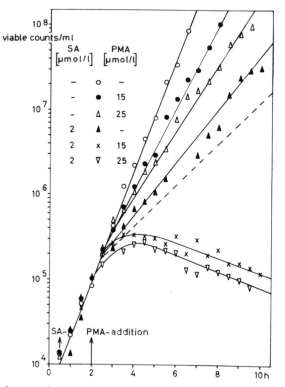

Fig. 16. Typical generation rate curves of *Escherichia coli* (mutaflor) at 37 °C in the presence of 2 μmol/l SMX and 15 or 25 μmol/l PMA alone and in combination. PMA was added five generations (1.5 h) later when SMX-affected steady state was obtained. The dashed line is the calculated generation rate curve for the combination of 20 μmol/l SMX and 15.0 μmol/l PMA using Eq. 4; $k_{app} = 1.53 \times 10^{-4}$ for phase I inhibition and $k_{app} = 0.94 \times 10^{-4}$ for phase II inhibition; curves are as follows:

	SMX (μmol/l)	PMA (μmol/l)	k_{app} (s^{-1})
Open circles	0.0	0.0	3.83×10^{-4}
Full circles	0.0	15.0	3.11×10^{-4}
Upward open triangles	0.0	25.0	2.47×10^{-4}
Full triangles	2.0	0.0	1.98×10^{-4}
Crosses	2.0	15.0	-4.74×10^{-5}
Downward open triangles	2.0	25.0	-5.40×10^{-5}

Seydel and Wempe (1975)

4. Sufficient solubility of the sulfonamide and its metabolites, especially under the varying pH conditions of the urine

5. pK_a not too acidic (≥ 7) because of less influence on half-life of changes in the urinary pH and because of better permeation properties.

Criterion 5 can be demonstrated by results published by Winningham and Stamey (1970). The permeation of sulfonamides into the prostatic fluid increases with a de-

Table 7. Antibacterial effect (*Escherichia coli*) of combinations of TMP derivatives (see Table 1) with sulfonamides. (SEYDEL and WEMPE 1980)

No.	TMP derivative (µmol/l)	k_0 (s⁻¹) × 10⁻⁴	Reduction in growth rate compared with control rate (%)	Sulfonamides (µmol/l)	Reduction (%)	Sulfonamide +TMP derivative Reduction (%)	k_{app} (s⁻¹) × 10⁻⁴ Kill rate (viable count)
II	0.75	3.56	34.1	0.05 SMX	0	66.6	
	0.75	3.56	34.1	0.10	3.0	83.0	
	1.5	3.45	64.5	2.0	44	>100	−0.53
	2.5	3.45	78.8	2.0	44	>100	−0.61
III	0.5	3.98	35.4	0.01 SMX	0	40	
	0.5	3.98	35.4	0.02	0	45.2	
	0.5	3.80	35.0	0.01	0	44	
	0.5	3.80	35.0	0.02	0	47.6	
	0.5	4.48	37.8	0.04	0	51.4	
	0.5	4.48	37.8	0.06	2.2	57.0	
	0.5	3.64	33.2	0.05	0	55	
	0.5	3.64	33.2	0.1	2.0	81	
	0.5	4.24	39.4	0.08	2.4	72.2	
	0.5	4.24	39.4	0.10	3.5	77.3	
	1.7	4.12	60.0	40 SDZ	90.0	>100	−1.64
	1.7	3.36	52	40	87.6	>100	−1.72
	1.7	3.36	52	5	52	>100	−1.78
	3.0	3.63	89	40	90.6	>100	−1.59
	3.0	3.72	>100	40	90.0	>100	−2.43
IV	0.2	3.59	24.0	0.05 SMX	<1.0	51	
	0.2	3.59	24.0	0.10	5.0	71	
	0.9	3.21	45.0	5.0	40	>100	−0.58
	1.8	3.21	61.7	5.0	40	>100	−0.68
	1.8	3.43	57.1	7.0	56	>100	−2.20
	3.6	3.43	100	7.0	56	>100	−2.18
	5.0	3.66	96.0	7.0	56	>100	−0.91
	0.75	3.63	20.0	0.05 SMX	0	45	
	0.75	3.63	20.0	0.10	2.8	64	
	5.0	3.66	66.0	7.0	56	>100	−0.58

crease in the ionized fraction of the sulfonamide. A regression analysis resulted in the following equation:

$$\log \mathrm{PF/P} = (0.48 \pm 0.06)\mathrm{p}K_a - 4.08 \tag{6}$$

$n = 16$, $r = 0.91$, $s = 0.2$, $F = 71$.

PF/P gives the quotient of the concentration of prostatic fluid to the concentration in the plasma, n is the number of compounds studied, r the regression coefficient, s the standard deviation, and F is the decision statistic of the F test of significance. The equation describes an increase in the concentration in the prostatic fluid with increase in $\mathrm{p}K_a$ of the compound. The lipophilicity is probably another important

Table 8. Antibacterial activity (*Escherichia coli*) and some physico-chemical and pharmacokinetic data of various sulfonamides and TMP

Compound[a]	pK_a	Water solubility 37 °C (mg/l)		Lipid solubility[b] $\log P$ pH 7.4	Biologic half-life (h)	Protein binding[c]		Average acetylated drug found in urine (%)
		≈pH 5	≈pH 7			K_{diss} (µmol/l)	Bound drug (%)	
SMX	5.67	631	4,757	−0.704	10 (8–14)	536	≈80	61
N⁴–Ac–SMX	5.10	129	3,029	−0.582	7.6–19.7			
SDMO	7.15	1,549	4,442	−0.241	11 (8–14)	348	≈90	47
N⁴–Ac–SDMO	6.69	165	260	0.205				
SDZ	6.44	127	678	−0.742	~12	720	≈50	30
N⁴–Ac–SDZ	5.86	198	2,595	−0.427				
SM	5.03	1,160	26,720 (pH 6.7)	−1.239	7		≈78	78
N⁴–Ac–SM	≈4.5	800	31,660 (pH 6.7)					
SIMD	7.36	3,600	11,000		7		80	20
N⁴–Ac–SIMD		1,900	4,900					
TMP	7.2		350 (20 °C)	0.73	8–12		35–45	
Tetroxoprim	≈7.2		2,650 (30 °C)	0.34	≈ 5		13	

[a] Ac indicates acetyl derivative at N^4

[b] P is the partition coefficient of the drugs between octanol and water

[c] K_{diss} is the dissociation constant for the albumin–drug complex

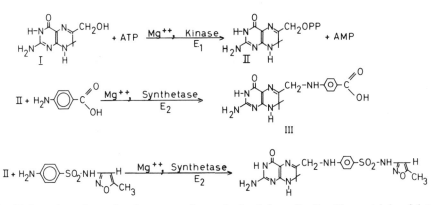

Fig. 17. Reaction scheme for the enzymatic synthesis of the sulfanilamide-containing folate analog. (SEYDEL 1975)

parameter. By the criteria for judgment listed, SMX seems not to be the optimal sulfonamide in every respect for combination with a dihydrofolate inhibitor such as TMP (see also KASS 1976). Sulfonamides such as SDMO, sulfisomidine (SIMD), and sulfadiazine (SDZ) seem to have certain advantages compared with SMX. Pharmacokinetic and physicochemical properties of some TMP derivatives and sulfonamides are listed in Table 8.

V. Mode of Action of Sulfonamides, TMP, and Their Combinations

1. Sulfonamides

Recognition of the importance of p-aminobenzoic acid (pABA) in folic acid metabolism and the ability of certain folate derivatives and/or products to reverse the effect of sulfonamides and sulfones has led to a general theory of sulfonamide. In principle, this theory states that sulfonamides are comparative inhibitors of the enzymatic incorporation of pABA into folic acid (ROGERS et al. 1964). The sequential pathway of folic acid synthesis has been evaluated by JAENICKE and CHAN (1960), BROWN (1962), SHIOTA et al. (1964), and ORTIZ and HOTCHKISS (1966), and is given in Fig. 17a, b (line 1+2). It has also been shown that bacterial (WOLF and HOTCH-KISS 1963; ORTIZ and HOTCHKISS 1966; MILLER et al. 1972; BOCK et al. 1974), plant (MITSUDA and SUZUKI 1969), and plasmodial (FERONE 1973) cell-free folate synthesizing extracts are inhibited by sulfonamides. Later, it has been found that sulfonamides not only compete with pABA for enzymatic binding sites, but form reaction products with the dihydropteridine pyrophosphate which leads to dihydropteroic acid analogs (Fig. 17c; MILLER et al. 1972; BOCK et al. 1974). This has been confirmed by FERONE (1973). The rate-determining step for various sulfonamides in this reaction, however, is the result of the affinity for the receptor site and is not due to the formation of a dihydropteroic acid analog of the sulfonamide (see Fig. 17; SEYDEL and SCHAPER 1980). The ionized and un-ionized form of the sulfonamide are bound to the enzyme protein, the affinity of the ionized form, however, is 30 times greater (SEYDEL and SCHAPER 1980).

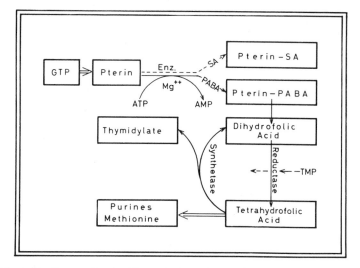

Fig. 18. Schematic diagram for the biosynthetic pathway of tetrahydrofolic acid and for the interference of sulfonamides (SA) and TMP. (SEYDEL et al. 1972)

Table 9. Inhibition constants K_i of sulfonamide for *Escherichia coli* dihydrofolate reductase and *E. coli* dihydropteroate synthetase. (POE 1976)

Compound	K_i (mol/l)		K_i^{2} [a]
	Dihydropteroate synthetase	Dihydrofolate reductase	
Sulfaquinoxaline		1.3×10^{-4}	$1.7 \pm 0.4 \times 10^{-4}$
4,4'-Diaminodiphenylsulfone		1.8×10^{-4}	$3.0 \pm 1.1 \times 10^{-4}$
Sulfamerazine	4.0×10^{-6}	4.0×10^{-4}	$6.3 \pm 2.2 \times 10^{-4}$
Sulfapyridine	1.3×10^{-5}	5.7×10^{-4}	$1.7 \pm 1.2 \times 10^{-3}$
Sulfathiazole	2.3×10^{-6}	7.4×10^{-4}	$9.6 \pm 4.8 \times 10^{-4}$
Sulfamethoxazole		2.0×10^{-3}	$2.3 \pm 0.3 \times 10^{-3}$
Sulfinilic acid	8.3×10^{-6}	3.5×10^{-3}	$6.5 \pm 0.8 \times 10^{-3}$
Sulfaguanidine	1.7×10^{-5}	3.9×10^{-3}	5.6×10^{-1}
Sulfisoxazole		6.5×10^{-3}	$3.0 \pm 0.3 \times 10^{-3}$
Sulfanilamide	6.7×10^{-5}	2.4×10^{-2}	$1.3 \pm 0.7 \times 10^{-2}$

[a] K_i^{2} gives the synergism constant of the sulfonamide when used in combination with pyrimethamine ($K_i = 1.3 \times 10^{-8}$ M)

2. TMP

2,4-Diaminopyridines and related structures have a high affinity for the enzyme dihydrofolate reductase (HITCHINGS et al. 1948; HITCHINGS 1961; HITCHINGS and BURCHALL 1965). HITCHINGS and BUSHBY (1961), and ROTH et al. (1962) have been able to modify these structures in such a way that compounds with selective toxicity (affinity) for folate reductase of a given bacterium and/or animal species have been found. It has been shown that one of these compounds, TMP, has a very high

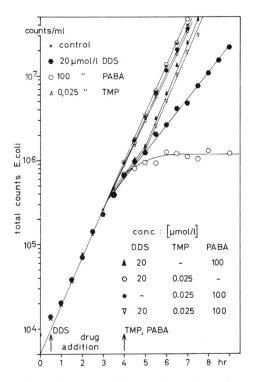

Fig. 19. Typical generation rate curves of *Escherichia coli* (mutaflor) at 37 °C in the presence of DDS, pABA, and TMP alone and in combination; curves are as follows:

	DDS (μmol/l)	TMP (μmol/l)	pABA (μmol/l)
Crosses	0.0	0.0	0.0
Full hexagons	20.0	0.0	0.0
Open circles	0.0	0.0	100.0
Upward open triangles	0.0	0.025	0.0
Full triangles	20.0	0.0	100.0
Open hexagons	20.0	0.025	0.0
Full circles	0.0	0.025	100.0
Downward open triangles	20.0	0.025	100.0

SEYDEL et al. (1980)

affinity for bacterial folate reductase and a low affinity for mammalian folate reductase (65,000: 1; HITCHINGS 1969; BURCHALL 1969). As a consequence of this selective binding, the bacterial synthesis of tetrahydrofolic acid is diminished and a reduction in the synthesis of essential purines, thymidine, and some amino acids results. Because of the oxidation of the tetrahydrofolate to the dihydro form during synthesis of thymidine, it is expected that this step would be especially critical for bacterial reproduction. The inhibitory effect of TMP can partly be antagonized by thymidine (SEYDEL et al. 1972).

3. Combination of Sulfonamides and TMP

Combinations of sulfonamide and TMP are therefore postulated to act at different sites of the same sequential pathway of folic acid synthesis (HITCHINGS and BURCHALL 1965; Fig. 18). The results with sulfonamides are wholly in accord with this mode of action (MILLER et al. 1972; BOCK et al. 1974; SEYDEL et al. 1972; SEYDEL and SCHAPER 1980). Many of the results with TMP and TMP derivatives may also be explained by the aforementioned mechanism of action. The bacterial dihydrofolate reductase has been purified and X-ray analysis has been performed (MATTHEWS et al. 1978) so that the specific binding sites for TMP can be discussed.

The mechanism of the observed synergism of combinations of sulfonamides, sulfones, and TMP or TMP derivatives is still not fully understood. The synergism may be due to inhibition of a cyclic pathway by TMP (WEBB 1963). HARVEY (1978) has derived a mathematical model by which the observed synergism can be described. POE (1976) has made another proposal to explain synergistic behavior of the combination. He assumes that sulfonamides and sulfones such as diamino-diphenylsulfone (DDS) act not only at the enzyme, dihydropteroic acid synthetase (Figs. 17 and 18), but also at the dihydrofolate reductase. The published K_i values (see Table 9) for various sulfonamides and DDS acting on dihydrofolate reductase show, however, that they are at least two orders of magnitude larger than the inhibition constants observed for inhibition of dihydropteroic acid synthetase. This argument has also been put forward by BURCHALL (1977). Another argument is the observed totally antagonistic effect of pABA on the synergism of TMP/sulfonamide combinations (THEN 1977). Another possibility could be an affinity to the dihydrofolate reductase of the sulfonamide or DDS analogs formed in the synthetase-catalyzed reaction (see Fig. 17). An experiment was designed where pABA was added after 4 h to a culture inhibited by DDS. During these 4 h, a certain amount of analog has been enzymatically synthesized in the bacterial cells. A possible inhibitory action of the analog should not be antagonized by pABA, which has no affinity to the dihydrofolate reductase. The analog could then show a synergistic or additive effect in combination with TMP. The results are summarized in Fig. 19, together with the curves obtained in the presence of DDS alone, and in a mixture with TMP. It is clearly demonstrated that, at least in case of *E. coli*, the DDS inhibitory activity can be totally antagonized by pABA; i.e. there seems to be no additional activity of the DDS analog or DDS at the dihydrofolate reductase level (SEYDEL et al. 1980).

References

Baker BR, Bang-Thong H (1964) Differential inhibition of dihydrofolic reductase from different species. J Pharm Sci 53:1137–1138

Bock L, Miller GH, Schaper K-J, Seydel JK (1974) Sulfonamide structure-activity relationship in a cell-free system. II. Proof for the formation of a sulfonamide containing folate analogue. J Med Chem 17:23–28

Böhni E (1969) Vergleichende bakteriologische Untersuchungen mit der Kombination Trimethoprim/Sulfamethoxazol in vitro und in vivo. Chemotherapy [Suppl] 14:1

Böhni E (1976) Bacteriostatic and bactericidal activity of two trimethoprim-sulfonamide combinations. Chemotherapy 22:262–273

Brown GM (1962) The biosynthesis by sulphonamides. J Biol Chem 237:536–540

Burchall JJ (1969) Comparative studies of dihydrofolate reductase. Postgrad Med J [Suppl] 45:29–32

Burchall JJ (1977) Synergisms between trimethoprim and sulfamethoxazole. Science 197:1300–1301

Bushby SRM (1970) Trimethoprim and sulphonamides. Laboratory studies. S Afr Med J [Aug Suppl] 3–10

Bushby SRM, Barnett M (1967) Trimethoprim-sulphonamides – in vitro sensitivity of 384 strains of bacteria. In: 5th Int Congr Chemother. Abstracta, Part 1, Verlag der Wiener Medizinischen Akademie, Wien

Bushby SRM, Hitchings GH (1968) Trimethoprim, a sulphonamide potentiator. Br J Pharmacol Chemother 33:72–90

Dornbusch K (1971) Regression line analysis of the synergistic effect for the combination of TMP/sulphamethoxazole. Chemotherapy 16:229–238

Ferone R (1973) The enzymatic synthesis of dihydropteroate and dihydrofolate by plasmodium berghei. J Protozool 20:459–464

Fowle ASE (1970) National use of trimethoprim and sulphamethoxazole for one year – problems and solutions. S Afr Med J [Aug Suppl] 15–20

Garrett ER (1958) Classification and evaluation of combined antibiotic activity. Antibiot Chemother 8:8–20

Garrett ER (1966) The use of microbial kinetics in the quantification of antibiotic action. Arzneim Forsch 16:1364–1369

Garrett ER (1971) Drug action and assay by microbial kinetics. Drug Res 15:271–353

Garrett ER, Brown MRW (1963) The action of tetracycline and chloramphenicol alone and in admixture on the growth of E. coli. J Pharm Pharmacol [Suppl] 15:185 T–191 T

Garrett ER, Miller GH (1965) Kinetics and mechanism of action of antibiotics on microorganisms. III. Inhibitory action of tetracycline and chloramphenicol on Escherichia coli established by total and viable counts. J Pharm Sci 54:427–431

Garrett ER, Wright OK (1967) Kinetics and mechanism of action of drugs on microorganisms. VII. Quantitative adherence of sulfonamide action on microbial growth to a receptor-site model. J Pharm Sci 56:1576–1585

Garrod LP (1971) Evaluations on new drugs. Trimethoprim-sulphamethoxazole. Drugs 1:8–53

Greenwood D, O'Grady F (1976) Activity and interaction of trimethoprim and sulphamethoxazole against Escherichia coli. J Clin Pathol 29:162–166

Harvey RJ (1978) Interaction of two inhibitors which act on different enzymes of a metabolic pathway. J Theor Biol 74:411–437

Hirsch J (1943) Die „parasitropen" Eigenschaften der Sulfanilamide. Schweiz Med Wochenschr 73:1470–1477

Hitchings GH (1961) A biochemical approach to chemotherapy. Trans NY Acad Sci 23:700–708

Hitchings GH (1969) Species differences among dihydrofolate reductases as a basis for chemotherapy. Postgrad Med J [Suppl] 45:7–10

Hitchings GH, Burchall JJ (1965) Inhibition of folate biosynthesis and function as a basis for chemotherapy. Adv Enzymol 27:417–468

Hitchings GH, Bushby SRM (1961) 5-Benzyl-2,4-diaminopyrimidines, a new class of systematic antibacterial agents. 5th Int Congr Biochem Abstr. Pergamon Press Ltd, Oxford, p 165

Hitchings GH, Elion GB, Vanderwerff H, Falco EA (1948) Pyrimidine derivatives as antagonists of pteroylglutamic acid. J Biol Chem 174:765–766

Jaenicke L, Chan PC (1960) Die Biosynthese der Folsäure. Angew Chem 72:752–753

Jawetz E, Gunnison JB (1953) Antibiotic synergism and antagonism. An assessment of the problem. Pharmacol Rev 5:175–192

Jawetz E, Gunnison JB, Bruff JA, Coleman VR (1952) Studies of antibiotic synergism and antagonism. Synergism among seven antibiotics against various bacteria in vitro. J Bacteriol 64:29

Kass E (1976) Design and achievements in chemotherapy. Scientific Medical Publishing Co, Library of Congress 76–13370, Washington

Knothe H (1975) The antibacterial efficacy of two trimethoprim-sulphonamide combinations. Chemotherapy 22:62–69

Kohn HI, Harris JS (1941) On the mode of action of sulphonamides. I. Action on E. coli. J Pharmacol Exp Ther 73:343–361

Kuhne J, Kohlmann FW, Seydel JK, Wempe E (1976) Pharmakokinetik der Kombination Sulfamoxol/Trimethoprim (CN 3123) bei Tier und Mensch. Arzneim Forsch 26:561–657

Matthews DA, Alden RA, Bolin JT et al. (1978) Dihydrofolate reductase from Lactobacillus casei. J Biol Chem 253:6946

Miller GH, Doukas PH, Seydel JK (1972) Sulfonamide structure-activity relationships in a cell-free system. Correlation of inhibition of folate synthesis with antibacterial activity and physicochemical parameters. J Med Chem 15:700–706

Mitsuda H, Suzuki Y (1969) Enzymatic pyrophosphorylation of 2-amino-4-hydroxy-6-hydroxymethyl-7,8-dihydropteridine by cell-free extracts of Escherichia coli. Biochem Biophys Res Commun 36:1–6

Nolte H (1973) Beispiel für die Untersuchung eines chemotherapeutischen Kombinationspräparates. Arzneim Forsch 23:1654–1657

Ortiz PJ, Hotchkiss RD (1966) The enzymatic synthesis of dihydrofolate and dihydropteroate in cell-free preparations from wild-type and sulfonamide-resistant pneumococcus. Biochemistry 5:67–74

Poe M (1976) Antibacterial synergism: a proposal for chemotherapeutic potentiation between trimethoprim and sulfamethoxazole. Science 194:533–535

Rogers EF, Clark RL, Becker HJ et al. (1964) Antiparasitic drugs. V. Anticoccidial activity of 4-amino-2-ethoxybenzoic acid and related compounds (29616). Proc Soc Exp Biol Med 117:488–492

Roth B, Falco EA, Hitchings GH (1962) 5-benzyl-2,4-diaminopyrimidines as antibacterial agents. I. Synthesis and antibacterial activity in vitro. J Med Pharm Chem 5:1103–1123

Seydel JK (1975) Physicochemical factors in drug-receptor interactions demonstrated on the example of the sulfanilamide. Top Infect Dis 1:25–43

Seydel JK, Miller GH (1973) Quantification of the antibacterial action of trimethoprim (TMP) alone and in combination with sulphonamides (SA) by bacterial growth kinetics (E. coli). In: Bernstein LS, Salter AJ (eds) Trimethoprim/sulphamethoxazole in bacterial infections. Churchill Livingstone, Edinburgh, pp 17–29

Seydel JK, Schaper K-J (1978) Bakterienwachstumskinetik, ein Modell zur Bestimmung thermodynamisch definierter Aktivitätsparameter sowie zur Differenzierung von synergistischen, antagonistischen oder additiven Effekten von Chemotherapeutica. In: Franke R (ed) Symposium über Beziehungen zwischen chemischer Struktur und biologischer Wirkung – Quantitative Ansätze. Akademie-Verlag, Berlin, pp 373–386

Seydel JK, Schaper K-J (1980) Quantitative structure-activity relationships as applied to enzyme inhibitors. In: Sandler M (ed) Enzyme inhibitors as drugs. Macmillan, London, pp 53–71

Seydel JK, Wempe E (1975) Kinetics and mechanism of action of "folate synthesis inhibitors," alone or in combination, on Escherichia coli. III. Pyrimethamine, trimethoprim and sulfamethoxazole. Chemotherapy 21:131–145

Seydel JK, Wempe E (1977) Untersuchungen zum synergistischen Verhalten und zur Pharmakokinetik von Sulfonamid-Trimethoprim-Kombinationen. IV. Eine vergleichende Untersuchung zur Potenzierung der Trimethoprim-Wirkung durch verschiedene Sulfonamide und eine kritische Betrachtung ihrer Dosierung. Arzneim Forsch 27:1521–1532

Seydel JK, Wempe E (1978) Potentiation of trimethoprim action with various sulfonamides: a comparison using bacterial growth kinetic techniques (Escherichia coli). Curr Chemother 658–660

Seydel JK, Wempe E (1979) Synergistic antibacterial activity in vitro of trimethoprim and sulphonamides and the importance of pharmacokinetic properties for optimal therapy. Infection [Suppl 4] 7:313–320

Seydel JK, Wempe E (1980) Bacterial growth kinetics of E. coli in the presence of various trimethoprim derivatives alone and in combination with sulfonamides. V. Chemotherapy 26:361–371

Seydel JK, Wempe E, Miller GH, Miller L (1972) Kinetics and mechanism of trimethoprim and sulfonamides, alone or in combination, upon *E. coli*. Chemotherapy 17:217–258

Seydel JK, Wempe E, Miller GH, Miller L (1973) Quantification of the antibacterial action of trimethoprim alone and in combination with sulfonamides by bacterial growth kinetics. J Infect Dis 128:S463–S469

Seydel JK, Richter M, Wempe E (1980) Mechanism of action of folate blocker diaminodiphenylsulfone (Dapsone, DDS) studied in *E. coli* cell-free enzyme extracts in comparison to sulfonamides (SA). Int J Lepr 48:18–29

Shiota T, Disraely MN, McCann MP (1964) The enzymatic synthesis of folate-like compounds from hydroxy-methyl-dihydropteridine pyrophosphate. J Biol Chem 239:2259–2266

Then R (1973) Influence of sulfonamide antagonists on the synergism of sulfamethoxazole/ trimethoprim in *Escherichia coli*. Zentralbl Bakteriol [Orig A] 225:34–41

Then R (1977) Synergism between trimethoprim and sulfamethoxazole. Science 197:1301

Then R, Angehrn P (1973) Nature of the bactericidal action of sulfonamides and trimethoprim, alone and in combination. J Infect Dis [Suppl] 128:S498–S501

Tiesler E (1970) Wirksamkeit einer Sulfonamid-Trimethoprim-Kombination gegen einige gramnegative Stäbchen und grampositive Kokken im Agardiffusionstest. Med Klin 65:1825–1828

Webb JL (1963) Enzyme and metabolic inhibitors, vol 1. Academic Press, New York

Winningham D, Stamey T (1970) Diffusion of sulphonamides from plasma into prostatic fluid. J Urol 104:559–563

Wolf B, Hotchkiss RD (1963) Genetically modified folic acid synthesizing enzymes of pneumococcus. Biochemistry 2:145–150

Disposition and Metabolism of Trimethoprim, Tetroxoprim, Sulfamethoxazole, and Sulfadiazine

C.W. Sigel

A. Introduction

Since the antibacterial sulfonamides and their potentiators are used extensively in both human and veterinary medicine, detailed pharmacokinetic and biotransformation studies in both humans and animals were conducted during preclinical and clinical trials. As a necessary adjunct to these studies, sensitive and specific analytical procedures had to be devised. The methods most often used and the results of disposition studies in laboratory and domestic animals for trimethoprim (TMP), tetroxoprim (TXP), sulfamethoxazole (SMX), and sulfadiazine (SDZ) are reviewed in this chapter. Metabolic pathways in the various species including humans are also summarized. The pharmacokinetic profile for co-trimoxazole (TMP/ SMX in the ratio 1:5) in humans is described in more detail in Chap. 10.

B. Drug Disposition

I. Drug Absorption

Studies in rats (Meshi and Sato 1972), dogs (Kaplan et al. 1970; Preslar et al. 1980; Lazaro et al. 1980), and humans (Schwartz and Ziegler 1969; Kaplan et al. 1973a; Welling et al. 1973; Andreasen et al. 1978) have shown that TMP is completely absorbed following oral administration. Peak concentrations in blood are reached in 1–2 h for most species. TXP is also rapidly absorbed by rats (Vergin and Fritschi 1979), dogs (Preslar et al. 1980), and humans (Reeves et al. 1979). The absolute bioavailability for TXP in the rat was estimated to be 100% by Vergin and Fritschi (1979); however, in the dog (Preslar et al. 1980) the absolute bioavailability was 61%, which is suggestive of either incomplete absorption or extensive first-pass metabolism.

The sulfonamides are absorbed well after oral administration, but the rate of absorption is slower than for the benzylpyrimidines. After an oral dose, peak blood concentrations of SMX are generally observed within 1 h in the rat (Fujihara et al. 1975), and 4 h in the dog (Lazaro et al. 1980), calf (Kovacs et al. 1976), and human (Kaplan et al. 1973a). The absolute bioavailability of SMX in humans was estimated to be approximately 85% by Reber et al. (1963) and 80% for the dog by Lazaro et al. (1980). SDZ reaches peak blood levels within 1 h in the rat (Vergin and Fritschi 1979), 4 h in the dog (Sigel et al. 1981b), and human (Andreasen et al. 1978; Reeves et al. 1979). Männistö et al. (1973) presented evidence that the absolute bioavailability for SDZ in humans is 100%, based upon the excretion pattern during maintenance therapy. Subsequently, Reeves et al. (1979) reported 94.3% ± 9.7% of the SDZ dose administered to human subjects was excreted in the urine.

II. Distribution into Biologic Fluids and Tissues

1. Physicochemical Properties that Influence Distribution

The passive diffusion of compounds across biologic membranes into various tissue compartments is influenced by several physicochemical properties including molecular size, extent of ionization, lipophilicity, and degree of binding to plasma proteins and tissue components. Because organs and tissues account for varying percentages of total body weight in different animals, the pattern of distribution is species dependent. TMP, a weak organic base with moderate lipophilicity (Table 1), is widely distributed throughout body tissues. The apparent volumes of distribution (V_d) range from 1.1 l/kg in cows (Davitiyananda and Rasmussen 1974a), to 1.4 l/kg in humans (Schwartz and Rieder 1970), and 1.6–1.8 l/kg in dogs (Kaplan et al. 1970). TXP which is more hydrophilic than TMP (Table 1) has a relatively low V_d of 0.4 l/kg in humans (Reeves et al. 1979).

As weak organic acids, SDZ, SMX, and other sulfonamides have V_d values in the intermediate range. The V_d values for SDZ range from 0.36 l/kg in humans (Andreasen et al. 1978), to 0.75 l/kg in cows (Nielsen and Rasmussen 1977), and 1.19 l/kg in dogs (Sigel et al. 1981b). SMX, which is more lipophilic than SDZ and slightly more acidic, has somewhat lower V_d values (e.g., 0.28 l/kg in humans: Rieder and Schwartz 1975, and 0.30 l/kg in cows: Nielsen and Rasmussen 1977).

Literature values for the extent of protein binding for these compounds vary considerably, depending upon the technique utilized and the species studied. Some representative values are reported in Table 1. The extent of protein binding for TXP is reported as 13% for humans by Vergin and Fritschi (1979). TMP is more extensively bound with a mean value of 45% reported by Hansen (1979). Nielsen and Rasmussen (1977) measured the extent of protein binding in bovine plasma for 11 sulfonamides and reported that relative to the other compounds, SDZ was the least extensively bound (mean value in vivo was 14%). SMX was 62% protein bound. Anton (1973) has reported that the extent of protein binding of SDZ varies considerably in different species, e.g., monkey 35%; dog 17%; cat 13%; rat 45%; mouse 7%; rabbit 55%; and chicken 16%. The extent of protein binding for TMP is not influenced significantly by the presence of sulfonamide and vice versa (Schwartz and Ziegler 1969; Davitiyananda and Rasmussen 1974b).

2. Relationship Between Plasma and Tissue Concentrations

The relatively high V_d for TMP indicates that the compound is distributed extensively into tissue compartments. In contrast, concentrations of SMX and SDZ in tissues are consistently lower than in plasma. The tissue distribution of TMP in rats was investigated by Schwartz and Rieder (1970), Schulz (1972), and Meshi and Sato (1972); TMP and SMX in rats by Yoshikawa et al. (1975). The tissue distribution of SDZ in the rat was studied by Woolley and Sigel (1979). These experiments showed that relative to plasma, high concentrations of TMP (total

Table 1. Physicochemical properties for trimethoprim, tetroxoprim, sulfadiazine, and sulfamethoxazole

Compound	Molecular weight (daltons)	pK_a	Reference	Partition coefficient [a] (log P)	Reference	Protein binding Serum or plasma	Method	Binding (%)	Reference
Trimethoprim	290	7.1	[1]	0.89	[4]	Human plasma (50–1,600 ng/ml)	Equilibrium dialysis	44–46	[5]
						Human plasma (50–1,600 ng/ml)	Ultrafiltration	42–45	[5]
Tetroxoprim	334	8.25	[2]	0.25–0.54 [b]	[2]	Human serum albumin	Ultrafiltration	10–14	[2]
Sulfadiazine	250	6.15	[3]	−0.092	[3]	Human serum	Ultrafiltration	58	[6]
						Bovine plasma	Ultrafiltration	14	[7]
Sulfamethoxazole	253	5.81	[3]	0.890	[3]	Human serum	Ultrafiltration	72	[6]
						Bovine plasma	Ultrafiltration	62	[7]

[a] Partition coefficient of un-ionized form between n-octanol and water, unless stated otherwise
[b] Partition coefficients were determined in n-octanol/buffer systems over a range of pH values

[1] ROTH and STRELITZ (1969)
[2] VERGIN and FRITSCHI (1979)
[3] MORISHITA et al. (1973)
[4] ROTH et al. (1980)
[5] SCHWARTZ and ZIEGLER (1969)
[6] ÖRTENGREN et al. (1979)
[7] NIELSEN and RASMUSSEN (1977)

Table 2. Mean concentration[a] in serum and tissue (μg/g or μg/ml) of trimethoprim (TMP) and sulfamethoxazole (SMX) at equilibrium following infusion of the combination to four monkeys

	TMP	SMX	Quotient SMX/TMP
Serum	1.9 (1.2– 2.5)	78.43 (62.4–100.4)	42.4
Kidney	21.1 (15.4–24.2)	29.40 (24.8– 33.4)	1.4
Liver	12.6 (7.9–16.7)	11.75 (9.0– 15.8)	1.0
Lung	4.3 (2.7– 5.2)	20.8 (18.3– 24.5)	5.1
Heart	3.1 (1.8– 4.2)	22.5 (19.4– 25.8)	7.7
Muscle	2.7 (2.0– 3.4)	10.2 (8.8– 11.9)	3.8
Brain	1.1 (0.8– 1.4)	7.4 (5.8– 8.9)	7.0
Pancreas	7.1 (4.4– 8.0)	11.1 (6.3– 15.0)	1.6
Thyroid	4.9 (3.1– 8.4)	11.2 (6.1– 16.3)	2.4
Adrenal	4.9 (1.6– 9.0)	12.1 (7.1– 18.1)	3.0
Spleen	6.1 (3.7– 8.0)	7.4 (6.0– 8.6)	1.3
Intestine	4.7 (2.6– 6.6)	9.4 (7.3– 12.9)	2.1
Skin	1.4 (1.0– 1.8)	6.1 (4.1– 7.9)	4.6
Fat	1.1 (0.6– 1.4)	8.5 (6.1– 13.0)	8.2

[a] Data from Craig and Kunin (1973); range in parenthesis

radioactivity) were found in lung, kidney, liver, skin, and spleen. Heart and muscle had similar TMP concentrations to plasma, but brain had concentrations about one-tenth the plasma level. For the first 24 h following administration of SMX ^{14}C to the rat, total radioactivity concentrations were highest in plasma (Yoshikawa et al. 1975). Lung, kidney, and liver SMX concentrations were 30%–60%, and muscle and brain less than 30%, of the corresponding plasma concentrations. Craig and Kunin (1973) determined tissue concentrations of TMP and SMX during constant intravenous (i.v.) infusion of the combination to four monkeys. The distribution patterns (Table 2) were similar to those reported for the rat, although significant TMP penetration into the brain relative to plasma was observed. Tissue distribution studies in other large animals, e.g., sheep (Atef et al. 1978) and goats and a cow (Nielsen and Rasmussen 1975a), showed brain concentration of TMP that approached plasma concentrations also. Fujihara et al. (1975) studied the transport of TMP ^{14}C and SMX ^{14}C into the cerebrospinal fluid (CSF) of rabbits. Peak concentrations of both drugs occurred within 2 h, but the CSF: plasma ratios continued to increase for up to 6 h after treatment. At 6 h, the CSF: plasma ratios were 0.15:1.0 and 0.17:1.0 for TMP and SMX, respectively.

Vergin and Fritschi (1979) reported that TXP had rapid and high tissue penetration into muscle, liver, and kidney, but not into brain. Compared with serum concentrations, TXP levels 0.5 h after intramuscular (i.m.) administration (24 mg/kg) were 3.3 times higher in muscle, 6.9 in liver, and 6.4 in kidney (Table 3). When the serum concentration was 28.6 μg/ml in serum 1 h after an i.m. dose of 48 mg/kg, tetroxoprim was not detected (< 2.5 μg/g) in brain tissue.

Piercy (1978) compared TMP and SDZ plasma and extravascular tissue fluid concentrations, since he believed that approach was more relevant to providing a basis for the treatment of infections. He implanted subcutaneously "tissue cages," which produced an inflammatory reaction and a highly vascularized fibrous membrane surrounding the cage. Fluid in the cage resembled interstitial fluid. Piercy

Table 3. Tissue distribution[a] of tetroxoprim (TXP) in guinea pigs after i.m. administration

Tissue	Tissue concentration of TXP (μg/ml or μg/g)	
	0.5 h after i.m. dose (24 mg/kg)	1 h after i.m. dose (48 mg/kg)
Serum	7.0 ± 2.4	28.6 ± 11.9
Muscle	23.1 ± 9.4	51.3 ± 25.4
Liver	48.3 ± 13.9	51.6 ± 30.2
Kidneys	44.8 ± 14.4	100.1 ± 72.3
Brain	< 2.5	< 2.5

[a] Data from VERGIN and FRITSCHI (1979)

concluded that tissue fluids provide a TMP reservoir which is available for potentiation of the more slowly eliminated sulfonamide.

In a similar study, MAIGAARD et al. (1979) implanted tissue chambers in the upper and lower pole of each kidney of several dogs. They also collected hilar lymph by cannulation of vessels in other dogs. They found that the renal interstitial fluid TMP concentrations averaged 0.32 times the corresponding plasma concentration, while the lymph: plasma ratio averaged 1.24: 1.00. Since urine concentrations were generally 20 times the plasma concentrations, these authors concluded that plasma concentrations are more meaningful than urine concentrations for estimating renal interstitial concentrations.

To establish a scientific basis for the use of TMP combinations in treating chronic urethritis in women and chronic prostatitis in men, numerous model studies on the distribution into canine vaginal, urethral, and prostatic fluid secretions have been conducted. REEVES and GHILCHEK (1970) showed that the TMP concentration in prostatic fluid was 2–3 times higher than the corresponding serum concentration, while the SMX concentration was about one-fourth of the serum concentration. Subsequently, STAMEY et al. (1973), using progressive i.v. loading of TMP in dogs, reported that the average prostatic fluid: plasma TMP concentration ratio varied from 5.9: 1.0 to 7.0: 1.0. These observations were repeated by MADSEN et al. (1976), but in addition, they showed that high concentrations of TMP relative to plasma were found in the prostates of patients undergoing transurethral resection of the prostate. More recently FAIR et al. (1979) have disputed the relevance of the observations in dogs based on the failure of TMP to eradicate prostatic infections in a majority of their patients. They speculated that the reason for a poor response in men was that normal human prostatic fluid has pH 7.28 ± 0.04, which is much higher than for canine prostatic fluid, and during bacterial prostatitis the pH of prostatic fluid is even increased considerably. In 14 patients with prostatitis the mean pH was 8.32 ± 0.07.

FRIMODT-MÖLLER et al. (1979) compared the SDZ and SMX prostatic fluid concentrations after constant i.v. infusion of TMP/SMX combinations to the dog. SDZ concentrations were 3.6 times higher than SMX concentrations in urine, but

SMX prostatic fluid: serum ratios were higher than for SDZ. HOYME et al. (1978) reported that during constant i.v. infusion of TMP to dogs, the vaginal and urethral secretion: plasma ratios ranged from 0.95:1.00 to 4.04:1.00 and 1.34:1.00 to 2.87:1.00, respectively, over a 4-h period. This observation led to the recommendation that TMP should be investigated clinically for treatment of bacterial urethritis and vaginitis. Additional tissue distribution data derived from clinical trials in humans are summarized in Chap. 10.

III. Excretion

TMP, TXP, and the sulfonamides are excreted mainly by the kidney. BERGAN and BRODWALL (1972) reported a close relationship between creatinine and TMP clearance in humans for creatinine clearance values above 10 ml/min. In contrast, in domestic animals, NIELSEN and RASMUSSEN (1975b) found that the renal clearance of TMP by pigs varied between 32% and 141% of the creatinine clearance and in cows, DAVITIYANANDA and RASMUSSEN (1974) found it varied between 8% and 150% of the creatinine clearance. All three studies indicated that in addition to filtration, active tubular secretion and back-diffusion are involved in the excretion of TMP, and that urinary pH plays an important role in establishing the renal clearance. At low urine pH values, TMP will be ionized in the tubular lumen, and it is more likely to be excreted. At high urine pH values, back-diffusion is pronounced. In species that typically have high urinary pH values because of dietary composition, extensive back-diffusion occurs. DAVITIYANANDA and RASMUSSEN (1974) and ANDREASEN (1978) reported also that the rate of renal clearance of TMP increases as the blood concentration decreases. Urine flow rate does not appear to be a very significant factor in establishing TMP clearance. Because of similar physicochemical properties to TMP, renal clearance of TXP should be governed by the same factors. For TXP significant enterohepatic circulation has been noted (REEVES et al. 1979).

The renal clearance of SMX is fairly low, irrespective of the creatinine clearance. Most of the filtered SMX is reabsorbed by the tubules (BERGAN and BRODWALL 1972). As a result the half-life for SMX in human patients is not influenced markedly by renal function. Excretion of SMX is influenced by urinary pH; however, since it is a weak acid, it is affected in the opposite way from TMP. At low pH values the sulfonamide is un-ionized and reabsorption is extensive. VREE et al. (1978) reported that under acidic urine conditions (pH < 5.5–6.0), the net compound excreted unchanged was < 10%. When the urine was alkaline (pH 7–8), 30%–40% of the SMX dose was excreted unchanged.

The excretion of TMP and the sulfonamides into milk is also highly dependent upon pH. TMP, as a weak base, generally has concentrations 1–5 times higher in milk than in plasma, while SDZ, for example, will have concentrations in milk about one-fifth those in plasma (NIELSEN and RASMUSSEN 1974).

DU SOUICH et al. (1978) have observed nonlinear pharmacokinetics for SDZ and have conducted studies to determine the causes. In their work with rabbits, the mean plasma half-life increased from 60.1 min after a 20 mg/kg dose to 82.8 min after a 40 mg/kg dose. There were no statistically significant changes found in the renal clearance of SDZ or its major metabolite, N-acetyl-SDZ, indicating that metabolic or renal mechanisms were probably not involved. The dose-dependent increase in the half-life appeared more likely to be related to an increase in the volume of distribution, which resulted from decreased protein binding at the higher serum concentrations. The elimination rates for the sulfonamides and benzylpyrimidines vary considerably in different species. Half-life data for various species are summarized in Table 4.

IV. Metabolism

1. Trimethoprim

Using TMP ^{14}C, SCHWARTZ et al. (1970) studied the excretion and biotransformation of TMP by rats, dogs, and humans. For all three species, most of the administered radioactivity was excreted in the urine. Within 3 days, rats excreted 66% of the dose in urine, dogs 78%–88%, and humans 80%. Rats extensively metabolized TMP; only 21% of the radioactivity in the cummulative 24-h urine was found to be the parent compound. In contrast, 66.19% and 77.5% of the radioactivity in human and canine urine collected for 24 h after the dose was due to TMP. The same four metabolites, shown in Fig. 1 are: TMP-1-oxide (V), α-hydroxy-TMP (II), and 3- (III) and 4-desmethyl-TMP (IV); they were formed in the three species, but there were significant quantitative differences in the excretion patterns.

TMP-1-oxide and α-hydroxy-TMP metabolites were excreted unconjugated while the desmethyl metabolites were excreted as conjugates, mainly glucuronides. For the rat, the major metabolic pathway appeared to be 0-demethylation followed by conjugation; however, a significant portion (38%) of the radiocarbon in urine remained in a water-soluble fraction which was not further characterized. MESHI and SATO (1972) reported a similar metabolic pattern for TMP in the rat, but also discovered an additional minor metabolite, shown to be α-carbonyl-TMP (I, Fig. 1). The excretion of TMP and metabolites by rats (MESHI and SATO 1972) or human (SCHWARTZ et al. 1970) was not significantly influenced by simultaneous administration of SMX.

Studies on the excretion and biotransformation of TMP in animals of agricultural importance revealed that TMP was extensively metabolized by pigs, goats, and cows with only 15%, 2%, and 3% excreted as unchanged drug in urine (NIELSEN and RASMUSSEN 1975 b). Only trace to minor amounts of the α-hydroxy-TMP and the TMP-1-oxide metabolite were detected in pig (NIELSEN and RASMUSSEN 1975 b) or goat urine (NIELSEN and RASMUSSEN 1976). As for the rat, the major metabolic pathway was 0-demethylation; however, in both of these species a significant part (56%–65%) of the radiocarbon in urine was characterized as "other water-soluble metabolites." Following isolation by gel filtration and paper chromatography, NIELSEN and DALGAARD (1978) showed that most of the unidentified polar fraction was the sulfate conjugate of the 3-desmethyl compound. The isolated metabolite was shown to be stable to enzymatic hydrolysis with sulfatase. 3-Desmethyl-TMP could be isolated, however, by boiling the conjugate for a few seconds in dilute HCl, followed by precipitation of the liberated sulfate by Ba^{2+}.

Additional data on the biotransformation of TMP in humans were reported by SIGEL and BRENT (1973) and SIGEL et al. (1973), who studied the urinary concen-

Table 4. Half-lives $t_{1/2}$ of trimethoprim, tetroxoprim, sulfadiazine, and sulfamethoxazole in various species

Species	Trimethoprim Dose/route	$t_{1/2}$ (h)	Tetroxoprim Dose/route	$t_{1/2}$ (h)	Sulfadiazine Dose/route	$t_{1/2}$ (h)	Sulfamethoxazole Dose/route	$t_{1/2}$ (h)	Reference
Human	200 mg, p.o.	16.1			800 mg, p.o.	15.2			KAPLAN et al. (1970)
	160 mg, p.o.	7.4							ANDREASEN et al. (1978)
	160 mg, p.o.	8.8					800 mg, p.o.	7.7	ÖRTENGREN et al. (1979)
			200 mg, p.o.	6.3	500 mg, p.o.	11.7			VERGIN and FRITCHI (1979)
	400 mg, p.o.	14.5					2 g, p.o.	11	KAPLAN et al. (1973)
	160 mg, p.o.	8.6					800 mg, p.o.	9	SCHWARTZ and RIEDER (1970) KAPLAN et al. (1970)
Dog	5.7 mg/kg, i.v.	3.1							PRESLAR et al. (1980)
	5 mg/kg, p.o.	2.01	5 mg/kg, p.o.	0.98					SIGEL et al. (1981b)
	5 mg/kg, p.o.	2.51			25 mg/kg, p.o.	9.84	80 mg/kg, p.o.	12	LAZARO et al. (1980)
Rat	50 mg/kg, i.v.	1.26							SCHULZ (1972)
			1.43 mg/kg, p.o.	5–8.9	7.16 mg/kg, p.o.	7.4–12.8			VERGIN and FRITCHI (1979)
							100 mg/kg, p.o.	~ 4	KITAKAZE et al. (1973)
Rabbit	40 mg/kg, i.v.	0.7							LADEFOGED (1977)
			1.43 mg/kg, p.o.	3.6–5.2	7.16 mg/kg, p.o.	1.7–2.2			VERGIN and FRITCHI (1979)
							40 mg/kg, p.o.	~ 2	FUJIHARA et al. (1975)
	8 mg/kg, i.v.	1							DAVITIYANANDA and RASMUSSEN (1974)

Species	Dose, route	Value	Dose, route	Value	Dose, route	Value	Reference
Cow	5 mg/kg, i.v.	4.89	60–100 mg/kg, i.v.	2.5	60–100 mg/kg, i.v.	2.3	Nielsen and Rasmussen (1977)
			130–180 mg/kg, i.v.	5.43			Atef et al. (1979)
Calf	10–22 mg/kg, i.v.	2–2.25			25 mg/kg, i.v.	3.1	Kovacs et al. (1976)
Pig	10 mg/kg, i.v.	3.06–3.59			50 mg/kg, p.o.	2.84–3.27	Nielsen and Rasmussen (1975)
	20 mg/kg, p.o.	3.20					Romvary and Horvay (1976b)
							Ladefoged (1979)
Goat	10 mg/kg, i.v.	0.5–0.66					Nielsen and Rasmussen (1975)
Horse	5 mg/kg, p.o.	2.4	25 mg/kg, p.o.	7.4			Sigel et al. (1981a)
	5.6 mg/kg, i.v.	3.8					Alexander and Collett (1975)
Goose	14 mg/kg, p.o.	2.37			70 mg/kg, p.o.	3.08	Romvary and Horvay (1976a)

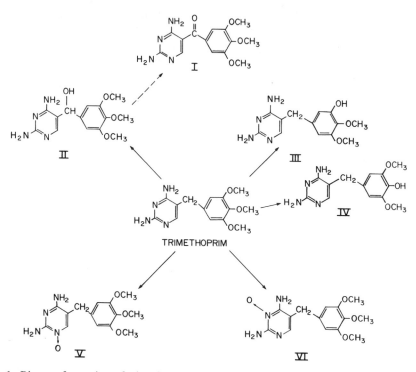

Fig. 1. Biotransformation of trimethoprim by various species. The 3- and 4-desmethyl metabolites are shown as free metabolites, but they are excreted mainly as sulfate or glucuronide conjugates. I 2,4-diamino-5-(3,4,5-trimethoxybenzoyl)pyrimidine; II α-(2,4-diamino-5-pyrimidyl)-3,4,5-trimethoxybenzyl alcohol; III 2,4-diamino-5-(3-hydroxy-4,5-dimethoxybenzyl)pyrimidine; IV 2,4-diamino-5-(4-hydroxy-3,5-dimethoxybenzyl)pyrimidine; V 2,4-diamino-5-(3,4,5-trimethoxybenzyl)pyrimidine-1-oxide; VI 2,4-diamino-5-(3,4,5-trimethoxybenzyl)pyrimidine-3-oxide

trations of TMP and metabolites in six healthy volunteers following oral administration of 160 mg TMP and 800 mg SMX. They found that α-hydroxy-TMP was a minor metabolite and barely detectable in the urine of some individuals. A new metabolite, the TMP-3-oxide (VI, Fig. 1), was identified and quantitated. Their results showed that in male adults, 48% (range 29%–70%) of the TMP administered was excreted as unchanged drug in the first 24 h. Small quantities of free and conjugated metabolites were found; each of the N-oxides accounted for about 2% of the dose and the desmethyl metabolites (as conjugates) from 2% to 6% (Table 5).

A second study in humans explored whether the pattern of TMP metabolism remained the same during repeated treatment (Sigel et al. 1975a). During a 10-day period of treatment with TMP/SMX, 24-h urine samples from five male patients (ages 13–30 years) were collected on days 2, 5, 7, and 10. Although there was considerable variation between individuals, on the average, a high percentage (76% ±10%) of the TMP-related material in urine was unchanged drug (Table 6). The metabolites accounted for 1.9% (1-oxide), 2.5% (3-oxide), 8.5% (3-desmethyl), and 10.9% (4-desmethyl) of the TMP-related material in urine. For each individual, the relative amounts of TMP or metabolites did not vary significantly during

Table 5. Average cumulative urinary excretion (24 h) of TMP and metabolites[a] for six healthy male subjects following a single oral dose of TMP (160 mg)/SMX (800 mg)

Subject	TMP	3-Desmethyl	4-Desmethyl	1-Oxide	3-Oxide	Total excreted (%)	Fraction excreted as intact TMP (%)
1	56.5	6.1	1.3	1.9	2.6	68.4	82.6
2	35.6	8.0	1.5	1.3	1.6	48.0	74.0
3	28.9	4.7	3.0	1.8	1.7	40.1	72.1
4	70.4	6.5	3.1	1.3	1.1	82.4	85.4
5	50.6	7.9	4.3	1.5	1.3	65.6	77.1
6	47.7	4.4	1.4	2.0	2.5	58.0	82.2
Average	48.2 ± 14.8	6.3 ± 1.5	2.4 ± 1.2	1.6 ± 0.3	1.8 ± 0.6	60.3 ± 15.1	78.9 ± 5.3

[a] Data from SIGEL et al. (1975a)

Table 6. Average cumulative urinary excretion for 24 h urine collections[a] on four separate days for five male patients receiving TMP/SMX during a 10-day course of therapy

Patient	TMP	3-Desmethyl	4-Desmethyl	1-Oxide	3-Oxide
MT–57	89.2 ± 1.7	3.9 ± 0.6	3.4 ± 0.7	1.8 ± 0.4	1.5 ± 0.4
MT–37	89.9 ± 2.6	4.3 ± 0.3	7.6 ± 2.3	2.0 ± 0.2	3.2 ± 0.6
MT–67	64.8 ± 5.0	17.4 ± 2.0	14.0 ± 2.8	1.8 ± 0.4	1.9 ± 0.4
MT–68	68.9 ± 6.1	8.6 ± 1.9	15.4 ± 5.2	2.9 ± 0.9	4.5 ± 2.4
MT–33	74.8 ± 4.8	8.5 ± 0.8	14.4 ± 4.6	0.75 ± 0.3	1.6 ± 0.3
Average	76.1 ± 10	8.5 ± 5.0	10.9 ± 5.0	1.86 ± 0.8	2.5 ± 1.3

[a] Data from SIGEL et al. (1975a)

the 10 days of therapy (mean relative standard deviation was 5.6% for TMP). Thus, in this study there was no evidence that repeated administration of TMP induced or altered its own metabolism.

The TMP metabolites have been tested for antibacterial activity. When assayed in vitro against *Escherichia coli*, streptococci, and staphylococci, the 3- and 4-desmethyl TMP metabolites and the 1-oxide showed about the same activity as TMP (RIEDER 1973). The α-hydroxy metabolite was inactive, and the 3-oxide was not tested. The 1-oxide metabolite and 4-desmethyl-TMP also showed some activity against *E. coli* in a mouse model (RIEDER 1973). Demonstration of activity in vivo for the 1-oxide can be explained by the observations of HUBBELL et al. (1978) that rats dosed orally with either TMP-1-oxide or TMP excrete a similar pattern of urinary metabolites. Thus, the 1-oxide is apparently reduced extensively in vivo to TMP, which is metabolized via its usual pathway. The possible role of gut flora has not been studied.

2. Tetroxoprim

A pharmacokinetic study with TXP (Fig. 2) in the dog indicated that the absolute bioavailability was 61%, which was suggestive of either incomplete absorption or

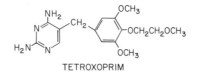

TETROXOPRIM

Fig. 2. Tetroxoprim, 2,4-diamino-5-[3,5-dimethoxy-4-(2-methoxyethoxy)benzyl] pyrimidine

extensive first-pass metabolism (PRESLAR et al. 1980). In that study, following administration of TXP (5 mg/kg) to three dogs, the mean recovery of unmetabolized drug in the 24-h cummulative urine was $10.6\% \pm 1.23\%$. In contrast, after oral administration of TXP ^{14}C (200 mg) to human volunteers, 60.9% of the dose was excreted into the urine. About 91% was unmetabolized TXP and 9% was an unidentified polar metabolite designated UH-1 (KORN et al. 1979).

REEVES et al. (1979) compared antipyrine half-lives in two volunteers before and after 8 days of treatment with TXP and found no evidence for induction of metabolism. In the same study, the quantities of unchanged TXP excreted daily in the urine were shown to remain reasonably constant. Evidence for formation of a single metabolite (UR-1) by the rat was reported by VERGIN and FRITSCHI (1979).

3. Sulfamethoxazole

Although the biotransformation of SMX has been the subject of several studies in rats and humans, all of this work was done without the use of radioisotopes. Consequently, complete animal balance or detailed metabolism data for SMX have not been reported. The extent of metabolism of SMX by the rat was studied by KITAKAZE et al. (1973). SMX was administered alone and with TMP orally to male rats. In the first 48 h after a 100 mg/kg dose of SMX, 73.8% of the dose was excreted in urine; N^4-acetyl-SMX (I), SMX and a glucuronide metabolite (Fig. 3) accounted for 39.3%, 26.8%, and 7.7% of the excreted drug, respectively. When TMP (20 mg/kg) was administered with SMX, the fraction of the dose found in urine collected 0–48 h after the dose was increased to 82.3%; most of the additional SMX-related material was unmetabolized SMX.

The biotransformation of SMX in humans has been studied more extensively than in other animals (UEDA et al. 1972; RIEDER 1973). UEDA determined the amount of parent drug and each of the metabolites excreted in 72 h following oral doses of 1 g SMX to four subjects. The mean fraction of the dose excreted in 72 h was 86.5% of which $18.63\% \pm 3.99\%$ was intact drug. The major metabolite was the N^4-acetyl compound, which represented 61% of the total drug excreted. About 15% of the drug-related material in urine consisted of N-glucuronides. Two of these have been shown (Fig. 3) to be the N^1-glucuronide (V, 11.6%) and the ring N-glucuronide (VI, $\sim 2\%$). It is uncertain whether N^4-conjugates are formed. UEDA et al. (1971) also identified a minor urinary metabolite as 5-hydroxymethyl-3-sulfanilamidoisoxazole (III, Fig. 3).

RIEDER (1973) isolated the same metabolites, but in addition, found two minor metabolites, which were partially characterized. Subsequently, while analyzing urinary calculi that were shown by infrared spectral analysis to contain TMP/SMX-

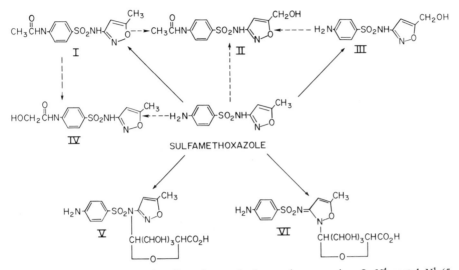

Fig. 3. Biotransformation of sulfamethoxazole by various species. I N^4-acetyl-N^1-(5-methyl-3-isoxazolyl)sulfanilamide; II N^4-acetyl-N^1-(5-hydroxymethyl-3-isoxazolyl)sulfanilamide; III N^1-(5-hydroxymethyl-3-isoxazolyl)sulfanilamide; IV N^4-glycolyl-N^1-(5-methyl-3-isoxazolyl)sulfanilamide; V N^1-(5-methyl-3-isoxazolyl)sulfanilamide-N^1-glucuronide; VI N^1-(5-methyl-3-isoxazolyl)sulfanilamide-2'-glucuronide

related material, WOOLLEY et al. (1980 b) isolated and identified two novel SMX metabolites that had similar properties to the compounds described by RIEDER (1973). In addition to N^4-acetyl-SMX, which accounted for 65% of the mass of the crystalline material, they found SMX, the 5-hydroxymethyl metabolite and two new metabolites, N^4-glycolyl-SMX (IV) and the N^4-acetyl-5-hydroxymethyl metabolite (II, Fig. 3). The last four compounds each accounted for <2% of the mass of the calculi. Of the known SMX metabolites, the 5-hydroxymethyl metabolite is the only compound that may contribute to the bacteriostatic activity (RIEDER 1973).

4. Sulfadiazine

The metabolism of SDZ by humans and other animals has been the subject of many studies since 1940 when the compound was first synthesized, but until 1978 all of the work was done without the use of radioisotopes. In the earlier work, UNO et al. (1963) and UNO and SEKINE (1966) established that the major metabolite of SDZ in human urine was N^4-acetyl-SDZ (III, Fig. 4). In addition, they identified small amounts of the N^4-glucuronide (VIII), N^4-sulfonate (VII), and sulfanilamide. ATEF and NIELSEN (1975) studied the biotransformation of SDZ in goats, and established that a major metabolite was 2-sulfanilamido-4-hydroxypyrimidine (I, Fig. 4, ~15% in urine).

In the first study reported using radiolabeled drug, WOOLLEY and SIGEL (1979) elucidated the metabolic pathway for SDZ administered to the rat, alone or along with TMP. Following a single oral dose (30 mg/kg) of SDZ ^{35}S/TMP (5/1, W/W),

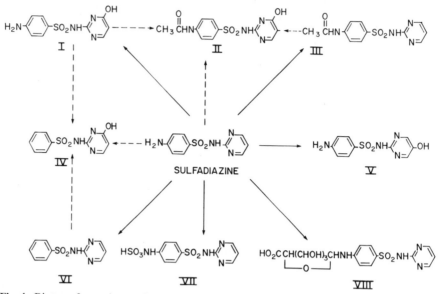

Fig. 4. Biotransformation of sulfadiazine by various species. I N^1-2-(4-hydroxy-pyrimidinyl)sulfanilamide; II N^4-acetyl-N^1-2-(4-hydroxypyrimidinyl)sulfanilamide; III N^4-acetyl-N^1-2-pyrimidinylsulfanilamide; IV N^1-2-(4-hydroxypyrimidinyl)benzenesulfon-amide; V N^1-2-(5-hydroxypyrimidinyl)sulfanilamide; VI N^1-2-pyrimidinylbenzenesulfon-amide; VII N^4-sulfonate-N^1-2-pyrimidinylsulfanilamide; VIII, N^4-glucuronide-N^1-2-pyrimidinylsulfanilamide

87% of the radioactivity was found in urine and 15% in feces. SDZ and N^4-acetyl-SDZ accounted for 56% and 19% of the radioactivity in urine in the first 24 h after the dose. The only other major metabolite (> 5% of the radioactivity in urine) was the N^4-glucuronide. In addition, three minor metabolites were identified as N^4-acetyl-2-sulfanil-amido-4-hydroxypyrimidine (II, Fig. 4), 2-sulfanilamido-4-hy-droxypyrimidine, and 2-sulfanilamido-5-hydroxypyrimidine (V, Fig. 4). The pres-ence of TMP did not significantly alter the excretion pattern for SDZ or its metab-olites.

Disposition studies with SDZ ^{14}C in the neonatal calf by WOOLLEY et al. (1980c) revealed a novel pathway for biotransformation of sulfonamides. Two healthy male calves ($\sim$40 kg) received oral doses of SDZ ^{14}C (1 g) and TMP (0.2 g) for 5 days consecutively. The calves were killed 14 days after the last dose. Analysis of tissue, plasma, and urine extracts established the presence of SDZ, N^4-acetyl-SDZ, 4-hydroxy-SDZ, and N^4-acetyl-4-hydroxy-SDZ and two novel deaminated metabolites shown to be 2-benzenesulfonamidopyrimidine (VI, Fig. 4) and 2-ben-zenesulfonamido-4-hydroxypyrimidine (IV, Fig. 4). It was found that 87% of the dose was excreted in the urine, with SDZ and N^4-acetyl-SDZ accounting for 16% and 42% of the dose. The other four metabolites accounted for < 5% of the dose.

Perhaps the most important observation in the study was that even though the amount of desamino-SDZ excreted in urine represented less than 1% of the SDZ dose, it accounted for most of the solvent-extractable radioactivity when total SDZ ^{14}C residues approached tolerance levels. Thus, in this case, most of the residue would not be detected by the widely used Bratton–Marshall surveillance method for sulfonamides, which is based upon the presence of the aromatic amino group. The relevance of this observation was underscored by the identification of desaminosulfamethazine as a minor metabolite in muscle from pigs killed 24 h after receiving a single oral dose of sulfamethazine ^{14}C, one of the most widely used sulfonamides in animal husbandry (PAULSON and STRUBLE 1980).

C. Drug Assay Methods

Several analytical procedures have been reported that are applicable to the measurement of TMP, related benzylpyrimidines, or sulfonamide concentrations in biologic samples. The most commonly used procedures are outlined in this section, and reference is made to some additional methods.

I. Trimethoprim and Related Benzylpyrimidines

1. Spectrofluorometric Methods

Analytical procedures based upon spectrofluorometric measurements are probably the most widely used methods for measuring TMP. The first procedure was reported by SCHWARTZ and ZIEGLER (1969) and involved a chloroform extraction of TMP from biologic fluids at an alkaline pH, followed by back-extraction into dilute sulfuric acid and oxidation of TMP to trimethoxybenzoic acid with alkaline permanganate. The trimethoxybenzoic acid is extracted into chloroform, and the fluorescence of the resulting solution is measured in a spectrofluorometer. The limit of sensitivity is about 50 ng/ml plasma. The method is not absolutely specific since TMP metabolites can contribute to the fluorescence. A semiautomated spectrofluorometric method based upon this procedure has been reported by KAPLAN et al. (1973 b). LICHTENWALNER et al. (1979) simplified the procedure by eliminating the potassium permanganate oxidation and extended the method so that SMX concentrations could be measured in the same samples. They found that TMP concentrations in the range of 0.5–40 µg/ml serum could be measured directly in the initial chloroform extract by irradiating the sample with an excitation wavelength of 295 nm and measuring the emitted fluorescence at 330 nm. To measure SMX concentrations, the aqueous fraction was adjusted to pH 2 and extracted with butyl chloride. The quantity of SMX (over the range of 1–400 µg/ml serum) in the organic extract is measured by fluorometry by exciting the sample at 295 nm and measuring the relative intensity at 330 nm.

2. Quantitative Thin Layer Chromatography

TMP and its major metabolites can be determined with thin layer chromatography (TLC) spectrodensitometry by measuring either the absorbance immediately after development of the TLC plate (SIGEL et al. 1974), or the fluorescence that appears on the plate after it is exposed to air and light (SIGEL and GRACE 1973). Quantities of TMP and metabolites above 0.2 µg can be scanned in about 24 h after application to the plate. For smaller amounts, 2–5 days are required for the intensity of fluorescence to reach a sufficient level for quantitation. The lower limits of detection for either measurement, fluorescence or absorbance, are comparable (0.01 μg), but fluorescence is more specific and is utilized for determinations of intact drug or metabolites extracted from urine or tissue. Following minor modifications of the TLC method for TMP, specific assays for other benzylpyrimidines, including TXP, have been developed and utilized for pharmacokinetic studies (ROTH et al. 1981).

3. High Pressure Liquid Chromatographic Methods

Several sensitive and specific assays using high pressure liquid chromatography (HPLC) for quantitation of TMP in biologic fluids have been reported. GAUTAM et al. (1978) and KLIMEK et al. (1980) extracted alkalinized plasma or urine samples with chloroform: 2-propanol (95: 5) or chloroform, respectively, evaporated the extracts, and analyzed portions of the residues by reversed-phase chromatography with fluorescence detection. KLIMEK et al. (1980) used procainamide as an internal standard and applied the method to determination of TMP concentrations in middle ear fluid as well. The lower limit of detection for both procedures was about 0.1 μg/ml. ASCALONE (1980) reported a similar HPLC method using a reversed-phase column and internal standardization, but he extended the procedure to include quantitation of SMX and N^4-acetyl-SMX following a single extraction with ethyl acetate of plasma or urine that had been adjusted to pH 6.8. WEINFELD and MACASIEB (1979) reported ten-fold greater sensitivity (~ 0.01 μg/ml blood, plasma, or urine) by HPLC of a chloroform extract on a microparticulate silica column with UV monitoring at 280 nm. Quantitation was accomplished using the peak height ratio of TMP to a reference standard, 2,4-diamino-5-(3,5-dimethoxy-4-methylbenzyl)pyrimidine.

4. Gas-Liquid Chromatographic Analysis

A method for determination of TMP concentrations in plasma and urine was reported by LAND et al. (1978). Following evaporation of a chloroform extract, the residue was analyzed by GLC using a nitrogen detector. 2,4-Diamino-5-(3,4-dibromophenyl)-6-methylpyrimidine was used as an internal standard. The lower limit of sensitivity is 1 ng TMP, and the method can be used routinely to measure plasma or urine concentrations down to 0.1 μg/ml.

5. Microbiologic Procedures

Known amounts of a suitably diluted TMP-bearing sample are pipetted into wells punched into a culture plate of agar medium inoculated with *Bacillus pumilus* (BUSHBY and HITCHINGS 1968). After incubation for 18 h at 28 °C, diameters of zones of inhibition resulting from the activity of the drug are measured and used for calculation of the quantity of TMP by comparison with zones obtained in the presence of TMP standards. The lower limit of quantitation for this method is about 0.02 μg/ml.

6. Other Methods

Additional procedures for assaying TMP are based upon spectrophotometry (Bushby and Hitchings 1968), differential pulse polarography (Brooks et al. 1973), and a combination of TLC and the microbiologic assay (Moncalvo et al. 1972).

II. Sulfonamides

Numerous analytical methods for measuring the quantities of the antibacterial sulfonamides in biologic samples have been reported. The most widely used procedures for SMX and SDZ are emphasized in this section.

1. Spectrophotometric Methods

Many adaptations of a colorimetric procedure based upon the Bratton–Marshall (BM) reaction have been reported (Bratton and Marshall 1939). Briefly, a diazonium derivative of the sulfonamide is prepared. The diazonium cation is reacted with a chromogenic coupling reagent, and the colored azo product is measured by absorption spectrophotometry. In general, BM procedures are nonspecific and measure the sulfonamides or metabolites that are not substituted at N-4. Rieder (1972) introduced a modification to the general procedure, which provides an estimate that more closely approximates the bacteriostatically active fraction; the BM reaction is run directly in an ethyl acetate extract of the nonhydrolyzed body fluid. The Rieder method is generally applicable to the routine determination of sulfonamide concentrations in body fluids and can be automated as described by Falk and Kelley (1965), Bye and Fox (1974), and Weinfeld and Lee (1979). With the latter method, 40 samples/h can be processed with a sensitivity limit of 2 µg/ml. Methods based upon the BM reaction are also widely used for surveillance of sulfonamide residues in milk and edible tissues (e.g., Tishler et al. 1968). As discussed previously, Lichtenwalner et al. (1979) have reported a method for extraction and measurement of SMX concentration in serum by spectrofluorometric detection without derivative formation.

2. Quantitative Thin Layer Chromatography

Concentrations of sulfonamides in biologic fluids and tissues can be measured specifically by simple and direct scanning spectrodensitometric methods (Sigel and Woolley 1979). Extracts of the biologic fluid or tissue are applied to a TLC plate, and following separation, the quantity of sulfonamide is determined by measuring the absorbance of the compound on the plate irradiated with UV light (Sigel et al. 1974). Quantities as low as 5 ng can be detected. Reaction of SDZ on the plate with fluorescamine furnishes a fluorescent compound that can be measured down to 0.2 ng (Sigel et al. 1975b). The latter technique has been useful for detection and quantitation of sulfonamide residues in the edible tissues of food-producing animals (Woolley et al. 1980a).

3. High Pressure Liquid Chromatographic Methods

The use of HPLC has been extensively studied for the determination of the concentrations of sulfonamides and their N^4-acetylated metabolites in biologic fluids and tissues. JOHNSON et al. (1975) reported an assay procedure for measurement of residues of sulfamethazine in bovine kidney, liver, muscle, and fat tissue. The method, which involved chromatographic separation of an extract on a Porasil B/C_{18} Bondapak column and UV detection, had a lower limit of sensitivity of 0.04 parts/10^6. SHARMA et al. (1976) reported a similar method that was useful for the separation and quantitative determination of sulfamethazine, sulfamerazine, sulfathiazole, and their N^4-acetylated metabolites isolated from cattle urine. GEOHL et al. (1978) extended the range of applications by reporting a method useful for the simultaneous determination of SDZ, sulfamerazine, and sulfamethazine in human serum. After precipitation of serum proteins with trichloroacetic acid, an aliquot of the supernatant was chromatographed using a reversed-phase microparticulate column. A linear calibration curve in the 1–30 µg/ml range was reported. SALVESEN and NORDBO (1979) reported a similar method for the measurement of the individual components in a triple sulfa combination and also conditions for simultaneous determination of SMX and its N^4-acetyl metabolite.

D. Conclusion

As discussed elsewhere (Chap. 1) TMP and the sulfonamides are synergistic as a result of inhibiting two different enzymatic reactions in the synthesis of tetrahydrofolic acid. Although in vitro, optimal TMP: sulfonamide concentration ratios can be determined for various pathogens, as long as both drugs are present at the infection site, synergism occurs. This observation has great practical significance because it means that bioavailability assessments based on serum concentrations alone give a limited indication of chemotherapeutic potential. It is important that both drugs reach the infection to achieve an additive effect, but it is not necessary or practical to match pharmacokinetic profiles to achieve specific concentration ratios. Because of the different distribution characteristics of TMP and the sulfonamides, the ratio of components in the dosage form or the serum concentration profiles do not provide an indication of the ratio of each component at the infection site. TMP, a weak base with moderate lipophilicity, has a relatively high volume of distribution, while the acidic and more polar sulfonamides are mainly central compartment drugs. As a consequence, tissue fluids provide a TMP reservoir which makes TMP available for potentiation of the more slowly eliminated sulfonamide. These observations have provided a rational basis for devising treatment schedules and extending clinical indications for this extremely useful chemotherapeutic combination.

References

Alexander F, Collett RA (1975) Trimethoprim in the horse. Equine Vet J 7:203–206

Andreasen F, Elsborg L, Husted S, Thomsen O (1978) Pharmacokinetics of sulfadiazine and trimethoprim in man. Eur J Clin Pharmacol 14:57–67

Anton AH (1973) Increasing activity of sulfonamides with displacing agents: a review. Ann NY Acad Sci 226:273–292

Ascalone V (1980) Assay of trimethoprim, sulfamethoxazole and its N_4-acetyl metabolite in biological fluids by high-pressure liquid chromatography. J High Res Chrom and Chrom Comm 3:261–264

Atef M, Nielsen P (1975) Metabolism of sulphadiazine in goats. Xenobiotica 5:167–172

Atef M, Al-Khayyat AA, Fahd K (1978) Pharmacokinetics and tissue distribution of trimethoprim in sheep. Zentralbl Veterinaermed 25(7):579–584

Atef M, Salem AA, Al-Samarrae SA, Zafer SA (1979) Ruminal and salivary concentration of some sulphonamides in cows and their effect in rumen flora. Res Vet Sci 27:9–14

Bergan T, Brodwall EK (1972) Kidney transport in man of sulfamethoxazole and trimethoprim. Chemotherapy 17:320–333

Bratton AC, Marshall EK (1939) A new coupling component for sulfanilamide determination. J Biol Chem 128:537–550

Brooks MA, de Silva JAF, D'Arconte LM (1973) Determination of 2,4-diamino-5-(3,4,5-trimethoxybenzyl)-pyrimidine (trimethoprim) in blood and urine by differential pulse polarography. Anal Chem 45:263–266

Bushby SRM, Hitchings GH (1968) Trimethoprim a sulfonamide potentiator. Br J Pharmacol Chemother 33:72–90

Bye A, Fox AFJ (1974) Modification of an automated method for measurement of sulfamethoxazole and its major metabolite in biological fluids. Clin Chem 20:288–293

Craig A, Kunin CM (1973) Distribution of trimethoprim-sulfamethoxazole in tissues of Rhesus monkeys. J Infect Dis [Suppl] 128:S575–S579

Davitiyananda D, Rasmussen F (1974a) Half-lives of sulfadoxine and trimethoprim after a single intravenous infusion in cows. Acta Vet Scand 15:356–365

Davitiyananda D, Rasmussen F (1974b) Mammary and renal excretion of sulfadoxine and trimethoprim in cows. Acta Vet Scand 15:340–355

Du Souich P, McLean AJ, Lalka D, Vicuna N, Chauhuri E, McNay JL (1978) Sulfadiazine handling in the rabbit. II. Mechanisms of nonlinear kinetics of elimination. J Pharmacol Exp Ther 207(1):228–235

Fair WR, Crane DB, Schiller N, Heston WDW (1979) A re-appraisal of treatment in chronic bacterial prostatitis. J Urol 121:437–441

Falk HB, Kelley RG (1965) An automated method for the determination of sulfonamides in plasma. Clin Chem 11:1045–1050

Frimodt-Möller H, Maigaard S, Madsen PO, Naber KG (1979) Co-trimazine distribution in the canine prostate. Infection [Suppl 4] 7:345–348

Fujihara M, Meshi T, Joh K, Yoshikawa M, Takahashi T, Sato Y (1975) Studies on sulfamethoxazole/trimethoprim transport of drugs into cerebrospinal fluid of rabbits. Pharmacometrics (Tokyo) 10:485–491

Gautam SR, Chungi VS, Bourne DWA, Munson JW (1978) HPLC assay for trimethoprim in plasma and urine. Anal Lett B 11:967–973

Goehl TJ, Mathur LK, Strum JD et al. (1978) Simple high-pressure liquid chromatographic determination of trisulfapyrimidines in human serum. J Pharm Sci 67:404–406

Hansen I (1979) Pharmacokinetic properties of co-trimoxazole. In: van der Waaij D, Verhoef J (Eds) New criteria for antimicrobial therapy. Excerpta Medica, Amsterdam, pp 158–164

Hoyme U, Baumueller A, Madsen PO (1978) Antibiotics excretion in canine vaginal and urethral secretions. J Pharm Sci 16:35–38

Hubbell JP, Henning ML, Grace ME, Nichol CA, Sigel CW (1978) N-oxide metabolites of the 2,4-diaminopyrimidine inhibitors of dihydrofolate reductase, trimethoprim, pyrimethamine, and metoprine. In: Garrod JW (ed) Biological oxidation of nitrogen. Elsevier/North-Holland Biomedical, Amsterdam, p 177

Johnson KL, Jeter DT, Claiborne RC (1975) High pressure liquid chromatographic determination of sulfamethazine in bovine tissue. J Pharm Sci 64:1657–1660

Kaplan SA, Weinfeld RE, Cotler S, Abruzzo CW, Alexander K (1970) Pharmacokinetic profile of trimethoprim in dog and man. J Pharm Sci 59:358–363

Kaplan SA, Weinfeld RE, Abruzzo CW, McFaden K, Jack ML, Weissman L (1973a) Pharmacokinetic profile of trimethoprim-sulfamethoxazole in man. J Infect Dis [Suppl] 128:547–555

Kaplan SA, Weinfeld RE, Lee TL (1973 b) Semiautomated spectrophotofluorometric determination of trimethoprim in biological fluids. J Pharm Sci 62:1865–1870

Kitakaze T, Ito K, Ogaway (1973) Absorption, distribution, excretion, and metabolism of sulfamethoxazole in rats. Chemotherapy 21:224–228

Klimek JJ, Nightingale C, Lehman WB, Quintiliani R (1980) Penetration characteristics of trimethoprim-sulfamethoxazole in middle ear fluid of patients with chronic serious otitis media. In: Nelson JD, Grassi C (eds) Current chemotherapy and infectious disease. American Society for Microbiology, Washington, DC, p 1146

Korn A, Ferber H, Hitzenberger G, Vergin H (1979) Biotransformation of tetroxoprim in man. J Antimicrob Chemother [Suppl B] 5:139–147

Kovacs J, Romvary A, Horvay MS (1976) Pharmacokinetics of various trimethoprim-sulphonamide combinations in newborn calves. Acta Vet Acad Sci Hung 26:73–93

Ladefoged O (1977) Pharmacokinetics of trimethoprim (TMP) in normal and febrile rabbits. Acta Pharmacol Toxicol (Copenh) 41:507–514

Ladefoged O (1979) Pharmacokinetics of antipyrene and trimethoprim in pigs with endotoxin-induced fever. J Vet Pharmacol Ther 2:209–214

Land G, Dean K, Bye A (1978) The gas-liquid chromatographic analysis of trimethoprim in plasma and urine. J Chromatogr 146:143–147

Lazaro A, Queralt J, Castells I, Ruiz J (1980) Comparative blood kinetics of trimethoprim and sulfamethoxazole in the beagle after intramuscular and oral administration of two different formulations. Drug Exp Clin Res 6:15–19

Lichtenwalner DM, Suh B, Lorber B, Sugar AM (1979) Rapid assay for determination of trimethoprim and sulfamethoxazole levels in serum by spectrofluorometry. Antimicrob Agents Chemother 16:579–583

Madsen PO, Kjaer TB, Baumueller A (1976) Prostatic tissue and fluid concentrations of trimethoprim and sulfamethoxazole. Urology 8(2):129–132

Männistö P, Tuomisto J, Saris N-E, Lehtinen T (1973) Pharmacokinetic studies with trimethoprim and different doses of sulfadiazine in healthy human subjects. Chemotherapy 19:289–298

Maigaard S, Frimodt-Möller N, Naber KG, Madsen PO (1979) Renal lymph and interstitial fluid concentration of co-trimazine: an experimental study in dogs. Infection [Suppl 4] 7:S 349–S 353

Meshi T, Sato Y (1972) Studies on sulfamethoxazole/trimethoprim. Absorption, distribution, excretion, and metabolism of trimethoprim in rat. Chem Pharm Bull 20:2079–2090

Moncalvo F, Bernareggi V, Bugada G, Cassola A, Levi G (1972) The pharmacokinetics of the sulphamethoxazole-trimethoprim combination in man: New method of determination and isolation. Gazz Med Ital 131:176

Morishita T, Yamazaki M, Yata N, Kamada A (1973) Studies on absorption of drugs. VIII. Physicochemical factors affecting the absorption of sulfonamides from the rat small intestine. Chem Pharm Bull 21:2309–2322

Nielsen P, Dalgaard L (1978) A sulfate metabolite of trimethoprim in goats and pigs. Xenobiotica 8:657–664

Nielsen P, Rasmussen F (1974) Relationships between molecular structure and excretion of drugs. Life Sci 17:1495–1512

Nielsen P, Rasmussen F (1975 a) Concentration of trimethoprim and sulphadoxine in tissues from goats and a cow. Acta Vet Scand 16:405–410

Nielsen P, Rasmussen F (1975 b) Half-life and renal excretion of trimethoprim in swine. Acta Pharmacol Toxicol (Copenh) 36:123–131

Nielsen P, Rasmussen F (1976) Elimination of trimethoprim, sulphadoxine and their metabolites in goats. Acta Pharmacol Toxicol (Copenh) 38:104–112

Nielsen P, Rasmussen F (1977) Half-life, apparent volume of distribution and protein-binding for some sulphonamides in cows. Res Vet Sci 22:205–208

Örtengren B, Magin L, Bergan T (1979) Development of sulfonamide-trimethoprim combinations for urinary tract infections. Infection [Suppl 4] 7:371–381

Paulson G, Struble C (1980) A unique deaminated metabolite of sulfamethazine [4-amino-N-(4,6-dimethyl-2-pyrimidinyl)benzenesulfonamide] in swine. Life Sci 27:1811–1817

Piercy DWT (1978) Distribution of trimethoprim/sulphadiazine in plasma, tissue and synovial fluids. Vet Rec 102:523–524

Preslar D, Grace ME, Sigel CW (1980) Pharmacokinetic studies in dogs with antibacterial 2,4-diaminobenzylpyrimidines, tetroxoprim, ethanesulfonate derivatives of trimethoprim, and related compounds. In: Nelson JD, Grassi C (eds) Current chemotherapy and infectious disease. The American Society for Microbiology, Washington, DC, p 428

Reber H, Wild F, Paris J (1963) Experimentelle Daten über das neue Sulfonamid 5-Methyl-3-Sulfanilamidoisoxazole (Ro 4-2130) beim Erwachsenen. Chemotherapia 6:273–284

Reeves DS, Ghilchek M (1970) Secretion of the antibacterial substance trimethoprim in the prostatic fluid of dogs. Br J Urol 42:66–72

Reeves DS, Boughall JM, Bywater MJ, Holt HA, Vergin H (1979) Pharmacokinetics of tetroxoprim and sulphadiazine in human volunteers. J Antimicrob Chemother [Suppl B] 5:119–138

Rieder J (1972) Quantitative determination of the bacteriostatically active fraction of sulfonamides and the sum of their inactive metabolites in the body fluids. Chemotherapy 17:1–21

Rieder J (1973) Metabolism and technique for assay of trimethoprim and sulfamethoxazole. J Infect Dis [Suppl] 128:567–573

Rieder J, Schwartz DE (1975) Pharmakinetik der Wirkstoffkombination Trimethoprim + Sulfamethoxazol bei Leberkranken im Vergleich zu Gesunden. Arzneim Forsch 25:656–666

Romvary A, Horvay MS (1976a) On the pharmacokinetics of sulphonamide + trimethoprim combination orally administered to geese. Acta Vet Acad Sci Hung 26:173–182

Romvary A, Horvay MS (1976b) Data on the pharmacokinetics of sulfonamid-trimethoprim combinations in sucking pigs. Zentralbl Veterinaermed [A] 23:781–792

Roth B, Strelitz JZ (1969) The protonation of 2,4-diaminopyrimidines. I. Dissociation constants and substituent effects. J Org Chem 34:821–836

Roth B, Strelitz JZ, Rauckman BS (1980) 2,4-Diamino-5-benzylpyrimidines and analogues as antibacterial agents. 2. C-Alkylation of pyrimidines with Mannich bases and application to the synthesis of trimethoprim and analogues. J Med Chem 23:379–384

Roth B, Aig E, Rauckman BS et al. (1981) 2,4-Diamino-5-benzylpyrimidines and analogues as antibacterial agents 5. 3',5'-dimethoxy-4'-substituted benzyl analogues of trimethoprim. J Med Chem 24:933–941

Salvesen B, Nordbo P (1979) HPLC determination of sulphanilamides and their acetyl metabolites in blood. Midd Norsk Farm Selsk 41:15–27

Schulz R (1972) Distribution and elimination of trimethoprim in pregnant and newborn rats. Naunyn-Schmiedebergs Arch Pharmacol 272:369–377

Schwartz DE, Rieder J (1970) Pharmacokinetics of sulfamethoxazole + trimethoprim in man and their distribution in the rat. Chemotherapy 15:337–355

Schwartz DE, Ziegler WH (1969) Assay and pharmacokinetics of trimethoprim in man and animals. Postgrad Med J [Suppl] 45:32–37

Schwartz DE, Vetter W, Englert G (1970) Trimethoprim metabolites in rat, dog, and man: qualitative and quantitative studies. Arzneim Forsch 20:1867–1871

Sharma JP, Perkins EG, Bevill RF (1976) High-pressure liquid chromatographic separation, identification, and determination of sulfa drugs and their metabolites in urine. J Pharm Sci 65:1606–1608

Sigel CW, Brent DA (1973) Identification of trimethoprim 3-oxide as a new urinary metabolite of trimethoprim in man. J Pharm Sci 62:694–695

Sigel CW, Grace ME (1973) A new fluorescence assay of trimethoprim and metabolites using quantitative thin-layer chromatography. J Chromatogr 80:111–116

Sigel CW, Woolley JL (1979) Sulfonamides. In: Touchstone JC, Sherma J (ed) Densitometry in thin layer chromatography. Wiley Interscience, New York, p 677

Sigel CW, Grace ME, Nichol CA (1973) Metabolism of trimethoprim in man and measurement of a new metabolite: a new fluorescence assay. J Infect Dis [Suppl] 128:580–583

Sigel CW, Grace ME, Nichol CA, Hitchings GH (1974) Specific TLC determination of trimethoprim and sulfamethoxazole in plasma. J Pharm Sci 63:1202–1205

Sigel CW, Grace ME, Nichol CA (1975a) Trimethoprim metabolism in man during repeated treatment with Septrin. 9th Int Congr Chemother, London 1975

Sigel CW, Woolley JL, Nichol CA (1975b) Specific TLC tissue residue determination of sulfadiazine following fluorescamine derivatization. J Pharm Sci 64:973–976

Sigel CW, Byars DVM, Divers TJ, Murch O, Preslar D (1981a) Serum concentrations of trimethoprim and sulfadiazine following oral paste administration to the horse. Am J Vet Res 42:2002–2005

Sigel CW, Ling GV, Bushby SRM, Woolley JL, Preslar D, Eure S (1981b) Pharmacokinetics of trimethoprim and sulfadiazine in the dog: Urine concentrations after oral administration. Am J Vet Res 42:996–1001

Stamey TA, Bushby SRM, Bragonje J (1973) The concentration of trimethoprim in prostatic fluid: nonionic diffusion or active transport. J Infect Dis [Suppl] 128:S686–S690

Tishler F, Sutter JL, Bathisk JN, Hagman HE (1968) Improved method for determination of sulfonamides in milk and tissues. J Agric Food Chem 16:50–53

Ueda M, Takegoshi I, Koizumi T (1971) Studies on metabolism of drugs. X. New metabolite of sulfisomezole in man. Chem Pharm Bull 19:2041–2045

Ueda M, Orita K, Koizumi T (1972) Studies on the metabolism of drugs. XIII. Quantitative separation of metabolites in human urine after oral administration of sulfisomezole and sulfaphenazole. Chem Pharm Bull 20:2047–2050

Uno T, Sekine Y (1966) Studies on the metabolism of sulfadiazine. II. Quantitative separation of excrements in the human urine after administration of sulfadiazine. Chem Pharm Bull 14:687–691

Uno T, Yasuda H, Sekine Y (1963) Metabolism of sulfadiazine. I. Separation and identification of products in human urine after its oral administration. Chem Pharm Bull 11:872–875

Vergin H, Fritschi E (1979) Pharmacokinetics of tetroxoprim and sulphadiazine in various species. J Antimicrob Chemother [Suppl B] 5:103–118

Vree TB, Hekster YA, Baars AM, Damsma JE, van der Kleijn E (1978) Pharmacokinetics of sulfamethoxazole in man: Effects of urinary pH and urine flow on metabolism and renal excretion of sulfamethoxazole and its metabolite N_4-acetylsulphamethaxozole. Clin Pharmacokinet 3:319–329

Weinfeld RE, Lee TL (1979) Simultaneous automated determination of free and total sulfisoxazole and sulfamethoxazole in plasma and urine. J Pharm Sci 68:1387–1392

Weinfeld RE, Macasieb TC (1979) Determination of trimethoprim in biological fluids by high-performance liquid chromatography. J Chromatogr 164:73–84

Welling PG, Craig WA, Amidon GL, Kunin CM (1973) Pharmacokinetics of trimethoprim and sulfamethoxazole in normal subjects and in patients with renal failure. J Infect Dis [Suppl] 128:S556–S566

Woolley JL, Sigel CW (1979) Metabolism and disposition by the rat of ^{35}S-sulfadiazine alone and in the presence of trimethoprim. Drug Metab Dispos 7(2):94–99

Woolley JL, Grace ME, Sigel CW (1980a) Surveillance of sulfonamide residues in food-producing animals. In: Touchstone JC, Rogers D (eds) Thin layer chromatography: quantitative environmental and clinical applications. Wiley Interscience, New York, pp 517–535

Woolley JL, Grace ME, Sigel CW (1980a) Surveillance of sulfonamide residues in food-producing animals. In: Touchstone JC, Rogers D (eds) Thin layer chromatography: quantitative environmental and clinical applications. Wiley Interscience, New York, pp 517–535

Woolley JL, Ragouzeous A, Brent DA, Sigel CW (1980b) Sulfonamide crystalluria: Isolation and identification of sulfamethoxazole and four metabolites in urinary calculi. In: Nelson JD, Grassi C (eds) Current chemotherapy and infectious disease. The American Society for Microbiology, Washington, DC, p 552

Woolley JL, Sigel CW, Wels CM (1980c) Novel deaminated sulfadiazine metabolites in neonatal calf tissue, plasma, and urine following oral treatment with ^{14}C-sulfadiazine. Life Sci 27:1819–1826

Yoshikawa M, Endo H, Takahashi T, Sato Y (1975) Sulfamethoxazole and trimethoprim. Studies on sulfamethoxazole/trimethoprim retention of drugs in rats. Pharmacometrics 10(3):475–483

Preclinical Toxicity Testing of Co-trimoxazole and Other Trimethoprim/Sulfonamide Combinations

A.D. DAYAN

A. Introduction

The early development of co-trimoxazole, the 1:5 combination of trimethoprim (TMP) and sulfamethoxazole (SMX), was in the late 1950's and early 1960's, before much of today's formalisation of a rigid pattern of toxicity testing of a new medicine. Initial interest lay in co-trimoxazole itself, and in its separate components, trimethoprim and sulfamethoxazole, but there have subsequently been studies of trimethoprim combined with other sulfonamides. It is not surprising, therefore, that the reports of toxicity tests are complex, nor that they are sometimes incomplete according to the standards of the 1980's, more reliance having been placed on observations in the target species, such as humans and domestic animals, rather than on the contrived circumstances of laboratory experiments.

For convenience, the available information has been divided according to the major categories of toxicity testing that would now be applied to a new medicinal substance: general pharmacodynamic actions, acute, subacute, and chronic toxicity tests, fertility, fetal toxicity, and teratology experiments, and mutagenicity. Most attention has been paid to results from laboratory animals, but relevant information from domestic animals has been included where it illuminates particular points. Preference has been given, too, to data already available in the scientific literature, and unpublished reports have been cited only when no other reference source was available.

B. General Pharmacodynamic Actions

I. Trimethoprim

Trimethoprim has little pharmacodynamic activity. For example, in the anaesthetised cat, only the very large dose of 100 mg/kg injected intravenously as a bolus produced severe hypotension and respiratory arrest, and smaller doses had no important effect on sympathetic or parasympathetic function (BUSHBY and HITCHINGS 1968). These actions were probably secondary to mechanical obstruction of the capillary bed by deposition of crystals of trimethoprim. No analgesic, mydriatic or sedative action was detected after subcutaneous injection of 5 mg/kg in mice. In isolated organ bath experiments, trimethoprim 10 µg/ml produced slight inhibition of the responses of isolated rat intestinal and uterine smooth muscle preparations to acetylcholine, histamine, and 5-hydroxytryptamine, but the response of rabbit colon to adrenaline was not affected (BUSHBY and HITCHINGS 1968).

Trimethoprim has recently been shown to depress the post-neural functional responsiveness in vitro of guinea-pig ileum and rabbit colon, but only at the very high concentration of approximately 50 µg/ml (LEES and PERCY 1981).

II. Trimethoprim and Sulfamoxole

The findings in a detailed set of pharmacodynamic investigations of trimethoprim and sulfamoxole (1:5) have been published by GRIES et al. (1976). Oral doses of 50 mg/kg of the combination caused diuresis and natriuresis in the rat, and some prolongation of barbiturate-induced sedation. Oral doses of the order of 50–100 mg/kg in the guinea-pig reduced heart rate and the force of cardiac contraction, and in the dog they lowered arterial blood pressure. None of these effects was large.

C. Acute Toxicity

There is little difference between the acute toxicity of trimethoprim and various sulfonamides in clinical use, either in terms of the median lethal dose (LD_{50}, Table 1) or in the pattern of clinical signs produced. Information about co-trimoxazole may be taken as a good guide to combinations of trimethoprim with sulfonamides other than sulfamethoxazole.

I. Trimethoprim, Sulfamethoxazole, and Co-trimoxazole

Brief numerical details are reported by BUSHBY and HITCHINGS (1968), ANON (1971), and a fuller clinical account by HONDA et al. (1973). In the acute toxicity studies of trimethoprim, lethal doses killed mice within 24 h after oral administration and within 35 min of intraperitoneal injection (HONDA et al. 1973). At autopsy, congestion of the lungs was seen. After subcutaneous injection there was some delayed loss of weight, and drug was seen still to be present at the injection site, even after 7 days. Effects in the rat were comparable, although there was definite depression and sedation of the animals shortly after high oral and intraperitoneal doses (HONDA et al. 1973).

Sulfamethoxazole in large oral or intraperitoneal doses produced depression, both of mice and rats, and extension of the limbs. At the highest dose level, respiratory difficulties and convulsions were sometimes seen. Autopsy revealed only congestion of the lungs and the presence of unabsorbed drug at the site of subcutaneous injection (HONDA et al. 1973).

The combination of trimethoprim and sulfamethoxazole (1:5) produced similar effects in rats and mice (HONDA et al. 1973). After very high doses, there was general depression, some animals lay prone with extension of their limbs, and occasionally, in higher dose groups, trembling or spasmodic muscle-jerking was seen. Death occurred within 24 h of oral administration, and about 3 h after intraperitoneal injection. Animals surviving beyond those times recovered and regained weight. Congestion of the lungs was found at necropsy of rats and mice that died after oral or intraperitoneal dosing.

Table 1. LD$_{50}$ of trimethoprim (TMP), sulfamethoxazole (SMX), co-trimoxazole (TMP:SMX 1:5), and for comparison, TMP/sulfamethoxypyrazine

Preparation	Species	Route[a]	LD$_{50}$ (mg/kg)[b]		References
			Males	Females	
TMP	Mouse	p.o.	> 2,000 mg/kg		BUSHBY and
		i.v.	~ 200 mg/kg		HITCHINGS (1968)
		p.o.	5,200 (4,200–6,400)	5,400 (4,500–6,500)	HONDA et al.
		i.p.	1,870 (1,520–2,480)	2,200 (1,500–3,220)	(1973)
		s.c.	> 5,000	> 5,000	
		p.o.	4,400 (3,140–6,150)		DE PASCALE et al. (1977)
	Rat	p.o.	2.1 g/kg		ANON (1971)
		p.o.	1,670 (1,390–2,005)	1,670 (1,360–2,060)	HONDA et al.
		i.p.	1,530 (1,300–1,805)	1,460 (1,227–1,737)	(1973)
		s.c.	> 5,000	> 5,000	
		p.o.	2,800 (2,380–3,290)		DE PASCALE et al. (1977)
SMX	Mouse	p.o.	3,900 (3,223–4,719)	3,471 (2,650–4,540)	HONDA et al.
		i.p.	2,300 (1,980–2,660)	2,450 (2,060–2,920)	(1973)
		s.c.	> 5,000	> 5,000	
	Rat	p.o.	8,640 (7,024–10,627)	8,400 (6,829–10,332)	HONDA et al.
		i.p.	2,790 (2,405–3,236)	2,690 (2,319–3,120)	(1973)
		s.c.	> 5,000	> 5,000	
TMP:SMX	Mouse	p.o.	> 1,000 mg/kg		BUSHBY
1:2	Rat	p.o.	> 1,000 mg/kg		(1970)
1:5	Mouse	p.o.	7,200 (5,950–8,700)	6,400 (5,420–7,550)	HONDA et al.
		i.p.	2,010 (1,890–2,140)	2,197 (2,000–2,420)	(1973)
		s.c.	> 3,000	> 3,000	
	Rat	p.o.	7,300 (6,600–8,074)	7,200 (5,420–7,550)	HONDA et al.
		i.p.	2,450 (2,130–2,818)	2,840 (1,414–2,392)	(1973)
		s.c.	> 3,000	> 3,000	
Sulfamethoxy-pyrazine	Mouse	p.o.	1,830 (1,520–2,200)		DE PASCALE
	Rat	p.o.	> 6,000		et al. (1977)
TMP:Sulfa-methoxy-pyrazine 5:4	Mouse	p.o.	3,500 (2,990–4,090)		DE PASCALE
	Rat	p.o.	3,550		et al. (1977)

[a] Abbreviations: i.p. = intraperitoneal; i.v. = intravenous; p.o. = oral; s.c. = subcutaneous
[b] Figures in parentheses are 95% confidence limits

II. Trimethoprim and Sulfamethoxypyridazine

For comparison, information about this combination (5:4) is included. Its clinical effects in oral and parenteral LD$_{50}$ tests were comparable to those of co-trimoxazole (DE PASCALE et al. 1977).

D. Subacute and Chronic Toxicity Tests

Toxicity tests of trimethoprim alone and in combination with various sulfonamides have been reported in several standard laboratory species, and some work in domestic animals has also been described.

I. Trimethoprim

The first account by BUSHBY and HITCHINGS in 1968 summarised studies subsequently reported in more detail by UDALL (1969). Additional data have subsequently become available (ITO et al. 1972a; HONDA et al. 1973).

1. Rats

Conventional studies have been described in Wistar rats, to whom trimethoprim 100 and 300 mg/kg was administered daily by gavage, for up to 6 months, to groups of ten males and females, in comparison with controls given only the inert vehicle (UDALL 1969). The animals received a conventional laboratory diet and were housed on grid bottom cages, which prevented coprophagy. The diet, as was common practice at that time, would probably have been formulated to contain folic acid approximately 1–2 mg/kg, but in practice it might have contained less, owing to breakdown on storage. The animals were 21 days old when treatment commenced, i.e. shortly after weaning, so they were exposed to very high doses of trimethoprim throughout most of the period of active growth.

There was no effect on growth or food consumption. Terminally, the peripheral blood picture was normal, including assessment of total erythrocyte, leucocyte, and platelet counts, the morphological appearances of blood cells and the differential white cell count. Blood chemistry, too, was not affected [electrolytes, glucose, urea, alanine transferase (ALT, formerly called SGOT), aspartate transferase (AST, formerly called SGPT), alkaline phosphatase, total protein, albumin and bilirubin]. At necropsy after 1 month, there was a possible slight change towards megaloblastic haemopoiesis in the bone marrow (BUSHBY and HITCHINGS 1968), but this was not confirmed at 6 months, when no abnormality related to treatment was found in the appearance and weight of the viscera, or in a very extensive histopathological survey of all the major organs and tissues.

A comprehensive experiment was done in which trimethoprim 30, 100, 200, 450, and 600 mg/kg was administered to Wistar rats, ten males and ten females in each group, daily by gavage for 30 days (HONDA et al. 1973). In addition to measurement of body weight and food consumption, urine and blood were examined terminally, followed by necropsy and histological survey of major organs. Survival, weight gain and food utilisation were generally similar in control and treated animals. The results of urinalysis and of a wide range of haematological and clinical chemistry tests did not show any consistent effect of treatment, only occasional abnormalities not related to dose. The suggestion by the authors, that trimethoprim had had a significant effect on red blood cells, is not supported by their own quantitative data in Table 2 of HONDA et al. (1973). At autopsy, there was a slight decrease in the absolute and relative weight of the liver in male and female rats given trimethoprim 450 mg kg^{-1} day^{-1}, but as there was no difference between animals given trimethoprim 600 mg kg^{-1} day^{-1} and the controls, this cannot be attributed to treatment. The histological appearances of the major organs and tissues were normal.

In a larger experiment of similar design, generally comparable results were obtained, but with certain additional, largely negative findings (ITO et al. 1972a). Trimethoprim 34.7, 69.5, 139, or 278 mg/kg was administered to Wistar rats, 6 days a week for 6 months; five rats in each group were bled for laboratory tests and killed after 12 weeks, and a further five in each group were kept without treatment for a further month at the end of the experiment, to study recovery from the effects seen. In addition to regular measurement of body weight and food consumption, urine was examined terminally, and extensive haematological and clinical chemical tests on blood were done, as well as necropsy and a limited histological survey of the principal viscera. Detailed results are given.

Growth and food consumption in the treated and control animals were similar, except that during the final recovery period rats in the 69.5 and 278 mg kg^{-1} day^{-1} dose groups did not show any gain in weight. However, as animals in the 139 mg kg^{-1} day^{-1} group did grow at the same rate as the controls, and as the differences were small, this is more likely to represent biological variation than a consequence of treatment. Scattered differences from controls were detected at various times in urine pH and electrolyte content, but there was no consistent pattern of abnormality.

A similar picture of occasional abnormalities in the haematological results was reported after 3 and 6 months of treatment, but none were consistent or related to dose, and a comparably disparate set of variations was found in recovery animals. Clinical chemical findings, too, fluctuated from time to time, but they also appeared to represent only random variation.

Bone marrow smears from all groups, taken at 3 and 6 months, and from recovery animals, all appeared normal. Of the findings at autopsy, the only consistent change was a small increase in the weight of the seminal vesicles in rats in the 278 mg kg^{-1} day^{-1} group, killed at 6 months, and after the recovery period. Histological examination showed only isolated abnormalities in a few animals, including controls, and so were not attributable to treatment. In conclusion, trimethoprim appears remarkably non-toxic in the rat, even after oral administration for up to 6 months, of up to 300 mg kg^{-1} day^{-1}. There has been no evidence of the usual consequences of disturbed folate metabolism.

2. Monkeys

Conventional toxicity tests lasting up to 6 months have been done in patas monkeys *(Erythrocebus patas)*, and there have been shorter term studies in that species and in rhesus monkeys *(Macaca mulatta)*, all giving similar results (BUSHBY and HITCHINGS 1968; UDALL 1969). All these animals received a conventional pelleted died, supplemented with fresh fruit. The pellets were formulated to contain folate up to 6 mg/kg, although the concentration on consumption was probably less. The fruit should have provided some additional folate.

Daily oral administration of trimethoprim up to 100 mg/kg, for up to 6 months, had no effect on general behaviour, survival or growth of patas monkeys, nor did it cause changes in the peripheral blood in a broad range of haematological and clinical chemistry tests. At autopsy, the appearances and weights of organs were normal. The sole consistent histopathological change at this dose level was in bone marrow smears, which showed slight maturation arrest, but no definite megaloblastic change. In the case of trimethoprim 50 mg kg^{-1} day^{-1} for 6 months, there was no effect, not even on bone marrow. However, trimethoprim 300 mg kg^{-1} day^{-1} caused generalised depression of haemopoiesis, which was manifested after 14 days by severe anaemia and pancytopenia in peripheral blood, and by hypoplasia of the bone marrow. Some animals were so severely affected that they died, probably because of their impaired defences against infection, and bleeding due to thrombocytopenia, but survivors recovered after four weeks without treatment (UDALL 1969).

The principal toxic effect of the high doses of trimethoprim was considered probably to respresent an effective state of folate deficiency, because of the known inhibition by trimethoprim of folate reductase, and the similarity of its effects to those of classical inhibitors of folate reductase. This mechanism was proved by an experiment in the patas monkey involving co-administration of trimethoprim and leucovorin (dihydrofolate or folinate; UDALL 1969). Four patas monkeys receiving trimethoprim 300 mg kg^{-1} day^{-1} alone survived a mean of 17.5 days before dying with bone marrow depression. Of four monkeys given trimethoprim 300 mg kg^{-1} day^{-1} plus leucovorin 2 mg kg^{-1} day^{-1} orally, the mean survival period was 56 days, and one monkey lived to the end of the experiment at 90 days. There was considerable protection and prevention of bone marrow suppression by leucovorin, which strongly suggests that the toxic effect of the high dose of trimethoprim was due to inhibition of folate reductase.

3. Other Species

There is little information. Oral trimethoprim 45 mg kg^{-1} day^{-1}, 6 days a week for 3 months, had no harmful effect in the dog, but trimethoprim 135 mg/kg in the same regimen caused inhibition of haemopoiesis and a fall in the red and white cell counts, haemoglobin and platelets (BUSHBY and HITCHINGS 1968).

II. Trimethoprim and Sulfamethoxazole

Most toxicity tests have employed trimethoprim and sulfamethoxazole (TMP/SMX) in the 1:5 ratio employed in co-trimoxazole, but some work has been done with different proportions. As the findings have been so similar, they have all been combined.

1. Rats

In the initial work by UDALL (1969), Wistar rats were dosed by gavage with TMP/SMX, in 1:2 or 1:5 ratio, daily for up to 6 months. As described in Sect. D.I.1, trimethoprim up to 300 mg kg^{-1} day^{-1} had no effect on growth, and sulfamethoxazole up to 1,200 mg/kg caused only slight retardation in weight gain after 1 month.

The combination of these two compounds (trimethoprim 300 mg kg^{-1} day^{-1} and sulphamethoxazole 1,200 mg kg^{-1} day^{-1}) produced definite retardation in weight gain after 14 days. The oestrus cycle became irregular after administration of this dose for 3 months. There was no change in the results of conventional clinical chemistry screening of the blood. On haematological examination, however, even after 1 month, the total leucocyte count and the fraction of polymorphs were reduced; the platelet count was not affected. Treatment for 6 months at this dose level caused a fall both in the erythrocyte and the platelet counts. At autopsy, the sole change in relative organ weight was enlargement of the thyroid, with loss of colloid and a tall follicular epithelium, and some fatty change in the liver.

A few differences were noted in a subsequent experiment in Wistar rats (HONDA et al. 1973), given TMP/SMX up to 450 + 2,250 mg kg^{-1} day^{-1} orally for 30 days. This dose caused death of males in 3 weeks and marked retardation of weight gain by females, whereas the next lowest dose level (300 + 1,500 mg kg^{-1} day^{-1}) produced only marked slowing of the growth of both sexes. This, but no lower daily dose, led to a slight fall in the terminal haemoglobin concentration and haematocrit, both in males and females. There was no change in the clinical chemistry screening, or in the results of urinalysis. At autopsy, a number of organs had abnormal absolute and relative weights in one or more groups, but there was no consistent pattern or trend with dose, except for significant enlargement of the thyroid (up to five-fold in males and females of the top dose group), and slight enlargement of the liver and suprarenals and slight shrinkage of the thymus and spleen in the same animals. Histologically, the thyroid appeared very active, with a tall columnar epithelium in the follicles and almost no visible colloid. In the pituitary there was a corresponding reduction in acidophils as stained by haematoxylin and eosin. The kidney, liver, bone marrow and other major viscera appeared normal.

A formal 6-month experiment in the rat has also been described (ITO et al. 1972b). Male Sprague–Dawley rats were dosed orally, 6 days a week for 6 months, with TMP/SMX (1:5) up to 1,200 mg/kg. A "recovery" group was included, members of which were left for 4 weeks without treatment at the end of the experiment.

Again, there was no striking effect of the treatment, but there were some differences in the findings, which may reasonably be attributed to biological variation. Thus, weight gain, even by the top dose group animals was transiently retarded. In those animals the red cell count, haemoglobin and haematocrit were slightly reduced after 6 months, but the bone marrow cell population was unaffected by treatment. There was no biochemical abnormality in the blood. Urine from top dose rats showed a slight tendency to a higher pH and a greater sodium concentration. Organ weights at necropsy were not consistently different from controls, except for some enlargement of the thyroid and liver in the top dose group. The only important histological finding was a reduction in the number of small follicles and of the general colloid content of the thyroid, i.e. appearances consistent with greater activity. An inconsistent scatter of changes was described in the recovery group of rats.

A further test in rats has been described (WISLAWSKA-ORLOWSKA et al. 1977), in which particular attention was paid to haematological and bone marrow changes in male Wistar rats given TMP/SMX (1:5 total amount 60, 600, and 1,950 mg kg^{-1} day^{-1}) by gavage daily for 30 days. There was no change in any of the haematological variables conventionally assayed in peripheral blood, nor in the differential white cell count or in the appearance of cells in stained blood films. A few megaloblasts (4%) were seen in femoral bone marrow from four of seven rats in the top dose group.

2. Rabbits

In a parallel haematological study to that in the rat, rabbits were given the same doses of co-trimoxazole for 30 days (Wislawska-Orlowska et al. 1977). Again, the only changes seen were trivial. It is interesting that sulfamethoxazole on its own had a similar effect on bone marrow and the thyroid in the rat when the high dose of 1,800 mg kg^{-1} day^{-1} was administered for 30 days (Honda et al. 1973).

3. Monkeys

In studies of patas (E. patas) and rhesus (M. mulatta) monkeys, with comparable doses and a similar experimental design to that employed in the rat, Udall (1969) noted some depression of bone marrow activity on prolonged administration of high doses of TMP/SMX (1:5), together with reduced mitotic activity in splenic germinal centres and slight fatty liver. There was no laboratory or pathological evidence of abnormality of the thyroid, bone marrow or kidneys, not even after daily oral treatment for 6 months.

E. Combinations of Trimethoprim and Other Sulfonamides

The overall toxicological pattern has been similar in all the available reports, and has been dominated by the sulfonamide moiety.

I. Trimethoprim and Sulfafurazole

The earliest account (Bushby and Hitchings 1968) notes death of monkeys owing to neutropenia and lymphopenia, and fatal pancytopenia in rats, given oral trimethoprim plus sulfafurazole: monkeys 100 + 400 mg/kg, rats 300 + 1,200 mg/ kg, daily for up to 6 months. The monkeys died after 50 days, but the rats survived for 6 months. Lower doses had no particular effect.

II. Trimethoprim and Sulfadiazine

Toxicity tests on the combination of trimethoprim and sulfadiazine in the ratio 1:5 have been reported for the dog and cat (Craig and White 1976). Dogs were given a total dose of 300 mg/kg/day, i.e. ten times the recommended therapeutic dose, for 20 consecutive days, using tablets administered just before the morning feed. Four 2-month-old puppies and four adult dogs were used. Intensive clinical observation and monitoring of peripheral blood for haematological and chemical changes did not reveal any effect, and the puppies grew at a normal rate.

In a further test in the dog, doses of 15 and 45 mg kg^{-1} day^{-1} were administered orally for 8 weeks (Lording and Bellamy 1978). The low dose had no toxic effect clinically or in multiple laboratory tests, but the high dose produced moderate pancytopenia and uraemia after about 4–6 weeks, returning towards normal after a treatment-free recovery period of 5 weeks. At all times, the bone marrow appeared normal.

This combination was more toxic in the cat (CRAIG and WHITE 1976). Three 5-month-old cats were given total doses of 43–57, 97–104, or 300 mg kg^{-1} day^{-1} for 20–30 days, and three adult cats were given 30–37 mg kg^{-1} day^{-1} for 30 days. The toxic effects of lethargy and anorexia were seen only in the animals receiving 300 mg kg^{-1} day^{-1}, from about the fourth dose onwards. One adult cat died from viral pneumonia on day 17, but two others survived the full 20 days of treatment, after which they rapidly recovered. All three animals showed progressive anaemia and leucopenia in the last week of treatment, with falls in haemoglobin and total leucocyte count of 30%–60%, and a four-fold rise in serum urea. In the two survivors, all these variables had returned to normal after 16 days without treatment.

III. Trimethoprim and Sulfamoxole

The results of standard toxicity tests of the 1:5 combination have been described (LAGLER et al. 1976). It has low acute toxicity; LD$_{50}$ oral > 12,000 mg/kg in the mouse > 14,000 mg/kg in the rat and > 1,000 mg/kg in the dog; intraperitoneal LD$_{50}$ in rat and mouse 2,000 mg/kg.

In a 4-week oral toxicity test in Wistar rats, only the top dose (total 600 mg kg^{-1} day^{-1}) caused marked slowing of weight gain. Haematological and clinical chemistry screening tests on blood did not reveal any abnormality. The sole pathological finding was of hyperactivity of the thyroid and anterior pituitary thyrotroph cells, again only in animals in the highest dose group. The changes disappeared after a 6 week recovery period.

In beagles, 180 mg kg^{-1} day^{-1} orally for 4 weeks led to loss of weight and to a slight increase in serum alkaline phosphatase and ALT, and the 600 mg kg^{-1} day^{-1} dose had the same effects, but to a greater degree. Histological examination showed similar changes in the thyroid and pituitary, and in the highest dose group, small necrotic foci in the liver.

The changes both in rat and dog were identical to those produced by the same dose of sulfamoxole on its own. Similarly designed 6-month experiments in the rat and beagle are also described (LAGLER et al. 1976). Rats given 600 mg kg^{-1} day^{-1} showed severe reduction in weight gain (recoverable in animals kept without treatment after 6 months), an increase in serum ALT, and thrombocytopenia. Of the 30 animals at this dose level, 2 died prematurely. Lower doses had no toxicological effect. The anticipated pathological changes in the thyroid and anterior pituitary were seen.

In the dog, treatment with 180 mg kg^{-1} day^{-1} again led to a rise in serum alkaline phosphatase after 18 weeks and increased thyroid activity. The dose of 600 mg kg^{-1} day^{-1} caused premature death of all five animals, loss of weight, pancytopenia, generalised abnormalities in liver function tests, increased serum urea, histological features of grossly disturbed thyroid function, necrosis, and fatty change in the liver, and a small reduction in the weight of the testes.

IV. Trimethoprim and Sulfamethoxypyrazine

Like the other combinations, daily administration for 6 months of more than a certain dose (ratio 5:4, 135 mg/kg total) to the rat produced enlargement of the thyroid (DE PASCALE et al. 1977). Non-specific degeneration of the liver also occurred after administration of 450 mg kg^{-1} day^{-1}. Diverse haematological and clinical chemistry tests did not show consistent abnormalities.

Following a comparable experimental protocol, Göttingen minipigs (starting weight 15 kg) were dosed orally with the combination for 6 months. The dose of 36 mg kg^{-1} day^{-1} had no harmful effects on growth, the results of haematological and clinical chemistry tests or on the findings at autopsy. The higher dose of 120 mg kg^{-1} day^{-1} caused progressive failure of growth after 5 months, and 360 mg/kg led to severe weight loss and death after 6–7 weeks. There were variable haematological changes, with a tendency to anaemia and especially to leucopenia, most marked in top dose animals, and a striking rise in AST in the two higher dose groups – up to an eight-fold increase by 120 days in pigs given 120 mg kg^{-1} day^{-1}. The principal findings at autopsy in animals given either 120 or 360 mg kg^{-1} day^{-1}, were widespread haemorrhages in the viscera, attributed to thrombocytopenia, hyperactivity of the thyroid, which was enlarged, and non-specific hepatic damage.

F. Special Studies of the Thyroid and Trimethoprim/Sulfonamide Combinations

A consistent finding in all species given large doses of trimethoprim plus a sulfonamide has been an increase in the weight of the thyroid, histological signs of hyperactivity, namely, loss of colloid and unusually tall columnar cells lining the follicles, and sometimes hyperplasia of thyrotroph cells in the anterior pituitary (e.g. UDALL 1969; KOBAYASHI et al. 1973; SWARM et al. 1973; DE PASCALE et al. 1977; LAGLER et al. 1976; LORDING and BELLAMY 1978). Most or all of this effect may be attributed to the sulfonamide component.

The production of dose-related thyroid hyperplasia, which sometimes progressed to frank nodule formation and even to metastasising thyroid carcinoma, has been described in the rat (SWARM et al. 1973) after administration of sulfamethoxazole 300–600 mg kg^{-1} day^{-1}. Hyperplasia was apparent after 13 weeks, and it became progressively more severe up to the end of the experiment at 52–60 weeks. Co-administration of trimethoprim (1:5 ratio) had no apparent effect on this phenomenon. Regression of the hyperplasia occurred after 7–20 weeks of a treatment-free regime.

In the rhesus monkey, TMP/SMX (60 + 300 mg kg^{-1} day^{-1}) for up to 52 weeks had no effect on thyroid weight, or on its histological appearance (SWARM et al. 1973). There is extensive evidence that the goitrogenic activity of sulfonamides is only seen in certain species, e.g. rat, mouse and dog, and not in others, e.g. guinea-pig and monkey (reviewed by SWARM et al. 1973). Humans, too are relatively insensitive to this activity. The species differences may reflect variation in the pharmacokinetics of the sulfonamides, but other factors may be involved, too, probably including the innate properties of thyroidal enzyme systems. In the majority of instances this effect has been attributed to the well-known effect of sulfonamides of blocking normal thyroidal iodine metabolism, so diminishing release of thyroxine (KOBAYASHI et al. 1973), and causing an increase in pituitary thyroid-stimulating hormone (TSH) output and consequent stimulation of thyroid epithelial cells.

Trimethoprim itself has not usually been considered to affect the thyroid. In a direct experiment, the effect of twice daily subcutaneous injection for 14 days in Wistar rats of trimethoprim 6 mg, sulfamethoxazole (15 or 30 mg) or the combination, on thyroidal iodine metabolism and hormone output was examined (KOBAYASHI et al. 1973). The sulfonamide alone and the combination caused a marked increase in thyroid weight and decreased ratio-iodine uptake by about 30% and 50%, respectively. Trimethoprim did not affect the weight of the thyroid, but it did increase that of the adrenals, and thyroidal radio-iodine uptake was diminished by about 15%. Further studies of the combination showed that the trimethoprim component had some additive effect on the action of the sulfonamide in inhibiting uptake and organification of iodine, possibly by enhancing blockade of thyroidal peroxidase by sulfonamides (KOBAYASHI et al. 1973).

G. Other Actions of Trimethoprim Alone or Combined with Sulfonamides

I. Co-trimoxazole and Immunosuppression

There is a brief report that co-trimoxazole can inhibit the incorporation of thymidine-^{3}H into DNA in phytohaemagglutinin-stimulated human lymphocytes in vitro (GAYLARDE and SARKANY 1972). Based on this work, it was claimed in a small study that clinical treatment of humans could slightly reduce the antibody response to tetanus toxoid (ARVILOMMI et al. 1972). There is also an unconfirmed report that co-trimoxazole 1 g/kg, either daily for 22 days, or on alternate days for 22 days, produced significantly prolonged survival of skin grafts from R strain to Wistar rats (GARAS et al. 1974). All these actions have been attributed to the "antifolate" effect of the combination, although without any direct evidence to support the hypothesis.

II. Local Effects of Intramuscular Injection of Trimethoprim and Various Sulfonamides

The local irritancy of intramuscular injections of proprietary brands of trimethoprim on its own, and combined with sulfadiazine or sulfadoxine, dissolved in glycerol formal, were compared in Landrace pigs by RASMUSSEN and SVENDSEN (1976). There was no particular difference between the effects of the different preparations or of the solvent alone. Residues of the active drugs were present at the injection site after 6 days, but after 30 days only sulfonamides were found there.

III. Co-trimoxazole and Renal Failure

It has been suggested that co-trimoxazole may affect renal function (KALOWSKI et al. 1974), although kidney damage in experimental animals has only been observed after administration of extremely high doses for a prolonged period (UDALL 1969). To investigate this suggestion, co-trimoxazole 13.8 and 27.6 mg kg^{-1} day^{-1} was administered for 7 days to male Wistar rats, in half of whom uraemia had previously been induced by surgical removal of $1^1/_3$ to $1^1/_2$ kidneys (ROBINSON et al. 1977). The treatment had no effect on plasma urea (controls 5.5, low dose group 12.3, high dose 15.4 mmol/l).

H. Reproductive Toxicology

During the development of co-trimoxazole, a number of experiments was done to examine the effects of trimethoprim and sulfamethoxazole, alone and in various combinations, on fertility, organogenesis and the growth and development of embryos and neonates born to treated rats and rabbits. Like the general toxicity testing, the nature of the studies was guided by scientific judgement and understanding of the action of TMP/SMX rather than by the detail of regulatory requirements, as the latter were only devised after much of the work had been completed. It is still convenient, however, to consider the results under the now conventional headings of fetal toxicity and fertility tests.

Tests of the combination of trimethoprim and alternative sulfonamides will also be described, as well as other related experiments.

I. Fetal Toxicity Tests

1. Rats

Many experiments were done to explore the effects of trimethoprim and sulfamethoxazole, alone and in various combinations, on fetal development. The results obtained by Dr. P. FRASER, who was responsible for much of the early work, are summarised in the following discussion and in Table 2 (FRASER 1968, 1969).

The experiments were of a conventional type, in which groups of ten or more pregnant Wistar rats, fed on a conventional diet of rat cake, were dosed by gavage on days 6–18 of gestation, or on the selected days of maximal sensitivity (days 8–11), with trimethoprim or sulfamethoxazole, alone or in combination. On day 20 of gestation, dams were killed, their uteri examined for implantation sites, etc. and the fetuses were examined externally, internally and for skeletal malformations.

It was shown that oral administration of low doses of trimethoprim or sulfamethoxazole throughout gestation had no harmful effect, but that extremely high doses produced a proportionate increase in the fetal death rate, and in a characteristic pattern of cleft palate, beaking of the snout, short or curly tail and sometimes limb malformations. The morphological pattern of the harmful effects resembled that produced by known antifolates, such as aminopterin and methotrexate (TUCHMANN-DUPLESSIS et al. 1959), which suggested that the effects of trimethoprim and sulfamethoxazole were due to their known, principal pharmacological activity of inhibition of dihydrofolate reductase.

Table 2. Fetal toxicity of orally administered TMP and SMX, alone or in combination, in Wistar rats, and effects of oral co-administration of leucovorin (folinic acid) (FRASER 1968, 1969)

	Control	TMP $(mg\,kg^{-1}/day^{-1})$ Days 8–16			SMX $(mg\,kg^{-1}/day^{-1})$ Days 8–16			TMP:SMX (1:5) $(mg\,kg^{-1}/day^{-1})$ Days 8–16			TMP 2,000 mg/kg + Leucovorin 2 mg/kg, day 11	+ 8 mg/kg	SMX 2,000 mg/kg + Leucovorin 8 mg/kg, days 11–13	TMP:SMX (1:5) 2,400 mg/kg + Leucovorin 8 mg/kg, days 11–13
		133	200	300	384	512	800	328	510	800				
Mean maternal weight gain (g)	106	99	81	66	91	84	76	90	100	79	69	77	68	76
Mean no. implantations	11	12	10	10	11	11	11	10	11	11	9	11	9	10
Mean no. normal fetuses	10	11	9	1	11	10	5	10	11	9	3	12	3	5
Deformed fetuses (%)	0	0	2	81	0	6	53	0	1	14	68	0	45	41
Fetal loss (%) (dead and deformed and resorptions)	6	4	2	86	0	1	48	5	5	19	71	3	70	47
Fetuses with cleft platate (%)	0	0	3	58	0	0	0	0	0	16	67	0	45	41
Beaked snout	0	0	2	40	0	0	0	0	0	2	60	0	0	0

This was explored by concurrent administration of folinic acid (leucovorin), which resulted in dose-related prevention of the fetotoxic effects of trimethoprim, as shown in Table 2, and considerable diminution in the effects of the combination of trimethoprim and sulfamethoxazole (1:5). Interestingly, the addition of leucovorin to a high dose of sulfamethoxazole may even have enhanced its fetotoxic action.

A preliminary assessment was also made of the role of dietary "folate" in counteracting the consequences of putative inhibition of dihydrofolate reductase by treatment with co-trimoxazole. The rat cake on which the animals were fed was known to be formulated with a nominal content of "total folates" of about 1 mg/kg, some of which might have been destroyed during manufacture. In several small tests, giving rats fresh grass ad libitum in addition to the normal diet greatly diminished the teratogenic effect of a high dose of co-trimoxazole, as did feeding them solely on a rabbit diet, which contained a higher concentration of total folate (probably 4–6 mg/kg).

A subsequent report by HELM et al. (1976) describes the effect of trimethoprim in a fetal toxicity test in the Wistar rat. Trimethoprim 100 mg kg^{-1} day^{-1} on days 8–15 of gestation led to a small increase in the number of resorptions and of fetal abnormalities, but 250 mg kg^{-1} day^{-1} resulted in a striking increase in resorptions and a mean incidence of abnormal fetuses of 20.5%. The principal malformations affected the maxillary and intermaxillary bones.

2. Rabbits

Work in New Zealand White rabbits involved natural mating, administration of test compounds by gavage on days 6–18 of pregnancy, and on day 28 autopsy of the dams, followed by external and internal examination of fetuses, and assessment of some of them as skeletal preparations (FRASER 1968). Only a very high dose of trimethoprim (62.5 mg kg^{-1} day^{-1}) or sulfamethoxazole (500 mg kg^{-1} day^{-1}) had a toxic effect, causing decreased maternal weight gain (Table 3). The 1:5 combination, in corresponding doses, had no fetotoxic action (Table 3).

II. Fertility Tests

1. Rats

Co-trimoxazole up to 600 mg kg^{-1} day^{-1} was administered orally to young male and female Wistar rats, daily for 60 days. Dosed animals were then mated with each other, and treatment of the females was continued throughout gestation and until 3 weeks post-partum (UDALL and WALDRON 1970a). Treatment had no effect on oestrus cycling. Qualitative assessment of the number and appearances of spermatozoa in vaginal smears after natural mating suggested a slight reduction in sperm count in females mated with males given 600 mg kg^{-1} day^{-1}, but not in those given 200 mg kg^{-1} day^{-1}; as the pregnancy rate in both groups was identical to that in the controls, this was not considered biologically important. Litter size and composition were similar in controls and dosed animals, but in the high dose group (600 mg kg^{-1} day^{-1}) there was a possible slight incrase in the number of still-born fetuses. Subsequent survival and development of the neonates up to weaning was normal.

Table 3. Fetal toxicity test in the New Zealand White Rabbit of orally administered TMP and SMX, alone and in 1:5 combination. (Fraser 1968)

	Con-trols	Treatment							
		TMP (mg kg^{-1}/day^{-1})			SMX (mg kg^{-1}/day^{-1})			TMP:SMX (1:5) mg kg^{-1}/day^{-1}	
		31.25	62.5	125	125	250	500	156	312
Mean weight gain (kg)	0.36	0.21	0.38	0.32	0.27	0.39	0.06	0.36	0.48
Mean no. implantations	11	8	12	10	10	9	7	10	10
Deformed fetuses (%)	4	3	9	0	2	2	5	0	1
Fetal loss (%)	11	24	25	16	43	18	38	13	16
Maternal death due to treatment (%)	0	0	0	0	0	17	50	0	0

2. Rabbits

In a comparable experiment in New Zealand White rabbits, co-trimoxazole 200 mg kg^{-1} day^{-1} was administered orally from 60 days before mating to 6 weeks post-partum (Udall and Waldron 1970b). Treatment had no effect on pregnancy rate, maternal weight gain, the numbers and composition of the litters, or on survival of the young.

3. Hamsters

Groups of ten female hamsters (species not stated) were given TMP/SMX (1:5) 16 or 32 mg/kg on day 8 of pregnancy, or 10 mg/kg on days 6, 8, and 10 (Haliniarz and Sikorski 1979). They were all killed on day 14, the numbers of live and dead fetuses were counted, and the fetuses were examined externally, as skeletal preparations and the kidney, liver, lungs, and brain were evaluated histologically. All three doses were considered to produce slight retardation of bodily development, and a reduction in the number of ossification centres in the occipital bone. All the changes, however, were slight, and their importance remains uncertain in the absence of any information about the pharmacokinetics and metabolism of trimethoprim and sulfamethoxazole in the hamster, and the lack of information about dietary folate intake by the dams.

4. Conclusions

Extremely high doses of co-trimoxazole (more than 1,000 mg kg^{-1} day^{-1}), or of its separate components, were able to cause maternal and fetal toxicity and a teratogenic effect in the rat. The morphological pattern of the fetal abnormalities, and their reversal by co-administration of leucovorin, or by dietary manipulation, strongly suggest that they are a consequence of inhibition of dihydrofolate reductase. In the rabbit, the sole effect of high dose treatment was maternal toxicity due to sulfamethoxazole. In neither species did co-trimoxazole affect fertility, or growth or development of neonates up to weaning.

5. Other Related Information

RONZONI et al. (1972), using groups of ten animals, administered co-trimoxazole 30 mg/kg to 60-day-old Sprague–Dawley rats by gavage daily for 14 days. At the end of treatment one testicle was removed and weighted, and after a further 10 days without treatment, the other testicle was similarly treated. Both testicles were examined histologically for relative activity of the different stages of spermatogenesis.

There was no change in the mean testicular weight after treatment, but some delay in spermatogenic maturation was claimed, as there appeared to be an excess of intermediate forms of spermatozoa. Complete recovery occurred after cessation of treatment. This report should be viewed in the light of several factors, including the failure to observe any such effect in previous studies, in which much larger quantities of co-trimoxazole were administered for longer periods, the lack of any effect in the more severe test of a fertility study, and employment of suboptimal histological technique, namely formalin fixation.

III. Reproductive Toxicity of Trimethoprim Combined with Other Sulfonamides

1. Trimethoprim and Sulfamoxole

The 1:5 combination was administered orally to Sprague–Dawley and Wistar rats, and to New Zealand White rabbits, in comprehensively described, conventional fetal toxicity tests (HELM et al. 1976). Standard fertility and peri-natal and postnatal development tests in the rat are also reported in the same paper. The rats were given the Altromin 1323 diet, or Eggersmann pellets, and the rabbits received "Ssniff" pellets. The sensitive period of organogenesis in the fetal toxicity tests was considered to be days 8–15 in the rat, and days 8–14 in the rabbit. During those periods administration of the combination up to 180 mg kg^{-1} day^{-1} had no effect. Doses of 420 mg kg^{-1} day^{-1} in Sprague–Dawley rats, and 600 mg kg^{-1} day^{-1} in Wistar rats, caused increased resorptions, reduced fetal weight gain, and a very significant incidence of morphological abnormalities in surviving fetuses, as well as diminished maternal weight gain. The fetal abnormalities comprised cleft palate, micrognathia and shortened limbs.

As similar effects were produced by trimethoprim 100 mg kg^{-1} day^{-1}, but not by sulfamoxole 500 mg kg^{-1} day^{-1}, it was concluded that the changes were secondary to inhibition of folate reductase by the trimethoprim moiety of the combination. In the rabbit, administration of the combination 600 mg kg^{-1} day^{-1} had no teratogenic action, although it did produce a slight increase in resorptions.

There was no effect on fertility in the Sprague–Dawley rat of oral administration of the combination up to 420 mg kg^{-1} day^{-1} for 10 weeks. Up to 600 mg kg^{-1} day^{-1} administered in the last 5 days of pregnancy and for the weeks of lactation had no effect on fetal and post-natal survival, and caused only minimal slowing of fetal growth.

2. Trimethoprim and Sulfamethoxypyrazine

A detailed account has been published of experiments in which Sprague–Dawley rats were dosed orally for 42 days before, to 6 days after mating, on days 6–15 of gestation, and from day 15 of gestation to the end of weaning. New Zealand White rabbits were treated on days 6–18 of pregnancy (DE PASCALE et al. 1979). The studies followed the conventional pattern of numbers of animals, methods of examination, etc.

In the fertility test, the most important effects of the 5:4 combination were produced by the highest dose employed, i.e. 450 mg kg^{-1} day^{-1}: slight reduction in weight gain by the males, and significant effects on fetuses, shown by a decreased number of corpora lutea and implantations, an increase in resorptions and general features of fetal immaturity.

The high dose of 350 mg kg^{-1} day^{-1} in the fetal toxicity test also produced diminution of fetal weight gain in the rat, and a low incidence of skeletal and visceral anomalies, and of cataract. The same dose had no particular harmful effect in the peri-natal and post-natal study. In the rabbit, only the top dose of 600 mg kg^{-1} day^{-1} caused a definite reduction in the number of viable fetuses.

J. Mutagenicity

Studies in bacteria and in human patients have been reported.

I. Point Mutation Tests in Bacteria

No effect of trimethoprim at up to a toxic concentration was found in standard Ames spot and plate tests, with and without Aroclor-induced S-9 hepatic microsomes, using *Salmonella typhimurium* TA 1535, 1537, 1538, 98, and 100 (GENTHER et al. 1977). In the same report trimethoprim was claimed to have produced mutations to folic acid independence and to rifampicin resistance in a strain of *Streptococcus faecium (faecalis)* (ATCC 8043) used to assay folate and antifolate activity in biological media. This suggestion cannot be accepted for several reasons, including failure to substantiate the mutagenic nature of the change in behaviour of the bacteria, and so to exclude phenocopying or some other impermanent effect, the lack of information about a dose–response relationship, and the implication that such a mutation, being a reverse change, would require the naturally occurring folate-dependent *S. faecium* to be at a selective disadvantage in nature. It appears more likely that, if the effect of trimethoprim had been fully characterised, it would have been found not to represent a true point mutation.

II. Human Cytogenetic Studies

Chromosomes from lymphocytes of patients treated with co-trimoxazole for various periods have been examined. No abnormality was seen in metaphase preparations, even after treatment for several years (Gebhart 1975; Stevenson et al. 1973). Very recently, an increased number of micronuclei was reported on examination of bone marrow cells from 12 patients treated with co-trimoxazole for urinary tract infection (Sørensen and Jensen 1981). Metaphase preparations made simultaneously from the same specimens of marrow did not show a significant increase in the number of structural aberrations.

It is difficult to evaluate the results, because of the paucity of essential information, but it should be noted that an abnormal incidence of micronuclei was found only in the 2 oldest of the 12 patients examined, the others appearing normal, and that no information is provided to exclude other possible causes of micronuclei, such as diagnostic X-rays or concurrent drug therapy. Because of the very irregular occurrence of the lesion, the discordance between micronuclear and chromosomal changes, the impossibility of excluding other causes and the lack of supporting evidence from other experiments, it appears quite improbable that the effect was a consequence of conventional co-trimoxazole therapy.

References

Anon (1971) Trimethoprim – sulphamethoxazole. Drugs 1:8–53

Arvilommi H, Vuori M, Salmi A (1972) Immunosuppression by co-trimoxazole. Br Med J 3:761–762

Bushby SRM (1970) Trimethoprim and sulphonamides: laboratory studies. S Afr Med J [Suppl] 44:3–10

Bushby SRM, Hitchings GH (1968) Trimethoprim, a sulphonamide potentiator. Br J Pharmacol Chemother 33:72–90

Craig GR, White G (1976) Studies in dogs and cats dosed with trimethoprim and sulphadiazine. Vet Rec 93:82–86

De Pascale V, Bamonte F, Craveri F, Crema A, Perucca E, Teggia-Droghi M (1977) Studio tossicologico dell associazione trimethoprim-sulfametossipirazine. Boll Chim Farm 116:155–170

De Pascale V, Crema A, Craveri F, Mandelli V (1979) Effetti dell associazione trimethoprim-sulfametossipirazine sulla riproduzione nel ratto e nel coniglio. Farmaco [Sci] 34:279–294

Fraser P (1968) Effects of trimethoprim, sulphamethoxazole and 1:2 and 1:4 mixtures of trimethoprim and sulphamethoxazole in pregnant animals. Wellcome Found Rep, P 6155. Wellcome Foundation, Beckenham, UK

Fraser P (1969) The effects of leucovorin on the teratogenicity of trimethoprim, sulphamethoxazole and a 1:5 mixture of trimethoprim and sulphamethoxazole in the primipara rat. Wellcome Found Rep P 6758. Wellcome Foundation, Beckenham, UK

Garas J, Economides F, Besbeas F, Fassoulaki A, Sirmakeshian T (1974) Septrin: effect on survival of skin allografts in rats. IRCS Med Sci Libr Compend 2:1247

Gaylarde PM, Sarkany I (1972) Suppression of thymidine uptake of lymphocytes by co-trimoxazole. Br Med J 3:144–146

Gebhart E (1975) Chromosomenuntersuchungen bei Bactrim-behandelten Kindern. Z Kinderheilkd 119:47–52

Genther CS, Schoeny RS, Loper JC, Smith CC (1977) Mutagenic studies of folic acid antagonists. Antimicrob Agents Chemother 12:84–92

Gries J, Kretzschmar R, Kuhne J, Neumann W, Osterloh G, Scherschlicht R, Worstmann W (1976) Pharmakologische Untersuchungen zur Verträglichkeit der Kombination Sulfamoxol/Trimethoprim (CN 3123), eines neuen Breitbandchemotherapeutikums. Arzneim Forsch 26:623–633

Haliniarz W, Sikorski R (1979) Evaluation of the embryotoxicity of Biseptol-Polfa on pregnant hamsters (in Polish). Ginekol Pol 50:481–486

Helm F, Kretzschmar R, Leuschner F, Neumann W (1976) Untersuchungen über den Einfluß der Kombination Sulfamoxol/Trimethoprim (CN 3123) auf Fertilität und Embryonalentwicklung an Ratten und Kaninchen. Arzneim Forsch 26:643–651

Honda K, Matuyama D, Mitarai H, Nakamura T, Ota E, Tejima Y (1973) Toxicological studies on sulpha-methoxazole-trimethoprim combination – acute and subacute toxicities (in Japanese). Chemotherapy 21:175–186

Ito R, Toida S, Matsuura S, Sasaki T, Tanihata T, Hidano T (1972a) Chronic toxicity of trimethoprim (in Japanese). J Med Soc Toho Univ 19:505–511

Ito R, Toida S, Matsuura S, Sasaki T, Tanihata T, Hidano T (1972b) Chronic toxicity of sulphamethoxazole-trimethoprim (5:1 mixture) in rats (in Japanese). Toho Igakkai Zasshi 19:673–679

Kalowski S, Nanra RS, Mathew TH, Kincaid-Smith P (1974) Deterioration in renal function in association with co-trimoxazole therapy. Prog Biochem Pharmacol 9:129–140

Kobayashi R, Harada A, Kanno Y, Yamada T (1973) Potentiation of goitrogenic action of sulfonamide by trimethoprim. Proc Soc Exp Biol Med 142:776–780

Lagler F, Kretzchmar R, Leuschner F, Foitzik E, Kiel H, Kuhne J, Neumann W (1976) Toxicologische Untersuchungen der Kombination Sulfamoxol/Trimethoprim (CN 3123), eines neuen Breitbandchemotherapeutikums. Arzneim Forsch 26:634–643

Lees GM, Percy WH (1981) Antibiotic-associated colitis: an in vitro investigation of the effects of antibiotics on intestinal motility. Br J Pharmacol 73:535–547

Lording PM, Bellamy JEC (1978) Trimethoprim and sulfadiazine: adverse effects of long-term administration in dogs. J Am Anim Hosp Assoc 14:410–417

Rasmussen F, Svendsen O (1976) Tissue damage and concentration at the injection site after intramuscular injection of chemotherapeutics and vehicles in pigs. Res Vet Sci 20:55–60

Robinson MF, Campbell GR, Craswell PR (1977) Co-trimoxazole in chronic renal failure – a controlled experiment in Wistar rats. Clin Toxicol 10:411–415

Ronzoni G, Grassetti F, Ngalikpima V, Alcini A, Alma R (1972) Arresto della spermatogenesi dopo somministrazione di alcuni antibiotici e chemioterapici comunemente usati in urologia. Chir Patol Sper 20:107–114

Sørensen PJ, Jensen MK (1981) Cytogenetic studies in patients treated with trimethoprim-sulphamethoxazole. Mutat Res 89:91–94

Stevenson AC, Clarke G, Patel CR, Hughes DTD (1973) Chromosomal studies in vivo and in vitro of trimethoprim and sulphamethoxazole (co-trimoxazole). Mutat Res 17:255–260

Swarm RL, Roberts GKS, Levy AC, Hines LR (1973) Observations on the thyroid gland in rats following the administration of sulphamethoxazole and trimethoprim. Toxicol Appl Pharmacol 24:351–363

Tuchmann-Duplessis H, Lefebvre-Boisselot J, Mercier-Parot L (1959) L'action teratogène de l'acide X-méthyl-folique sur diverses éspèces animales. Arch Fr Pediatr 15:509

Udall V (1969) Toxicology of sulphonamide-trimethoprim combinations. Postgrad Med J [Suppl] 45:42–45

Udall V, Waldron MM (1970a) Effects of trimethoprim-sulphamethoxazole (1:5 mixture) on reproduction in the rat. Wellcome Found Rep Pathol 70. Wellcome Foundation, Beckenham, U.K.

Udall V, Waldron MM (1970b) Effects of trimethoprim-sulphamethoxazole (1:5 mixture) on reproduction in the rabbit. Wellcome Found Rep Pathol 71. Wellcome Foundation, Beckenham, U.K.

Wislawska-Orlowska B, Polkowska-Kulesza K, Robak T, Mikuta M (1977) Effect of biseptol on the haematopoietic system of experimental animals (in Polish). Bromatol Chem Toksykol 10:181–185

Clinical Pharmacology

CHAPTER 9

Adverse Effects of Co-trimoxazole

D.H. LAWSON

A. Introduction

Although there is a large body of information available on the subject of adverse drug reactions, much of it is based on anecdotal case reports or uncontrolled studies of drug recipients. These studies often come to unwarranted conclusions or at least to conclusions which are difficult to interpret fully, resulting in considerable differences of opinion even amongst acknowledged experts (KOCH-WESER et al. 1977). In an attempt to circumvent some of the ambiguities inherent in many of the reports of adverse drug effects FEINSTEIN and his colleagues have proposed using a stepwise decision process for their operational assessment (KRAMER et al. 1979; HUTCHINSON et al. 1979; LEVENTHAL et al. 1979). Unfortunately such developments have little bearing on the present report since it is not possible using this technique to assess retrospectively the validity of most published studies of adverse reactions. Nevertheless it is to be hoped that approaches such as advocated by this group will be adopted in the future, so as to render interpretation of case reports of adverse reactions a much easier task.

The type of research strategy best suited to detecting and quantitating common adverse drug effects occurring shortly after exposure to a selected drug is the randomised controlled clinical trial with total event recording, i.e. where cohorts of recipients and non-recipients are followed until a definable end point is reached and records are kept of all events which occur in both groups during the period of observation. When a possible undesired effect is delayed, infrequent or occurs only after prolonged exposure to the study drug, this method of approach is unlikely to prove helpful and different techniques involving uncontrolled cohort studies, case-control studies or spontaneous reports to registries may be of greatest value (for general discussion of this topic see JICK 1977; LAWSON 1979).

In this chapter I shall place particular weight on the few studies which have incorporated control subjects; the anecdotal nature of many of the other studies cited should be appreciated fully. Greatest weight will be assigned to information which provides both numerator (reactor) and denominator (number exposed) data together with a reference population. Less valuable but often acceptable are frequency data, i.e. numerator and denominator figures in uncontrolled groups, and of least value is the situation where only numerator information is available without any clear idea of the denominator. I shall deal primarily with the most frequently used trimethoprim/sulfonamide combination – co-trimoxazole. A similar problem of adverse reactions is seen with other trimethoprim/sulfonamide combinations; any differences being solely due to toxicity resulting from the particular sulfonamide chosen.

The principal adverse effects attributed to trimethoprim/sulfamethoxazole (co-trimoxazole) in the early clinical trials and for the ensuing few years after marketing were alimentary upsets (involving mainly the upper gastrointestinal tract), skin reactions (usually mild but occasionally more severe as for example Stevens–Johnson syndrome and toxic epidermal necrolysis – Lyell's syndrome), and haematological upsets of varying severity (FRISCH 1973a; KOCH-WESER et al. 1971). In his report FRISCH, representing one of the major manufacturers of this drug combination, concluded that "clinical experience with the combination of trimethoprim-sulfamethoxazole does not give cause for any undue concern about its safety in the recommended dose." Since then a substantial body of experience in the use of this combination has been developed and at the same time incidents such as the practolol affair (FELIX and IVE 1974) and the undesired effects of hormone replacement therapy (ZIEL and FINKL 1975) have focused greater attention on adverse drug effects, particularly those of major severity occurring after long-term use of drugs. In keeping with this changing attitude the independent review tabloid *Drug and Therapeutics Bulletin* questioned whether this combination of sulfamethoxazole and trimethoprim, which had by 1977 attained world-wide sales of approximately 600 million standard treatment courses, may be "too toxic for minor infections?" (DRUGS AND THERAPEUTICS BULLETIN 1979). This chapter aims to review critically the published evidence on co-trimoxazole toxicity and provide a basis for conclusions as to the risks associated with this form of treatment.

Between 1968 and 1977, details of 1,419 adverse effects attributed to co-trimoxazole in 1,062 patients had been notified to one of the principal manufacturers of this compound (A.D. MUNRO-FAURE and D. RYCROFT 1979, personal communication). These reactions were collected mainly from the United Kingdom and Australasia and refer to unpublished case reports. The most frequent reactions reported were skin lesions (542 lesions in 434 patients), and haematological upsets (177 in 164 patients). Other conditions such as glossitis (49 patients), renal disorders (30 patients), jaundice (29 patients), and goitre (1 patient) were reported much less frequently.

More recently this compound has become available in Japan where a hospital-based 3-year surveillance programme has been undertaken on all newly marketed compounds. This study is being conducted in over 1,500 hospitals. During the period under review some 69,000 patients received co-trimoxazole of whom 7,340 reported some form of adverse effect (10%). The most frequent effects in this study of short-term co-trimoxazole use were upper alimentary symptoms (7.4%), diarrhoea (0.7%), skin rashes (1.1%), haematological disorders (0.1%), and hepatic disorders (0.1%). In this series 53 patients developed leucopenia and 6 thrombocytopenia. No patients developed toxic epidermal necrolysis but two had Stevens–Johnson syndrome (MINISTRY OF HEALTH AND WELFARE 1979).

Another source of information on reactions attributed to co-trimoxazole is the *Annual Report of the New Zealand Committee on Adverse Drug Reactions* (MCQUEEN 1974, 1975, 1976, 1977, 1978). Although this is a spontaneous reporting system and therefore provides only incomplete numerator data, strong efforts are made to encourage reporting, especially of serious reactions and reactions attributed to newly marketed products. Consequently the completeness of reporting in New Zealand appears to be somewhat higher than elsewhere. Over the period

1965–1977 the Committee received an average of 500 reports of adverse reactions annually. Since 1973, eight deaths have been associated with co-trimoxazole and a further 260 non-fatal reactions have been notified (some 44 annually). The principal causes of co-trimoxazole-attributed fatalities have been severe skin lesions (3), thrombocytopenia/pancytopenia (3), agranulocytosis (1), and disseminated intravascular coagulation (in a patient with underlying cancer). Most of the non-fatal cases reported have been allergic skin rashes, with signs of bone marrow depression infrequent (11 cases), and other conditions appearing rarely: angioneurotic oedema (6 patients), jaundice (2 patients), and anaphylaxis (2 patients).

In Sweden, all adverse drug reactions should be reported to the Adverse Drug Reaction Committee. During the years 1965–1975 a total of 11,596 reactions were reported (BÖTTIGER et al. 1979 a) in this country of 8.25 million inhabitants. The annual number of reports increased from 600–1,600 over the study interval. However the annual number of fatal reactions, 274 in all, has remained consistent at 25–30. Antibacterials comprised 21% of the fatal reactions attributed to drugs in this period, two fatal reactions being attributed to co-trimoxazole therapy.

B. Gastrointestinal Disorders

Alimentary upsets are commonly attributed to a wide variety of medications. Indeed in one Irish drug surveillance programme studying hospital subjects, some 30% of the reported reactions were related to the alimentary tract (HURWITZ and WADE 1969).

I. Upper Gastrointestinal Symptoms

The most frequent reaction attributed to co-trimoxazole is one of nausea and vomiting. These entities are extremely difficult to evaluate, being influenced by factors such as diet, stress, surroundings, illness, and presentation of medication (colour, taste, capsules, or tablets, etc.). Nevertheless they are important since they may influence a patient to continue or abandon an advised course of treatment. Because of the wide inter- and intra-individual variations in factors which predispose to nausea or vomiting, no precise quantitation of the risks of its occurring in any individual can easily be made. Sulfonamide mixtures are not amongst the list of drugs most likely to precipitate upper gastrointestinal symptoms. On average such symptoms were reported in about 1%–4% of patients in the early clinical trials. When it occurs the nausea does not appear to be centrally mediated and usually disappears rapidly even if treatment is continued.

In a prospective study of 649 hospitalised co-trimoxazole recipients participating in the Boston Collaborative Drug Surveillance Program, LAWSON and JICK (1978) reported an incidence of nausea, vomiting, and anorexia of 3.4%; such reactions being approximately twice as common in females than males and almost all occurring within the first 72 h of treatment. Glossitis, which was once noted regularly in co-trimoxazole recipients (FRISCH 1973 b) is now much less frequently reported; whether this is due to a true fall in incidence, a change in formulation or some other factor is unclear. It may occur as part of the rare Stevens–Johnson syndrome (see Sect. C) or in debilitated patients who develop oral candidiasis, a condition which has rarely been attributed to co-trimoxazole as to virtually all other antibacterial substances.

II. Lower Gastrointestinal Symptoms

Diarrhoea is a much rarer problem with co-trimoxazole than is nausea or vomiting. In the series cited the prevalence was 0.6%, a figure in accordance with that seen in the early clinical trial material and only one-sixth the prevalence of upper gastrointestinal tract symptomatology. The diarrhoea is rarely severe and need not warrant discontinuation of drug treatment. Superinfection particularly involving the alimentary tract and so presenting as diarrhoea, also appears rare in co-trimoxazole recipients. A severe bowel upset presenting with copious diarrhoea, pseudomembranous colitis, has been attributed to therapy with certain antibiotics, notably lincomycin and clindamycin. Cases of this disorder have been attributed to co-trimoxazole (ANDREJAK 1976; CAMERON and THOMAS 1977; RODDIS 1978). In 1978 *Clostridium difficile* and its toxin were found in patients suffering from pseudomembranous colitis (BARTLETT et al. 1978) and it is now generally accepted that this is the causative agent of the condition. It seems likely that any antimicrobial drug may suppress normal gut flora and so facilitate the growth of *C. difficile* if it is present in the local environment. There is a wide spectrum of severity of symptoms, the condition being most frequent in elderly hospitalised subjects. It may occur up to 4 weeks or more after even a short course of antibacterial therapy and is best treated with oral vancomycin and cessation of other antibacterial therapy. Since 1978 cases of pseudomembranous colitis have been attributed to virtually all antibacterial drugs in common use. To date there is no evidence to suggest that co-trimoxazole is associated with this condition more frequently than other antibiotics (EDITORIAL 1981).

C. Skin Disorders

A variety of skin lesions have been attributed to co-trimoxazole since its first release in 1968. Before attempting to review the evidence linking this drug with skin disease, it is appropriate to define clearly the types of skin lesions which have been described. These cover a wide spectrum of severity. In addition to the expected problem of relating drug exposure to skin event, we have the additional problem of inconstancy of nomenclature for skin eruptions. The major types of skin eruption attributed to trimethoprim-sulfonamide combinations are as follows:

1. *Exanthemata.* A spectrum of conditions varying from mild to potentially lethal (see Figs. 1–5).
a) Toxic erythema. A measles-like maculopapular or diffuse eruption (Fig. 1) which occurs early during treatment with a wide variety of drugs and is probably due to the Arthus reaction occurring in skin blood vessels. It is usually transient and fades within a few days. Pruritus is a moderately common accompaniment. Transient proteinuria may occur during the erythematous phase, indicating that the condition is not solely a skin lesion.

b) Erythema nodosum. A reaction of dermal blood vessels usually presenting as raised tender indurated lesions on the shins. The lesions enlarge, gradually turn purple and then involute, lesions at several stages being present at any one time. The condition may last up to 3 weeks or more. Although occurring in sarcoidosis and in streptococcal and tuberculous infections, drug-related cases are perhaps now the most common. The drugs frequently incriminated include sulfonamides and oral contraceptives.

c) Fixed drug eruption. A circumscribed erythematous lesion occurring at a fixed site whenever a particular drug is given to a susceptible individual.

d) Erythema multiforme. Multiple erythematous maculopapular eruptions most common on extensor surfaces of limbs. These are often self-limiting after 2–6 weeks and occur in association with many infections, both bacterial and viral. Drugs incriminated include barbiturates, hydantoins, and sulfonamides. If the lesions of erythema multiforme extend to become confluent and are associated with toxic symptoms of pyrexia and mucous membrane ulceration, particularly involving buccal mucosa but also genitalia and occasionally the conjunctiva, the conditions is sometimes referred to as the Stevens–Johnson syndrome (Fig. 2). This is frequently associated with urticaria and occasionally the bullae become haemorrhagic.

e) Lyell's syndrome. In this condition, variously described as acute epidermal necrolysis or scalded skin syndrome, the skin appears red and tender and the surface loosens to peel off in sheets (Fig. 3). The epidermis may strip if rubbed gently by an examining finger (Nikolski's sign). The affected area is usually extensive and although toxic accompaniments are common the condition often heals in a few days. Several factors have been incriminated in this condition (LYELL 1979), one of which is exposure to drugs, including barbiturates, phenylbutazone, sulfonamides, and penicillins. Less than one-third of cases seem to be drug-related.

2. Urticaria. Acute urticaria is usually manifest as wheals on any part of the body (Fig. 4). In its severest form it affects the neck and face and is referred to as angioneurotic oedema. It may be drug related or may occur for unknown reasons in viral infections where drugs are not given or indeed it may be idiopathic.

3. Exfoliative Dermatitis. This is a serious condition in which the entire skin surface becomes red and scaly and peels (Fig. 5). If severe, toxic manifestations which can progress to hypothermia and cardiac failure may occur. This condition is commoner in atopic subjects, in psoriatics and in subjects with lymphoproliferative disease. Many drugs including sulfonamides, phenylbutazone, and heavy metals have been incriminated in its aetiology.

4. Photodermatitis. Eczematous or urticarial eruptions on light-exposed surfaces which occur in porphyria and after use of certain drugs, including sulfonamides, diuretics, and oral contraceptives. The lesions are often persistent.

5. Necrotising Vasculitis. Purpuric, ulcerated or haemorrhagic blisters occurring in dependent or pressure areas and often thought to have an immunological basis. This condition may be quite persistent, even after putative causes have been removed.

Although in all these conditions, sulfonamides in general, including co-trimoxazole, have been incriminated as aetiological factors, all can occur spontaneously in the absence of drug therapy. Most can occur during the course of infections

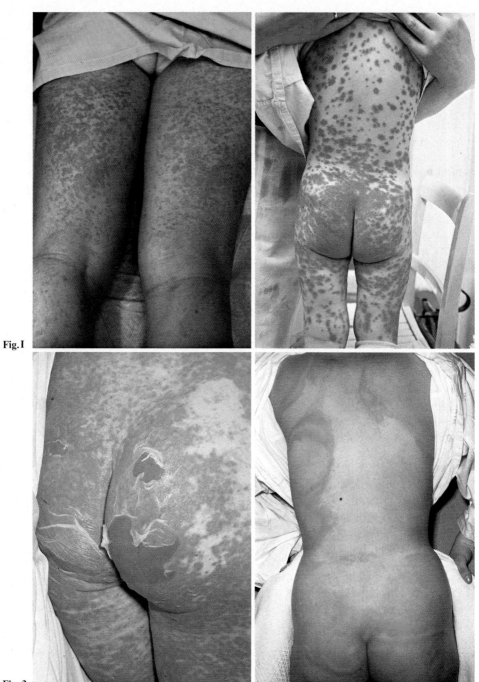

Fig. I

Fig. 1

Fig. 3

Fig.

Fig. I belongs to p. 280, Chap. 12

Fig. 1. Toxic erythema showing widespread maculopapular rash, most extensive on buttocks

Fig. 2. Stevens–Johnson syndrome showing involvement of buccal mucosa in ulcerative process with early crusting

Fig. 3. Toxic epidermal necrolysis (Lyell's syndrome) showing involvement primarily of buttocks against a background of toxic erythema. The tendency of the epidermis to peel off in sheets is clearly demonstrated

Fig. 4. Urticaria showing widespread wheals on buttocks and back

Fig. 5. Exfoliative dermatitis showing red scaly peeling skin

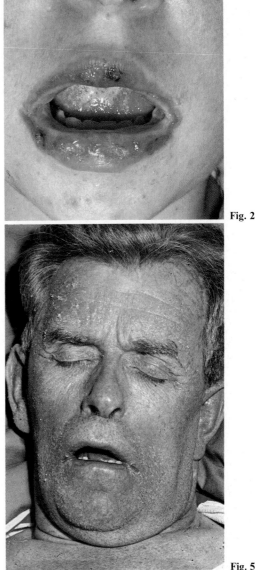

Fig. 2

Fig. 5

(usually viral) when drugs are not administered. No useful tests have been devised to aid in the search for the aetiology of such lesions. The most reliable guide is of course rechallenge with the suspect drug, but this may be dangerous even when the original lesion is mild. It is usually inadvisable and even when performed may prove unhelpful. Thus in attempting to assess whether a drug has a causative link with any skin eruption one is left to rely on

The history of previous contact or reactions to the agent involved

The timing of the reaction in relation to the drug's administration

The course of the reaction after withdrawal or continuation of the drug

A review of other concurrent and recently discontinued therapy

An understanding of the condition for which the drug therapy was initially commenced

In addition to the difficulties in attributing individual skin lesions to administered drugs, it should also be appreciated that any single drug can produce a wide variety of skin reactions in individual recipients. A good example of this is that described by BERGOEND et al. in 1968. These workers, faced with a large epidemic of cerebrospinal meningitis in Morocco, decided to give prophylactic sulfonamides to some 110,000 residents of Marrakech and Rabat, approximately one-third receiving only a single dose of sulfomethoxine and the remaining two-thirds receiving several doses. The risk of skin rashes in this population related to dose and duration of therapy; there being 997 reactions in 72,485 persons receiving multiple doses. Reactions to this sulfonamide were most common in the third week of treatment and showed a wide range from mild toxic erythema, through severe erythema multiforme, alone or with associated mucus membrane abnormalities (Stevens–Johnson syndrome), to toxic epidermal necrolysis (Lyell's syndrome). Moreover in some patients with severe skin lesions, the clinical appearances varied from day to day so that at one time or in one site the lesion appeared more like erythema multiforme while at another areas of epidermal necrolysis were observed. This study demonstrated convincingly that these lesions can all be caused by exposure to a single drug and that, although "allergic" phenomena account for a large proportion of the rashes, other factors must also play significant roles in their development.

I. Toxic Erythema

In the initial clinical trials of co-trimoxazole, toxic erythema, manifest usually as morbilliform rashes, has been reported in approximately 1% of those exposed. The frequency of such reactions detected in cohort studies such as the Boston Collaborative Drug Surveillance Program and other similar studies also varies between 1%–4% of those exposed (KOCH-WESER et al. 1971; LAWSON and MACDONALD 1977). In the Boston study LAWSON and JICK (1978) reviewed data on some 649 individuals and observed that erythematous rashes occurred in 3.5% of recipients. Rashes were twice as common in females as in males and usually occurred in the first few days following treatment; there being no secondary peak of rashes occurring 10 days or more after the first use of the drug, such as has been reported with ampicillin (SHAPIRO et al. 1969).

The Boston study collects details mainly of drug-attributed events. Nevertheless since skin rashes are highly likely to be attributed to one or more of the drugs a patient receives in hospital, most rashes occurring in the study cohort will be notified. Under these circumstances, more detailed analyses of the data are possible. By ignoring the drugs actually incriminated by the attending physician and using prior assessments of risks of reactions with known allergens, individual drugs can be revealed which are temporally associated with at least two-fold greater frequencies of rashes than expected in this population. Details of the exact methodology used in this type of analysis have been published elsewhere (ARNDT and

JICK 1976). When the 507 allergic skin reactions reported in 22,227 consecutive in-patients were subjected to this type of analysis, co-trimoxazole appeared to be one of the drugs most frequently associated with toxic erythematous rashes (along with blood and blood products, ampicillin, and the semisynthetic penicillins). Neverthe-less at the time the study was undertaken only 169 co-trimoxazole recipients had been monitored and accordingly the calculated reaction rate of 59/1,000 recipients is an unstable figure having 95% confidence intervals lying between 24/1,000 and 95/1,000 recipients. By similar methods applied to the 649 recipients reported by LAWSON and JICK (1978), calculated 95% confidence intervals for the rate of skin reactions likely to be due to co-trimoxazole were 21/1,000 and 49/1,000 recipients. Rashes were not of major significance as regards prolonging the patients' stay in hospital and usually cleared rapidly upon discontinuation of therapy and admin-istration of antihistamines. By contrast, data from the various national adverse drug reaction registries, for example the Committee on Safety of Medicines in the United Kingdom or the Committee on Adverse Reactions in New Zealand, record much lower prevalences of mild skin reactions to drugs in general, including co-trimoxazole. This is due to under-reporting of such mild reactions to the agencies and does not indicate over-estimation of risk in the data cited previously.

II. Other Skin Reactions

While it is possible to give approximate risks of toxic erythematous skin rashes in co-trimoxazole recipients, no such information is available for the more severe types of reactions defined above. In no large cohort study has a measurable frequency of these events been recorded. We can therefore conclude that they are very rare events.

Information on these rare reactions is available only from sources such as case reports to journals or to regulating agencies where it is often difficult to ascertain whether or not the reaction is indeed truly attributable to the drug in question. If the assumptions are made that the reported reactions are likely to be drug related and that the likelihood of severe reactions being reported is substantially higher than for non-severe reactions, some idea of the magnitude of the risks can be ob-tained most easily from the reports of the New Zealand Committee on Adverse Reactions. During the six years 1971–1977 a total of 166 skin reactions were at-tributed to co-trimoxazole of which three were fatal – one case of exfoliative der-matitis, one of erythema multiforme and one of Lyell's syndrome (McQUEEN 1974, 1975, 1976, 1977, 1978).

Similarly, FRISCH (1973a) reviewed all cases of severe skin reactions reported between 1968 and 1971 to one manufacturer of co-trimoxazole. He calculated that during the time covered by the review some 20 million standard 5-day courses of co-trimoxazole had been sold. Eight cases of severe skin lesions, four described as Lyell's syndrome and four as Stevens–Johnson syndrome were reported. Three of the former group died but none of the latter.

By 1978, a review of information reported to the Committee on Safety of Medicines in the United Kingdom, the Canadian Health Protection Board, the Australian Committee on Adverse Reactions, the New Zealand Committee on Ad-verse Reactions and published case reports or studies from all countries revealed

60 cases of erythema multiforme, 57 cases of Stevens–Johnson syndrome, 29 of Lyell's syndrome and 27 of exfoliative dermatitis attributed to co-trimoxazole (D. Langford 1979, personal communication), whereas the terminology is not necessarily uniform in these cases, i.e. some confusion exists between Stevens–Johnson syndrome, extensive erythema multiforme and Lyell's syndrome, this total adds up to 173 cases reported during a decade when world sales approximated to 600 million recommended treatment courses (i.e. two tablets twice daily for 5 days). If one assumes (arbitrarily) a degree of under-reporting of approximately 30-fold, the frequency of serious skin lesions possibly related to co-trimoxazole may be of the order of 1/100,000 standard 5-day treatment courses. It seems possible that the true frequency may be lower than this. Because of this extreme rarity it is difficult to indicate whether certain subgroups of the population are at greater than average risk of serious skin lesions. We do not know if these risks are increased with long-term use, and although females appear to have a greater susceptibility to toxic erythema, we have insufficient information available to know whether this applies also to rare conditions such as Stevens–Johnson syndrome or Lyell's syndrome. Urticaria has been reported infrequently after co-trimoxazole therapy, some 66 cases notified to the U.K. Committee on Safety of Medicines between 1968 and 1971 (Girdwood 1976).

III. Sulfamethoxazole or Trimethoprim?

Although most prospective studies, both controlled and uncontrolled, point to a frequency of toxic erythema lying somewhere between 1% and 4% of co-trimoxazole recipients, it is not clear which component of this drug mixture is causing the rashes. Comparative data with other sulfonamides is not available readily since most were released prior to the realisation of the need for detailed collection of adverse reaction information. Isolated case reports involving rechallenge with one component (Halpern 1972) have raised the possibility that trimethoprim is as likely to cause a toxic erythematous rash as the sulfonamide which has previously been regarded as the prime suspect. However interpretation of such experiments is difficult and subject to many variables. Until reliable information is published on the frequency of rashes following the use of trimethoprim alone this subject will remain controversial. To date insufficient numbers of individuals have been treated with trimethoprim alone to warrant any clear conclusions as to its role in the aetiology of toxic erythema after co-trimoxazole therapy (Kasanen et al. 1978).

D. Renal Disorders

Drug-induced renal disease is a well recognised, if rare, entity. Diagnosis depends upon the clinical recognition of its presence together with biochemical evidence of renal dysfunction. The latter usually is present only when substantial renal damage has occurred. Thus for example the blood urea concentration is only elevated above normal levels when glomerular filtration rates have fallen to around 30 ml/min (from a normal value of 100–120 ml/min). Since many independent factors affect blood urea concentrations, the serum creatinine concentration is more frequently measured to provide a reasonably accurate estimate of glomerular function. It is unfortunate therefore that trimethoprim interferes with creatinine handling and so renders interpretation of serum creatinine concentrations difficult. Creatinine is filtered at the glomerular level and in addition a small amount is secreted by the tubules. Trimethoprim interferes with this latter secretory pathway by competing with creatinine for the available secretory sites (BERGLUND et al. 1975). Moreover, trimethoprim interferes to a minor degree with the common method of estimating creatinine by autoanalysis technique. Thus elevations of serum creatinine in patients without coincidental elevations in urea concentrations or fall in glomerular filtration rates as measured by inulin (HORN and COTTIER 1974; KALOWSKI et al. 1973) merely reflect this competition and/or interference which is of no serious clinical significance.

Two main types of renal dysfunction have been reported with sulfonamides. The relatively insoluble early sulfonamides such as sulfadiazine were frequently given in high dosage and were occasionally reported to cause crystalluria – the deposition of crystalline sulfonamides throughout the nephron and pelvis of the kidney. This resulted in acute renal failure (BULL et al. 1958; WINTERBORN and MANN 1973). Trimethoprim does not affect the solubility of sulfamethoxazole or its acetylated derivative nor does it affect their renal handling (APPEL and NEU 1977). Crystalluria has been reported following co-trimoxazole use (SIEGEL 1977; BUCHANAN 1978), and sulfamethoxazole and some of its metabolites have been found in urinary tract calculi (WOOLEY et al. 1980). Nevertheless this complication is extremely rare and can be avoided by maintaining an adequate fluid intake during co-trimoxazole therapy.

Acute interstitial nephritis is rare and usually occurs after treatment with some of the semisynthetic penicillins (methicillin, nafcillin, oxacillin). Within 2 weeks after starting treatment, patients develop fever, rash, eosinophilia, and general malaise associated with microscopic haematuria, the syndrome appearing to have an immunological basis (BORDER et al. 1974). This condition is readily reversible upon stopping administration of the causative agent and may recur following rechallenge. Interstitial nephritis has been reported after sulfonamide therapy and RICHMOND et al. (1979) described four co-trimoxazole recipients who had coincidental occurrence of a hypersensitivity type of rash and acute renal failure in which renal biopsy showed features of acute interstitial nephritis. All were elderly subjects who, in the opinion of the authors, had received excessive doses of co-trimoxazole in the presence of mild to moderate renal impairment. It seems possible therefore that very rarely co-trimoxazole can cause acute interstitial nephritis.

Despite initial concern (KALOWSKI et al. 1973), it seems likely that co-trimoxazole can be given to patients with chronic renal failure, in reduced dosage if the glomerular filtration rate is less than 10 ml/min, without fear of reduction in renal function (TASKER et al. 1975; BENNETT and RAVEN 1976).

In the series of 649 consecutive co-trimoxazole recipients already cited (LAWSON and JICK 1978) there was no case in which deterioration of function attributed to co-trimoxazole was observed. One patient, a 44-year old female with rheumatoid arthritis developed renal tubular acidosis which disappeared upon discontinuation of co-trimoxazole and was attributed to this preparation by the attending physician.

E. Haematological Disorders

One of the principal concerns of the manufacturer when the combination of trimethoprim/sulfamethoxazole was released onto the market was to establish whether there was a substantial risk of haematological toxicity. Such concern is present to a certain extent when any new drug is marketed, but was particularly acute with this combination, containing as it does an antifolate drug.

I. Folic Acid Deficiency

Sulfamethoxazole inhibits conversion of p-aminobenzoic acid to dihydrofolate. Trimethoprim inhibits dihydrofolate reductase. Despite the fact that the latter action is vastly more marked on the bacterial cell than on human cells, the combination was suspected to have potential for inducing megaloblastic states. Such potential has been realised only very infrequently; 4 years after release of the combined preparation, GIRDWOOD (1973) was unable to trace a single convincing instance of megaloblastic anaemia attributable to the combination and concluded that in normal individuals such an event was likely to be a rarity. Overall, some 24 cases of megaloblastic anaemia attributed to co-trimoxazole have been reported. In many of these predisposing factors were apparent. Thus for example, folate deficiency can be induced rapidly in healthy volunteers fed a folate-depleted diet. Therefore care should be exercised when prescribing more than a short course of co-trimoxazole to patients who are likely to have deficient folate intake, such as elderly debilitated individuals, those suffering from malabsorption or alcoholism, those taking other antifolate drugs or those who are pregnant (KAHN et al. 1968). With these caveats, it seems unlikely that co-trimoxazole therapy will be associated with measurable risks of megaloblastosis.

By contrast co-trimoxazole has been reported to delay substantially response to specific haematinic therapy in patients with pre-existing vitamin B_{12} or folic acid deficiency megaloblastic anaemia (CHANARIN and ENGLAND 1972). Such reports, although plausible, are difficult to prove conclusively since the delay in response may be due to the underlying infection which caused co-trimoxazole use; rather than to the drug itself. At the present time, to be safe neither co-trimoxazole nor trimethoprim alone should be used to treat infections in patients suffering from acute megaloblastic states, even when under active therapy with vitamin B_{12} or folic acid.

In response to concern about the development of folic acid deficiency in co-trimoxazole recipients, some workers have monitored serum folate levels using the *Lactobacillus casei* method. This is inappropriate unless a trimethoprim-resistant strain is used since it will lead to erroneous results arising from the therapeutic concentrations of trimethoprim present in the plasma, inhibiting growth of this organism (HJORTSHOJ et al. 1978).

II. Leucopenia/Agranulocytosis

Leucopenia is said to occur when the total white cell count falls below 3,000 mm^{-3}. In the case of agranulocytosis, the reduction in total white cell count is due primarily to a fall in number or complete absence of polymorphonuclear leucocytes. Agranulocytosis has often been attributed to drugs, perhaps the most commonly incriminated being the phenylbutazone group (GIRDWOOD 1974; INMAN 1977). Leucopenia may however occur in response to severe infection. If such patients then receive antibacterial therapy, there is a likelihood that the blood dyscrasia may be attributed erroneously to the drug rather than the infection which caused the initial prescription of the drug. In 1977 INMAN, reviewing the data of the Committee on Safety of Medicines, reported a strong association between fatal aplastic anaemia and phenylbutazone or oxyphenbutazone treatment. During the course of his analysis he also observed an association between fatal agranulocytosis and co-trimoxazole and concluded that this drug was the most common cause of agranulocytosis in the United Kingdom. No comparison population was provided to assess whether other antibacterial agents appeared to be equally commonly taken by these patients. This conclusion was disputed by LAWSON and HENRY (1977) who emphasised that insufficient evidence was produced to justify the claims; exposure to co-trimoxazole within 12 months of the diagnosis of agranulocytosis, being deemed causal. Were co-trimoxazole to be causally associated with death from agranulocytosis, these workers argued that vital statistics data obtained from death certificates should show a rise during the period when co-trimoxazole use became frequent. No such rise is apparent. Therefore further information from the Committee on Safety of Medicines in the United Kingdom is required before INMAN's data can be accepted as showing that co-trimoxazole is associated with a clinically significant risk of fatal agranulocytosis.

In a 10-year review of drug-related blood dyscrasias in Sweden, BÖTTIGER et al. (1979 b) noted that the prevalence of reports was reasonably constant at 1,600/year or around 10% of all reported drug-induced disease in Sweden. There were 63 deaths from agranulocytosis in this period and 26 from aplastic anaemia. Sulfonamides were the drugs most commonly associated with both these conditions; the types of sulfonamide used in Sweden included co-trimoxazole, sulfasalazine, and sulfamethoxypyridazine. As with the data of INMAN (1977) it should be emphasised that the Swedish group are working with uncontrolled case reports in which doctors have linked clinical events to drug therapy in a manner which could be quite appropriate but could also reflect biases for or against a particular type of drug or drug combination. Thus their data have to be viewed cautiously.

A similar problem lies with the World Health Organization data in Switzerland (and now Sweden), where spontaneous reports to national agencies are collated. Reviewing the data collected between 1968 and 1973, the late Professor DE-GRUCHY (1975) noted that co-trimoxazole had been incriminated in 76 cases of leucopenia/agranulocytosis, whereas phenylbutazone was incriminated only in 64, chlorpromazine in 55 and chloramphenicol in 36. Apart from issues of confidence in these individual reports and lack of knowledge of the numbers of patients exposed to the drugs in question, a major factor in producing this type of information is that the co-trimoxazole combination was *introduced* during this time interval and so was subjected to quite different scrutiny as compared with the other drugs. The frequency of such reports are therefore not comparable from drug to drug.

III. Thrombocytopenia

Drug-induced thrombocytopenia is a well-recognised entity which is usually due to peripheral destruction of the platelets or to their impaired production. Drugs which can cause leucopenia or marrow aplasia are often involved in the development of thrombocytopenia. Sulfonamides have been incriminated in the development of thrombocytopenia and co-trimoxazole is no exception. The mechanism whereby this effect occurs is not clearly understood. Clinical consequences of thrombocytopenia depend upon its severity, presence of potential haemorrhagic lesions and co-administration of ulcerogenic drugs. Of the original 15 cases of thrombocytopenia attributed to co-trimoxazole, 3 were fatal (FRISCH 1973a). Drug-induced thrombocytopenia has been reported more frequently in females than males for reasons as yet unclear (BÖTTIGER and WESTERHOLM 1972; DICKSON 1978). Co-trimoxazole-induced thrombocytopenia is undoubtedly rare, however its true incidence is unknown.

By 1978, some 230 cases of co-trimoxazole-attributed instances of leucopenia/agranulocytosis, 146 of thrombocytopenia and 10 of pancytopenia had been reported in the literature; with a total of 78 fatalities. Many of these reports gave insufficient details to permit independent evaluation. In others, it was obvious that the basic pathology could have been associated with the development of the condition and the effect of co-trimoxazole was if any, marginal. In no large cohort of co-trimoxazole recipients, followed over a definite period, have drug-related haematological disorders appeared with a measurable frequency.

IV. Haemolytic Anaemia

Early sulfonamides were thought to cause haemolytic anaemia. Drugs may cause haemolysis either in genetically predisposed individuals with underlying red cell or haemoglobin abnormalities, e.g. glucose-6-phosphate dehydrogenase (G6PD) deficiency or as a result of immunological mechanisms (e.g. penicillin, methyldopa). Occasional instances of haemolysis have been attributed to sulfonamides, most frequently in individuals with G6PD deficiency. Theoretically this may occur even after a small dose of sulfonamide which should be avoided in such patients, where possible. Despite widespread use, only an occasional case of co-trimoxazole-induced haemolysis in a G6PD-deficient individual has been reported. Thus while it would seem advisable to avoid co-trimoxazole in patients with known G6PD deficiency except where no suitable alternative is available, the risks of precipitating a haemolytic crisis seem small.

On balance, it would seem that co-trimoxazole may infrequently be causally related to the development of leucopenia/thrombocytopenia/agranulocytosis. This occurs most often in elderly or debilitated individuals and is usually of mild degree. The frequency with which co-trimoxazole induces these reactions is unknown but is likely to be extremely low, at least during short-term (conventional) therapy. Fatal aplasia has been reported with a world-wide frequency of 1/year since release of the drug for marketing. This is likely to be an underestimate of the true frequency but the extent of the under-reporting is unknown.

F. Jaundice

I. Liver Damage

Hepatic problems caused by drug treatment are notoriously difficult to evaluate. Major liver damage can occur before clinical manifestations will have become apparent to even the most attentive physician. Thus estimates of the prevalence of liver damage secondary to drug exposure are often based upon the results of serial blood samples taken for enzyme assays. These parameters may be affected by a variety of factors such as diet, alcohol consumption, other drugs, underlying disease processes, in addition to the drug under study. In the prospective clinical trials where serial liver enzyme results were available, co-trimoxazole has rarely been associated with abnormal results. In the 10 years since its release, several single cases of jaundice attributed to this combination have been reported in the literature. Where liver biopsies have been performed, an appearance of cholestatic jaundice has been observed. Several of the reported cases have occurred in patients who have previously suffered from some form of "infective" hepatitis, although the reason for this apparent link has not been elucidated (SALTER 1973). Overall, it would appear unlikely that liver damage secondary to co-trimoxazole therapy is other than an extremely rare phenomenon.

II. Hyperbilirubinaemia of the Newborn

Unconjugated bilirubin is strongly bound to albumin in the plasma. It can be displaced by several drugs of which sulfonamides are amongst the most frequently administered. When displaced, the unconjugated bilirubin may precipitate kernicterus in the newborn (ODELL et al. 1969). For this reason (amongst others, see Sect. G), co-trimoxazole should be avoided during pregnancy. However to date there are no substantiated reports in the literature of co-trimoxazole precipitating kernicterus in the newborn, nor are there any unpublished reports of its occurrence to the Committee on Safety of Medicines in the United Kingdom at the present time.

G. Pregnancy

Co-trimoxazole should not be given to pregnant patients. This advice is based on concern, first that the drug may be teratogenic and second that it may predispose to hyperbilirubinaemia of the newborn.

The folic acid antagonists as a group are amongst the most potent teratogens known and indeed for a time were used as abortifacients in humans (THIERSCH 1952). Their use during early pregnancy usually results in intra-uterine death and when the foetus survives between 20% and 35% have major malformations, the nature of which reflect the time of administration rather than any specific group of organ defects. The antifolate activity of trimethoprim is however substantially less than that of the antifolates used to treat malignant disease. In rats, trimethoprim shows teratogenic effects only when given in doses some 50-fold greater on a weight basis than the maximum recommended dose in humans. By contrast, sulfamethoxazole given in doses of 600 mg/kg to rats between 8 and 16 days pregnant has been associated with the development of cleft palate in the foetus.

Extrapolation of animal data to the human setting is however notoriously difficult. WILLIAMS and co-workers (WILLIAMS 1969) gave co-trimoxazole for the treatment of bacteriuria of pregnancy to 120 subjects, 10 of whom were less than 16 weeks pregnant at the time. No abnormal births were noted in these patients. Several subsequent workers have given this drug for short periods during pregnancy, with no deleterious effects noted. Thus there is no conclusive evidence that co-trimoxazole is teratogenic in humans (SMITHELLS 1978). Both constituents cross the human placenta to enter the foetal bloodstream (REID et al. 1975). This combination therefore should be avoided in early pregnancy in order to minimise the risk of teratogenicity. In late pregnancy the main risk is hyperbilirubinaemia and its catastrophic sequel, kernicterus. This condition is extremely rare in the United Kingdom and no cases attributable to sulfonamides given during pregnancy has been reported to the Committee on Safety of Medicines.

H. Miscellaneous

A variety of other rare or non-specific effects have been attributed to co-trimoxazole therapy. Subjective symptoms such as headaches, depression and more infrequently, visual or aural hallucinations, have been reported after commencing co-trimoxazole therapy. Such symptoms do however occasionally accompany chest or urinary infections and may merely reflect the underlying illness rather than the drug used to treat it. They are usually mild and transient, and do not necessitate discontinuation of therapy. Occasional reports of effects on immunosuppression due to trimethoprim appear to be of no clinical significance (SALTER 1973).

A statistically significant fall in serum triiodothyronine has been observed in volunteers taking co-trimoxazole (COHEN et al. 1979). The fall however was of doubtful clinical significance, except in so far as it might possibly invalidate tests of thyroid function in patients taking this combination. Although sulfonamides have been reported to cause goitres in humans, only one such report in which thyroid enlargement has been attributed to co-trimoxazole or sulfamethoxazole has been reported to the manufacturers during the 10 years to the end of 1977 (A.D. MUNRO-FAURE and D. RYCROFT 1979, personal communication).

J. Drug Interactions

I. Pyrimethamine

In patients taking pyrimethamine for malaria prophylaxis, the risks of developing megaloblastic anaemia are enhanced by co-administration of co-trimoxazole. This is due to an additive effect on folate metabolism between the trimethoprim and pyrimethamine, which is particularly apparent when the latter is given in weekly doses exceeding 25 mg (ANSDELL et al. 1976).

II. Azathioprine

Use of co-trimoxazole in azathioprine-treated renal transplant recipients has been reported to cause more than the expected degree of leucopenia (HULME and REEVES 1971), but such reports have not been supported by other workers (HALL 1974).

III. Warfarin

Several isolated reports of interactions between co-trimoxazole and warfarin have appeared in recent years (BARNETT and HANCOCK 1975; HASSALL et al. 1974). Theoretically, warfarin handling could be affected either directly by alterations in protein binding, volume of distribution or elimination, or indirectly by effects on vitamin K production by the intestinal flora. In practice, sulfamethoxazole has been shown in vitro to displace warfarin from binding to plasma albumin (TILSTONE et al. 1977), but the magnitude of the effect is such as to preclude clinical relevance except in patients receiving high doses of warfarin who have relatively low plasma albumin concentrations – an unusual combination. More recently, O'REILLY (1980) showed that co-trimoxazole has a stereoselective interaction with the separated enantiomorphs of racemic warfarin in humans. There is a significant augmentation of both plasma concentration of warfarin and its hypoprothrombinaemic effect when co-trimoxazole is given to subjects receiving S-warfarin which is not present in those receiving R-warfarin. Since S-warfarin is approximately four times more potent than R-warfarin in humans (O'REILLY 1974), this could account for a small increase in anticoagulant effect in subjects receiving standard racemic warfarin. The magnitude of this effect is however small. No evidence has been produced to substantiate an interaction due to reduced vitamin K production by endogenous bacteria. Thus although co-trimoxazole and warfarin can be prescribed together, clinical impressions are that excessive warfarin effects are extremely rare. Patients receiving both drugs should ensure that a regular watch is kept on their prothrombin activity, but the risks associated with use of this combination appear to be of a low order and in most instances may be due as much to the underlying infection as to the co-trimoxazole therapy.

IV. Phenytoin

In a recent review of trimethoprim/sulfamethoxazole in the United States (WORMSER and KEUSCH 1979), an interaction between sulfamethoxazole and phenytoin was reported; the sulfonamide prolonging the half-life of phenytoin by inhibiting its metabolic clearance. Further details of such an interaction are required before its clinical significance can be assessed and the mode of action clarified. Interactions involving alterations in metabolic clearance of phenytoin are particularly troublesome to elucidate adequately, since this drug is subject to saturable metabolism at doses which are commonly prescribed. Another potential method of interaction between these drugs is via an additive effect on impairing folate metabolism. This seems of theoretical rather than immediate clinical relevance provided therapy with co-trimoxazole is not given on a long-term basis.

V. Hypoglycaemic Agents

All sulfonamides, including sulfamethoxazole, may rarely potentiate the hypoglycaemic effects of sulfonylurea drugs such as tolbutamide and chlorpropamide,
usually by displacement of the sulfonylurea from its binding sites on plasma albumin (Mihic et al. 1975).

K. Conclusions

Despite recent increased attention being directed towards undesired effects of drug
treatment, the present review does not give rise to substantial concern about
reactions to co-trimoxazole. At present the pattern of adverse effects attributed to
co-trimoxazole is essentially similar to that described shortly after its release by
Frisch (1973 a). The principal common adverse effects are those of upper gastrointestinal symptoms, mild transient erythematous rashes and headaches. All are of
minor severity. Severe reactions are rare. The most troublesome are extensive skin
lesions (such as erythema multiforme, Stevens–Johnson syndrome and Lyell's syndrome) and haematological upsets. Severe skin lesions appear to occur with a
frequency which could be of the order of 1 in 100,000 exposed to a standard 5-day
course of treatment. Agranulocytosis and thrombocytopenia are the most frequent
of the haematological disorders attributed to co-trimoxazole. The former is reported approximately twice as often as the latter in the world literature. Assuming that
all reported cases are indeed drug-induced and that under-reporting of such cases
is very frequent, the prevalence of co-trimoxazole-induced agranulocytosis and
thrombocytopenia could be of similar magnitude to that of severe skin lesions,
namely 1 in 100,000 exposed to a 5-day treatment course.

Other side effects such as jaundice and renal disease are infrequently reported
and do not appear to constitute a significant risk as far as co-trimoxazole therapy
is concerned. Co-trimoxazole can be given safely in chronic renal insufficiency but
the dose should be reduced when the creatinine clearance falls below 10 ml/min.
This drug is best avoided in early and late pregnancy and in the neonatal period,
in patients with untreated megaloblastic states and in patients with glucose-6-phos-
phate dehydrogenase deficiency, unless the indications for its use are pressing. Particular care should be exercised when prescribing co-trimoxazole to patients who
are receiving warfarin, azathioprine, pyrimethamine, and hypoglycaemic agents.

Acknowledgments. The author wishes to acknowledge the assistance of Dr. Alan Lyell
in providing Figs. 1–3 for this chapter.

References

Andrejak M (1976) Colite aigue iatrogene au sulphamethoxazole-trimethoprim. Nouv
    Presse Med 5:1998–1999
Ansdell VE, Wright SG, Hutchinson DBA (1976) Megaloblastic anaemia associated with
    combined pyrimethamine and cotrimoxazole administration. Lancet 2:1257
Appel GB, Neu HC (1977) The nephrotoxicity of antimicrobial agents. N Engl J Med
    296:784–787
Arndt KA, Jick H (1976) Rates of cutaneous reactions to drugs. JAMA 235:918–923
Barnett DP, Hancock BW (1975) Anticoagulant resistance: an unusual case. Br Med J
    I:608–609

Bartlett JG, Chang TW, Gurwith M, Gorbach SL, Onderdonk AB (1978) Antibiotic-associated pseudomembranous colitis due to toxin-producing clostridia. New Engl J Med 298:531–534

Bennett WM, Raven R (1976) Urinary tract infections with severe renal diseases. JAMA 236:946–948

Berglund F, Killander J, Pompeius R (1975) The effect of trimethoprim-sulphamethoxazole on the renal excretion of creatinine in man. J Urol 114:802–808

Bergoend H, Loffler A, Amar R, Maleville J (1968) Reactions cutanees survenues au cours de la prophylaxie de masse de la meningite cerebro-spinale par un sulfamide long-retard (A propos de 997 cas). Ann Dermatol Syphiligr 95:481–490

Böttiger LE, Westerholm B (1972) Thrombocytopenia: II. Drug-induced thrombocytopenia. Acta Med Scand 191:541–548

Böttiger LE, Furhoff AK, Holmberg L (1979a) Fatal reactions to drugs. Acta Med Scand 205:451–456

Böttiger LE, Furhoff AK, Holmberg L (1979b) Drug induced blood dyscrasias. Acta Med Scand 205:457–461

Border WA, Lehman DH, Egan JD, Sass HJ, Glode JE, Wilson CB (1974) Renal failure and interstitial nephritis. N Engl J Med 291:381–384

Buchanan N (1978) Sulphamethoxazole, hypoalbuminaemia, crystalluria and renal failure. Br Med J 2:172

Bull GM, Joekes AM, Lowe KG (1958) Acute renal failure due to poisons and drugs. Lancet 1:134–136

Cameron A, Thomas M (1977) Pseudomembranous colitis and co-trimoxazole. Br Med J 1:1321

Chanarin T, England JM (1972) Toxicity of trimethoprim-sulphamethoxazole in patients with megaloblastic hemopoiesis. Br Med J 1:651–653

Cohen HN, McIntyre H, Beastall GH, Ratcliffe W, Kennedy JS, Thomson JA (1979) The antithyroid effects of trimethoprim/sulphonamide preparations in man and rodents. Scott Med J 24:255

De Gruchy GC (1975) Drug-induced blood disorders. Blackwell Scientific, Oxford

Dickson HG (1978) Trimethoprim-sulphamethoxazole and thrombocytopenia. Med J Aust 2:5–7

Drugs and Therapeutics Bulletin (1979) Co-trimoxazole – too toxic for minor infections? Drug Ther Bull 17:66–68

Editorial (1981) Antibiotic-associated colitis – the continuing saga. Br Med J 282:1913–1914

Felix RH, Ive FA (1974) Skin reactions to practolol. Br Med J 2:333

Frisch JM (1973a) Clinical experience with adverse reactions to trimethoprim-sulphamethoxazole. J Infect Dis [Suppl] 128:S607–S611

Frisch JM (1973b) Trimethoprim/sulphamethoxazole in bacterial infections. In: Bernstein LS, Salter AJ (eds) Churchill Livingstone, London, pp 227–234

Girdwood RH (1973) Trimethoprim/sulphamethoxazole: long-term therapy and folate levels. Med J Aust [Suppl] 1:34–36

Girdwood RH (1974) Death after taking medicaments. Br Med J 1:501–504

Girdwood RH (1976) The nature of possible adverse reactions to co-trimoxazole. Scand J Infect Dis [Suppl] 8:10–17

Hall CL (1974) Co-trimoxazole and azathioprine: a safe combination. Br Med J 4:15–16

Halpern GM (1972) Unusual reaction to trimethoprim in combined therapy. Br Med J 1:691

Hassall C, Feetham CL, Leach RH, Meynell MJ (1974) Potentiation of warfarin by co-trimoxazole. Br Med J 2:684

Hjortshoj A, Elsborg L, Jensen E (1978) Folate status during long-term therapy with trimethoprim and sulphadiazine. Chemotherapy 24:327–331

Horn B, Cottier P (1974) Serum creatinine concentration before and during treatment with co-trimoxazole. Schweiz Med Wochenschr 104:1809–1812

Hulme B, Reeves DS (1971) Leucopenia associated with trimethoprim-sulphamethoxazole after renal transplantation. Br Med J 3:610–612

Hurwitz N, Wade OL (1969) Intensive hospital monitoring of adverse reactions to drugs. Br Med J 1:531–536

Hutchinson TA, Leventhal JM, Kramer MS, Karch FE, Lipman AB, Feinstein AR (1979) An algorithm for the assessment of adverse drug reactions: II. Demonstration of reproducibility and validity. J Am Med Assoc 242:633

Inman WHW (1977) Study of fatal bone marrow depression with special reference to phenylbutazone and oxyphenbutazone. Br Med J 1:1500–1505

Jick H (1977) The discovery of drug-induced illness. N Engl J Med 296:481–485

Kahn SB, Fein SA, Brodsky I (1968) Effect of trimethoprim on folate metabolism in man. Clin Pharmacol Ther 9:550–560

Kalowski S, Nanra RS, Matthew TH, Kincaid-Smith P (1973) Deterioration in renal function in association with co-trimoxazole therapy. Lancet 1:394–397

Kasanen A, Antilla M, Elfving R et al. (1978) Trimethoprim. Ann Clin Res [Suppl 22] 10:5–39

Koch-Weser J, Sidel VW, Dexter H, Parish C, Finer DC, Kanarek P (1971) Adverse reactions to sulfisoxazole, sulfamethoxazole, and nitrofurantoin. Arch Intern Med 128:399–404

Koch-Weser J, Sellers EM, Zacest R (1977) The ambiguity of adverse drug reactions. Eur J Clin Pharmacol 11:75–78

Kramer MS, Leventhal JM, Hutchinson TA, Feinstein AR (1979) An algorithm for the operational assessment of adverse drug reactions. JAMA 242:623–632

Lawson DH (1979) Detecting adverse drug reactions. Br J Clin Pharmacol 7:13–18

Lawson DH, Henry DA (1977) Fatal agranulocytosis attributed to co-trimoxazole therapy. Br Med J 2:316

Lawson DH, Jick H (1978) Adverse reactions to co-trimoxazole in hospitalised medical patients. Am J Med Sci 275:53–57

Lawson DH, MacDonald S (1977) Antibiotic therapy in medical wards. Postgrad Med J 53:306–309

Leventhal JM, Hutchison TA, Kramer MS, Feinstein AR (1979) An algorithim for the operational assessment of adverse drug reactions. III. Results of tests among clinicians. JAMA 242:1991–1994

Lyell A (1979) Toxic epidermal necrolysis (the scalded skin syndrome) a reappraisal. Br J Dermatol 100:69–86

McQueen EG (1974) New Zealand committee on adverse drug reactions: ninth annual report. NZ Med J 80:305–311

McQueen EG (1975) New Zealand committee on adverse drug reactions: tenth annual report. NZ Med J 82:308–309

McQueen EG (1976) New Zealand committee on adverse drug reactions: eleventh annual report. NZ Med J 84:450–453

McQueen EG (1977) New Zealand committee on adverse drug reactions: twelfth annual report. NZ Med J 86:248–250

McQueen EG (1978) New Zealand committee on adverse drug reactions: thirteenth annual report. NZ Med J 89:145–149

Mihic M, Mautner LS, Feness JZ, Grant K (1975) Effect of trimethoprim sulphamethoxazole on blood insulin and glucose concentrations in diabetics. Can Med Assoc J 112:S80–S82

Ministry of Health and Welfare (1979) Adverse reactions of sulphamethoxazole-trimethoprim compounds. Nihon Iji Shinpo (Jpn Med J) 242:1991–1994

Odell GB, Cohen SN, Kelly PC (1969) Studies in kernicterus. J Pediatr 74:214–217

O'Reilly RA (1974) Studies of the optical enantiomorphs of warfarin in man. Clin Pharmacol Ther 16:348–354

O'Reilly RA (1980) Stereoselective interaction of trimethoprim-sulfamethoxazole with the separated enantiomorphs of racemic warfarin in man. New Engl J Med 302:33–35

Reid DWJ (1975) Maternal and transplacental kinetics of trimethoprim and sulphamethoxazole. Can Med Assoc J [Suppl] 112:67S

Richmond JM, Whitworth JA, Fairley KF, Kincaid-Smith P (1979) Co-trimoxazole nephrotoxicity. Lancet 1:493

Roddis MJ (1978) Antibiotic associated colitis: a retrospective study of fifteen cases. Age Ageing 7:182–188

Salter AJ (1973) The toxicity profile of trimethoprim/sulphamethoxazole after four years of independent use. Med J Aust [Suppl] 1:70–74

Shapiro S, Slone D, Siskind V, Lewis GP, Kick H (1969) Drug rash with ampicillin and other penicillins. Lancet 2:969–972

Siegel WH (1977) Unusual complications of therapy with sulphamethoxazole-trimethoprim. J Urol 117:397

Smithells RW (1978) Drugs, infections, and congenital abnormalities. Arch Dis Child 53:93–99

Tasker PRW, MacGregor GA, de Wardener HE, Thomas RD, Jones NF (1975) Use of co-trimoxazole in renal failure. Lancet 1:1216–1218

Thiersch JB (1952) Therapeutic abortions with a folic acid antagonist 4-aminopteroylglutamic acid (4-amino PGA) administered by the oral route. Am J Obstet Gynecol 63:1298–1304

Tilstone WJ, Gray JMB, Nimmo-Smith RH, Lawson DH (1977) Interaction between warfarin and sulphamethoxazole. Postgrad Med J 53:388–390

Williams JD (1969) The treatment of bacteruria in pregnant women with sulphamethoxazole and trimethoprim. Postgrad Med J [Suppl 71]:45

Winterborn MH, Mann JR (1973) Anuria due to sulphadiazine. Arch Dis Child 48:915–917

Wooley JL, Ragouzeous A, Brent DA, Sigel CW (1980) Sulfonamide crystalluria: Isolation and identification of sulfamethoxazole and four metabolites in urinary calculi. Curr Chemother Inf Dis 552–554

Wormser GP, Keusch GT (1979) Trimethoprim-sulphamethoxazole in the United States. Ann Intern Med 91:420–429

Ziel HK, Finkle WD (1975) Increased risk of endometrial carcinoma amongst users of conjugated oestrogens. N Engl J Med 293:1167–1170

CHAPTER 10

Clinical Pharmacokinetics of Co-trimoxazole

I. HANSEN

A. Introduction

Co-trimoxazole is a combination drug of trimethoprim (TMP) and sulfamethoxazole (SMX) in a 1:5 ratio. This combination interferes with two consecutive steps in the normal bacterial metabolism of folinic acid. All sulfonamides competitively inhibit the utilization of p-aminobenzoic acid (pABA) in the synthesis of dihydrofolic acid. Since humans do not synthesize dihydrofolic acid but depend on dietary sources for their needs, this inhibition occurs only in the microorganism. TMP blocks the conversion of dihydrofolic acid to tetrahydrofolic acid (folinic acid) by inactivating the enzyme dihydrofolate reductase. This reaction occurs both in humans and in microorganisms, but the enzyme system of the microorganism is 10,000–50,000 times more sensitive than the corresponding mammalian system (Chap 1). The synergistic, bactericidal effect of the combination TMP/SMX has been demonstrated (BÖHNI 1969; DARELL et al. 1968; DORNBUSCH 1971; SCHWARTZ and RIEDER 1970) in a wide variety of gram-positive and gram-negative organisms. The effect is maximal at a TMP/SMX ratio between 1:5 and 1:40, depending on the parasite involved (see also Chap. 4).

In the first and most widely distributed commercial TMP/sulfonamide combination, SMX was chosen as the sulfonamide component since it exhibited kinetic behavior which on essential points was in good agreement with the kinetics of TMP. Thus, both drugs are characterized by first-order elimination kinetics, with plasma half-lives ($t_{1/2}$) of the same magnitude.

TMP/SMX is given by mouth only. Preparations for parenteral administration are being developed, but at present available only in restricted quantities and for controlled trials. (However, see Chap. 19.)

B. Absorption and Biologic Half-Lives

After *oral administration*, TMP is almost completely absorbed from the gastrointestinal tract in the course of 2–3 h (KAPLAN et al. 1970; SCHWARTZ and ZEIGLER 1969). Studies by REBER et al. (1963) comparing the effects of intravenous and oral administration, have suggested that approximately 85% of ingested SMX is absorbed, in the course of 2–3 h. Using the same technique, the absorption rate for both substances was found to be 85%–90% within 8 h after intake (KORN et al. 1972). Values for the invasion constant (absorption constant) for active SMX and active TMP were found by RIEDER et al. (1974c) to be 1.014 and 2.070 h^{-1}, respec-

Table 1. Pharmacokinetic characteristics of SMX_a, SMX_t, and TMP

	SMX_a	SMX_t	TMP
Single dose, oral administration (160 mg TMP + 800 mg SMX)			
Absorption rate (%)		85–90	85–90
Invasion (absorption) constant (h^{-1})		1.014	2.070
Invasion half-life (min)		80	60
Peak blood level (µg/ml)	25–60	35–65	1.2–1.9
Peak blood level is obtained after (h)	2–4	2–4	2–4
Volume of distribution (l)		13 (10–16)	100 (69–138)
Protein binding (%)		58–66	45
Elimination constant (h^{-1})	0.080	0.060	0.060
Elimination half-life (h)	9	10–12	10–12
Organs of excretion		Kidney	Kidney
pK_a	5.8		7.3
Twice daily oral administration (160 mg TMP + 800 mg SMX)			
Minimum plasma concentration (µg/ml)	32–63	50–80	1.3–2.8
Average plasma level at equilibrium (µg/ml)	55 (27–96)	110 (87–135)	2.6 (2.1–3.0)
Steady state is obtained after (days)	3	3	3

tively. DONIKE et al. (1977) has found invasion half-lives of 60 min for TMP and 80 min for SMX.

After taking 160 mg TMP + 800 mg SMX as a single dose, significant levels of both drugs appear within 1 h, and after 2–4 h, plasma peak levels are reached for TMP, total SMX (active + metabolized) and active SMX of 1.2–1.9, 35–65, and 25–60 µg/ml, respectively (Table 1; BACH et al. 1973; BERGAN and BRODWALL 1972a; CRAIG and KUNIN 1973; KREMERS et al. 1974; NOLTE and BÜTTNER 1973; NOLTE and BÜTTNER 1974; RIEDER and SCHWARTZ 1975; SCHWARTZ and RIEDER 1970).

An effective plasma concentration is maintained for 6–8 h, of an order of magnitude such that the MIC (minimum inhibitory concentration) is exceeded for the majority of bacteria isolated from clinical infections (BÖHNI 1969; DARELL et al. 1968; DORNBUSCH 1971; SCHWARTZ and RIEDER 1970). A single dose of 400 mg TMP and 2,000 mg SMX gives a TMP peak level of 3.5 µg/ml and a SMX_a peak level of 55 µg/ml (KAPLAN et al. 1973); 8 h after a single, large oral dose of 720 mg TMP and 3,600 mg SMX the blood concentration of TMP and SMX_t is 6 µg/ml for TMP and 100 µg/ml for SMX. After 24 h, a concentration of 2.2 µg/ml for TMP and 32 µg/ml for SMX_t is achieved (YOSHIKAWA and GUZE 1976). On repeated administration, equilibrium is achieved by the third day. The dose usually recommended (160 mg TMP/800 mg SMX), twice daily, gives a minimum plasma concentration (C_{min}) of TMP, SMX_t, and SMX_a of 1.3–2.8, 50–80, and 32–63 µg/ml, respectively (KREMERS et al. 1974; NOLTE and BÜTTNER 1973; NOLTE and BÜTTNER 1974). Repeated intake of 240 mg TMP and 1,200 mg SMX, twice daily, results in a C_{min} (average) of 1.84 µg/ml for TMP and 98 µg/ml for SMX_t (KOCH et al. 1973).

Equilibrium and long-term studies by KAPLAN et al. (1973) with repeated administration of 160 mg TMP/800 mg SMX three times daily, gave a C_{min} (6 h after last intake) of 2.95 µg/ml for TMP and 53 µg/ml for SMX. The results of the afore-mentioned studies demonstrated no accumulation of the drugs. At equilibrium, after administration of 160 mg TMP/800 mg SMX three times daily, administrated by *rectal application*, the average plasma levels of TMP and SMX_a are about 70% and 80%, respectively, of the concentration achieved at steady state after oral intake of 160 mg TMP/800 mg SMX twice daily (LIEDTKE and HAASE 1979).

The plasma concentrations obtained after *intravenous infusion* of TMP/SMX were twice as high as the peak plasma concentrations after oral administration of the same dose. After 4 days therapy with 160 mg TMP and 800 mg SMX three times daily, a peak plasma concentration of 8–9.5 µg/ml for TMP and 95–115 µg/ml for SMX_a was achieved, while the C_{min} values observed were 5–6 µg/ml for TMP and 65–75 µg/ml for SMX_a. Compared with administration by the oral route, intravenous administration is characterized, not only by a greater and immediate presence of the drugs in the circulation, but also by a more rapid decrease of the plasma concentration. Thus the half-lives found for TMP and SMX were about 2 and 1 h shorter, respectively, than the half-lives at oral administration (ARDATI et al. 1979; GROSE et al. 1979; KREMERS et al. 1975).

C. Distribution

The two components in the commercially available preparation are present in the ratio 1:5 (TMP:SMX). Their distribution in fluids and tissues is discussed in the following sections.

I. Plasma

After absorption has been completed, the ratio in plasma of active, non-protein-bound TMP to active, non-protein-bound SMX, lies between 1:5 and 1:40 (KAPLAN et al. 1973; KREMERS et al. 1974, 1975; RIEDER et al. 1974c; SCHWARTZ and RIEDER 1970). This ratio, from a bacteriologic point of view the most useful range, also appears to hold in slightly reduced renal function and at all times following the drug administration (BACH et al. 1973; RIEDER et al. 1974c). The rather considerable change in the ratio between TMP and SMX after absorption has been completed may to a high degree be ascribed to differences in the respective volumes of distribution. The apparent volume of distribution for TMP is around 100:1 (69–138 l) but only around 13 l (10–16 l) in the case of SMX, which indicates a far greater tissue (cell) penetration for TMP than for SMX (BERGAN and BRODWALL 1972a; BÜNGER et al. 1961; NOLTE and BÜTTNER 1973, 1974; REBER et al. 1963; RIEDER and SCHWARTZ 1975; SCHWARTZ and RIEDER 1970). In agreement with this, equilibration with interstitial fluid is achieved much more rapidly for TMP than for SMX, and at a higher percentage level (CHISHOLM et al. 1973). In reduced renal function, the volume of distribution is increased, especially in the case of SMX_a, presumably as a secondary feature to reduced protein binding (BAETHKE et al. 1972; BÜTTNER et al. 1964; RIEDER et al. 1974c; WELLING et al. 1973) and to qualitative and quantitative changes in the body fluids (RIEDER et al. 1974c). Possibly the *N*-acetyl derivative competes with the native compound for protein binding sites (RIEDER 1963).

The bacteriologically active (diffusible) concentration present in plasma water depends on the degree of protein binding of the drugs. The proportion of drug bound to plasma was found to be 45% for TMP and 58%–66% for SMX. The addition of TMP did not appear to change the degree of protein binding of SMX (KORN et al. 1972; SCHWARTZ and ZEIGLER 1969). HALL (1961) showed that 64% of unconjugated and about 84% of the conjugated SMX was bound to plasma proteins.

II. Cerebrospinal Fluid

Some 12 h after oral administration – as well as after intravenous administration – the levels of TMP and SMX in the cerebrospinal fluid (CSF) were 30%–60% and about 20%–50%, respectively, of the plasma concentrations (ARDATI et al. 1979; BACH et al. 1973; BOGER and GAVIN 1960; FRIEDRICH and HÄNSEL 1977; FRIES et al. 1975; KAUFMANN and HENNES 1973; LAFAIX et al. 1972). A satisfactory ratio of TMP:SMX of around 1:10 is thus maintained. Taking into account the slight protein binding in the CSF, it is seen that the ratio between CSF and plasma of active, freely diffusible concentrations of the two drugs approaches 1:1. According to the bacterial MIC, these CSF concentrations are in the range of therapeutic effectiveness. Several successful clinical studies confirm this (FARID et al. 1976; LAFAIX et al. 1972; MORZARIA et al. 1969; ROY 1971; SABEL and BRANDBERG 1975). The TMP penetration into the CSF seems to be independent of age and of the state of the CSF (FRIES et al. 1975). Correspondingly, SMX in the CSF is found to be about one-quarter of the plasma concentration in both the presence and absence of meningitis (BOGER and GAVIN 1960; KAUFMANN and HENNES 1973). Others, however, have found that SMX and TMP have almost a two-fold greater power of penetration in meningitis (LAFAIX et al. 1972; TOSCANO and PASCHETTA 1972).

III. Aqueous Humor

Studies of the penetration of SMX into the aqueous humour (aq.h.) in noninflamed eyes all show for SMX an aq.h.:plasma ratio of 1:4. The results for TMP are more discordant. Average values of the aq.h.:plasma ratio are found to be 0.15:1.00, 0.30:1.00, and 0.80:1.00 (overall range 0.10–1.00:1.00; (POHJANPELTO et al. 1974; RIEDER et al. 1974a; SALMON et al. 1975). In the dosage regimen usually employed, TMP/SMX is presumably present in therapeutic concentrations and a satisfactory mutual ratio.

IV. Breast Milk

The concentration of TMP in breast milk exceeds the plasma concentration by 25%. On the contrary, the concentration of SMX in milk is only one-tenth of the corresponding plasma concentration. The ratio TMP/SMX in milk is found to be 1:2 (MILLER and SALTER 1973). The daily intake of TMP:SMX by the breast-fed infant results in such small serum concentration (1–2 µg/ml SMX) that it may be concluded that the administration of TMP/SMX to women who are breast-feeding represents a negligible risk to the infant.

V. Prostatic and Seminal Material

It has been shown, both theoretically and to some extent experimentally, that only lipid-soluble bases with a high pK_a can pass through the prostatic epithelium (with its high pH gradient) and become concentrated in the acini (STAMEY et al. 1970; WINNINGHAM et al. 1968). In contrast to SMX, TMP is a lipid-soluble base with a pK_a value of 7.3. In agreement with this, TMP in the dose usually recommended has been shown to have a ratio for noninflamed prostatic fluid: plasma of 1.5–2:1 (FOWLE and BYE 1972; NIELSEN and HANSEN 1972). At equilibrium, the ratio of TMP in noninflamed prostatic tissue to that in plasma varied from 2.0 to 2.3, while values for SMX_a varied from 0.3 to 0.5. The TMP/SMX ratio in prostatic tissue is 1:2 to 1:6 (BERGMANN et al. 1979; DABHOIWALA et al. 1976; OOSTERLINCK et al. 1976). When the MIC was determined for isolated, common urinary pathogens, employing nonoptimal ratios of TMP:SMX (1:1 and 1:2), a synergistic action was demonstrated (BUSHBY and BUSHBY 1976). In accordance with these results, the drug concentration found in prostatic tissue and prostatic fluid have in fact a therapeutic, synergistic effect. In seminal fluid, the TMP concentration was found to be equal to the concentration in blood plasma (FOWLE and BYE 1972; GNARPE and FRIBERG 1976; MALMBORG et al. 1976; see also Chap. 18).

VI. Vaginal Fluid

The pH gradient between blood plasma and vaginal fluid is much greater than that between plasma and prostatic fluid. In the light of the physicochemical aspects of drug penetration into prostatic fluid, as mentioned, good penetration of TMP into vaginal fluid would be expected, and poor penetration of SMX. STAMEY and CONDY (1975) have confirmed this suggestion. They found bactericidal concentrations of TMP in vaginal fluid which often exceeded the serum level many-fold. SMX was either undetectable or present only in fractional concentrations. Colonization of the vaginal introitus by Enterobacteriaceae was cleaned up dramatically.

VII. Placental and Fetal Material

After a single dose of the combined drug, the amniotic fluid levels of the individual drugs during the first few hours are about 5%–10% of the peak levels in the maternal plasma. During the next few hours, the levels slowly rise, and the peak levels of TMP and SMX in the amniotic fluid of 15% and 25%, are reached after 14 and 10 h, respectively (YLIKORKALA et al. 1973). At equilibrium, the concentrations of TMP in amniotic fluid, cord blood, and fetal tissues were found to be 75%, 57%, and about 50%, respectively, of the corresponding maternal plasma concentrations. The corresponding values for SMX in the same order were found to be 45%, 70%, and 4% (REID et al. 1975).

VIII. Bile Fluid

In bile fluid, the TMP content exceeds the corresponding plasma value by an average factor of two, while the SMX_a content is found to be 40%–70% of the plasma concentration. A nonoptimal ratio of TMP to SMX in bile is compensated by the low level of protein binding, and the TMP:SMX ratio appears suitable for curing infection of the biliary system caused by bacteria sensitive to these drugs (Neuman et al. 1972; Rieder et al. 1974b; Sharpstone et al. 1972).

IX. Erythrocytes

Erythrocytes showed a TMP content equal to that of plasma. The SMX content was 25%–50% of the plasma concentration (Bach et al. 1973; Pullin et al. 1972).

X. Bone

Clinical studies with TMP/SMX in cases of osteomyelitis indicate good therapeutic effects (Craven et al. 1970; McAllister 1974). In agreement with this, spongy bone and bone marrow from noninfected bone have been shown to have a TMP content of about two-thirds the simultaneous plasma concentration (I. Hansen et al. 1975). For technical reasons, due to the analytical method, the concentrations found must be regarded as minimal. In compact bone, concentrations were found which were either undetectable or below effective levels. In another study, using the same technique of homogenization but including infected bone, the content of TMP found in the bone compared with the corresponding plasma concentration shows such considerable variation that final evaluation is difficult. However, in a number of cases, the concentrations exceed the MIC (Klapp et al. 1973).

XI. Other Tissues and Organs

In lung tissue, normal as well as inflamed, the TMP content is found to be 2–6 times that of plasma. The concentration in bronchial secretion is somewhat lower, but still exceeds the corresponding plasma concentration (I. Hansen et al. 1973a, b; Hughes et al. 1972). The SMX content in lung tissue has been determined in animal studies, which showed a value only about 30% of that of plasma (Schwartz and Rieder 1970). The same studies showed a great accumulation of TMP in liver tissue (between six and seven times that of plasma), spleen (about twice), *skin* (twice), and *kidney* (seven times), confirming the earlier results of Bushby and Hitchings (1968). On the contrary, the SMX content in these tissues only amounts to 20%–50% of the plasma concentration. It is therefore probable that an unfavorable TMP/SMX ratio exists in these tissues. The TMP concentration in muscle tissue equals the simultaneous plasma concentration, while the SMX content is about 15% of this (I. Hansen et al. 1973a, b; Schwartz and Rieder 1970).

D. Metabolism

Six metabolites of TMP have been identified. They account for approximately 10%–15% of the total plasma TMP concentration. In urine, the percentage of TMP metabolites amounts to 20%. Metabolites II and III are found unconjugated both in plasma and urine, whereas I, IV, and V are conjugated and excreted in the urine, essentially in the form of glucuronides. Some metabolites are bacteriostatically inactive, and some show only a lesser degree of activity (RIEDER 1973; SCHWARTZ and RIEDER 1970; SCHWARTZ et al. 1970; SIGEL et al. 1973). Only very small amounts of TMP metabolites are determined by the specific spectrofluorometric procedure normally employed (SCHWARTZ et al. 1969). All TMP values quoted, therefore, are to be considered as values of active, nonmetabolized TMP. The metabolism of SMX in humans includes several metabolites, of which only two are of importance quantitatively: N^4-acetyl-SMX and N^1-glucuronide-SMX. The metabolites are considered to be bacteriostatically inactive (RIEDER 1973). Of the total SMX urinary excretion, the SMX metabolites amount to 60%–70%, mainly the N^4-acetyl derivative (KAPLAN et al. 1973; KREMERS et al. 1974; KUHNE et al. 1976; REBER et al. 1963). At equilibrium, the metabolites of SMX in plasma account for 20%–35% of the total SMX (KREMERS et al. 1974; KUHNE et al. 1976; NOLTE and BÜTTNER 1974). (See also chap. 7.)

E. Elimination

In intact renal function, the plasma $t_{1/2}$ of SMX and TMP are 10–12 h, while the $t_{1/2}$ of SMX_a is somewhat lower, 9 h (BERGAN and BRODWALL 1972a; BUSHBY and HITCHINGS 1968; BÜNGER et al. 1961; CRAIG and KUNIN 1973; KAPLAN et al. 1973; KREMERS et al. 1974; NOLTE and BÜTTNER 1973, 1974; RIEDER and SCHWARTZ 1975; SCHWARTZ and RIEDER 1970). In slightly or moderately impaired kidney function ($C_{CR} > 10$ ml/min), the $t_{1/2}$ of TMP shows no great change. (C_{CR} is the amount of creatinine excreted in unit time divided by the average plasma concentration; similar expressions, e.g., C_{TMP} for the excretion of TMP, $C_{SMX(a)}$ for the excretion of SMX_a, occur in the following discussion). Below this clearance value, the $t_{1/2}$ increased 2- to 3-fold. Even in cases with the most severe kidney damage and in patients with bilateral nephrectomy, there is a slow elimination of active TMP. The plasma $t_{1/2}$ of SMX_a is only slightly increased with impaired renal function. The fact that SMX_a is eliminated from plasma of patients with renal insufficiency, extending to total failure at practically the same rate as in subjects with normal kidney function, indicates that extrarenal biotransformation is the essential process that determines the disappearance of the active SMX from the blood. Conversely, the $t_{1/2}$ of SMX_t (active and metabolized) at a clearance of endogenous creatinine (C_{CR}) below 25 ml/min increased 3- to 5-fold, and when C_{CR} is less than 5 ml/min, $t_{1/2}$ rises to infinity (BAETHKE et al. 1972; BERGAN and BRODWALL 1972a; CRAIG and KUNIN 1973; RIEDER et al. 1974c).

The corresponding constants of elimination (K_e) for TMP, SMX_t, and SMX_a are found to be 0.060 h^{-1} (decreasing to 0.035 h^{-1} at $C_{CR} < 5$ ml/min), 0.060 h^{-1} (decreasing to 0.015 h^{-1} at $C_{CR} < 5$ ml/min), and 0.080 h^{-1} (decreasing to 0.065 h^{-1} at $C_{CR} < 5$ ml/min), respectively. Reflecting the elimination pattern, the average plasma level of SMX_a in the steady state ($\bar{C}$) varies around a fairly constant mean over the entire scale of creatinine clearance. $\bar{C}$ for the total SMX rises to almost twice the value at a C_{CR} between 30 and 10 ml/min, and when C_{CR} drops below 10 ml/min, in some patients $\bar{C}$ becomes infinite. It appears that in such cases a danger of intoxication may arise. The average plasma level of TMP ($\bar{C}$) remains approximately unaltered at C_{CR} between normal and about 30 ml/min (average 2.6 µg/ml), and when C_{CR} is below 10 ml/min, $\bar{C}$ attains a value of 3.6 µg/ml (BAETHKE et al. 1972; NOLTE and BÜTTNER 1973, 1974; RIEDER et al. 1974c).

After the steady state is achieved, further accumulation of the drugs is not observed after long-term treatment, in conditions of normal kidney function (FOWLE 1973; KAPLAN et al. 1973; KREMERS et al. 1974). As mentioned previously, SMX_t in particular (owing to the metabolic products of SMX) and to a less degree TMP, accumulates in impaired renal function (when C_{CR} is below 30 ml/min). Reflecting the values for $t_{1/2}$, $\bar{C}$, and K_e in reduced renal sufficiency, the total clearance of SMX_t and TMP shows direct proportionality to the C_{CR} values, while this is not the fact for SMX_a. However, the rate of decline of C_{TMP} is less than that of the creatinine clearance in impaired renal function. This indicates that the active TMP and the prevailing part of the SMX metabolites, predominantly the N^4-acetyl derivative, are eliminated from the body, chiefly by the renal route, whereas a considerable fraction of the active sulfonamide may be eliminated by extrarenal processes, such as metabolism and excretion into the bile (BAETHKE et al. 1972; RIEDER et al. 1974c; SHARPSTONE 1969).

The renal clearance of SMX_a is increased by higher urine flow rate and alkaline urine (VREE et al. 1978). The rate C_{SMXa}/C_{CR} is below 1, indicating tubular reabsorption in the kidneys. The increase in clearance with rising urine flow rate suggests that the tubular reabsorption is a passive process. It is suggested that TMP is subjected to passive, nonionic tubular diffusion. Acid urine generally results in net tubular secretion, whereas an alkaline urine involves net tubular reabsorption (BERGAN and BRODWALL 1972b; CRAIG and KUNIN 1973; SHARPSTONE 1969).

After a single dose of the combined drug, the cumulative urinary recovery after 72–96 h amounts to 70%–85% and 80%–95% of the dose for total TMP and SMX_t, respectively. The amount of active SMX recovery is about 30%. The urinary concentrations of the drugs depend on the urine flow rate, urine pH, and the time of collection. The approximate urine concentration for TMP is 100 times the plasma concentration, for SMX the level is 5 times the concentration in plasma. The active SMX content in urine is equal to the plasma concentration. Decrease in the ratio SMX:TMP is counteracted by the high content of TMP in the urine (BAETHKE et al. 1972; CRAIG and KUNIN 1973; KAPLAN et al. 1973; KREMERS et al. 1974; KUHNE et al. 1976; NOLTE and BÜTTNER 1973; RIEDER et al. 1974c; SCHWARTZ and RIEDER 1970). Decreasing renal function reduces the cumulative recovery in urine, most marked for TMP, and the ratio SMX:TMP becomes more favorable. Despite the decreased recovery of the drugs from the urine, urinary concentrations were usually obtained above the minimum inhibitory concentration of each drug for most urinary pathogens (BAETHKE 1972; BERGAN and BRODWALL 1972b; CRAIG and KUNIN 1973; RIEDER et al. 1974c).

The removal of TMP by dialysis does not add significantly to its spontaneous clearance from the blood. As to the SMX metabolites, they appear to be retained in patients, in spite of regular dialysis treatment. Only the active SMX can be cleared by hemodialysis (BAETHKE 1972; HITZENBERGER et al. 1971).

In view of the cumulative urinary recovery of the two drugs, it is seen that the kidneys are the organs of excretion. Extrarenal excretion amounts to only a few percent. Some 4% of the ingested TMP dose is detected in the faces (SCHWARTZ

Table 2. Preliminary dosage schedule for combination of SMX and TMP in adults with impaired renal function

Criteria of kidney function			Recommended dosage regimens (1 standard dose for adults = 2 tablets containing together 160 mg TMP + 800 mg SMX)
C_{cr} (ml/min)	Serum creatinine (mg-%)[a]		
> 25	Men Women	< 3.0 < 2.0	Dosage as for patients with normal functions, i.e., 1 standard dose every 12 up to 14 days, later on $^1/_2$ standard dose every 12 h
25–15	Men Women	3.0–7.0 2.0–4.5	1 standard dose every 12 h for 2 days, later on 1 standard dose every 24 h as long as allowed by control analyses[b]
< 15	Men Women	> 7.0 > 4.5	$^1/_2$–1 standard dose may be administered every 24 h as long as allowed by control analyses[c]

[a] The serum creatinine can be used as the basis for dosing only in cases of chronic renal impairment, not for acute or subacute kidney failure

[b] The concentration of SMX should be measured in plasma samples obtained 12 h after every third day of treatment. Treatment should be stopped if at any time the determined plasma level of SMX exceeds 150 µg/ml. As soon as the value of total SMX again drops below 120 µg/ml, treatment can be continued as recommended

[c] Control analyses in the same manner as mentioned in [b], but with plasma SMX_t determinations every second day, as a minimum

and ZEIGLER 1969). In saliva, TMP exceeds the plasma concentration 2- to 8-fold, while SMX gains access to the saliva only in trace amounts (BECK 1971; I. HANSEN et al. 1973a; QUAYLE and HAILEY 1973). In one study, however, the TMP content in saliva equals the corresponding plasma concentration (EATMAN et al. 1977).

On the basis of the aforementioned pharmacokinetic results, the following preliminary dosage schedule for the combination SMX/TMP in adults with impaired renal function is recommended by RIEDER et al. (1974c), slightly modified by the author (Table 2). The $t_{1/2}$ of SMX in infants who are less than 10 days old is longer than in adults. It then rapidly decreases during the next 2 weeks of life, and ultimately reaches a level approximately one-half of that in adults by the time the infant is 1 year old. This situation persists until the child is 6–8 years old, at which time the $t_{1/2}$ begins to lengthen, until it reaches that of the normal adult. This $t_{1/2}$ pattern is clinically important because the indicated dosage of the mixture in children more than 6 weeks old but less than 8 years old is frequently proportionally greater than that for an adult (FOWLE et al. 1975; SCHIFFMAN 1975; see also Chap. 14).

Several studies have documented unaffected pharmacokinetic behaviour, regardless of whether the drugs are administered singly or combined (KAPLAN et al. 1973; NOLTE and BÜTTNER 1974; WELLING et al. 1973). In cases of impaired hepatic function, the peak levels of SMX_a and TMP in plasma were lower by an average factor of 1.5–2.0 (RIEDER and SCHWARTZ 1975).

The combination sulfadiazine (SDZ) and TMP deviates from TMP/SMX by a relatively larger portion of active SDZ than SMX excreted in the urine. There-

fore, the ratio TMP: sulfonamide in the urine is more favorable in the case of TMP/
SDZ (Andreasen et al. 1978; Bergan et al. 1977; Männistö et al. 1973; Ohnhaus
and Spring 1975).

F. Interactions

TMP/SMX increases activity of oral coumarin anticoagulants, phenytoin, and oral
hypoglycemic agents of the sulfonylurea type, partly by displacing the agents from
plasma protein binding sites and partly by enzyme competition in the liver drug
metabolism (Christensen et al. 1963; J. Hansen et al. 1975; Hassall et al. 1975;
Lumholtz et al. 1975). The activity of methotrexate (folic acid antagonist) may be
increased in concomitant TMP/SMX administration (Burchall 1969). SMX
forms insoluble compounds in the urine, when hexamethylentetramine is given simultaneously.

References

Andreasen F, Elsborg L, Husted S, Thomsen O (1978) Pharmacokinetics of sulfadiazine and
  trimethoprim in man. Eur J Clin Pharmacol 14:57–67
Ardati KO, Thirumoorthi MC, Dajani AS (1979) Intravenous trimethoprim-sulfamethoxazole in the treatment of serious infections in children. J Pediatr 95:801–806
Bach MC, Gold O, Finland M (1973) Absorption and urinary excretion of trimethoprim,
  sulfamethoxazole, and trimethoprim-sulfamethoxazole: results with single doses in normal young adults and preliminary observations during therapy with trimethoprim-sulfamethoxazole. J Infect Dis [Suppl] 128:584–598
Baethke R, Golde G, Gahl G (1972) Sulphamethoxazole/trimethoprim: pharmacokinetic
  studies in patients with chronic renal failure. Eur J Clin Pharmacol 4:233–240
Beck H (1971) Etude pharmacocinetique des constituants du bactrim. Rev Med Liege
  23:1437
Bergan T, Brodwall EK (1972a) Human pharmacokinetics of a sulfamethoxazole-trimetho-
  prim combination. Acta Med Scand 192:483–492
Bergan T, Brodwall EK (1972b) Kidney transport in man of sulfamethoxazole and
  trimethoprim. Chemotherapy 17:320–333
Bergan T, Vik-Mo H, Ånstad U (1977) Kinetics of a sulfadiazine-trimethoprim combina-
  tion. Clin Pharmacol Ther 22:211–224
Bergmann M, Lederer B, Takacs (1979) Zur Bestimmung der Gewebskonzentration von
  Sulfametrol-Trimethoprim in der menschlichen Prostata. Urologe [A]18:335–337
Böhni E (1969) Vergleichende bakteriologische Untersuchungen mit Kombination Trime-
  thoprim/Sulfamethoxazol in vitro and in vivo. Chemotherapy [Suppl] 14:1–21
Boger WP, Gavin JJ (1960) Sulfamethoxazole: comparison with sulfisoxazole and sulfacthi-
  dole and cerebrospinal fluid diffusion. Antibiot Chemother 10:572
Bünger P, Diller W, Führ J, Krüger-Thimer E (1961) Vergleichende Untersuchungen an
  neueren Sulfanilamiden. Arzneim Frosch 11:247–255
Büttner H, Portwich F, Manzke E, Staudt N (1964) Zur Pharmakokinetic von Sulfonami-
  den unter pathologischen Bedingungen. Klin Wochenschr 42:103–108
Burchall JJ (1969) Discussion on interaction between trimothoprim and methotrexate. Post-
  grad Med J [Suppl] 45:51
Bushby SRM, Bushby MB (1976) Trimethoprim/sulfamethoxazole synergy and prostatis.
  In: Williams JD, Geddes AM (eds) Proc 9th Congr Chemother, London. Plenum, New
  York, pp 383–388
Bushby SRM, Hitchings GH (1968) Trimethoprim, a sulphonamide potentiator. Br J Phar-
  macol Chemother 33:72–90

Chisholm D, Waterworth PM, Calnan JS, Garrod LP (1973) Concentration of antibacterial agents in interstitial tissue fluid. Br Med J I:569–573

Christensen LK, Hansen JM, Kristensen M (1963) Sulphaphenazole-induced hypoglycaemic attacks in tolbutamide-treated diabetics. Lancet II:1298–1301

Craig WA, Kunin CM (1973) Trimethoprim-sulfamethoxazole: pharmacodynamic effects of urinary pH and impaired renal function. Ann Intern Med 78:491–497

Craven JL, Pugsley DJ, Blowers R (1970) Trimethoprim-sulphametoxazole in acute osteomyelitis due to penicillin-resistant staphylococci in Uganda. Br Med J III:201–203

Dabhoiwala NF, Bye A, Claridge M (1976) A study of concentrations of trimethoprim-sulphamethoxazole in the human prostate gland. Br J Urol 48:77–81

Darell JH, Garrod LP, Waterworth PM (1968) Trimethoprim: laboratory and clinical studies. J Clin Pathol 21:202–209

Donike M, Lücker PW, Simon B (1977) Klinisch-pharmakologische Untersuchungen zur Pharmakokinetik einer Trimethoprim/Sulfamethoxazol-Zubereitung an gesunden Versuchspersonen. Arzneim Forsch 27:2373–2377

Dornbusch K (1971) Regression line analysis of the synergistic effect for the combination of trimethoprim/sulphamethoxazole. Chemotherapy 16:229–238

Eatman FB, Maggio AC, Pocelinko R et al. (1977) Blood and salivary concentrations of sulfamethoxazole and trimethoprim in man. J Pharmacokinet Biopharm 5:615–624

Farid Z, Girgis NI, Yassin W, Edman DC, Miner WF (1976) Trimethoprim-sulfamethoxazole and bacterial meningitis. Ann Intern Med 84:50–51

Fowle ASE (1973) Aspect of the pharmacokinetic behaviour of trimethoprim and sulphamethoxazole. In: Bernstein LS, Salter AJ (eds) Trimethoprim/sulphamethoxazole in bacterial infections. Churchill Livingstone London, pp 63–72

Fowle ASE, Bye A (1972) Concentration of trimethoprim and sulphamethoxazole in human prostate fluid. Adv Antimicrob Antineoplast Chemother I/2:1289–1290

Fowle ASE, Bye A, Hariri F, Middlemiss D, Naficy K (1975) The dosage of Co-trimoxazole in childhood. Eur J Clin Pharmacol 8:217–222

Friedrich H, Hänsel G (1977) Liquorspiegel-Untersuchungen einer Trimethoprim-Sulfamethoxazol-Kombination im Ventrikelliquor bei neurochirurgischen Patienten. Acta Neurochir (Wien) 37:271–280

Fries N, Keuth U, Braun JS (1975) Untersuchungen zur Liquorgängigkeit von Trimethoprim im Kindesalter. Fortschr Med 93:1178–1183

Gnarpe H, Friberg J (1976) The penetration of trimethoprim into seminal fluid and serum. Scan J Infect Dis [Suppl] 8:50–52

Grose WE, Bodey GP, Ti Li Loo (1979) Clinical pharmacology of intravenously administered trimethoprim-sulfamethoxazole. Antimicrob Agents Chemother 15:447–451

Hall PW (1961) Renal secretory T_m for sulfonamide. Clin Res 9:248

Hansen I, Nielsen ML, Bertelsen S (1973 a) Trimethoprim in human saliva, bronchial secretion and lung tissue. Acta Pharmacol Toxicol (Copenh) 32:337–344

Hansen I, Nielsen ML, Heerfordt L, Henriksen B, Bertelsen S (1973 b) Trimethoprim in normal and pathological human lung tissue. Chemotherapy 19:221–234

Hansen I, Nielsen ML, Nielsen JB (1975) A new method for homogenization of bone exemplified by measurement of trimethoprim in human bone tissue. Acta Pharmacol Toxicol (Copenh) 37:33–42

Hansen JM, Siersbaek-Nielsen K, Skovsted L, Kampmann JP, Lumholtz B (1975) Potentiation of warfarin by Co-trimoxazole. Br Med J II:684

Hassall C, Feetan CL, Leach RH, Meynell MJ (1975) Potentation of warfarin by Co-trimoxazole. Lancet II:1155–1156

Hitzenberger G, Korn A, Kotzaurek R, Schmidt P, Deutsch E (1971) Pharmakokinetik von Trimethoprim und Sulfamethoxazol bei Patienten mit schwerster renaler Eliminationsstörung und Haemodialyse. In: Renal elimination of drugs. VIII. Symp Nephrol Assoc, Aachen

Hughes DTD, Bye A, Hodder P (1972) Levels of trimethoprim and sulphamethoxazole in blood and sputum in relation to treatment of chest infections. Adv Antimicrob Antineoplast Chemother I/2:1105–1106

Kaplan SA, Weinfeld RE, Cotler S, Abruzzo CW, Alexander K (1970) Pharmacokinetic profile of trimethoprim in dog and man. J Pharm Sci 59:358–363

Kaplan SA, Weinfeld RE, Abruzzo CW, MacFaden K, Jack ML, Weissman L (1973) Pharmacokinetic profile of trimethoprim-sulfamethoxazole in man. J Infect Dis [Suppl] 128:547–555

Kaufmann S, Hennes R (1973) Klinische Erfahrungen und pharmakokinetische Untersuchungen mit Bactrim „Roche" bei Meningitis. Med Welt 24:1903–1906

Klapp F, Baldauf G, Braun JS, Poeplau P, Hertel P (1973) Nachweis von Trimethoprim in gesundem und entzündetem Knochengewebe. Med Welt 24:944–945

Koch UJ, Schumann KP, Küchler R, Kewitz H (1973) Efficacy of trimethoprim sulfamethoxazole and the combination of both in acute urinary tract infection. Chemotherapy 19:314–321

Korn A, Hitzenberger G, Jaschek I (1972) Pharmacokinetics of the combination of trimethoprim with sulfamethoxazol. Adv Antimicrob Antineoplast Chemother I/1:21–24

Kremers P, Duvivier J, Heusghem C (1974) Pharmacokinetic studies of co-trimoxazole in man after single and repeated doses. J Clin Pharmacol 14:112–117

Kremers P, Claessens H, Heusghem C (1975) Comparative pharmacokinetics in man of parenterally and orally administered CO-trimoxazole. Medikon 4:19–21

Kuhne J, Kohlmann FW, Seydel JK, Wempe E (1976) Pharmakokinetic der Kombination Sulfamoxol/Trimethoprim (CN 3123) bei Tier und Mensch. Arzneim Forsch 26:651–657

Lafaix C, Pechere JC, Zarouf M, Neto JPA, Rey M (1972) The therapeutic of septic meningitis with sulfamethoxazole-trimethoprime. Adv Antimicrob Antineoplast Chemother I/2:1227–1229

Liedtke R, Haase W (1979) Steady-state pharmacokinetics of sulfamethoxazole and trimethoprim in man after rectal application. Arzneim Forsch 29:345–349

Lumholtz B, Siersbaek-Nielsen K, Skovsted L, Kampmann JP, Hansen JM (1975) Sulphamethizole-induced inhibition of dephenylhydantoin, tolbutamide, and warfarin metabolism. Clin Pharmacol Ther 17:731–734

Männistö P, Tuomisto J, Saris N-E, Lehtinen T (1973) Pharmacokinetic studies with trimethoprim and different doses of sulfadiazine in healthy human subjects. Chemotherapy 19:289–298

Malmborg A, Dornbusch K, Eliasson R, Lindholmer C (1976) Concentration of antibacterials in human seminal plasma. In: Williams JD, Geddes AM (eds) Proc 9 th Congr Chemother, London. Plenum, New York, pp 53–59

McAllister TA (1974) Treatment of osteomyelitis. Br J Hosp Med 12:535–545

Miller RD, Salter AJ (1973) The passage of trimethoprim/sulphamethoxazole into breast milk and its significance. Proc 8 th Congr Chemother, Athens, Vol 1, pp 687–691

Morzaria RN, Walton IE, Pickering D (1969) Neonatal meningitis treated with trimethoprim and sulfamethoxazole. Br Med J II:511

Neuman M, Kazmierczak A, Charbonnier A (1972) Etat fonctionnel du foie et pouvoir antibactérien de l'association triméthoprime-sulfaméthazole dans le sang, la bile et les urines chez l'homme. Therapie 27:1069–1080

Nielsen ML, Hansen I (1972) Trimethoprim in human prostatic tissue and prostatic fluid. Scand J Urol Nephrol 6:244–248

Nolte H, Büttner H (1973) Pharmacokinetics of trimethoprim and its combination with sulfamethoxazole in man after single and chronic oral administration. Chemotherapy 18:274–284

Nolte H, Büttner H (1974) Investigations on plasma levels of sulfamethoxazole in man after single and chronic oral administration alone and in combination with trimethoprim. Chemotherapy 20:321–330

Ohnhaus EE, Spring P (1975) Elimination kinetics of sulfadiazine in patients with normal and impaired renal function. J Pharmacokinet Biopharm 3:171–179

Oosterlinck W, Defoort R, Renders G (1976) The concentration of sulphamethoxazole and trimethoprim in human prostate gland. Chemotherapy 6:389–393

Pohjanpelto PEJ, Sarmela TJ, Raines T (1974) Penetration of trimethoprim and sulphamethoxazole into the aqueous humour. Br J Ophthalmol 58:606–608

Pullin C, Bye A, Fowle ASE (1972) The distribution of trimethoprim in total body water. Adv Antimicrob Antineoplast Chemother I/1:25–26

Quayle AA, Hailey DM (1973) Antimicrobial substances in saliva: sulphamethoxazole and trimethoprim (CO-trimoxazole). Br J Oral Surg 1:60–65

Reber H, Wild F, Paris J (1963) Experimentelle Daten über das neue Sulfonamid 5-Methyl-3-sulfanilamido-isoxazol (Ro 4-2130) beim Erwachsenen. Chemotherapia 6:273–284

Reid DWJ, Caille G, Kaufmann NR (1975) Maternal and transplancental kinetics of trimethoprim and sulfamethoxazole, separately, and in combination. Can Med Assoc J 112:67–72

Rieder J (1963) Physikalisch-chemische und biologische Untersuchungen an Sulfonamiden. Arzneim Forsch 13:81–88

Rieder J (1973) Metabolism and techniques for assay of trimethoprim and sulfamethoxazole. J Infect Dis [Suppl] 128:567–573

Rieder J, Schwartz DE (1975) Pharmakokinetik der Wirkstoffkombination Trimthoprim + Sulfamethoxazol bei Leberkranken im Vergleich zu Gesunden. Arzneim Forsch 25:656–666

Rieder J, Ellerhorst B, Schwartz DE (1974 a) Übergang von Sulfamethoxazol und Trimethoprim in das Augenkammerwasser beim Menschen. Graefes Arch Ophthalmol 190:51–61

Rieder J, Schwartz DE, Zangaglia O (1974 b) Passage of sulfamethoxazole and trimethoprim into the bile in man. Chemotherapy 20:65–81

Rieder J, Schwartz DE, Fernex M et al. (1974 c) Pharmacokinetics of the antibacterial combination sulfamethoxazole plus trimethoprim in patients with normal or impaired kidney function. Antibiot Chemother 18:148–198

Roy LP (1971) Sulphamethoxazole-trimethoprim in infancy. Med J Aust 1:148–149

Sabel KG, Brandberg Å (1975) Treatment of meningitis and septicemia in infancy with a sulphamethoxazole/trimethoprim combination. Acta Paediatr Scand 64:25–32

Salmon JD, Fowle ASE, Bye A (1975) Concentrations of trimethoprim and sulphamethoxazole in aqueous humour and plasma from regimes of CO-trimoxazole in man. J Antimicrob Chemother 1:205–211

Schiffman DO (1975) Evaluation of an anti-infective combination. JAMA 231:635–637

Schwartz DE, Rieder J (1970) Pharmacokinetics of sulfamethoxazole + trimethoprim in man and their distribution in the rat. Chemotherapy 15:337–355

Schwartz DE, Zeigler WH (1969) Assay and pharmacokinetics of trimethoprim in man and animals. Postgrad Med J 45:32–37

Schwartz DE, Koechlin BA, Weinfeld RE (1969) Spectrofluorimetric method for the determination of trimethoprin in body fluids. Chemotherapy [Suppl] 14:22–29

Schwartz DE, Vetter W, Englert G (1970) Trimethoprim metabolites in rat, dog and man: qualitative and quantitative studies. Arzneim Forsch 20:1867–1871

Sharpstone P (1969) The renal handling of trimethoprim and sulphamethoxazole in man. Postgrad Med J [Suppl] 45:38–42

Sharpstone P, Pickard J, Williams R (1972) Concentrations of trimethoprim and sulphamethoxazole in human bile. Proc 7th Congr Chemother, Prague. Adv Antimicrob Antineoplast Chemother I/2:1269–1971

Sigel CW, Grace ME, Nichol CA (1973) Metabolism of trimethoprim in man and measurement of a new metabolite: a new fluorescence assay. J Infect Dis [Suppl] 128:580–583

Stamey TA, Condy M (1975) The diffusion and concentration of trimethoprim in human vaginal fluid. J Infect Dis 131:261–266

Stamey TA, Meares EM, Winningham DG (1970) Chronic bacterial prostatitis and the diffusion of drugs into prostatic fluid. J Urol 103:187–194

Toscano F, Paschetta G (1972) Distribution of the sulfamethoxazole-trimethorpin combination in cerebro-spinal fluid. G Mal Infett Parassit 24:585

Vree TB, Hekster YA, Baars AM, Damsma JE, van der Kleijn E (1978) Pharmacokinetics of sulphamethoxazole in man: Effects of urinary pH and urine flow on metabolism and renal excretion of sulphamethoxazole and its metabolite N_4-acetylsulphamethoxazole. Clin Pharmacokinet 3:319–329

Welling PG, Craig WA, Amidon GL, Kunin CM (1973) Pharmacokinetics of trimethoprim and sulfamethoxazole in normal subjects and in patients with renal failure. J Infect Dis [Suppl] 128:556–566

Winningham DG, Nemoy NJ, Stamey TA (1968) Diffusion of antibiotics from plasma into prostatic fluid. Nature 219:139–143

Ylikorkala O, Sjöstedt E, Järvinen PA, Tikkanen R, Raines T (1973) Trimethoprim-sulfonamide combination administered orally and intravaginally in the first trimester of pregnancy: its absorption into serum and transfer to amniotic fluid. Acta Obstet Gynecol Scand 52:229–234

Yoshikawa TT, Guze LB (1976) Concentrations of trimethoprim-sulfamethoxazole in blood after a single, large oral dose. Antimicrob Agents Chemother 10:462–463

CHAPTER 11

Resistance: Genetics and Medical Implications

J.F. Acar and F.W. Goldstein

A. Introduction

Resistance to sulfonamides and/or trimethoprim (TMP) has been extensively documented in the last ten years. It is frequently overlooked or falsely reported in the clinical laboratory. Discs, containing the combination of sulfonamides and TMP as well as agar media unsuitable for the test are the major causes of errors in detecting resistance to TMP (BURCHALL 1973; BUSHBY 1973a; FERONE et al. 1975; SMITH 1980; STOKES and LACEY 1978).

B. Resistance to Sulfonamides

I. Definition

Resistance to sulfonamides can be defined on the basis of minimum inhibitory concentrations (MIC) exceeding 32 µg/ml. About 90% of the resistant strains display high level resistance to all the sulfonamides with MIC higher than 1,000 µg/ml. Only 10% of the resistant strains have lower MIC, between 64 and 512 µg/ml.

II. Natural Resistance

Among naturally resistant species, *Streptococcus faecalis* and lactobacilli are auxotrophic for folic acid and are not inhibited by sulfonamides (BUSHBY 1973a).

III. Acquired Resistance

Resistance to sulfonamides is very frequent among Enterobacteriaceae, and represents 40%–50% of the strains isolated from outpatients and 55%–65% of the strains isolated from hospitalized patients, in our experience, between 1975 and 1980. In the same period, resistance to sulfonamides represented only 13%–22% of the strains isolated in the United States (O'BRAIN et al. 1978). In the United Kingdom, percentages similar to those reported in France were observed (GRÜNEBERG 1976; HAMILTON-MILLER 1979).

C. Resistance to Trimethoprim

I. Definition

Resistance to TMP is defined as MIC > 2 µg/ml. Three groups of resistant strains, according to their MIC can be distinguished among Enterobacteriaceae isolated in

Paris from 1972 to 1979 (ACAR et al. 1973, 1977, 1980; GOLDSTEIN 1977). The first group, defined by MIC ranging from 4 to 32 μg/ml mostly includes *Klebsiella*, *Enterobacter*, and *Serratia*; it represents about 10%–30% of resistant strains. The second group, defined by MIC ranging from 64 to 512 μg/ml contains strains encountered less frequently (5% of resistant strains). In contrast, the third group, described as high level resistance to TMP (MIC > 1,000 μg/ml) represents more than 50% of resistant strains (GOLDSTEIN 1977; ACAR et al. 1973).

II. Natural Resistance

Many bacterial species are naturally resistant to TMP, at various levels (BLACK 1970; BUSHBY 1973a; THEN and ANGEHRN 1979; SMITH 1980; Table 1). *Streptococcus faecalis* is able under certain circumstances to use exogenous folates and to behave as if resistant to TMP (BUSHBY and HITCHINGS 1968).

III. Acquired Resistance

Despite the very large use of the combination of sulfonamides and TMP in France for 10 years, resistance to TMP does not exceed 10% among gram-negative bacteria isolated from outpatients and 22.5% from hospitalized patients. The resistance was observed in all the enterobacteria and can be related to mutation or plasmids.

D. Mechanisms of Acquired Resistance to Sulfonamides

Acquired resistance to sulfonamides was first reported in 1943 (LANDY et al. 1943), and several mechanisms of resistance have been documented since then. As for other antibiotics, acquired resistance can be due to mutational events or to the acquisition of an R factor.

I. Results of Mutations

1. Decreased Permeability

It is very difficult to produce evidence for an impermeability mechanism and often this mechanism is proposed to explain resistance which is not explained by another mechanism (AKIBA and YOKOTA 1962; PATO and BROWN 1963).

2. Hyperproduction of p-Aminobenzoic Acid

Many bacterial species have been reported to produce a 50- to 100-fold increased quantity of p-aminobenzoic acid (TILETT et al. 1943; WHITE and WOODS 1965a, b; RICHMOND 1966). This hyperproduction is stable and it is not related to the presence of sulfonamides in the media (LANDY and GERSTUNG 1944). According to RICHMOND, this resistance is due to a mutation in the regulating genes which results in a derepression of feedback control by the end products (RICHMOND 1966).

3. Altered Dihydropteroate Synthase

The existence of dihydropteroate synthase (DHPS) with decreased affinity for sulfonamides has been demonstrated in *Escherichia coli*, staphylococci, and pneumococci (DAVIS and MAAS 1952; WACKER et al. 1959; WOLF and HOTCHKISS 1963; WHITE and WOODS 1965a, b; PATO and BROWN 1969; SWEDBERG et al. 1979). In the case of pneumococci, the DHPS had an altered amino acid sequence responsible for the decrease in affinity for sulfonamides (WOLF and HOTCHKISS 1963).

Among several mutants of *E. coli* selected for resistance to sulfonamides, SWEDBERG et al. (1979) have found strains with a modified DHPS. The Michaelis constant (K_m) for sulfonamide of this modified DHPS was 150-fold higher than for the parent strain. The rate of mutation responsible for sulfonamide resistance through these different mechanisms and the chromosomal locations of these mutations have not been reported.

II. Acquisition of R Factors

R factor-mediated resistance to sulfonamides is very common and has been described since 1959, with the first plasmid isolated in Japan, where the resistance to sulfonamides was associated with other resistance markers (YOKOTA and AKIBA 1961). Today, sulfonamide-resistant plasmids have been found in almost all the gram-negative bacilli harboring resistance plasmids. In many cases, the sulfonamide resistance is linked to a resistance to streptomycin. Plasmid-mediated resistance governs the production of a DHPS which is highly resistant to sulfonamides and different from the chromosomal enzyme in molecular weight and heat sensitivity (SKÖLD 1976; WISE and ABOU-DONIA 1975).

Recently, SWEDBERG and SKÖLD (1980) have isolated two different classes of sulfonamide-resistant DHPS. In both cases, the sulfonamide-resistant DHPS was 10,000-fold less sensitive to sulfonamides than the chromosomal enzyme. The sulfonamide-resistant DHPS displayed a K_m value similar to the sulfonamide-sensitive chromosomal DHPS. These authors have also demonstrated the existence of a plasmid-borne resistance mechanism due to restricted penetration of sulfonamides in the bacteria, as suggested by previous studies (NAGATE et al. 1978).

E. Mechanism of Acquired Resistance to Trimethoprim

Acquired resistance to TMP has been documented since 1969, immediately after the combination TMP/sulfamethoxazole became available for clinical use. As with sulfonamides, acquired resistance to TMP can be due to mutational events or can be plasmid mediated.

I. By Mutation

1. Thymineless Organisms

Four mechanisms have been clearly shown to be responsible for chromosomally determined resistance to TMP.

a) Absolute

Thymine-less mutants lacking thymidylate synthetase require for growth an exogenous supply of thymine (50 µg/ml) or thymidine (5 µg/ml). Such mutants are easily obtained in vitro from various bacterial species with a mutation rate of 3×10^{-7} in $E.\,coli$. The gene governing this enzyme is located at 60' from the origin on the chromosome of $E.\,coli$ K_{12} (Bachmann et al. 1976).

b) Minimal Requirement

Some bacteria, which have undergone a second mutation on the structural genes deo B or deo C located at 99' from the origin on the $E.\,coli$ K_{12} chromosome have become low thymine requiring (Okada 1966; Harrison 1965; Lomax and Greenberg 1968; Dale and Greenberg 1972). As they can grow on most media except pure minimal salts agar, they are always overlooked in routine laboratory investigations.

c) Temperature-Sensitive Thymidylate Synthetase

A third group of thymineless strains have a temperature-sensitive thymidylate synthetase which recovers, at 27 °C a partial activity, sufficient to allow normal growth of the strains (Dale and Greenberg 1972).

d) Ribonucleoside Diphosphate Reductase Deficiency

Some bacteria require uridine diphosphate or any other compound belonging to the same metabolic chain for normal growth. Therefore, they can also be supplemented by thymidine and are always confused with the other thymineless bacteria (Fuchs and Neuhard 1973; Johnson et al. 1976). A thymineless strain which is no more able to synthetize folinic acid is always highly resistant to TMP, providing ample thymidine is available, since the site of action of TMP is bypassed by the direct incorporation of thymidine by the bacteria (Stacey and Simson 1965; Amyes and Smith 1974b, 1975).

2. Modification of Dihydrofolate Reductase

a) Quantitative

Hyperproduction of chromosomal dihydrofolate reductase (DHFR), between 3- and 80-fold has been reported in many species (Burchall and Hitchings 1968; McCuen and Sirotnak 1974; Sirotnak 1971; Viswanathan et al. 1970). The enzyme is still susceptible to TMP, but the amount of TMP necessary to inhibit the increased amount is much higher.

b) Qualitative

Reduced susceptibility of chromosomal DHFR to TMP is a frequent phenomenon in TMP-resistant bacteria, owing to a decrease in the affinity of TMP for the DHFR (Poe et al. 1972; Grey et al. 1979a; Sheldon 1977). The decrease in susceptibility can be more than 1,000-fold (R. Then 1980, personal communication). Interestingly, in some strains, the decreased susceptibility of the DHFR is associated with a hyperproduction of this altered DHFR and can explain the high level resistance (MIC > 1,000 µg/ml) observed in these strains (BREEZE et al. 1975). The genes governing the enzyme DHFR, called fol A and fol B, are located at 1' on the *E. coli* K$_{12}$ chromosome (BREEZE et al. 1975; BACHMAN et al. 1976). The mutation rate in *E. coli* or *Salmonella* is 3×10^{-10} (ARIOLI et al. 1977).

One-step mutants, resistant to TMP nalidixic acid, and chloramphenicol have been isolated in vivo and in vitro, in *Klebsiella*, *Enterobacter*, and *Serratia* (RONALD et al. 1976; TRAUB and KLEBER 1977; SMITH 1976). The frequency of this triple mutation in *Klebsiella* is 4×10^{-7}. The biochemical mechanism of this type of resistance is unknown.

II. Plasmid-Mediated Resistance

R plasmids, mediating high level (MIC > 1,000 µg/ml) resistance to TMP were first described by FLEMING et al. (1972). Such plasmids, all belonging to the incompatibility group W were isolated from *Klebsiella* and *E. coli*; in these strains, resistance to TMP and sulfonamides were always associated. A few months later, HEDGES et al. (1972) isolated a plasmid of the incompatibility group I harboring resistance to TMP alone.

Since these reports, R plasmids governing TMP resistance have been found in many countries. They were isolated from *E. coli*, *Salmonella*, *Shigella*, *Citrobacter*, *Klebsiella*, *Enterobacter*, *Serratia*, *Proteus*, *Providencia*, and *Vibrio cholerae* (El Tor) (ACAR et al. 1977, 1980; ROMERO and PERDUCA 1977; GOLDSTEIN et al. 1975; MANICARDI et al. 1979; AMYES et al. 1978 a, b; BANNATYNE et al. 1980; RICHARDS et al. 1978; THRELFALL et al. 1980 a; FLEMING 1973; JOBANAPUTRA and DATTA 1974; TOWNER et al. 1979; ELWELL et al. 1980; DATTA et al. 1980, GREY et al. 1979 a, b; KAYSER and MULLER 1978; M.E. PINTO 1980, personal communication). Recently, a transferable plasmid mediating TMP resistance has been isolated from *Acinetobacter calcoaceticus* (F.W. GOLDSTEIN et al., unpublished work).

In a study in Paris (F.W. GOLDSTEIN and J.F. ACAR 1980, unpublished work) it was shown that 48% of the high level TMP-resistant enterobacteria were able to transfer the TMP resistance marker into *E. coli* K$_{12}$. More surprisingly, resistance to TMP was associated with a chloramphenicol marker in 67%–83% of the isolated plasmids. Association with a metabolic marker was also observed in plasmids isolated from *Proteus* and *E. coli*. GOLDSTEIN et al. (1975) reported the isolation of 31 plasmids belonging to six different incompatibility groups: C, M, N, FII, B, I, as described later (ACAR et al. 1977).

During a 4-year survey from 1975 to 1978, the incompatibility group C was the most prevalent among classified plasmids, especially those of hospital origin. Group C represents 40% of the TMP-resistant plasmids. In Italy, the incompatibility groups characterized were FII, N, M, and S (ROMERO and PERDUCA 1977). Eight different incompatibility groups (C, FII, N, O, W, P, X, H$_2$) have found in Great Britain since 1972 (TOWNER et al. 1980; DATTA et al. 1980).

Two different transposons carrying the TMP resistance marker have been identified in several plasmids of human and animal origin: Tn 7 associated with resistance to streptomycin and very frequently identified in bacterial plasmids and chromosomes; and Tn 402 which has been shown to be capable of insertion into bacteriophage (Datta et al. 1979; Elwell et al. 1980; Barth et al. 1976; Shapiro and Sporn 1977; Richards et al. 1978; Barth and Datta 1977).

1. Transferable

The mechanism of R plasmid-induced resistance to TMP has been described by Amyes and Smith (1974a) and Sköld and Widh (1974). This resistance is due to the production of an additional highly resistant DHFR. Three types of TMP-resistant DHFR have been described already (Amyes and Smith 1976; Pattishall et al. 1977; Tennhammar-Ekman and Sköld 1979).

2. Nontransferable

Strains exhibiting high level (MIC > 1,000 µg/ml) nontransferable resistance to TMP have been isolated with an increased frequency (Acar et al. 1980, Towner et al. 1980). As high level TMP resistance may sometimes be due to mutational events, e.g., diploidy for DHFR, the physical presence of a TMP R plasmid should be documented in such strains. The reason why in some isolates the resistance markers cannot be transferred remains obscure. This may be due either to defective transfer factors or to the insertion of transposable elements mediating TMP resistance on a nontransferable plasmid or on the bacterial chromosome (Barth et al. 1976; Bukhari et al. 1977; Richards et al. 1978; Datta et al. 1979a; Shapiro and Sporn 1977; Elwell et al. 1980).

F. Medical Implications

The medical implications of resistance to sulfonamides and/or TMP raise three questions:

What is the consequence of the resistance to one drug in the combination?

What is the risk of emergence of a resistant strain in patients treated with the combination or with one of the drugs alone?

What are the present epidemiologic data about the plasmid-mediated resistance?

I. Sulfonamide-Resistant Strains

In sulfonamide-resistant and TMP-sensitive strains, the synergistic effect between the drugs persists in spite of the resistance to sulfonamides (Böhni 1969, 1974; Acar et al. 1973; Bushby 1973a; Bach et al. 1979; Grüneberg and Lorenzo 1966; Grüneberg 1975; Ekström et al. 1979; Grey et al. 1979b; Lacey 1979; Hamilton-Miller 1979; Sourander et al. 1972; Then 1978). Many controversial results have been published, in which the techniques used to check the synergistic effects were not comparable. The clinical significance of the synergistic effect in such strains has been the most disputed point (Grey et al. 1979b). The concentrations of sulfonamide and TMP displaying synergistic effects were widely distributed, depending upon the strains and exceeded, for certain strains, the level reachable in vivo.

In our experience, synergy between sulfonamides and TMP occurs in 78% of sulfonamide-resistant strains in the range of concentrations achievable in vivo. There are very few reports of the bactericidal activity of TMP combined with sulfonamides in sulfonamide-resistant strains (BÖHNI 1969; LORIAN and FODOR 1974). In a recent study (F.W.GOLDSTEIN and J.F.ACAR 1977, unpublished work) we have observed that when tested by the cellophane transfer method (CHABBERT and PATTE 1960) or on millipore filter membranes the combination of sulfonamide and TMP has a greater bactericidal effect than TMP alone. (See also Chap.6.)

II. Sulfonamide-Sensitive, Trimethoprim-Resistant Strains

When bacteria have a low level resistance to TMP (MIC < 64 μg/ml), synergy still occurs in more than 90% of the strains (GOLDSTEIN 1977). Most of the naturally resistant strains and TMP mutants have such a resistance level. The combination of sulfonamide and TMP is clinically effective and superior to TMP alone in the treatment of infections due to such strains (WORMSER 1978). With high level resistant strains naturally *(Pseudomonas aeruginosa)* or plasmid determined, synergy is not observed or is observed only with concentrations above the clinical levels.

III. Emergence of Resistant Strains During Therapy

TMP/sulfonamide may be given to patients for a short period of 5 days to treat an acute infection or therapy may cover a long period of months or years to prevent recurrent urinary tract infection (UTI). Resistant bacteria may be selected in the urinary tract or in the vaginal and fecal flora, which are the reservoirs of urinary pathogens. UTI with sulfonamide-resistant and TMP-resistant strains during or following therapy may be due either to relapse with a resistant variant of the initial strain or to reinfection with another strain.

One type of mutant selected by TMP is represented by the thymineless bacteria (MASKELL et al. 1979). Despite the widespread use of TMP/sulfonamide combinations, thymineless bacteria are not often isolated; this can be due partially to the absence of growth of these bacteria as well in vitro (in thymine-deficient media) as in vivo, where adequate amounts of thymine-like compounds are not always encountered (see also Chaps.3 and 4).

However, there are several reports of infections with thymineless bacteria (OKUBADEJO and MASKELL 1973; BARKER et al. 1972; TAPSALL et al. 1974; MASKELL et al. 1979).

In a study made between January 1976 and June 1979 in Paris, 444 patients with UTI were treated with TMP/sulfonamide for 10–45 days. In 15 cases (3.4%), reinfection with TMP-resistant strains occurred during treatment and in 24 cases (5.4%) between 1–4 weeks after the end of the treatment. A higher rate of TMP-resistant strains has been observed in patients receiving TMP/sulfonamide as prophylaxis twice a week for at least 3 months. In 184 patients, 44 (23.9%) reinfections were due to TMP-resistant strains. In all cases, the reinfecting organisms were *E. coli* (J. GUIBERT 1980, personal communication).

In patients treated for chronic UTI, with long-term low dosage of TMP/sulfonamide, TMP-resistant strains have been isolated in 21.8% of the patients. In 5.1%, the resistance was plasmid mediated (Towner et al. 1979). In another study made in Paris, TMP-resistant enterobacteria have been isolated in the fecal flora of hospitalized patients not receiving TMP/sulfonamide. Several other reports are much less disquieting. In most cases, there was a considerable reduction in the fecal coliform flora (Näff 1971; Winberg et al. 1973; Harding and Ronald 1974; Grüneberg 1976; Toivanen et al. 1976; Grüneberg et al. 1975; Stamey et al. 1977; Knothe 1979; Sietzen and Knothe 1978; Pancoast et al. 1980).

TMP-resistant strains could be easily isolated from rectal swabs in as much as 30% of children under low dosage TMP/sulfonamide therapy (Grüneberg et al. 1976). However, when treatment was withdrawn, TMP-resistant coliforms were no longer isolated and when reinfection occurred, the strains were sensitive to TMP. In another study by Pancoast et al. (1980), although TMP-resistant organisms were isolated from the fecal flora before initiating therapy, these organisms did not persist under treatment. Prophylactic studies undertaken in immunocompromized hosts show that the emergence of TMP-resistant bacteria was significantly more frequent in the presence of TMP alone (Gurwith and Trong 1980; McNaughton et al. 1980). In other studies, no increase of TMP-resistant strains has been observed in patients treated with TMP alone (Grüneberg et al. 1975; Pancoast et al. 1980; Lacey et al. 1980).

G. Epidemiologic Overview of Resistance to Trimethoprim

I. Gram-Positive Bacteria

There are very few available data concerning resistance to TMP in gram-positive bacteria. No strain of *Listeria monocytogenes* resistant to TMP has ever been described. Reports concerning *Staphylococcus aureus* are controversial and seem to be geographically determined. Less than 6% of the strains are resistant in England and Germany, contrasting with 25% of resistant strains in Switzerland (Chatto-padhyay 1977; Meyer-Rohn and Liehr 1974; Kayser and Muller 1978). Streptococci of groups A and B are only very rarely found to be resistant to TMP. There are few reports of TMP-resistant pneumococci (Sirotnak 1971; Howe and Wilson 1972). It is interesting to note that the multiresistant strains isolated in 1978 in Paris were also resistant to TMP (MIC = 100 µg/ml) (Peyrefitte et al. 1979), and TMP-resistance was also later claimed for the multiresistant strains isolated in 1976 in South Africa (Jacobs et al. 1978; Robins-Brown et al. 1979).

II. Gram-Negative Bacteria

Reports concerning *Hemophilus* spp. are extremely confusing (May and Davies 1972; Bushby 1973 c; Kirven and Thornsberry 1978). In a 6-year survey in Paris, 2,016 strains were isolated and only 2 were resistant to TMP (Goldstein et al. 1977). As multiresistant strains of *Hemophilus* are now being isolated, special care has to be taken when testing sulfonamides and TMP.

Most of the reports on TMP resistance concern enteric gram-negative bacteria. TMP resistance in gram-negative bacteria is a ubiquitous phenomenon; resistant strains have been isolated not only from humans but also from animals. As transmission from animals to humans has been demonstrated or strongly suggested, it is important to keep track of the TMP-resistant strains wherever they occur. Animal infection or colonization by TMP-resistant strains was very uncommon before 1977. The only report with a high percentage (23.3%) of TMP-resistant strains concerned coliforms isolated from freshwater mussels in Lake Rotoiti, New Zealand (COOKE 1976). A few *E. coli* with plasmid-mediated TMP resistance were isolated in 1972 from calves in Great Britain. These plasmids belonged to the incompatibility group I and, as demonstrated later, the resistance was determined by a transposon, called Tn 7 (FLEMING 1973; BARTH et al. 1976).

In a survey conducted in Great Britain since 1956, no TMP-resistant strains were isolated before 1976 in fecal specimens from pigs. Then, the rates increased very sharply and reached 78% of the specimens collected in 1979. In some cases, the entire *E. coli* flora appeared to consist of TMP-resistant organisms. 95% of these strains had a plasmid-mediated TMP resistance transferable to *E. coli* K_{12}. At least 12 different resistance patterns have been isolated, suggesting that resistance was not related to the spread of one plasmid (*W. Smith* 1980).

In another study in Melbourne, Australia, *E. coli* with plasmid-mediated resistance could be isolated from frozen chicken carcasses purchased from several retail stores. The plasmids belonged to the incompatibility group F_1, not described anywhere else in association with TMP (CAUDRY and STANISICH 1979). Multiresistant strains of *Salmonella typhimurium* appeared in calves and then in cattle in 1977 in Great Britain. The TMP resistance in these strains was also plasmid mediated; four different plasmids harboring the TMP-resistance marker could be identified: they belonged to the incompatibility groups I_1, I_2, and H_2 (THRELFALL et al. 1980 b).

In another study, in Great Britain, plasmid-determined TMP-resistant *Salmonella* of various serotypes have been isolated since 1975 from cattle, horses, gulls, poultry, and pigs. The plasmids belonged to the incompatibility groups $I\alpha$ and $I\delta$). It has been demonstrated that the resistance gene was carried on a transposon similar to Tn 7. The TMP associated with the streptomycin resistance marker could be transposed to other plasmids and to the *E. coli* chromosome. These strains have been responsible for 290 cases of food poisoning with 2 fatal cases (RICHARDS et al. 1978).

The number of TMP-resistant strains, isolated from human infections varies from country to country. At the Saint Joseph Hospital, in Paris, France, resistance to TMP in enterobacteria increased from 17.9% in 1972, to 22.5% in 1979. Highly resistant strains (MIC > 1,000 µg/ml) increased in the same period from 7.2% to 16.4%. In two surveys, in 1974–1975 and 1978–1979, respectively 31.2% and 48.3% of the highly resistant strains could transfer their resistance marker into *E. coli* K_{12}. In 1978, 12% of *E. coli* and *Proteus mirabilis* were resistant to TMP, compared with only 3% in a similar hospital in Boston, Massachusetts, United States.

In Great Britain, where the combination TMP/sulfonamide was first available for clinical use (in 1969), resistance to TMP has been carefully monitored. Resistant bacteria, especially *Klebsiella* had already been isolated long before its introduction (HAMILTON-MILLER and GREY 1975). Resistance was low in 1970 with only 2.5% of isolates from outpatients, mostly *Klebsiella* and *Enterobacter* (LACEY et al. 1972). After 2 years utilization, resistance to TMP increased in all the different surveys. In a multicenter study, resistance to TMP occurred in 7% of strains from outpatients and 12% from inpatients (MCALLISTER et al. 1971). In a London hospital, the incidence of TMP-resistant strains rose from 4% to 7% for outpatients and 17% to 24% for inpatients between 1971 and 1974. Lower rates were observed in two surveys from two London hospitals: from 1975 to 1977, the incidence of TMP-resistant strains increased from 8% to 10.8% (AMYES et al. 1978) in one study and from 11% in 1975 to 15% in 1979 in another study (DATTA et al. 1980). In both studies, however, an increase in strains harboring TMP-resistant plasmids was observed.

In another survey in Nottingham, England, the incidence of TMP-resistance showed a slight decrease from 4.8% in 1978 to 2.9% in 1979. However, there was a large increase, from 12.5% to 34.7% in the proportions of strains exhibiting a high level resistance to TMP, transferable or nontransferable (TOWNER 1979; TOWNER et al. 1980).

In Pavia, Italy, the incidence of TMP-resistant strains increased from 13% in 1973 to 30% in 1975, and the frequency of TMP R factors increased from 10% to 20% (ROMERO and PERDUCA 1977). In another study in Modena, TMP-resistant strains represented 9.4% of the isolates in 1976–1977. Of these strains, 18% had a TMP-resistant plasmid. About 20% of the strains isolated in Hamburg, Germany, between 1970 and 1973, and 8% of the strains isolated in Copenhagen, Denmark, were resistant to TMP (MEYER-ROHN and LIEHR 1974; FRUENSGAARD and KORNER 1974).

In Zürich, Switzerland, the incidence of TMP-resistant strains increased from 24% in 1974 to 28% in 1977. In 16% of these strains, the TMP-resistance was plasmid mediated (KAYSER and MULLER 1978). In Turku, Finland, plain TMP has been used since 1973, for UTI. In 1978, about 20% of isolates from outpatients and 40% from inpatients were resistant to TMP. Resistance was especially high in *Proteus mirabilis*: 52% of the strains isolated from outpatients and 76% of the strains isolated from inpatients were resistant. In contrast, the rate of resistant *Klebsiella* has been found to be higher when isolated from outpatients (56%) than when isolated from inpatients (41%) (HUOVINEN and TOIVANEN 1980). A comparison between enterobacteria isolated in 1978 from UTI in Finland and in France shows that 61.8% of the strains in Finland compared with 22.7% in France had low level TMP resistance, presumably chromosomally determined (ACAR et al. 1980).

In spite of heavy clinical use of TMP for a variety of clinical processes, bacterial resistance to TMP ordinarily remains low. However, some potential hazards are emerging:

1. The possible selection in vivo of TMP-resistant mutants in many bacterial species, especially in *Klebsiella*, *Enterobacter*, and *Serratia*.
2. The presence in many countries, and sometimes at high levels, of transferable R plasmids which may determine resistance to TMP and other antibiotics and thus be selected by TMP or by the other antibiotics.

References

Acar JF, Goldstein FW, Chabbert YA (1973) Synergistic activity of trimethoprim-sulphamethoxazole combination in Gram-negative bacilli. Observations in vitro and in vivo. J Infect Dis [Suppl] 128:470–477

Acar JF, Goldstein FW, Gerbaud GR, Chabbert YA (1977) Plasmides de résistance au tri-méthoprime: transférabilité et groupes d'incompabilité. Ann Inst Pasteur (Paris) 128 A:41–47

Acar JF, Goldstein FW, Pinto ME, Then RL, Toivanen P (1980) Comparison of trimetho-prim-resistant strains isolated from urinary tract infections in Finland and France. Proc 11 th ICC/19 th ICAAC, Boston. In: Nelson, JD, Grassi C (eds) Current chemotherapy and infectious diseases. American Society for Microbiology, Washington, DC

Akiba T, Yokota T (1962) Studies on the mechanism of transfert of drug resistance in bac-teria: 18: incorporation of 35 S sulphathiazole into cells of the multiple resistant strains and artificial sulfonamide-resistant strain of E. coli. Med Biol (Tokyo) 63:155–159

Amyes SGB, Smith JT (1974 a) R-factor trimethoprim resistance mechanism: an insuscep-tible target site. Biochem Biophys Res Commun 58:412–418

Amyes SGB, Smith JT (1974 b) Trimethoprim sensitivity testing and thymineless mutants. J Med Microbiol 7:143–153

Amyes SGB, Smith JT (1975) Thymineless mutants and their resistance to trimethoprim. J Antimicrob Chemother 1:85–89

Amyes SGB, Smith JT (1976) The purification and properties of the trimethoprim-resistant DHFR mediated by the R-factor R 388. Eur J Biochem 61:597–603

Amyes SGB, Smith JT (1978) R-factor mediated dihydrofolate reductase which confers trimethoprim resistance. J Gen Microbial 107:263–271

Amyes SGB, Emmerson AM, Smith JT (1978) R-factor mediated trimethoprim-resistance: result of two three months clinical surveys. J Clin Pathol 31:850–854

Arioli V, Berti M, Caniti G, Rossi E, Silvestri LG (1977) Interaction between rifampicin and trimethoprim in vitro and in experimental infections. J Antimicrob Chemother 3:87–94

Bachmann BJ, Brooks Low K, Taylor LA (1976) Recalibrated linkage map of Escherichia coli K12. Bacteriol Rev 40/1:116–167

Bannatyne RM, Toma S, Cheung R, Hu G (1980) Resistance to trimethoprim and other antibiotics in Ontario Shigellae. Lancet 1:425–426

Barker J, Healing D, Hutchinson JGP (1972) Characteristics of some co-trimoxazole resis-tant Enterobacteriacae from infected patients. J Clin Pathol 25:1086–1088

Barth PN, Datta N (1977) Transposons determining trimethoprim and streptomycin resis-tance that are indistinguishable from transposons 7. Proc Soc Gen Microbiol 4:99–100

Barth PT, Datta N, Hedges RW, Grinter NJ (1976) Transposition of a deoxyribonucleic acid sequence encoding trimethoprim and streptomycin resistance from R 483 to other replicons. J Bacteriol 125:800–810

Black WA (1970) Sensitivity of Nocardia to trimethoprim and sulfonamides in vitro. J Clin Pathol 23:423

Böhni E (1969) Vergleichende bakteriologische Untersuchungen mit der Kombination Tri-methoprim/Sulfamethoxazol in vitro and in vivo. Chemotherapy [Suppl] 14:1–21

Böhni E (1974) Co-trimoxazole in sulfonamide-resistant infections. Prog Chemother 2:204–210

Breeze AS, Sims P, Stacey KA (1975) Trimethoprim-resistant mutants of E. coli K 12: pre-liminary genetic mapping. Genet Res 25:207–214

Burchall JJ (1973) Mechanisms of action of trimethoprim sulfamethoxazole. II. J Infect Dis [Suppl] 128:S 437–S 441

Burchall JJ, Hitchings GH (1968) The role of metabolites and antimetabolites in the control of folate coenzyme synthesis. Adv Enzyme Regul 6:323–333

Bushby SRM (1973 a) Trimethoprim-sulphamethoxazole: in vitro microbiological aspects. J Infect Dis [Suppl] 128:442–462

Bushby SRM (1973 b) Sensitivity testing with trimethoprim/sulphamethoxazole. Med J Aust [Suppl] 1:10–18

Bushby SRM (1973 c) Haemophilus influenzae apparently resistant to trimethoprim. Br Med J 3/1:50–51

Bushby SRM, Hitchings GH (1968) Trimethoprim, a sulphonamide potentiator. Br J Phar-macol Chemother 33:72–90

Caudry SD, Stanisich VA (1979) Incidence of antibiotic-resistant Escherichia coli associated with frozen chicken carcasses and characterization of conjugative R-plasmids derived from such strains. Antimicrob Agents Chemother 16/6:701–709

Chabbert YA, Patte JC (1960) Cellophane transfer. Application to the study of activity of combinations of antibiotics. Appl Microbiol 8:193–197

Chattopadhyay B (1977) Co-trimoxazole resistant staphylococcus aureus in hospital practice. J Antimicrob Chemother 3:371–375

Cooke MD (1976) Antibiotic resistance among coliform and fecal coliform bacteria isolated from the freshwater mussel Hydridella menziesii. Antimicrob Agents and Chemother 9/6:885–888

Dale BA, Greenberg GR (1972) Effect of the folic acid analogue, trimethoprim, on growth, macromolecular synthesis and incorporation of exogenous thymine in E. coli. J Bacteriol 110:905–916

Datta N, Hugues VM, Nugent ME, Richards H (1979a) Plasmids and transposons and their stability and mutability in bacteria isolated during an outbreak of hospital infection. Plasmid 2:182–186

Datta N, Nugent M, Amyes SGB, McNeilly P (1979b) Multiple mechanisms of trimethoprim-resistance in strains of Escherichia coli from a patient treated with long term co-trimoxazole. J Antimicrob Chemother 5:399–406

Datta N, Dacey S, Hughes V et al. (1980) Distribution of genes for trimethoprim and gentamicin resistance in bacteria and their plasmids in a general hospital. J Gen Microbiol 118:495–508

Davis BD, Maas WK (1952) Analysis of the biochemical mechanisms of drug resistance in certain bacterial mutants. Proc Nat Acad Sci USA 38:775–785

Ekström B, Forsgren V, Ötengren B, Bergan T (1979) Development of sulphonamide-trimethoprim combinations for urinary tract infections, part I. Infection [Suppl 4] 7:359–366

Elwell LP, Fling M, Walton L, Dornbush K (1980) Plasmid-mediated trimethoprim-resistance: detection of the trimethoprim-resistance transposon Tn 7, and cloning and expression of plasmid-encoded reductase genes. Proc 11 th ICC/19 th ICAAC, Boston. In: Nelson JD, Grassi C (eds) Current chemotherapy and infectious diseases. American Society of Microbiology, Washington, DC

Ferone R, Bushby SRM, Burchall JJ, Moore WD, Smith D (1975) Identification of the Harper-Cawston factor as thymidine phosphorylase and removal from media of substances interfering with susceptibility testing to sulfonamides and diaminopyrimidines. Antimicrob Agents Chemother 7:91–98

Fleming MP (1973) Trimethoprim resistance and its transferability in E. coli isolated from calves treated with trimethoprim-sulphadiazine: a two-year study. J Hyg (Lond) 71:669–677

Fleming MP, Datta N, Grüneberg RN (1972) Trimethoprim resistance determined by R factors. Br Med J 1:726–728

Fruensgaard K, Korner B (1974) Alterations in the sensitivity pattern after use of trimethoprim/sulfamethoxazole for two years in the treatment of urinary tract infections. Chemotherapy 20:97–101

Fuchs JA, Neuhard J (1973) A mutant of Escherichia coli defective in ribonucleoside diphosphate reductase. I. Isolation of the mutants as a deoxyuridine auxotroph. Eur J Biochem 32:451–456

Goldstein FW (1977) Mécanismes de résistance aux sulfamides et au triméthoprime. Bull Inst Pasteur (Paris) 75:109–139

Goldstein FW, Acar JF, Gerbaud GR, Chabbert YA (1975) Transferable trimethoprim resistance mediated by plasmids of various incompatibility groups. Abstracts 15 th ICAAC, p 169

Goldstein FW, Boisivon A, Leclerc P, Acar JF (1977) Sensibilité d'Hémophilus sp. aux antibiotiques. Transfert de résistance à Escherichia coli. Pathol Biol (Paris) 25/5:323–332

Grey D, Hamilton-Miller JMT, Brumfitt W (1979a) Incidence and mechanisms of resistance to trimethoprim in clinically isolated Gram-negative bacteria. Chemotherapy 25:147–156

Grey D, Hamilton-Miller JMT, Brumfitt W (1979b) Combined action of sulphamethoxazole and trimethoprim against clinically-isolated sulphonamide-resistant bacteria. Chemotherapy 25:296–302

Grüneberg E, de Lorenzo WF (1966) Potentiation of sulfonamides and antibiotics by trimethoprim [(2,4-diamino-5 (3,4,5-trimethoxybenzyl) pyrimidine]. Antimicrob Agents Chemother: 430–433

Grüneberg RN (1975) The use of co-trimoxazole in sulphonamide-resistant Escherichia coli urinary tract infection. J Antimicrob Chemother 1:305–310

Grüneberg RN (1976) Susceptibility of urinary pathogens to various antimicrobial substances: a four-year study. J Clin Pathol 29:292–295

Grüneberg RN, Leakey A, Bendall MJ, Smellie JM (1975) Bowel flora in urinary tract infection: effect of chemotherapy with special reference to co-trimoxazole. Kidney Int [Suppl] 8 S:122–129

Grüneberg RN, Smellie JM, Leakey A (1976) Long-term low dosage co-trimoxazole in prophylaxis of childhood urinary tract infection: bacteriological aspects. Br Med J 2:206–208

Gurwith M, Trong K (1980) Comparison of prophylactic trimethoprim/sulfamethoxazole and trimethoprim alone in compromized hosts. Proc 17th ICC/19th ICAAC, Boston. In: Nelson JD, Grassi C (eds) Current chemotherapy and infectious diseases. American Society for Microbiology, Washington, DC

Hamilton-Miller JMT, Grey D (1975) Resistance to trimethoprim in Klebsiella isolated before its introduction. J Antimicrob Chemother 1:213–218

Hamilton-Miller JMT (1979) Mechanisms and distribution of bacterial resistance to diaminopyrimidines and sulphonamides. J Antimicrob Chemother [Suppl B] 5:61–73

Harding GKM, Ronald AR (1974) A controlled study of antimicrobial prophylaxis of recurrent urinary infection in women. N Engl J Med 291:597–601

Harrison AP Jr (1965) Thymine incorporation and metabolism by various classes of thymineless bacteria. J Gen Microbiol 41:321–333

Hedges RW, Datta N, Flemings MP (1972) R factors confering resistance to trimethoprim but not to sulfonamides. J Gen Microbiol 73:573–575

Howe JG, Wilson TS (1972) Co-trimoxazole resistant pneumococci. Lancet 2:184–185

Huovinen P, Toivanen P (1980) Trimethoprim-resistance in Finland after five years use of plain trimethoprim. Br Med J 280:72–74

Jacobs MR, Koornhof HJ, Robins-Browne RM et al. (1978) N Engl J Med 299:735–740

Jobanaputra RS, Datta N (1974) Trimethoprim R factors in enterobacteria from clinical specimens. J Med Microbiol 7:169–177

Johnson JR, Collins GM, Rementer ML, Hall ML (1976) Novel mechanism of resistance to folate analogues: ribonucleoside diphosphate reductase deficiency in bacteriophage T_4. Antimicrob Agents Chemother 9:292–300

Kayser FH, Muller I (1978) Resistance of bacteria to sulfamethoxazole/trimethoprim. Proc 10th Int Congr Chem 1:657–658

Kirven LA, Thornsberry C (1978) Minimum bactericidal concentration of sulfamethoxazole-trimethoprim for Haemophilus influenzae: correlation with prophylaxis. Antimicrob Agents Chemother 14/5:731–736

Knothe H (1979) The effect of trimethoprim-sulphonamide, trimethoprim and sulfonamide on the occurence of resistant Enterobacteriacae in human intestinal flora. Infection [Suppl 4] 7:321–323

Lacey RW (1979) Mechanism of action of trimethoprim and sulphonamides: relevance to synergy in vivo. J Antimicrob Chemother [Suppl B] 5:75–83

Lacey RW, Gillespie WA, Bruten DM, Lewis EL (1972) Trimethoprim-resistant coliforms. Lancet 1:409–411

Lacey RW, Lord VL, Gunasekera HKW, Leiberman PJ, Luxton DEA (1980) Comparison of trimethoprim alone with trimethoprim-sulfamethoxazole in the treatment of respiratory and urinary infections with particular reference to selection of trimethoprim resistance. Lancet 1:1270–1273

Landy M, Gerstung RB (1944) Para-aminobenzoic acid synthesis by Neisseria gonorrhoeae in relation to clinical and cultural sulfonamides resistance (note). J Bacteriol 47:448

Landy M, Larkum NW, Oswald EJ, Streighitoff F (1943) Increased synthesis of para-aminobenzoic acid associated with the development of sulfonamide resistance in Staphylococcus aureus. Science 97:265

Lomax MS, Greenberg GR (1968) Characteristics of the deo operon: role in thymine utilization and sensitivity to deoxyribonucleosides. J Bacteriol 96:501–514

Lorian V, Fodor G (1974) Technique for determining the bacterial effect of drug combinations. Antimicrob Agents Chemother 6:630–633

Manicardi G, Bondi M, Ferrari L, Neglia R, Quaglio GP, Eabio U (1979) Classification of trimethoprim resistance plasmids. In: Brumfitt W, Cucio L, Silvestri L (eds) New perspectives in clinical microbiology, vol 2. Martinus-Nijhoff, The Hague

Maskell R, Okubadejo OA, Payne RH, Plad L (1979) Human infections with thymine requiring bacteria. J Med Microbiol 11:33–45

May JR, Davies J (1972) Resistance of Haemophilus influenzae to trimethoprim. Br Med J 3:376–377

McAllister TA, Alexander JG, Dulake C, Percival A, Boyce JMH, Normald PJ (1971) The sensitives of urinary-pathogens – a survey. Multicentric study of sensitives of urinary tract pathogens. Postgrad Med J [Suppl] 47:7–14

McCuen RW, Sirotnak FM (1974) Hyperproduction of dihydrofolate reductase in Diplococcus pneumoniae by mutation in the structural gene. The absence of an effect on other enzymes of folate coenzyme biosynthesis. Biochim Biophys Acta 338:540–544

McNaughton RD, Riben P, Light B et al. (1980) Comparison of trimethoprim and trimethoprim/sulfamethoxazole prophylaxis in neutropenic patients: elimination of potential pathogens and emergence of resistance. Proc 17th ICC/19th ICAAC, Boston. In: Nelson JD, Grassi C (eds) Current chemotherapy and infectious diseases. American Society for Microbiology, Washington, DC

Meyer-Rohn, Liehr W (1974) Zur Resistenzentwicklung von Bacterien gegen Trimethoprim/Sulfamethoxazol (Eusaprim). Fortsch Med 92:121–126

Näff H (1971) Über die Veränderungen der normalen Darmflora des Menschen durch Bactrim. Pathol Microbiol 37:1–22

Nagate T, Inoue M, Inoue K, Mitsuhashi S (1978) Plasmid-mediated sulfonamide resistance. Microbiol Immunol 22:367–375

O'Brien TF, Acar JF, Medeiros AA, Norton RA, Goldstein FW, Kent RL (1978) International comparison of prevalence of resistance to antibiotics. JAMA 239/15:1518–1523

Okada T (1966) Mutational site of the gene controlling quantitative thymine requirement in E. coli K 12. Genetics 54:1329–1336

Okubadejo OA, Maskell RM (1973) Thymine-requiring mutants of Proteus mirabilis selected by co-trimoxazole in vivo. J Gen Microbiol 77:533–535

Pancoast SJ, Hyams DMeu HC (1980) Effect of trimethoprim-sulfamethoxazole on development of drug-resistant vaginal and fecal flora. Antimicrob Agents Chemother 17/2:263–268

Pato ML, Brown GM (1969) Mechanisms of resistance of E. coli to sulfonamides. Arch Biochem Biophys 103:443–448

Pattishall KH, Acar JF, Burchall JJ, Goldstein FW, Harvey RJ (1977) Two distinct types of trimethoprim-resistant dihydrofolate reductase specified by R. plasmids of different compatibility groups. J Biol Chem 252/7:2319–2323

Peyrefitte F, Galland A, Malhuret C, Goldstein FW, Bouvet A (1979) Les pneumocoques aussi sont résistants aux antibiotiques. Nouv Presse Med 8/11:872

Poe M, Greenfield NJ, Hirshfield JM, Williams MN, Hoogsteen K (1972) Dihydrofolate reductase purification and characterization of the enzyme from an amethopterin resistant mutant of E. coli. Biochemistry 11:1023–1030

Richards H, Datta N, Wray C, Sojka WJ (1978) Trimethoprim-resistance plasmids and transposons in Salmonella. Lancet 2:1194–1195

Richmond MH (1966) Structural analogy and chemical reactivity in the action of antibacterial compounds. Symp Soc Gen Microbiol 16:301–335

Robins-Brown RM, Gaspar MN, Ward JI, Wachsmuth IK, Koornhof HJ, Jacobs MR, Thornsberry C (1979) Resistance mechanisms of multiply resistant pneumococci: antibiotic degradation studies. Antimicrob Agents Chemother 15/3:470–474

Romero E, Perduca M (1977) Compatibility groups of R-factors for trimethoprim-resistance isolated in Italy. J Antimicrob Chemother [Suppl C] 3:35–38

Ronald AR, Cates C, Hoban S, Harding G (1976) The epidemiology of Nalidixic acid and or trimethoprim resistant Enterobacteria. Clin Res 24:678 B

Shapiro JA, Sporn P (1977) Tn 402: a new transposable element that inserts in bacterio-phage Lambda. J Bacteriol 129:1632–1635

Sheldon R (1977) Altered dihydrofolate reductase in fol regulatory mutants of Escherichia coli K 12. Mol Gen Genet 151:215–219

Sietzen W, Knothe H (1978) Effect of trimethoprim, trimethoprim/sulfamethoxazole and sulfamethoxazole on the occurence of drug resistant Enterobacteriacae in the human bowel flora. Curr Chemother 1:660–662

Sirotnak FM (1971) High dihydrofolate reductase levels in Diplococcus pneumoniae after mutation in the structural gene. J Bacteriol 106:318–324

Sköld O (1976) R-factor mediated resistance to sulfonamides by a plasmid-borne drug re-sistant dihydropteroate synthase. Antimicrob Agents Chemother 9:49–54

Sköld O, Widh A (1974) A new dihydrofolate reductase with low trimethoprim sensitivity induced by an R-factor mediating high resistance to trimethoprim. J Biol Chem 249:4324–4325

Smith HW (1976) Mutants of Klebsiella pneumoniae resistant to several antibiotics. Nature 259:307–308

Smith JT (1980) Some biochemical mechanisms of antibiotics acting together on bacterial folate metabolism. In: Williams JD (ed) Antibiotic interactions. Academic Press, New York London, pp 87–98

Smith W (1980) Antibiotic-resistant Escherichia coli in market pigs in 1956–1979: the emer-gence of organisms with plasmid-borne trimethoprim-resistance. J Hyg (Lond) 84:467–477

Sourander L, Saarimaa H, Arvilommi H (1972) Treatment of sulfonamide-resistant urinary tract infections with a combination of sulfonamide and trimethoprim. Acta Med Scand 191:1–3

Stacey KA, Simson E (1965) Improved method for the isolation of thymine requiring mu-tants of E. coli. J Bacteriol 90:554–555

Stamey TA, Condy M, Mihara G (1977) Prophylactic efficacy of nitrofurantoin macrocrys-tals and trimethoprim-sulfamethoxazole in urinary infections. Biologic effects on the vaginal and rectal flora. N Engl J Med 296:780–783

Stokes A, Lacey RW (1978) Effect of thymidine on activity of trimethoprim and sul-phamethoxazole. J Clin Pathol 31:165

Swedberg G, Sköld O (1980) Characterization of different plamid-borne dihydropteroate synthases mediating bacterial resistance to sulfonamides. J Bacteriol 142:1–7

Swedberg G, Cartensson S, Sköld O (1979) Characterization of mutationally altered dihy-dropteroate synthase and its ability to form a sulfonamide-containing dihydrofolate analog. J Bacteriol 137:129–136

Tapsall JW, Wilson E, Harper J (1974) Thymine dependent strains of E. coli selected by trimethoprim-sulfamethoxazole therapy. Pathology 6:161–167

Tennhammar-Ekman B, Sköld O (1979) Trimethoprim-resistance plasmids of different or-igin encode different drug-resistant dihydrofolate-reductases. Plasmid 2:334–346

Then R (1978) Synergism between trimethoprim and sulphamethoxazole. Science 197:1301

Then R, Angehrn P (1979) Low trimethoprim susceptibility of anaerobic bacteria due to in-sensitive dihydrofolate reductases. Antimicrob Agents Chemother 15/1:1–6

Threlfall EJ, Rowe B, Huq I (1980a) Plasmid-encoded multiple antibiotic resistance in Vi-brio cholerae El Tor from Bangladesh. Lancet I:1247–1248

Threlfall EJ, Ward LR, Ashley AS, Rowe B (1980b) Plasmid-encoded trimethoprim resis-tance in multiresistant epidemic Salmonella thyphimurium phage types 204 and 193. Br Med J 5:1210–1211

Tillet WS, Cambier MJ, Harris WH Jr (1943) Sulfonamide-fast pneumococci. Clinical re-ports of two cases of pneumonia together with experimental studies on the effectiveness of penicillin and tyrothricin against sulfonamide-resistant strains. J Clin Invest 22:249–255

Toivanen A, Kasanen A, Sundquist H, Toivanen P (1976) Effect of trimethoprim on the oc-curence of drug-resistant coliform bacteria in the faecal flora. Chemotherapy 22:97–103

Towner KJ (1979) Classification of transferable plasmids conferring resistance to trimetho-prim isolated in Great-Britain. FEMS Microbiol Lett 5:319–321

Towner KJ, Pearson NF, Cattell WR, O'Grady F (1979) Trimethoprim R plasmids isolated during long-term treatment of urinary tract infection with co-trimoxazole. J Antimicrob Chemother 5:45–52

Towner KJ, Pearson NJ, Pinn PA, O'Grady F (1980) Increasing importance of plasmid-mediated trimethoprim resistance in enterobacteria: two six-month clinical surveys. Br Med J 280/1:517–519

Traub WH, Kleber I (1977) Selected and spontaneous variants of Serratia marcescens with combined resistance against chloramphenicol, nalidixic acid and trimethoprim. Chemotherapy 23:436

Viswanathan G, Amin PM, Noronha JM (1970) Folate metabolism: α-aminopterin resistance in Escherichia coli. Indian J Biochem 7:226–230

Wacker A, Trebst A, Simon H (1959) Über den Stoffwechsel des Sulfanilamids S_{35} bei empfindlichen und resistenten Bakterien. Z Naturforsch [C] 12b:315–319

White PJ, Woods DD (1965a) The synthesis of para-aminobenzoic acid and folic acid by staphylococci sensitive and resistant to sulphonamides. J Gen Microbiol 40:243–253

White PJ, Woods DD (1965b) Biochemical properties of staphylococci sensitive and resistant to sulphonamides. J Gen Microbiol 40:255–271

Winberg J, Bergstoin T, Lincoln K (1973) Treatment trials in urinary tract infections with special reference to the effects of antimicrobials on the fecal and periurethral flora. Clin Nephrol 142–148

Wise EM Jr, Abou-Donia MM (1975) Sulfonamide resistance mechanisms in E. coli: R plasmids can determine sulfonamide-resistant dihydropteroate synthetases. Proc Natl Acad Sci USA 72:2621–2625

Wolf B, Hotchkiss RD (1963) Genetically modified folic acid synthetising enzymes of Pneumococcus. Biochemistry 2:145–150

Wormser GP (1978) Trimethoprim-sulfamethoxazole. II. Clinical studies. NY State J Med 78/13:2058–2067

Yokota T, Akiba T (1961) Studies on the mechanism of transfert of drug-resistance in bacteria. – IV. Biochemical aspects of the mechanism of resistance to sulfonamide in the sulfonamide-resistant and multiple-drug-resistant strains of E. coli. Med Biol (Tokyo) 58:151–154

Clinical Studies

CHAPTER 12

Trimethoprim Alone: Clinical Uses

D.W. Barry and K.H. Pattishall

A. Introduction

Trimethoprim (TMP) is an effective and potent antibacterial agent. Although academics and practitioners alike have been intrigued by the consistent enhancement of TMP's activity by sulfamethoxazole and have more recently been fascinated by its synergism with other sulfonamides as well as agents as disparate as polymyxin and rifampin, it would be unfortunate if this intellectual attraction were to prevent a critical examination of the potential use of TMP alone in certain infections. In this chapter, the accumulated clinical data on the use of TMP as a single entity will be reviewed so that the comparative safety and efficacy of this drug may be defined. We will also analyze those clinical situations in which its synergistic activity with sulfamethoxazole is required to cure the infection and those in which it is not. In addition, by examination of available in vitro, epidemiologic, and human experimental data, the risk and clinical relevance of the potential emergence of TMP-resistant organisms may be determined.

B. Microbiologic and Pharmacokinetic Properties

Before embarking on a review of clinical investigations with TMP, however, it is worthwhile to summarize briefly the appropriate microbiologic and pharmacologic aspects of the drug (see also Chaps. 4, 10). As shown in Table 1, the majority of aerobic gram-positive and gram-negative organisms are inhibited by less than 4 μg/ml TMP (Bushby and Hitchings 1968; Bushby 1969). Exceptions to this are *Mycobacterium tuberculosis, Nocardia asteroides, Pseudomonas aeruginosa*, and *Neisseria gonorrhoeae*, or *Neisseria meningitidis*, which are relatively insensitive. *Clostridium perfringens* and other strict anaerobes usually are not sensitive. Although these sensitivities may be improved 10- to 50-fold by the addition of 20 parts sulfamethoxazole for each part TMP, it might be expected that this enhanced inhibitory activity will be useful only in those tissues where the inhibitory level of TMP against the infecting bacterium cannot be achieved. Careful examination of the pharmacology of TMP will clarify the circumstances under which those conditions may occur.

As shown in Fig. 1, a single oral dose of 100 mg TMP will yield a peak plasma level of approximately 1 μg/ml (of which approximately 44% is protein bound) within 1–4 h after ingestion. A single 200 mg dose will yield levels approximately twice as high (Bach et al. 1973; Schwartz and Ziegler 1969). The half-life of TMP in the serum ranges from 8 to 14 h (Welling et al. 1973). TMP is moderately

Table 1. Sensitivity of bacterial strains to TMP

Organism	Minimum inhibitory concentration of TMP (µg/ml)
Gram-positive bacteria	
Staphylococcus pyogenes	0.2
Streptococcus pyogenes (Group A)	0.4
Streptococcus pneumoniae	1.0
Streptococcus viridans	0.25
Streptococcus faecalis (faecium) (Enterococcus, Group D)	0.5
Clostridium perfringens	50.0
Corynebacterium diphtheriae	0.4
Gram-negative bacteria	
Escherichia coli	0.2
Enterobacter (Aerobacter) spp.	3.0
Klebsiella pneumoniae	0.5
Citrobacter freundii	0.1
Proteus spp.	1.0
Salmonella typhi	0.4
Salmonella typhimurium	0.3
Shigella spp.	0.4
Neisseria gonorrhoeae	12.0
Neisseria meningitidis	8.0
Hemophilus influenzae	0.12
Bordetella pertussis	1.0 − 3.0
Vibrio cholerae	0.8
Pseudomonas aeruginosa	> 100.0
Miscellaneous	
Mycobacterium tuberculosis	250.0
Nocardia asteroides	10.0

[a] Compiled from data published by Bushby and Hitchings (1968) and Bushby (1969), see also Chap. 4

removed by hemodialysis (Rieder et al. 1974), but not by intraperitoneal dialysis (Hoppe-Seyler et al. 1974).

TMP is widely distributed in the body and, in fact, is concentrated in a number of tissues and organs, primarily as a result of its lipophilic properties (Craig and Kunin 1973). Figure 2 shows the ratio of tissue concentration to serum concentration for TMP in various organs of the rhesus monkey, and demonstrates that the drug is very significantly concentrated in the kidney, liver, lung, pancreas, thyroid, adrenal, spleen, and intestine. Less complete and primarily anecdotal data have been obtained in humans for a number of tissues and they are shown in Table 2. The general trend shows that for TMP, concentrations in the various tissues exceed the concentrations in plasma.

Data from other studies show that levels of TMP in sputum are equal to or greater than the corresponding blood level (Jordan et al. 1975; Hughes et al. 1977; Beck and Pechere 1970). In the cerebrospinal fluid, the drug

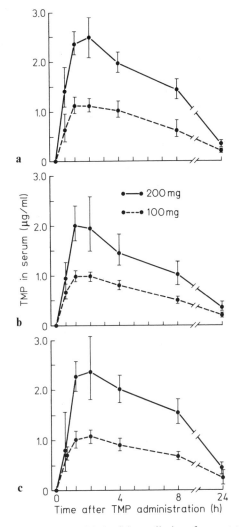

Fig. 1a-c. Geometric means and 95% confidence limits of concentrations of trimethoprim (TMP) in serum of normal young adults after single doses of TMP alone as determined by fluorometric assay [Hoffmann La Roche (**a**)] and two bioassays [Channing (**b**) and Burroughs Wellcome (**c**)]. BACH et al. (1973)

level achieved is approximately 40%–50% of the plasma level (FRIES et al. 1975; SABEL und BRANDBERG 1975; SVEDHEM and IWARSON 1979). TMP also may be found in the bile and breast milk (RIEDER 1973; ARNAULD et al. 1972). Levels of TMP in the uninflamed prostate (tissue and fluid) have been reported to be higher than corresponding serum levels (OOSTERLINCK et al. 1975; DABHOIWALA et al. 1976; LYKKEGAARD-NIELSEN and HANSEN 1972). The level of TMP has also been documented to equal or exceed the simultaneous plasma level in saliva (FOWLE 1973; EATMAN et al. 1977), vaginal secretions (STAMEY and CONDY 1975), intracellular fluid (FOWLE 1973), and fetal blood (REID et al. 1975), whereas lower,

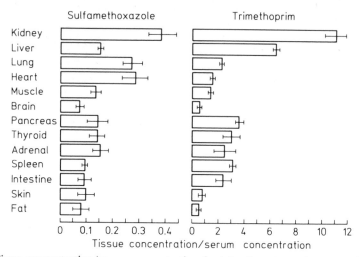

Fig. 2. Tissue concentration/serum concentration for trimethoprim and nonacetylated sulfamethoxazole in 13 types of tissue at equilibrium; mean values for four monkeys, with standard deviations. Craig and Kunin (1973)

but potentially therapeutic concentrations have been found in bone marrow, spongy and compact bone (Hansen et al. 1975), amniotic fluid (Ylikorkala et al. 1973), seminal fluid (Gnarpe and Friberg 1976), aqueous humor (Salmon et al. 1975; Pohjanpelto et al. 1974), and abscess cavity (Greene et al. 1975).

C. Relation of Sensitivities and Pharmacokinetics to Therapy of Urinary Tract Infections

I. General

Excretion of TMP occurs chiefly through glomerular filtration and renal tubular secretion, and thus extremely high levels of TMP are found in the urine (Sharpstone 1969); 50%–60% of the ingested dose is excreted by the kidneys within 24 h, 80% of which is in the unmetabolized form. After a single oral dose of 100 mg, 30–160 µg/ml TMP will be found in the urine during the first 4 h, and urinary levels of 18–91 µg/ml may be found in the 8–24 h collection sample (Bach et al. 1973). In renal insufficiency, the half-life of TMP is increased; however, the rate of decline of TMP clearance is less than that of creatinine clearance (Rieder et al. 1974).

It therefore becomes readily apparent that TMP alone might be expected to be effective in eradicating most *Enterobacteriaceae* from the urinary tract since TMP will be found in the urine at concentrations usually many times their inhibitory level listed on Table 1. Stamey and co-workers have previously demonstrated that the concentration of the antibacterial in the urine rather than the blood determines whether the organism will be eradicated and the patient cured of either cystitis or pyelonephritis (Stamey et al. 1965). Conversely, TMP alone might be expected to be ineffective if the patient is suffering from a septicemia caused, for example, by *Klebsiella pneumoniae* with a minimum inhibitory concentration (MIC) of 5 µg/ml

Table 2. Concentrations[a] of trimethoprim in tissues and body fluids

Patient	Tissue type	Tissue TMP (μg/g wet weight)	Plasma TMP (μg/ml)
1	Stomach	5.0	4.1
2	Stomach	3.0	5.3
3	Stomach	4.5	1.2
4	Colon	20.7	12.0
3	Colon	12.6	5.9
5	Gall bladder	7.1	3.0
6	Gall bladder	18.9	7.3
7	Gall bladder	13.8	8.2
8	Skin	13.5	2.7
9	Skin	5.6	5.0
10	Anal skin and hemorrhoid tissue	10.3	3.8
11	Anal skin and hemorrhoid tissue	7.0	4.4
12	Anal skin and hemorrhoid tissue	14.0	5.1
13	Thyroid tissue	12.2	7.9
14	Thyroid tissue	1.0	4.1
15	Thyroid tissue	4.2	6.0
16	Breast	7.2	5.3
17	Varicose veins	5.1	6.4
6	Varicose veins	6.5	7.5
18	Varicose veins	13.9	6.1
19	Lung	21.0	2.4
5	Aneurysmal wall	2.7	7.5
20	Aneurysmal wall	19.3	7.7
21	Right auricle	5.6	10.7
22	Uterus	6.0	2.0
23	Uterus	6.7	4.3
24	Uterus	3.3	3.2
25	Uterus	5.8	4.7
26	Uterus	2.8	4.8
27	Uterus	12.2	5.8
23	Salpinx	14.0	4.3
24	Salpinx	3.7	3.2
27	Salpinx	6.7	5.8
23	Ovary	8.0	4.3
24	Ovary	2.4	3.2

[a] Compiled from data on file, Burroughs Wellcome Company, Research Triangle Park, North Carolina, United States

if the patient is taking an oral dose of 100–200 mg TMP yielding serum levels of only 1–2 μg/ml. In this instance, the use of the combination drug, co-trimoxazole (TMP and sulfamethoxazole combined in a ratio of 1:5) might be more appropriate and effective because the synergistic activity afforded by the sulfonamide component would have reduced the MIC of TMP to a range of 0.15–0.5 μg/ml.

Based on these considerations, clinical investigations of the use of TMP alone have therefore been largely confined to the treatment of urinary tract infections. However, before evaluating the results of these studies, several factors must be kept in mind in order to prevent erroneous interpretation of the data. The first is that bacteriuria in significant numbers (greater than 100,000 organisms/ml urine) must be the sine qua non for establishing the diagnosis of urinary tract infection (KASS 1956, 1960). Likewise, the eradication of these bacteria is the hallmark for cure after the completion of therapy (KASS 1960). It must be noted that approximately 50% of women who have the classical symptoms of burning, frequency, urgency, and pain associated with urinary tract infection, in fact, do not have significant bacteriuria (BROOKS and MAUDAR 1972; GALLAGHER et al. 1965; MOND et al. 1965) and their illness has been called "the acute urethral syndrome" or "trigonitis" and variously attributed to *Chlamydia trachomatis* (STAMM et al. 1980), interstitial cystitis caused by small numbers of bacteria (MESSING and STAMEY 1978), viruses (STAMM et al. 1980), infection of the periurethral glands (GALLAGHER et al. 1965), trauma, perineal nerve hypersensitivity, or a variety of other causes. These symptoms usually disappear spontaneously or with minimal supportive therapy and thus it would be inappropriate to include them in studies on the efficacy of antibacterials in curing documented bacterial urinary tract infections. These patients are nonetheless commonly encountered in clinical practice and, if not properly recognized, their consistently positive response to any therapy (including antibiotics) might portray to the practitioner an overly optimistic view of the effectiveness of any antibacterial regimen.

It is well established that the symptoms of documented bacterial urinary tract infection, including fever, flank pain, and costovertebral angle tenderness, will disappear within a few days of appropriate therapy, but that rapid recurrence of bacteriuria and/or symptoms will occur if the organism has not been fully eradicated from the urinary tract (STAMEY 1978). Thus, unless otherwise indicated, the term "efficacy" in the studies reviewed will not be defined by symptomatic response, but rather by the fraction of patients whose significant bacteriuria before therapy disappeared after therapy. Usually the determination of eradication was made 7–14 days after the completion of therapy to ensure that any remaining antibacterial in the urine at the end of therapy was not merely suppressing small numbers of residual bacteria.

It should also be noted that the dosage of TMP varied in these studies from as low as 100 mg twice a day to as high as 250 mg twice a day and that the duration of therapy ranged from 5 to 14 days. Therefore, it may be difficult to compare the results of TMP therapy in one study with those in another. Furthermore, some of the studies did not analyze those patients whose organism was not initially sensitive in vitro to the antibacterial to be used. In effect, since only "sensitive" organisms were treated, the results of these studies often provide higher cure rates than may be expected by the practitioner, who often must initiate therapy before the sensitivity of the organism is known. The disparity between the results of these studies and those of the physician's own experience will therefore be proportional to the natural resistance of the common *Enterobacteriaceae* to the agent he or she uses. For some agents, such as the sulfonamides, this may be great because a significant fraction of strains of *Escherichia coli* are resistant, whereas for others, such as TMP, it may be minimal because natural resistance is uncommon among the gram-negative bacteria.

There was also little differentiation generally made in these studies between lower urinary tract infections (cystitis) and upper urinary tract infections (pyelonephritis). This latter distinction might prove to be impossible because the difficulty and the hazards of determining the site of infection have been well recognized (MUNDT and POLK 1979), whether this determination is based on symptoms (FAIRLEY et al. 1971), antibody coating (V. THOMAS et al. 1974; JONES et al. 1974), ureteral catheterization (STAMEY et al. 1965), or a number of other techniques (BRUN et al. 1965). This separation may also be somewhat artificial because, with few exceptions (FANG et al. 1978; RUBIN et al. 1980), clinical studies have not shown a difference in response to therapy if the infection is in the upper rather than lower urinary tract. It has been demonstrated, however, that response to therapy is substantially different if the infection is of an acute, uncomplicated nature rather than a repeatedly recurrent or chronic illness that may be complicated by anatomic abnormalities or lithiasis of the urinary tract (HOIGNÉ et al. 1970). Because of these variables, it is important to consider each study separately so that the type of patient and illness, the criteria for inclusion and cure, as well as the expected compliance of the patient with the regimen assigned, all remain relatively constant and therefore the cure rate produced by an accepted therapeutic alternative may be critically examined and allow the reader to place the study in appropriate perspective.

II. Uncomplicated Urinary Tract Infections

Table 3 summarizes the results of 12 controlled clinical studies on acute urinary tract infections where TMP was compared with an alternative antibacterial agent commonly used in clinical practice. The first reported study (HOIGNÉ et al. 1970) was designed to compare, as were a number of other studies, the effectiveness of the combination of TMP and sulfamethoxazole with its individual components in the treatment of acute, uncomplicated urinary tract infections. An attempt was made to adjust the dosage of each regimen so that the results would not be prejudiced in favor of the synergistic combination, which in vitro has many times the potency against infecting bacteria than either of the components. Thus, those receiving TMP alone received 500 mg/day whereas those receiving the lowest dose of the combination received 160 mg/day TMP in addition to 800 mg/day sulfamethoxazole. Likewise, those receiving sulfamethoxazole alone received 2,000 mg/day. In spite of the fact that the regimens were thus not entirely comparable and the number of patients was heavily weighted toward those who received the combination drug (because there were three different combination regimens), the results nevertheless clearly indicate that either of the single regimens was as efficacious as the combination in the treatment of acute, uncomplicated urinary tract infections and all induced cure rates in at least 90% of the patients.

BRUMFITT and PURSELL's (1972) double-blind study confirmed this observation, even though the dose of TMP for those receiving the combination more closely approximated the regimen of those patients receiving TMP alone and the patients were assigned to the various therapies without regard to the sensitivity of the in-

Table 3. Comparative studies in acute, uncomplicated urinary tract infections

Reference	Drug	Dosage[a]	Patients	Microbiologic Efficacy (%)
Hoigne et al. (1970)	TMP	250 mg bid × 7 days	15	93
	Sulfamethoxazole	1,000 mg b.i.d. × 7 days	10	90
	TMP/ sulfamethoxazole	80 mg/400 mg b.i.d. × 7 days to 250 mg/1,000 mg b.i.d. × 7 days (3 different regimens)	42	95
Brumfitt and Pursell (1972)	TMP	200 mg b.i.d. × 7 days	84	83
	TMP/sulfamethoxazole	160 mg/800 mg b.i.d. × 7 days	83	83
	Ampicillin	1 g b.i.d. × 7 days	88	73
	Cephalexin	1 g b.i.d. × 7 days	84	69
Koch et al. (1973)	TMP	240 mg b.i.d. × 5–10 days	23	96
	Sulfamethoxazole	1,200 mg b.i.d. × 5–10 days	13	92
	TMP/ sulfamethoxazole	240 mg/1,200 mg b.i.d. × 5–10 days	39	95
Männistö (1976)	TMP	200 mg b.i.d. × 14 days	12	100
	TMP/ sulfamethoxazole	160 mg/800 mg b.i.d. × 14 days	12	92
	Oxolinic Acid	750 mg b.i.d. × 14 days	11	91
Sander et al. (1980)	TMP	200 mg b.i.d. × 10 days	39	90
	Nitrofurantoin	50 mg q.i.d. × 10 days	54	87
Pancoast et al. (1980)	TMP	100 mg b.i.d. × 14 days	12	100
	TMP/ sulfamethoxazole	160 mg/800 mg b.i.d. × 14 days	14	100
Iravani et al. (1981)	TMP	100 mg b.i.d. × 10 days	107	97
	Sulfisoxazole	500 mg q.i.d. × 10 days	100	97
Kuhn and Celniker (1979, un-published work)	TMP	100 mg b.i.d. × 10 days	38	95
	Amoxicillin	250 mg b.i.d. × 10 days	29	72
Freid and Worthington (1979, un-published work)	TMP	100 mg b.i.d. × 10 days	39	97
	Sulfamethoxazole	1,000 mg b.i.d. × 10 days	39	97
Lacey et al. (1980)	TMP	100 mg b.i.d. × 5 days	22	59
	TMP/ sulfamethoxazole	100 mg/500 mg b.i.d. × 5 days	20	60
Mabeck and Vejlsgaard (1979)	TMP	200 mg b.i.d. × 7 days	341	79
	Sulfamethizole	1 g b.i.d. × 7 days	321	69
	TMP/ Sulfadiazine	90 mg/110 mg b.i.d. × 7 days	299	84

Table 3. continued

Reference	Drug	Dosage[a]	Patients	Microbiologic Efficacy (%)
IRAVANI et al.	TMP	200 mg q.d. × 10 days	84	98
(1982)	TMP	300 mg q.d. × 7 days	91	98
	Nitrofurantoin	100 mg q.i.d. × 10 days	83	96

[a] Abbreviations: b.i.d. twice a day; q.d. once a day; q.i.d. four times a day

fecting organism. The determination of cure or failure was based on observations made both at 1 week and at 4–6 weeks after the completion of therapy. These patients were fairly evenly distributed between those who were pregnant, those seen in general outpatient practice, and hospitalized patients. While the majority of them may have had acute uncomplicated urinary tract infections, it is possible that some of the patients may have had the more complicated or recurrent forms of this disease, thus accounting for the somewhat lower cure rate (83%) than may be noted in most of the other studies. Confirming this hypothesis is the observation that TMP alone cured 100% and TMP/sulfamethoxazole 91% of those patients seen as part of a domiciliary general practice. Unaccountably, there was a 38% failure rate when these patients were given cephalexin. KOCH et al. (1973) studied urinary tract infections occurring in women who had been routinely catheterized for gynecologic surgery. They found that, in those patients with sensitive bacteria, there was no apparent difference in the effectiveness of either TMP alone, sulfamethoxazole alone, or the combination in precisely equivalent doses, even though the number of patients again was fairly heavily skewed toward those receiving the combination because assignment to the treatment groups was based on in vitro sensitivity testing. The four failures in each group were attributed to occult chronic pyelonephritis. A double-blind study conducted in Finland (MÄNNISTÖ 1976) indicated an almost universal cure rate, although the number of patients treated was rather small. This paucity of patients also prevented any determination as to whether TMP alone or TMP/sulfamethoxazole might be superior to a 14-day course of oxolinic acid. In another double-blind study (SANDER et al. 1980), no significant difference was observed in the cure rates produced by 200 mg TMP twice a day for 10 days and by nitrofurantoin 50 mg four times a day for 10 days, even though a substantial number of patients was included in both regimens. It is noteworthy that the cure rate for TMP remained at 90% at both the 4-day and 1-month posttherapy evaluation, while the cure rate for nitrofurantoin fell from 87% to 77% during the same period.

PANCOAST and co-workers in Dr. H.C. NEU's laboratory in New York conducted a double-blind study in nonpregnant young females and reported that even lower doses of TMP alone, that is 100 mg twice a day, were universally effective as was an even higher dose of TMP (320 mg/day) combined with 1,600 mg sulfamethoxazole (PANCOAST et al. 1980). In three other studies (IRAVANI et al. 1981; KUHN and CELNIKER 1979; FREID and WORTHINGTON 1979) using this lower dosage

(100 mg twice a day for 10 days), 95%–97% of the patients were free of the initial symptoms and bacteriuria at the examination period occurring at least 7 days after the completion of their 10-day course of therapy. The appropriate alternative drug also generally produced high cure rates, as might be expected, because only those patients receiving a drug to which the organism was susceptible were included in the analysis. Investigators in Dr. G.A. Richard's clinic, for example, induced a similar cure rate with 500 mg sulfisoxazole four times a day (Iravani et al. 1981), and Freid and Worthington (1979, unpublished work) produced a 97% cure rate with sulfamethoxazole, 1,000 mg twice a day. Conversely, in Richard's study, only 50% (5/10) of the patients were cured by sulfamethoxazole if the infecting organism was sulfonamide resistant. Before therapy, 16.9% of the isolated pathogens were found to be sulfonamide resistant in his study, whereas only one of the 331 organisms were initially TMP resistant (Iravani et al. 1981). The only anomalous finding was the rather low cure rate of 72% in the study by Kuhn and Celniker (1979, unpublished work) when 250 mg amoxicillin was given twice a day.

Lacey et al. (1980) showed TMP to be comparable to co-trimoxazole in 42 patients with acute urinary tract infections. Low success rates of 60% were found for both groups which the investigators felt were "undoubtedly due to indwelling catheters" in 12 patients in each treatment group during the course of the study. Lacey and co-workers additionally treated 216 patients for respiratory infections with the two regimens with the efficacy of each regimen being similar. Mabeck and Vejlsgaard (1979) likewise treated patients with acute urinary infections with TMP alone, but with comparisons with sulfamethizole and TMP/sulfadiazine. The TMP and TMP/sulfadiazine regimens were deemed comparable, and statistically superior to the sulfamethizole regimen, 2 weeks after the initiation of 7 days therapy. Another study conducted by Iravani and co-workers indicated that 200 mg/day for 10 days in the treatment of uncomplicated urinary tract infections was as efficacious as 300 mg/day for 7 days, as well as nitrofurantoin 100 mg four times a day for 10 days (Iravani et al. 1982).

Several conclusions may therefore be reached concerning patients who receive TMP for their acute, uncomplicated urinary tract infections. The first is that the cure rate is high; 796 of the 907 patients (88%) who received any of the regimens of TMP alone were cured of their urinary tract infection. If one examines only those patients who received the lower dose – that is 100 mg twice a day or 200 mg once a day each for 5–10 days – 94% (285 of 302) were cured. The second conclusion that may be reached is that the regimen of 100 mg twice a day or 200 mg once a day for 10 days is at least as effective as commonly used alternatives for uncomplicated infections, such as sulfisoxazole, sulfamethoxazole, nitrofurantoin, and amoxicillin. Other TMP dosage regimens have also been shown to be at least as effective in treating uncomplicated infections as ampicillin, cephalexin, oxolinic acid, and nitrofurantoin. Third, in acute, uncomplicated infections, there appears to be no advantage in adding sulfamethoxazole to TMP; the cure rates for TMP alone appear to be essentially identical to those with appropriate dosages of the combination. This is not unexpected, both because the rates of cure with TMP alone were high, and because of theoretical considerations based on the microbiologic and pharmacokinetic data cited previously.

III. Complicated Urinary Tract Infections

If one examines the cure rates for complicated, recurrent, or chronic urinary tract infections, the results are somewhat at variance with those for uncomplicated infections and should be viewed in a different context. It must be remembered that the etiology and pathophysiology of these conditions are not only different from those of acute, uncomplicated urinary tract infections, but are also heterogeneous within any individual study. A multitude of factors, including persistent adhering bacteria, unhygienic toilet habits, sexual activity, anatomic abnormalities, stones, or foreign bodies in the collecting system, diabetes, prostatic hypertrophy, incomplete emptying of the bladder, as well as poorly understood mechanisms of renal parenchymal infection, all may lead to renal disease which is more difficult to treat (STAMEY 1978). The studies summarized in Table 4 include the full spectrum of these causes but, unfortunately, not in equal proportions. It is beyond the scope of this review to dissect fully each study to indicate which ones included more patients with stones, uncomplicated recurrences, foreign bodies and the like, and, in many instances, such factors were not specified. Therefore, interpretation and comparison of these studies once again can be made only with same caveats noted for those concerning acute, uncomplicated urinary tract infections.

Several salient points become evident when one examines the summary of these studies. As might be expected, cure rates are lower than those for acute, uncomplicated urinary tract infections. The overall cure rate for all regimens for the latter was approximately 88%–94% whereas only about two-thirds of those patients with chronic, recurrent, or complicated infections were cured. The second striking figure is the remarkably low cure rate induced by sulfamethoxazole alone. Only 164/344 (48%) of the patients were cured by the usual regimen of approximately 2 g/day sulfamethoxazole, compared with 238/359 (66%) for TMP alone and 398/485 (82%) for the combination. It should be noted, nevertheless, that in many of the studies the incidence of sulfonamide-resistant organisms was substantial, e.g., approximately 30% in the study by GLECKMAN (1973) and, in one study (SOURANDER et al. 1972), only patients with sulfonamide-resistant organisms were evaluated.

Not listed in Table 4 are several studies where a comparative drug was not used. SCHNEIDER et al. (1965), for example, conducted an uncontrolled study of chronic urinary tract infections in which 100–200 mg TMP were given four times a day for 4–24 days (mean = 8 days), and found that it cured 15/22 patients (68%). The most extensive uncontrolled study of patients with urinary tract infections was conducted by KASANEN et al. (1978), who found only 12/30 (40%) patients responded to 100 mg TMP twice a day for 10 days, while 36/40 (90%) and 45/51 (88%) responded to 150 mg twice a day or 250 mg twice a day, respectively, for the same duration of therapy. Although many of these patients had acute infections, a significant number were considered difficult treatment problems which required referral to a special university clinic and, thus, must be considered to have also had complicated disease.

More difficult to explain is the fact that in only some of the studies did the combination of TMP/sulfamethoxazole produce significantly better cure rates than did TMP alone. In some instances the relatively small numbers of patients in each

Table 4. Comparative studies in chronic (recurrent) urinary tract infections

Reference	Drug	Dosage[a]	Patients	Microbiologic Efficacy (%)
Sourander et al. (1967)	TMP	2.75 g total over 5 days	25	88
	Sulfisoxazole	46 g total over 5 days	15	33
	TMP/sulfisoxazole or Sulfamethoxazole	0.5–2.875 g/5–23 g total over 5 days	90	91
Cox and Montgomery (1969)	TMP	50 mg q.i.d. × 10–14 days	39	41
	Sulfisoxazole	1,000 mg q.i.d. × 10–14 days	80	51
	TMP/sulfisoxazole	50 mg/1,000 mg q.i.d. × 10–14 days	23	78
Hoigne et al. (1970)	TMP	250 mg b.i.d. × 7 days	65	74
	Sulfamethoxazole	1,000 mg b.i.d. × 7 days	35	43
	TMP/sulfamethoxazole	80 mg/400 mg b.i.d. × 7 days to 250 mg/1,000 mg b.i.d. × 7 days (3 different regimens)	108	78
Schnaars and Escher (1969)	TMP	750 mg, then 250 mg b.i.d. × 3 days	43	77
	Sulfamethoxazole	2,000 mg, then 1,000 mg b.i.d. × 3 days	39	39
	TMP/sulfamethoxazole	250 mg/1,000 mg q.d. × 3 days	10 ⎫ Acute and	60
	TMP/sulfamethoxazole	100 mg/1,000 mg q.d. × 3 days	22 ⎬ chronic	86
	TMP/sulfamethoxazole	160 mg/800 mg q.d. × 3 days	23 ⎭	83
Sourander et al. (1972)	TMP	160 mg b.i.d. × 15 days	19 ⎫ Sulfo-	42
	Sulfamethoxazole	800 mg b.i.d. × 15 days	12 ⎬ namide	8
	TMP/sulfamethoxazole	160 mg/800 mg b.i.d. × 15 days	24 ⎭ resistant	88
Gleckman (1973)	TMP	200 mg b.i.d. × 10 days	146	66
	Sulfamethoxazole	1,000 mg b.i.d. × 10 days	152	53
	TMP/sulfamethoxazole	160 mg/800 mg b.i.d. × 10 days	161	84
Seneca et al. (1974)	TMP	200 mg b.i.d. × 10 days	13	85
	Sulfamethoxazole	1,000 mg b.i.d. × 10 days	11	55
	TMP/sulfamethoxazole	160 mg/800 mg b.i.d. × 10 days	12	50
	Carbenicillin	1,000 mg q.i.d. × 10 days	30	67
Männistö (1976)	TMP	200 mg b.i.d. × 14 days	9	44
	TMP/sulfamethoxazole	160 mg/800 mg b.i.d. × 14 days	12	67
	Oxolinic Acid	750 mg b.i.d. × 14 days	12	75

[a] Abbreviations: b.i.d. twice a day; q.d. once a day; q.i.d. four times a day

treatment group, as, for example, the studies by MÄNNISTÖ (1976), SCHNAARS and ESCHER (1969), SENECA et al. (1974), and SOURANDER et al. (1972), precluded an adequate demonstration of the superiority of one regimen over another. In other studies, the brevity of the treatment period, 3 days in the trial by SCHNAARS and ESCHER (1969), or *widely* disparate dosages of the drugs employed prevented precise comparison of the two agents. The most complete study was the double-blind, multicenter trial reported by GLECKMAN (1973). The 84% cure rate (135/161) achieved by the combination was significantly better ($P < 0.015$) than the 66% cure rate (96/146) noted following the use of TMP alone. HOIGNÉ's trial did not demonstrate a significant difference between TMP alone and the combination; however, precise interpretation of this study is difficult because one of the combination dosage regimens employed was considerably lower than is commonly used in practice (HOIGNÉ et al. 1970). Both TMP and the combination were associated with cure rates significantly superior ($P < 0.05$) to that observed following the use of sulfonamide alone. The interpretation of COX and MONTGOMERY's (1969) study is clouded by the fact that all patients were first treated with a sulfonamide and only the failures went on to receive TMP alone. Although a significant superiority of the combination was not noted in all studies, the trend in that direction is fairly consistent, and the overall high cure rate (82%) achieved with the combination argues strongly for its use in these difficult infections.

D. Prophylaxis

I. Recurring Urinary Infection in Women and Children

One of the most difficult areas in medical therapeutics is the management of those patients with frequently recurring urinary tract infections. Such patients are usually young or middle-aged women who respond normally to a course of most antibacterials for their acute infection, but then go on to have another infection within a brief period of time. A complete urologic workup, including an intravenous pyelogram, retrograde visualization of the collecting system, as well as a voiding cytourethrogram, will often reveal no abnormalities and the cause for recurrence often remains cryptic. It is thought that these recurrences are related either to hygienic standards (ADATTO et al. 1979) or sexual activity (VOSTI 1975), or possibly even to unusually adherent and/or pathogenic bacteria (FOWLER and STAMEY 1977). A number of regimens have been developed over the years in an attempt to prevent these repeated infections and thus spare the patient the pain and risk of repeated urinary tract infections. These regimens usually consist of low dose therapy once a day or only following sexual intercourse (VOSTI 1975). Several studies have been conducted comparing low dose TMP with either placebo or accepted effective prophylactic therapy and they are summarized in Table 5. Because of the less common nature of this disease and the long duration of follow-up, the number of patients in these studies must necessarily be smaller than in those which deal with more acute illness. The usual regimen for TMP was 100 mg once a day for a number of months. While the actual rates of infection are difficult to compare between studies because of a different patient population and different methods of calculating recurrence rates, it is obvious that this regimen of TMP was as effective

Table 5. Comparative studies in prophylaxis of urinary tract infections

Reference	Drug	Dosage[b]	Patients	Total number of treatment months	Recurrences
HELLE (1975)	TMP	3 mg/kg × 6 months	22	123	0
	Sulfonamide[a]	100–200 mg/kg t.i.d. × 6 months	23	145	0
	Nitrofurantoin[a]	1–3 mg/kg t.i.d. × 6 months	23	145	0
MÄNNISTÖ (1976)	TMP	100 mg qd.	12	32	12.5[c]
	TMP/sulfamethoxazole	80 mg/400 mg qd.	15	32	22.5[c]
	Oxolinic acid	375 mg qd.	12	41	12.2[c]
KASANEN et al. (1978)	TMP	100 mg qd. × 3–14 months	14	34	11.7[d]
	TMP	100 mg b.i.d. × 3–14 months	14	39	12.8[d]
	Nitrofurantoin	100 mg b.i.d. × 3–14 months	14	47	10.6[d]
	TMP	100 mg qd. × 3–5 months	54	119	5.9[d]
	Nitrofurantoin	100 mg qd. × 3–5 months	55	122	6.6[d]
KASANEN et al. (1974)	TMP	100 mg qd. × 1–8 months	66	267	1.5[c]
	TMP/sulfamethoxazole	80 mg/400 mg qd. × 1–8 months	62	261	2.3[c]
	Nitrofurantoin	50 mg qd. × 1–8 months	61	264	3.8[c]
	Methenamine hippurate	1 g qd. × 1–8 months (average = 4 months)	58	236	4.7[c]
	TMP	100 mg qd. × 1 year	50	12	5 infections
IWARSON and LIDIN-JANSON (1979)	TMP	100 mg q.d. × 6–17 months (mean = 7 months)	14	92	1.1[c]
STAMM et al. (1980)	TMP	100 mg q.d. × 6 months	14	84	0.0[e]
	TMP/sulfamethoxazole	40 mg/200 mg q.d. × 6 months	13	78	0.15[e]
	Nitrofurantoin	100 mg q.d. × 6 months	13	78	0.14[f]
	Placebo	1 tablet × 6 months	13	78	2.8[f]

a Received alternate weeks

b Abbreviations: b.i.d. twice a day; q.d. once a day; t.i.d. three times a day

c Recurrences/treatment month (%)

d Recurrences/100 treatment months

e Recurrences/patient year

f Recurrences/treatment year; $P < 0.001$ for each drug compared with placebo as the usual prophylactic regimens of nitrofurantoin, oxolinic acid, sulfonamide (when given three times a day), and co-trimoxazole.

In the pediatric study by HELLE (1975), no infections were noted during the 6-month therapy period in those children receiving either TMP alone, or alternating weeks of sulfonamide and nitrofurantoin therapy. MÄNNISTÖ (1976), however, found that 12.5% of the patients would have a recurrence during each month of TMP therapy, a rate comparable to that found with oxolinic acid therapy. Many of these patients had anatomic abnormalities of the urinary tract, permanent ind-welling urethral catheters, or diabetes. In the series of prophylactic studies con-ducted by KASANEN in Finland which were performed in a more representative population of patients with recurrent urinary tract infection, the incidence of "breakthrough" was much lower for TMP (KASANEN et al. 1978). The data for the first two studies performed by him are expressed as the number of recurrent infec-tions per 100 months of treatment (even though the patients were treated for only 3–14 months) and they are thus difficult to extrapolate and compare with other studies. Nevertheless, it is apparent that the effectiveness of suppression is equiv-alent, whether one uses 100 or 200 mg/day TMP, or 100 mg/day nitrofurantoin. In a more extensive study, KASANEN et al. (1974) noted only a 1.5% recurrence rate per treatment month with 100 mg of TMP once a day, whereas higher rates were noted for TMP/sulfamethoxazole (2.3%), nitrofurantoin (3.8%), and methena-mine hippurate (4.7%). IWARSON also found that the infection rate was 1.1% per month during the use of an identical dose of TMP (IWARSON and LIDIN-JANSON 1979). Unfortunately, only one study (STAMM et al. 1980) compared any of these regimens with no regimen at all, that is, one placebo tablet per day. The results of this study (expressed as the number of infections per patient year) were impressive and indicated that many of these regimens could reduce the incidence of recurrent infections more than 20-fold.

Based upon these data, it would appear that TMP at a dose of 100 mg once a day might be the ideal drug to prevent recurrences in these patients. Because of its pharmacokinetic profile already described, as well as its relative lack of toxicity with long-term low dose therapy to be discussed subsequently, it would appear to have significant advantages over the other drugs commonly used in prophylaxis. One of the other effective drugs in these studies, nitrofurantoin, for example, can cause pulmonary, hepatic, gastrointestinal, and neurologic reactions, some of which (chronic active hepatitis, diffuse interstitial pneumonitis and pulmonary fi-brosis) are associated with long-term therapy (BLACK et al. 1980; SHARP et al. 1980). See also Chap. 14.

II. Immunosuppressed Patients

Trimethoprim alone has also been used as a prophylactic to prevent bacterial in-fections in patients who are severely granulocytopenic as a result of intensive can-cer chemotherapy. In a study from Dr. A. RONALD's clinical service (McNAUGH-TON et al. 1980), patients were given either 300 mg/day TMP alone for an average of 23 days or 320 mg/day TMP combined with 1,600 mg/day sulfamethoxazole for an average of 17 days. Although the combination was more efficient in eliminating resident pharyngeal and rectal flora, there was not a significant difference between the two regimens in the reduction of febrile episodes. Gurwith treated both adults and children who were granulocytopenic with either 320 mg/day TMP alone or 320 mg/day TMP plus 1,600 mg/day sulfamethoxazole in both the inpatient and outpatient setting (Gurwith and Troug 1980). There were 31 patients in the TMP group and 35 in the co-trimoxazole group. The average duration of therapy in these groups ranged from 89 to 214 days. Adult patients were hospitalized 40% of the time, whereas the children were outpatients 90% of the time. Once again, no difference in the rates of infection, as measured by "febrile granulocytopenic days," could be noted in the two groups, and one bacteremia occurred in each group. There were no bacteremias in the pediatric patients although there was a significant difference in favor of the combination in the "readmission for suspected infection" rates. The precise reason for and validity of this observation are not clear. Gurwith also noted that TMP was somewhat less effective in suppressing enteric flora than was co-trimoxazole.

E. Adverse Reactions and Safety

I. General

There are myriad sources of data available to us concerning the undesirable effects of most drugs and our reliance upon their validity must depend upon the precision and zeal with which these adverse reactions were sought, as well as their relevance to usual clinical practice. The most complete data come from carefully controlled comparative clinical studies in which the administration of the drug is carefully supervised, the patient is assiduously questioned about possible adverse reactions, and blood samples are frequently monitored for even minor changes in body chemistry or hematologic function. These observations, however, may not be completely applicable to the use of the drug in patients encountered in normal clinical practice because the subjects in the study are aware that they are receiving experimental medication and, therefore, may anticipate adverse reactions. Second, some of the abnormalities found on extensive hematologic analysis, while being statistically significant, may have little or no clinical relevance. Third, the number of patients in such studies must necessarily be limited, and rare adverse reactions, such as those which might occur at a frequency of 1 in 1,000 or even 1 in 100,000 recipients could not be expected to be encountered in clinical investigations where only a few hundred patients are under careful observation. Such rare reactions are often the most severe and would naturally be of more concern to the physician than would more common, but less bothersome reactions, such as an upset stomach or an inconsequential change in lymphocyte count.

To obtain reaction rates which occur at low frequencies, one must depend upon direct or indirect epidemiologic surveillance of the reported adverse reactions following widespread commercial use of the drug. Reliance on this information is also fraught with pitfalls because there is clearly underreporting of these reactions (Frisch 1973) and the number of courses of therapy prescribed or the number of tablets actually consumed by patients is never fully known. Thus, both the numerator and denominator of this equation can only be considered to be within a certain "range" and the quotient therefore can only be estimated. Furthermore, causality is usually difficult or impossible to establish because there is a certain baseline of dreadful events or physiologic responses which occur apparently spontaneously in the population at large and more commonly in people who are ill. When one of these events occurs in temporal relation to the ingestion of a drug, it is a natural human tendency to infer that the drug caused the reaction and thus we run the risk of overestimating the adverse reactions "caused" by the drug. It is only when this reaction occurs with some consistency that it can be attributed to the drug. Reliance on this primarily anecdotal information is particularly difficult in the case of TMP alone since the vast majority of the clinical use of TMP has been in associated with the simultaneous use of sulfamethoxazole. Adverse reactions associated with sulfonamides include rashes and blood dyscrasias, both of varying frequency and severity, gastrointestinal upset, as well as a variety of other miscellaneous reactions. It has therefore been almost impossible to determine which of the reactions noted following the use of the combination resulted from the sulfonamide and which from TMP. Theoretically, it should be possible to subtract the known adverse reactions caused by sulfonamides from those observed following the use of the combination (co-trimoxazole) and the remainder would be due to TMP. However, because of the imprecision of the numbers involved and the often extremely low frequency of the purported adverse reaction, this interpolation cannot be performed.

In only one country (Finland) has TMP alone been available on a commercial basis for a significant period of time. Investigators in that country feel that reactions seen following the generally low dose used for prophylaxis (100 mg once a day for a number of weeks to months) have been rare and that the overall incidence of rash, for example, at this dosage is in the range of 1.5% (KASANEN et al. 1978). They feel these rashes are mild, and the more severe reactions sometimes seen following the use of the combination, such as erythema multiforme, Stevens–Johnson syndrome or toxic epidermal necrolysis, have not been observed (see also Chap. 9).

With these caveats, several points must be noted in examining the data presented in Table 6. The first is that the rate of adverse reactions, when assiduously sought, was still generally low in relation to the rates of adverse reactions noted following the use of other marketed drugs in these studies. The most common reactions were dermatologic, gastrointestinal, or hematologic.

II. Dermatologic

The rates of dermatologic reaction varied considerably (from 0% to 24%), with the higher rates being seen more often in those patients who took a larger total dose (400 mg/day or more for at least 10 days). The rashes were usually erythematous or morbilliform, generally pruritic, but not urticarial or exfoliative. Neither Stevens–Johnson syndrome nor toxic epidermal necrolysis were observed. In some instances, the rashes were so mild that they were not noted by the patient, but instead were observed by a friend or the examining physician, and thus the innocuous nature of these rashes may account for the great variability in the reported rates. The causes of these rashes are unknown but appear not to be phototoxic or

Table 6. Side effects of trimethoprim therapy

Reference	Dosage[a]	Type of infection	Patients	Side effects
BRUMFITT and PURSELL (1972)	200 mg b.i.d. × 7 days	UTI	84	3.6% rash, 4.8% gastrointestinal, 3.6% miscellaneous
COX and MONTGOMERY (1969)	50 mg q.i.d. × 10–14 days	UTI	39	2.5% gastrointestinal
HOIGNE et al. (1970)	250 mg b.i.d. × 7 days	UTI	112	5% hematologic, <10% gastro-intestinal
KOCH et al. (1973)	240 mg b.i.d. × 5–10 days	UTI	23	26% gastrointestinal, 4% reversible leukopenia
SANDER et al. (1980)	200 mg b.i.d. × 10 days	UTI	57	11% rash, 11% gastrointestinal, 5% miscellaneous
GLECKMAN (1973)	200 mg b.i.d. × 10 days	UTI	146	2.0% rash and pruritus, 4.0% gastro-intestinal, <10% hematologic
MÄNNISTÖ (1976)	200 mg b.i.d. × 14 days	UTI	29	14.0% rash and itching, 10.3% gastro-intestinal, 7.0% miscellaneous
KASANEN et al. (1978)	100 mg or 250 mg b.i.d. × 10 days	UTI	121	<1% eczema, 2% nausea
	100 mg q.d. × 3–14 months	UTI prophylaxis	68	None
	200 mg b.i.d. × 3–14 months	UTI prophylaxis	14	None
	100 mg × 267 treatment months	UTI prophylaxis	66	1.5% rash
SCHNAARS and ESCHER (1969)	750 mg, then 250 mg b.i.d. × 3 days	UTI	43	Occasional nausea and vomiting
SCHNEIDER et al. (1965)	100–200 mg q.i.d. × 4–24 days (11 days average)	UTI	22	14% gastrointestinal
SENECA et al. (1974)	200 mg b.i.d. × 10 days	UTI	13	Few gastric complaints
MARTIN and ARNOLD (1968)	2 g qd. × ? days	Healthy?	20	Intolerable gastrointestinal distress, no other effects reported
KAHN et al. (1968)	0.5–1.5 g q.d. × 5–7 days	Malaria	19	None
	250 mg q.i.d. × 4 weeks	Healthy	10	Occasional nausea, several hematologic effects, 80% giant metamyelocytes in bone marrow
DUBACH et al. (1973)	320 mg × 1 day	Healthy	9	None
IRAVANI et al. (1981)	100 mg b.i.d. × 10 days	UTI	115	None
IRAVANI et al. (1982)	200 mg b.i.d. × 14 days	UTI	50	24% rash
	200 mg q.d. × 10 days	UTI	90	6.7% rash
	300 mg q.d. × 7 days	UTI	94	2% dizziness, 1% rash, 1% nausea

Reference	Dose	Indication	No.	Side effects
Kuhn and Celniker (1979, unpublished work)	100 mg b.i.d. × 10 days	UTI	46	2% rash
Fried and Worthington (1979, unpublished work)	100 mg b.i.d. × 10 days	UTI	60	7% rash, 4% gastrointestinal
Foster (1979, unpublished work)	100 mg b.i.d. × 10 days	UTI	21	10% rash
	200 mg b.i.d. × 14 days	UTI	36	~20% rash
Pancoast et al. (1980)	100 mg b.i.d. × 14 days	UTI	12	none
Guerrant et al. (1981)	100 mg b.i.d. × 14 days	UTI	13	7.7% rash
	200 mg b.i.d. × 14 days	UTI	26	7.7% rash
Sourander et al. (1972)	160 mg b.i.d. × 15 days	UTI	19	None reported, no change in serum folates
Arvilommi et al. (1976)	160 mg b.i.d. × 5 days	Healthy following vaccination against TAB, tetanus, mumps, polio	20	Antibody response partially suppressed
Kunin et al. (1978)	100 mg q.d. × 3 years	UTI prophylaxis in a uremic patient	1	Slight anemia
Iwarson and Lidin-Janson (1979)	100 mg q.d. × 6–17 months (mean 7 months)	UTI prophylaxis	14	6.7% pruritus and erythema
Stamm et al. (1980)	100 mg q.d. × 6 months	UTI prophylaxis	14	Skin burning with no rash in one patient
Lacey et al. (1980)	100 mg b.i.d. × 5 days	Respiratory	107	10% gastrointestinal, 1% rash, 7.5% miscellaneous
Mabeck and Vejlsgaard (1979)	200 mg b.i.d. × 7 days	UTI	22	None reported
		UTI	341	4.1% skin reactions, 6.5% gastrointestinal, 3.8% miscellaneous
Gurwith and Troug (1980)	160 mg b.i.d. × 89 days average in adults × 214 days average in children	Prophylaxis of infection in granulocytopenic patients	31[b]	3% gastrointestinal, 3% rash
McNaughton et al. (1980)	300 mg q.d. × 23 days average	Prophylaxis of infection in granulocytopenic patients	30	None reported
Koch et al. (1973)	240 mg b.i.d. × 5 days	UTI	23	26% gastrointestinal
Helle (1975)	3 mg/kg × 6 months average	UTI prophylaxis	22	None

[a] Abbreviations: b.i.d. twice a day; q.d. once a day; q.i.d. four times a day
[b] 14 adults and 17 children

photoallergic (C.K. Kaidbey and A. Kligman 1979, unpublished work) nor related to extraneous substances in the medication or changes in phenylalanine–tyrosine metabolism (data on file, Burroughs Wellcome Company, Research Triangle Park, North Carolina, United States). There is some evidence that the rash is allergic in nature because some individuals will manifest a rash within 1–2 h if they are rechallenged with TMP several weeks after experiencing the initial rash. Chapter 9 (Fig. I, p.212) contains an illustration of a typical dermatologic condition associated with TMP.

III. Gastrointestinal

Gastrointestinal upset occurred in 0%–11% of the patients and its occurrence was extremely variable. The unusual 20% incidence of gastrointestinal upset noted in the study by Koch et al. (1973) is accounted for by the fact that all of the patients in the study were recovering from recent gastrointestinal surgery. Only occasionally was nausea and vomiting noted and rarely did the gastrointestinal upset prove to be sufficiently severe to require discontinuation of the drug. In some instances, the patients were instructed to take their medication with meals, and it appeared that this resulted in a significantly lower incidence of gastrointestinal upset.

IV. Hematologic

Hematologic abnormalities noted in these prospective studies were generally mild and of little or no clinical consequence. As might be expected following the use of a dihydrofolate reductase inhibitor, megaloblastic changes of the marrow and occasional transient decreases in red cell, white cell, and platelet counts could be noted in patients receiving high doses for prolonged periods. These changes were usually quite mild, occurring infrequently, and often seen only in those patients who had marginal folate reserves. In one patient who had taken 100 mg TMP once a day for 3.5 years (Kunin et al. 1978), a slight anemia was noted; however, the patient was uremic. Subtle morphological changes and biochemical correlates of folate deficiency, such as excretion of formiminoglutamic acid, transient megaloblastosis, and elevated lobe counts of polymorphonuclear leukocytes can be observed in patients taking TMP. Kahn et al. (1968) and Koutts et al. (1973) have shown that TMP can cause a further deterioration of the defective deoxyribonucleic acid–thymidine synthesis; however, both studies would indicate that the changes are of no pathologic significance and may be easily reversed, either by discontinuation of the drug or by the administration of tetrahydrofolic acid (leucovorin). Even the inhibition of cell function (as determined by megaloblastic changes and arrest of S phase), observed in vitro when 0.8 and 8 mg/ml TMP are incubated with rapidly growing cultures of marrow cells infected with Friend erythroleukemia virus, could be reversed with 100 ng/ml leucovorin (Steinberg et al. 1980). Hjortshoj et al. (1978) found no effect on the marrow (or on folic acid absorption) when patients were given 320 mg/day TMP (as well as 1,600 mg sulfadiazine) for 8 weeks, but cautioned that the Lactobacillus casei method of folate determination should not be used since the drugs themselves inhibit the growth of the bacteria. It is not surprising that the effect of TMP on the bone marrow is minimal, because the affinity of TMP for mammalian dihydrofolate reductase is 10,000–60,000 times less than its affinity for the bacterial enzyme (BURCHALL and HITCHINGS 1965). Clinical studies by HUGHES et al. (1977) in patients who received TMP/sulfamethoxazole for the prevention and treatment of *Pneumocystis carinii* pneumonitis and who were also receiving methotrexate, a potent noncompetitive inhibitor of the enzyme, showed little change in the hematologic picture of these patients.

When extremely large doses (2 g/day) TMP were given as a single dose, the drug induced intolerable gastrointestinal distress. Nevertheless, when 0.5–1.5 g was given for 5–7 days for the treatment of malaria, no adverse reactions were noted in 19 patients (MARTIN and ARNOLD 1968). Other miscellaneous reactions that have been noted following the use of TMP are fever, elevation of serum transaminase and bilirubin, and increases in both blood urea nitrogen and serum creatinine. It should be noted, however, that the relationship of these reactions to the administration of drug are only temporal, and causality has not been established. Such changes are not uncommon in patients who are ill, particularly those with urinary tract infections.

If the patient has inadvertently or intentionally ingested several grams of TMP, signs of acute overdosage may appear and include nausea, vomiting, dizziness, headaches, mental depression, confusion, and bone marrow suppression. Treatment should be instituted immediately and should include gastric lavage and general supportive care. Acidification of the urine will increase renal elimination of the drug. Peritoneal dialysis has been shown not to be effective and hemodialysis only moderately effective (HOPPE-SEYLER et al. 1974; RIEDER et al. 1974; SHARPSTONE 1969). If bone marrow depression occurs, leucovorin, 3–6 mg intramuscularly daily for 3 days, should be given, or even larger amounts if the response has not been sufficient. One patient was reported to have managed without great difficulty after the ingestion of 8 g TMP which caused a peak serum level of 19.6 µg/ml TMP (HOPPU et al. 1980).

The safety of TMP therapy during pregnancy has not been definitely established. Although there are no large, well-controlled clinical studies of the use of TMP in pregnant women, BRUMFITT and PURSELL (1972) treated 186 pregnant women with bacteriuria with either co-trimoxazole or placebo. The outcome reported was an incidence of congenital abnormalities in 4.5% (3/66) of those patients receiving placebo, and 3.3% (4/120) of those receiving co-trimoxazole. In addition, 10 patients had received the drug during the first trimester, with no congenital abnormalities noted in the infants. The authors also reported no congenital abnormalities in 35 children whose mothers had received co-trimoxazole at the time of conception or shortly thereafter; these patients were part of a separate survey.

F. Bacterial Resistance

I. General

A major consideration in the selection of any antibacterial agent is whether the organism to be treated is resistant initially to the drug or whether the use of the drug may induce resistance which may be of clinical significance to the patient or of epidemiologic significance to future patients within the community. One of the reasons why physicians and academics alike have until recently avoided the use of TMP alone was the fear that its use without a sulfonamide would induce rapid and widespread resistance among initially sensitive bacteria. Because there was no evidence that TMP alone induced resistance any more readily than most other antibacterial agents (and certainly not to the degree and frequency of rifampin, for example), the fear of rapid resistance development was based on somewhat inverted logic. That is, the combination of a sulfonamide and TMP was clearly shown to limit the development of resistance in vitro (Bushby 1973; Darrell et al. 1968). Thus, it was thought that the absence of the sulfonamide would be associated with the rapid emergence of resistance. However, it is necessary to examine in some detail the accumulated epidemiologic and experimental data surrounding this question to determine whether these initial fears might be borne out in clinical experience.

It must be remembered that all antibacterial agents can induce resistance, often by a variety of mechanisms. The question is not whether TMP alone can induce resistance, because it has been repeatedly demonstrated that it can, as discussed in Chap. 11. We need to determine instead whether this resistance might occur more readily or rapidly than that induced by other single antibacterial agents or by the use of co-trimoxazole. If resistance does emerge, will it spread throughout the microbial community and be found in the bacterial pools (usually stools) of the population at large, including many individuals who have not had personal experience with TMP? Finally, can these resistant organisms cause disease and if so, with what frequency?

II. Finnish Experience

As in the consideration of adverse reactions, it must be noted here also that the best answers to these questions can be derived only from the observation of microbial pool dynamics in a large human population that has been exposed to the drug for a significant period of time. Thus, observations in Finland, the only country where such a circumstance can be found, must once again serve as a guide. Co-trimoxazole has been available in Finland since 1968 and is used extensively there. Trimethoprim alone, which has been used primarily for the prophylactic treatment of chronic and recurring urinary tract infections, became commercially available there in 1973 (Burman 1980). Five years after this introduction, there had been a total of 600,000 patient months of treatment with TMP (Kasanen et al. 1978). The extent of the use of the combination (co-trimoxazole) is not entirely clear, but it is thought to be at least quantitatively equal to the use of TMP alone and up to 3–4 times the use observed in the United States. At the Helsinki University Central Hospital, approximately 400 E. coli were examined between 1972 and 1977 and there appeared to be no change in the MIC values over that 5 year period, with only 1% of the E. coli having an MIC greater than 8 μg/ml in hospitalized patients (Kasanen et al. 1978). It has been stated that in the city of Turku, the use of TMP alone has been more extensive than in other parts of Finland (Kasanen et al. 1978) and in 1976, 3 years after the introduction of TMP alone, 7% of 1,038 E. coli isolated from urinary infections were found to be resistant to the combination of sulfonamide and TMP, a figure consonant with the general resistance rates found elsewhere in Europe. In a more extensive study conducted in Turku in 1978, HUOVINEN and TOIVANEN (1980) found an 11% incidence of resistance among E. coli in outpatients. Whether this slight increase over the 7% noted 2 years previously is clinically or epidemiologically significant cannot be determined. However, it should be noted that the authors found that the level of TMP resistance among Enterobacteriaceae was similar to that seen with other antibacterials and felt that these data and the limited side effects associated with the drug confirmed the usefulness of TMP alone for urinary tract infections.

It should be noted that in-hospital epidemics of resistant organisms (often of the Proteus and Klebsiella genera) have been noted in Finland (HUOVINEN and TOIVANEN 1980) where both TMP and co-trimoxazole are used extensively, just as they have been noted in other European countries where only co-trimoxazole has been available until recently (GRÜNEBERG et al. 1975). These microbial epidemics usually occur in circumstances where the population is confined and elderly, and where the level of hygiene is less than optimal and cross-contamination common (BENDALL and GRÜNEBERG 1979). Such an "epidemic" can be rapidly quelled by temporarily discontinuing the use of the drug to which resistance has occurred. A similar phenomenon has been noted in the United States and elsewhere, associated with the use of a number of antibiotics, including ampicillin (GRÜNEBERG and BENDALL 1979), gentamicin (F. THOMAS et al. 1977; O'BRIEN et al. 1980), and other antibiotics (CHOW et al. 1979). This phenomenon also serves as a strong lesson in the careful avoidance of the excessive use of any antibacterial, particularly in closed populations of debilitated individuals where the conditions of nosocomial contamination are optimal.

Because both co-trimoxazole and TMP alone have been available in Finland for a number of years, it is difficult to make the definitive statement that the availability of TMP alone will or will not lead to the more rapid development of resistance, because the prior availability of the combination drug may be a confounding factor in this analysis. It is fair to state, however, that the introduction of TMP alone into a population where co-trimoxazole had been available for a number of years did not seem to accelerate the development of resistance among the microbial population. The incidence of resistance to TMP of E. coli, Proteus, Klebsiella, Enterobacter, and even staphylococci appears to be similar in Finland to those rates observed in other European countries with comparable levels of medical care and co-trimoxazole usage (KASANEN et al. 1978).

Other more controlled experiments would also tend to support the concept that TMP alone does not accelerate the introduction of resistant pathogenic bacteria into the microbial population any more rapidly than does co-trimoxazole. The first would be an "experiment of nature." Although DARRELL et al. (1968) and BUSHBY (1973) both showed that the presence of sulfamethoxazole could delay the emergence of bacterial resistance to TMP, this was particularly true only if the organisms were sulfonamide sensitive. As the sensitivity to sulfonamide decreased, this ability to prevent the emergence of resistance also decreased so that, at extremely high levels of sulfonamide resistance, the presence of the sulfonamide had minimal to no effect in the emergence of bacteria resistant to TMP. Since a high level of sulfonamide resistance is extremely common among the resident flora of

Table 7. Rectal flora in patients treated with TMP compared with other drugs

Reference	Drug	Dosage[a]	Patients or volunteers	Results
GUERRANT et al. (1981)	TMP	100 mg b.i.d. × 4 weeks	15	No emergence of TMP-resistant coliforms in fecal flora, but predominance of *Pseudomonas* and *Acinetobacter* sp.
	TMP/sulfamethoxazole	160 mg/800 mg b.i.d. × 4 weeks	14	No change in anaerobic or thymidine-requiring bacteria with either group
				Slight increase in TMP-resistant non-*Enterobacteriaceae* with TMP alone group, but no persistence
LACEY et al. (1980)	TMP	100 mg b.i.d. × 5 days	6	Similar change in fecal flora with both regimens
	TMP/sulfamethoxazole	100 mg/500 mg b.i.d. × 5 days	5	No TMP-resistant coliform isolated
				Predominance of enterococci, *Staphylococcus albus*, and *Pseudomonas aeruginosa* in fecal flora
KASANEN et al. (1978)	TMP	100 mg q.d. × 6–36 months	20	38.5% of fecal coliforms resistant to TMP; higher MICs (< 8 µg/ml) in TMP group compared with methenamine group
	Methenamine hippurate	1 g q.d. × 6–36 months	20	10.4% of fecal coliforms resistant to methenamine
KASANEN et al. (1978)	TMP	100 mg q.d. × 3 weeks	10	TMP alone did not result in appearance of TMP-resistant coliforms in fecal flora
	TMP/sulfamethoxazole	80 mg/400 mg q.d. × 3 weeks	10	Only 1/633 coliforms resistant to TMP

Reference	Drug	Dose	No.	Comments
	Sulfamethoxydiazine/sulfamethoxazole	100 mg/250 mg q.d. × 3 weeks	10	Both TMP/sulfamethoxazole and sulfonamide groups induced increase in sulfonamide-resistant coliforms
PANCOAST et al. (1980)	TMP	100 mg b.i.d. × 2 weeks	12	No emergence of TMP-resistant coliforms in fecal flora
	TMP/sulfamethoxazole	160 mg/800 mg b.i.d. × 2 weeks	14	TMP- or TMP/sulfamethoxazole-resistant isolates found before therapy disappeared during therapy. Predominant flora were enterococci, anaerobes and *Candida albicans*
SIETZEN and KNOTHE (1978)	TMP	100 mg b.i.d. × 4 weeks	10	TMP did not favor appearance of TMP-resistant strains; there was no significant difference between TMP and TMP/sulfamethoxazole groups
	TMP/sulfamethoxazole	80 mg/400 mg b.i.d. × 4 weeks	10	TMP alone affected fecal flora the same as TMP/sulfamethoxazole
	Sulfamethoxazole	500 mg b.i.d. × 4 weeks	10	In only 1/20 persons was a resistant *Escherichia coli* selected which persisted; this person was treated with TMP/sulfamethoxazole
STAMM et al. (1980)	TMP	100 mg q.d. × 6 months	15	Increased isolation of enterococci with TMP, as well as TMP/sulfamethoxazole
	TMP/sulfamethoxazole	40 mg/200 mg q.d. × 6 months	15	
	Placebo	1 tablet q.d. × 6 months	15	1/316 rectal, urethral, or vaginal *E. coli* resistant to TMP
	Nitrofurantoin	100 mg q.d. × 6 months	15	Patient receiving TMP/sulfamethoxazole infected (UTI) with *E. coli* with MIC to TMP 0.15 µg/ml and to sulfamethoxazole 2.85 µg/ml

[a] Abbreviations: b.i.d. twice a day; q.d. once a day

the colonic tract (the largest group of organisms exposed to any antibiotic), it is quite clear that on a simple probability basis, large numbers of bacteria highly resistant to sulfonamide have in effect been exposed to TMP alone during the treatment of various infections with co-trimoxazole. Since the progressive development of resistance among fecal and other isolates has not been noted after a decade of exceedingly wide clinical use (over 1 billion courses of therapy of co-trimoxazole worldwide), except in those ephemeral in-hospital epidemics noted previously, it is unlikely that exposing sulfonamide-sensitive organisms to TMP alone would produce any different result. It should be also noted that Bushby viewed those organisms that were TMP resistant to be at an adaptive disadvantage in that they grew slowly, were antigenically changed and consisted of rough colonies (Bushby 1973). Infections with TMP-resistant organisms have been noted only rarely (Towner et al. 1979).

III. Effect on Fecal Flora

When the fecal flora of patients receiving TMP alone were examined, additional data were gathered to support the concept that TMP alone does not significantly promote the long-term emergence of resistance. Table 7 summarizes those studies in which patients' feces were cultured during and after treatment with either TMP or co-trimoxazole; only those studies where both drugs were employed are considered. Although TMP-resistant coliforms could be isolated transiently from both treatment groups, differences in rates were usually not striking and, more significantly, emergence of these resistant organisms was generally a very passing effect and they did not become the dominant bacteria of the bowel. After withdrawal of the drug, the return to normal flora without significant numbers of resistant organisms is probably related either to Bushby's (1973) observation of the adaptive disadvantage of these organisms or to Van der Waaij's (1972) concept of "colonization resistance." (It is thought that co-trimoxazole and by extension, TMP, would have little disturbing effect on normal bowel flora, and also prevent the subsequent infection with secondary pathogens, because the drugs have little effect against the anaerobic bacteria which make up to 90%–99% of the bacteria in the colon.)

G. Conclusion

It may be stated, therefore, that TMP resistance can be regularly induced in vitro or in various animal experimental systems. The rapid emergence of resistance, however, has not been observed in the population at large and infections with organisms that have become resistant to TMP are relatively uncommon. Nevertheless, we should not be complacent in thinking that clinically significant resistance will never emerge. We must continue to monitor the sensitivity of organisms to TMP as the single entity is introduced in countries with larger populations than Finland, such as England, Denmark, and the United States, and as the quantity and duration of its use increases.

References

Adatto K, Doebele KG, Galland L, Granowetter L (1979) Behavioral factors and urinary tract infection. JAMA 241:2525–2526

Arnauld R, Soutoul JH, Gallier J, Borderon JC, Borderon E (1972) A study of the passage of trimethoprim into the maternal milk. Ouest Med 25:959–964

Arvilommi H, Vuori M, Salmi A (1976) Sulfamethoxazole-trimethoprim: effect on antibody response in man. Chemotherapy 22:37–42

Bach MC, Gold O, Finland M (1973) Absorption and urinary excretion of trimethoprim, sulfamethoxazole, and trimethoprim-sulfamethoxazole: Results with single doses in normal young adults and preliminary observations during therapy with trimethoprim-sulfamethoxazole. J Infect Dis 128:S 584–S 598

Beck H, Pechere JC (1970) A combination of trimethoprim with sulfamethoxazole: pharmacodynamic activity in old men. In: Umezawa H (ed) Progress in antimicrobial and anticancer chemotherapy. Proc 6th Int Congr Chemother. Baltimore University Park Press, Baltimore, pp 663–667

Bendall MJ, Grüneberg RN (1979) An outbreak of infection caused by trimethoprim-resistant coliform bacilli in a geriatric unit. Age Ageing 8:231–236

Black M, Rabin L, Schatz N (1980) Nitrofurantoin-induced chronic active hepatitis. Ann Intern Med 92:62–64

Brooks D, Maudar A (1972) Pathogenesis of the urethral syndrome in women and its diagnosis in general practice. Lancet 2:893–898

Brumfitt W, Pursell R (1972) Double-blind trial to compare ampicillin, cephalexin, co-trimoxazole, and trimethoprim in treatment of urinary infection. Br Med J 2:673–676

Brun C, Raaschou F, Eriksen KR (1965) Simultaneous bacteriologic studies of renal biopsies and urine. In: Kass EH (ed) Progress in pyelonephritis. Davis, Philadelphia, pp 461–467

Burchall JJ, Hitchings GH (1965) Inhibitor binding analysis of dihydrofolate reductases from various species. Mol Pharmacol 1:126–136

Burman LG (1980) Resistance to trimethoprim. Lancet 1:1409

Bushby SRM (1969) Combined antibacterial action in vitro of trimethoprim and sulfonamides. Postgrad Med J 45:S 10–S 18

Bushby SRM (1973) Trimethoprim-sulfamethoxazole: in vitro microbiological aspects. J Infect Dis 128:S 442–S 462

Bushby SRM, Hitchings GH (1968) Trimethoprim, a sulphonamide potentiator. Br J Pharmacol Chemother 33:72–90

Chow AW, Taylor PR, Yoshikawa TT, Gruze LB (1979) A nosocomial outbreak of infections due to multiply-resistant *Proteus mirabilis*: role of intestinal colonization as a major reservoir. J Infect Dis 139:621–627

Cox CE, Montgomery WG (1969) Combined trimethoprim-sulfisoxazole therapy of urinary infections. Postgrad Med J 45:65–71

Craig WA, Kunin CM (1973) Distribution of trimethoprim-sulfamethoxazole in tissues of rhesus monkeys. J Infect Dis 128:S 575–S 579

Dabhoiwala NF, Bye A, Claridge M (1976) A study of concentrations of trimethoprim-sulfamethoxazole in the human prostate gland. Br J Urol 48:77–81

Darrell JH, Garrod LP, Waterworth PM (1968) Trimethoprim: laboratory and clinical studies. J Clin Pathol 21:202–209

Dubach UC, Forgo I, Bückert A (1973) Absence of a hypoglycemic effect of Bactrim in healthy subjects. Klin Wochenschr 51:1028–1029

Eatman FB, Maggio AC, Pocelinko R et al. (1977) Blood and salivary concentrations of sulfamethoxazole and trimethoprim in man. J Pharmacokinet Biopharm 5:615–624

Fairley KF, Carson NE, Gutch RC et al. (1971) Site of infection in acute urinary tract infection in general practice. Lancet 2:615–618

Fang LST, Tolokoff-Rubin NE, Rubin RH (1978) Efficacy of single-dose and conventional amoxicillin therapy in urinary tract infection localized by the antibody-coated bacteria technic. N Engl J Med 298:413–416

Fowle ASE (1973) Aspects of the pharmacokinetics behaviour of trimethoprim and sulphamethoxazole. In: Bernstein LS, Salter AJ (eds) Trimethoprim/sulphamethoxazole in bacterial infections – a Wellcome Foundation Symposium. Churchill Livingston, Edinburgh London, pp 63–72

Fowler JE, Stamey TS (1977) Studies of introital colonization in women with recurrent urinary infections: the role of bacterial adherence. J Urol 117:472–476

Fries N, Keuth U, Braun JS (1975) Studies of cerebrospinal fluid diffusion of trimethoprim in infants and children. Fortsch Med 93:1178–1183

Frisch JM (1963) Clinical experience with adverse reactions to trimethoprim-sulfamethoxazole. J Infect Dis 128:S 607–S 611

Gallagher DJA, Montgomerie JZ, North JDK (1965) Acute infections of the urinary tract and the urethral syndrome in general practice. Br Med J 1:622–626

Gleckman RA (1973) A cooperative controlled study of the use of trimethoprim-sulfamethoxazole in chronic urinary tract infections. J Infect Dis 128:S 647–S 651

Gnarpe H, Fridberg J (1976) The penetration of trimethoprim into seminal fluid and serum. Scand J Infect Dis 8:S 50–S 52

Greene BM, Thomas FE Jr, Alford RH (1975) Trimethoprim-sulfamethoxazole and brain abcess. Ann Intern Med 82:812–813

Grüneberg RN, Bendell MJ (1979) Hospital outbreak of trimethoprim resistance in pathogenic coliform bacteria. Br Med J 2:7–9

Grüneberg RN, Leakey A, Bendall MJ, Smellie JM (1975) Bowel flora in urinary tract infection: effect of chemotherapy with special reference to cotrimoxazole. Kidney Int 8:S 122–S 129

Guerrant RL, Wood SJ, Krongard L, Reid RA, Hodge RH (1981) Resistance among fecal flora of patients taking sulfamethoxazole-trimethoprim or trimethoprim alone. Antimicrob Agents Chemother 19:33–38

Gurwith M, Troug K (1980) Comparison of prophylactic trimethoprim/sulfamethoxazole and trimethoprim alone in compromised hosts. In: Nelson JD, Grassi C (eds) Current chemotherapy and infectious disease. Proc 11 th Int Congr Chemother and 19 th Intersci Conf Antimicrob Agents Chemother. The American Society for Microbiology, Washington, DC, pp 1446–1447

Hansen I, Lykkegaard Nielsen M, Nielsen JB (1975) A new method for homogenization of bone exemplified by measurement of trimethoprim in human bone tissue. Acta Pharmacol Toxicol (Copenh) 37:33–42

Helle M (1975) Trimethoprim in the long-term treatment of children's urinary tract infections (in Finnish). Lääkeuutiset 4:125–127

Hjortshoj A, Elsborg L, Jensen E (1978) Folate status during long-term therapy with trimethoprim and sulphadiazine. Chemotherapy 24:327–331

Hoigné R, Müller U, Schneider HR (1970) A comparison of chemotherapy in patients with urinary tract infections using trimethoprim alone and in combination with sulfamethoxazole (Gantanol). In: Umezawa H (ed) Progress in antimicrobial and anticancer chemotherapy. Proc 6 th Int Congr Chemother. University of Tokyo Press, Tokyo, pp 971–974

Hoppe-Seyler G, Schollmeyer P, Grandpierre B, Junkers K (1974) Behavior of trimethoprim and sulphamethoxazole in anuria in hemodialysis and peritoneal dialysis. Verh Dtsch Ges Inn Med 80:672–676

Hoppu K, Partanen S, Koskela E (1980) Trimethoprim poisoning. Lancet 1:778

Hughes WT, Kuhn S, Chaudhary S et al. (1977) Successful chemoprophylaxis for Pneumocystis carinii pneumonitis. N Eng J Med 297:1419–1426

Huovinen P, Toivanen P (1980) Trimethoprim resistance in Finland after five years' use of plain trimethoprim. Br Med J 280:72–74

Iravani A, Richard GA, Baer H (1981) Treatment of uncomplicated urinary tract infections with trimethoprim versus sulfisoxazole with special reference to antibody-coated bacteria and fecal flora. Antimicrob Agents Chemother 19:842–850

Iravani A, Richard GA, Baer H (1982) Once-a-day trimethoprim versus nitrofurantoin in treatment of acute urinary tract infections in young women, with special reference to periurethral, vaginal, and rectal flora. Rev Inf Dis 4:378–387

Iwarson S, Lidin-Janson G (1979) Long-term, low-dose trimethoprim prophylaxis in patients with recurrent urinary tract infections. J Antimicrob Chemother 5:316–318

Jones SR, Smith JW, Sanford JP (1974) Localization of urinary tract infections by detection of antibody-coated bacteria in urine sediment. N Engl J Med 290:591–593

Jordan GW, Krajden SF, Hoeprich PD, Wong GA, Peirce TH, Rausch DC (1975) Trimethoprim-sulfamethoxazole in chronic bronchitis. CMA J 112:91 S–95 S

Kahn SB, Fein SA, Brodksy I (1968) Effects of trimethoprim on folate metabolism in man. Clin Pharmacol Ther 9:550–560

Kasanen A, Kaarsalo E, Hiltunen R, Soini V (1974) Comparison of long-term, low-dosage nitrofurantoin, methenamine hippurate, trimethoprim, and trimethoprim-sulfamethoxazole on the control of recurrent urinary tract infection. Ann Clin Res 6:285–289

Kasanen A, Anttila M, Kahela P et al. (1978) Trimethoprim, pharmacology, antimicrobial activity and clinical use in urinary tract infections. Ann Clin Res 10:1–39

Kass EH (1956) Asymptomatic infections of the urinary tract. Trans Assoc Am Physicians 69:56

Kass EH (1960) The role of asymptomatic bacteriuria in the pathogenesis of pyelonephritis. In: Quinn EL, Kass EH (eds) Biology of pyelonephritis. Little Brown, Boston, pp 399–418

Koch UJ, Schumann KP, Küchler R, Kewitz H (1973) Efficacy of trimethoprim, sulfamethoxazole and the combination of both in acute urinary tract infection. Chemotherapy 19:314–321

Koutts J, Van der Weyden MB, Cooper M (1973) Effect of trimethoprim on folate metabolism in human bone marrow. Aust NZ J Med 3:245–250

Kunin CM, Craig WA, Uehling DT (1978) Trimethoprim therapy for urinary tract infection. JAMA 239:2588–2590

Lacey RW, Lord VL, Gunasekera HKW, Leiberman PJ, Luxton DEA (1980) Comparison of trimethoprim alone with trimethoprim/sulfamethoxazole in the treatment of respiratory and urinary infections with particular reference to selection of trimethoprim resistance. Lancet 1:1270–1273

Lykkegaard-Nielsen M, Hansen L (1972) Trimethoprim in human prostatic tissue and prostatic fluid. Scand J Urol Nephrol 6:244–248

Mabeck CE, Vejlsgaard R (1979) Treatment of urinary tract infections with sulfonamide and/or trimethoprim. Infection 7:S 414–S 415

Männistö PT (1976) Comparison of oxolinic acid, trimethoprim, and trimethoprim-sulfamethoxazole in the treatment of long-term control of urinary tract infection. Curr Ther Res 20:645–654

Martin DC, Arnold JD (1968) Treatment of acute falciparum malaria with sulfalene and trimethoprim. JAMA 203:476–480

McNaughton RD, Riben P, Light B et al. (1980) Comparison of trimethoprim and trimethoprim/sulfamethoxazole prophylaxis in neutropenic patients: elimination of potential pathogens and emergence of resistance. In: Nelson JD, Grassi C (eds) Current chemotherapy and infectious disease. Proc 11 th Int Congr Chemother and 19 th Intersci Conf Antimicrob Agents Chemother. The American Society for Microbiology, Washington, DC, pp 1444–1446

Messing EM, Stamey TA (1978) Interstitial cystitis: early diagnosis, pathology and treatment. Urology 12:381–392

Mond NC, Percival A, Williams JD, Brumfitt W (1965) Presentation, diagnosis, and treatment of urinary tract infections in general practice. Lancet 1:514–516

Mundt KA, Polk BF (1979) Identification of site of urinary tract infections by antibody-coated bacteria assay. Lancet 1:1172–1175

O'Brien TF, Ross DG, Guzman MA, Medeiros AA, Hedges RW, Botstein D (1980) Dissemination of an antibiotic resistance plasmid in hospital patient flora. Antimicrob Agents Chemother 17:537–543

Oosterlinck W, Defoort R, Renders G (1975) The concentration of sulfamethoxazole and trimethoprim in human prostate gland. Br J Urol 47:301–304

Pancoast SJ, Hyams DM, Neu HC (1980) Effect of trimethoprim and trimethophrim/sulfamethoxazole on development of drug-resistant vaginal and fecal floras. Antimicrob Agents Chemother 17:263–268

Pohjanpelto PE, Sarmelo TJ, Raines T (1974) Penetration of trimethoprim and sulfamethoxazole into the aqueous humour. Br J Ophthalmol 58:606–608

Reid DW, Caillé G, Kaufman NR (1975) Maternal and transplacental kinetics of trimethoprim and sulfamethoxazole, separately, and in combination. Can Med Assoc J 112:S 67–S 72

Rieder J (1973) Excretion of sulfamethoxazole and trimethoprim into human bile. J Infect Dis 128:S 574

Rieder J, Schwartz DE, Fernex M et al. (1974) Pharmacokinetics of the antibacterial combination sulfamethoxazole plus trimethoprim in patients with normal or impaired kidney function. Antibiot Chemother 18:148–198

Rubin RH, Fang LS, Jones SR et al. (1980) Single-dose amoxicillin therapy for urinary tract infection. JAMA 244:561–564

Sabel KG, Brandberg A (1975) Treatment of meningitis and septicemia in infancy with a sulfamethoxazole/trimethoprim combination. Acta Paediatr Scand 64:25–32

Salmon JD, Fowle AS, Bye A (1975) Concentrations of trimethoprim and sulfamethoxazole in the aqueous humour and plasma from regimens of co-trimoxazole in man. J Antimicrob Chemother 1:205–211

Sander J, Fellner H, Kalstad S et al. (1980) Treatment of urinary tract infections in outpatients: double-blind comparison between trimethoprim and nitrofurantoin. In: Nelson JD, Grassi C (eds) Current chemotherapy and infectious disease. Proc 11 th Int Congr Chemother and 19 th Intersci Conf Antimicrob Agents Chemother. The American Society for Microbiology, Washington, DC, pp 1299–1300

Schnaars P, Escher J (1969) Results of treating acute and chronic infections of the urinary tract with Bactrim or its individual components sulfamethoxazole and trimethoprim. Praxis 58:1279–1283

Schneider M, Schwarzenberg L, Cattam A, Schlumberger JR, Amiel JL, Mathé G (1965) Treatment of a number of proteus infections with trimethoprim. Presse Med 73:893–894

Schwartz DE, Ziegler WH (1969) Assay and pharmacokinetics of trimethoprim in man and animals. Postgrad Med J 45:S 32–S 37

Seneca H, Zinsser HH, Uson A (1974) Chronic urinary tract infections. NY State J Med 74:494–498

Sharp JR, Ishak KG, Zimmerman HJ (1980) Chronic active hepatitis and severe hepatic necrosis associated with nitrofurantoin. Ann Intern Med 92:14–19

Sharpstone P (1969) The renal handling of trimethoprim and sulphamethoxazole in man. Postgrad Med J 45:S 38–S 42

Sietzen W, Knothe H (1978) Effect of trimethoprim, trimethoprim/sulfamethoxazole and sulfamethoxazole on the occurrence of drug-resistant *Enterobacteriaceae* in the human bowel flora. In: Siegenthaler W, Luethy R (eds) Current chemotherapy. Proc 10 th Int Congr Chemother. The American Society for Microbiology, Washington, DC, pp 660–662

Sourander LB, Werner GE (1967) Efficacy and tolerance of sulfonamide-trimethoprim combinations in geriatric patients with bacteriuria. Proc 5 th Int Congr Chemother. Wiener Medizinische Academie, Vienna, pp 199

Sourander L, Saarimaa H, Arvilommi H (1972) Treatment of sulfonimide-resistant urinary tract infections with a combination of sulfonimide and trimethoprim. Acta Med Scand 191:1–3

Stamey TA, Govan DE, Palmer JM (1965) The localization and treatment of urinary tract infections: the role of bactericidal urine levels as opposed to serum levels. Medicine 44:1–36

Stamey TA, Condy M (1975) The diffusion and concentration of trimethoprim in human vaginal fluid. J Infect Dis 131:261–266

Stamey TA (1978) Urinary tract infections in women. In: Harrison JH, Gittes RF, Perlmutter AD, Stamey TA, Walsh PC (eds) Campbell's urology, 4 th edn. Saunders, Philadelphia, pp 451–479

Stamm WE, Counts GW, Wagner KF, Martin D, Gregory D, McKevitt M, Turck M, Holmes KK (1980) Antimicrobial prophylaxis of recurrent urinary tract infections. Ann Intern Med 92:770–775

Steinberg SE, Campbell CL, Rabinovitch PS, Hillman RS (1980) The effect of trimethoprim/sulfamethoxazole on Friend erythroleukemia cells. Blood 55:501–504

Svedhem A, Iwarson S (1979) Cerebrospinal fluid concentrations of trimethoprim during oral and parenteral treatment. J Antimicrob Chemother 5:717–720

Thomas FE, Jackson RT, Melly A, Alford RH (1977) Sequential hospitalwide outbreaks of resistant Serratia and Klebsiella infection. Arch Intern Med 137:581–584

Thomas V, Shelokov A, Forland M (1974) Antibody-coated bacteria in the urine and the site of urinary tract infection. N Engl J Med 290:588–590

Towner KJ, Pearson NJ, Cattell WR, O'Grady FO (1979) Trimethoprim R plasmids isolated during long-term treatment of urinary tract infection with co-trimoxazole. J Antimicrob Chemother 5:45–52

Van der Waaij D, Berghuis JM, Lekkarkerk JEC (1972) Colonization resistance of the digestive tract of mice during systemic antibiotic treatment. J Hyg (Camb) 70:605–610

Vosti KL (1975) Recurrent urinary tract infections: prevention by prophylactic antibiotics after sexual intercourse. JAMA 231:934–940

Welling PG, Craig WA, Amidon GL, Kunin CM (1973) Pharmacokinetics of trimethoprim and sulfamethoxazole in normal subjects and in patients with renal failure. J Infect Dis 128:S 556–S 566

Ylikorkala O, Sjöstedt E, Järvinen R, Raines T (1973) Trimethoprim-sulfonamide combination administered orally and intravaginally in the first trimester of pregnancy: its absorption into serum and transfer to amniotic fluid. Acta Obstet Gynecol Scand 52:229–234

CHAPTER 13

Inhibitors of Dihydrofolate Reductase as Antiprotozoal Agents

I.M. ROLLO

A. Introduction

The therapeutic potential of inhibitors of dihydrofolate reductase as selectively toxic agents was first realized in early studies involving laboratory species of the genus *Plasmodium*. These experiments were carried out initially with readily standardized infections of *Plasmodium gallinaceum* in chicks and *P. berghei* in mice. The stimulus for these studies arose from the observations that a large number of pyrimidine derivatives inhibited the growth of a folate-dependent strain of *Lactobacillus casei*. Of the many active compounds, a high degree of activity was found in 2,4-diamino-5-p-chlorophenoxypyrimidine (Fig. 1, I). At that time it was noted that there was a formal resemblance between the structure of I and that of chloroguanide (II), a substance developed in Britain during World War II and widely used for chemoprophylaxis and treatment of the human malarias. This resemblance suggested that the latter might be an antagonist of folic acid, and, conversely, that the former might have antimalarial activity. Subsequent work confirmed both properties, the pyrimidine was found to have antimalarial activity against *P. gallinaceum* of the same order as that of quinine; chloroguanide was found to have antifolate activity (FALCO et al. 1949).

In retrospect it was perhaps fortuitous that antifolate activity was found in chloroguanide. Its activity was demonstrable only at concentrations very much

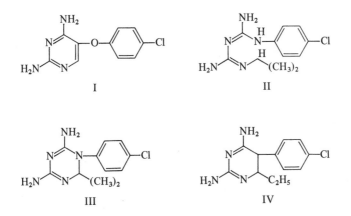

Fig. 1. I 2,4-diamino-5-p-chlorophenoxypyrimidine (an early member of the antimalarial series); II chloroguanide; III the dihydrotriazine metabolite of chloroguanide; IV pyrimethamine

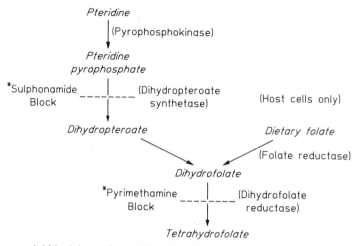

Fig. 2. Sequential block by sulfonamide and pyrimethamine of tetrahydrofolate biosynthesis

higher than those of the pyrimidine and was non-competitive in nature. In contrast, the pyrimidine was inhibitory at concentrations less than 1 µg/ml and its inhibition was characteristic of a classical pharmacological competitive antagonism. The answer to the apparent discrepancy was found however, when 2 years later, CARRINGTON et al. (1951) showed that the active form of chloroguanide in vivo is a dihydrotriazine (III), the cyclization brought about by biotransformation. This substance bears a striking resemblance to the pyrimidine, pyrimethamine (IV), which was eventually chosen as the most efficacious member of the several series of 2,4-diaminopyrimidine derivatives examined at that time. The original purely formal analogy which at least in part led to the search for clinically useful antimalarial substances, can now be regarded as a more firmly based functional as well as structural analogy.

Subsequent study has shown that clinically useful antimalarial activity depends upon a selective sensitivity of plasmodial dihydrofolate reductase compared with that from other sources. Like most bacteria, plasmodia are independent of an exogenous source of folate. The substrate for the enzyme is formed from dihydropteroate which in turn is formed from pteridine pyrophosphate (reviewed by SHERMAN 1979). It is this step, catalysed by the enzyme dihydropteroate synthetase, that is inhibited by sulfonamides (Fig. 2). This close approximation of two points of inhibition in the common pathway is responsible for the high degree of antimalarial potentiation observed when the two different agents are tested together, as discussed in Sect. C.VIII (ROLLO 1955).

The enzyme, dihydrofolate reductase, differs not only in size and shape, the relative molecular weights for plasmodial and mammalian enzymes being 190,000 and 20,000 daltons respectively, but also in susceptibility to inhibition by the pyrimidines. Some 50% inhibition of plasmodial enzyme is achieved by the very low concentration of 0.5 nM pyrimethamine while a 2,000-fold greater amount is required by the host erythrocyte enzyme (FERONE et al. 1969). The reason for the relatively large size of protozoal enzyme has been subject to further investigation

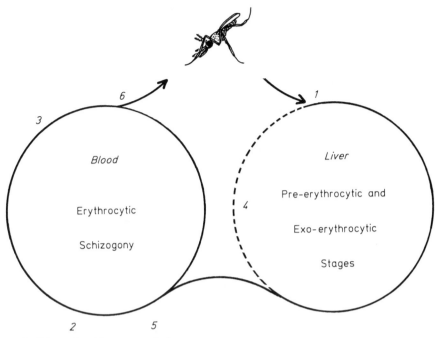

Fig. 3. Life-cycle of human malarias

by FERONE and ROLAND (1980). They have identified an association between protozoal dihydrofolate reductase and thymidylate synthetase either through a protein–protein association or through a bifunctional polypeptide. Such apposition could have been of considerable evolutionary advantage by enabling closer regulation and channelling of those reactions so important in rapidly dividing cells. Since this early discovery of antimalarial effectiveness of some diaminopyrimidines, pyrimethamine, and subsequently another analogue, trimethoprim, have been used world-wide in the suppression and treatment, first of malaria and then of several other protozoal pathogens.

B. Points of Possible Therapeutic Attack

In order to appreciate the intricacies of antimalarial chemotherapy it is necessary to have a basic understanding of the rather complex life cycle of the parasite. From the clinical point of view, greatest importance can be ascribed to the parasitaemia, that is the development of the asexual stages in the bloodstream. It is the continual multiplication within the red cell, lysis of the infected cell and subsequent infection of fresh red cells that give rise to the signs, symptoms, and hazards of clinical malaria. It is in this cycle also that sexually mature male and female gametocytes are found, which in themselves contribute nothing to the patient's disease but are responsible for the development within the mosquito of infective sporozoites. It is the injection of these sporozites in the feeding process of the infective mosquito that initiates the primary cycle of plasmodial development within the parenchymal cells

Table 1. Points of possible antimalarial attack

Chemotherapeutic Terminology[a]	Elaboration	Place for DHFR inhibitors
1. Causal prophylaxis	Kills parasites in pre-erythrocytic stage and prevents demonstrable infection	Yes/no
2. Suppression	Kills parasites at earliest erythrocytic development and prevents demonstrable infection	Yes
3. Clinical cure	Interrupts parasite development in the erythrocytes (schizogony) and terminates clinical attack; these agents are called schizontocides	Qualified yes
4. Radical cure	Eradicates not only erythrocytic parasites but also those persisting in the exoerythrocytic stages in the liver and responsible for relapse	No
5. Suppressive cure	Suppression (2), continues for a period longer than the natural life span of the infection	Yes
6. Gametocyticidal therapy	Destroys the sexual forms in the blood or prevents their development in the mosquito	Yes

[a] Reference to numbers in Fig. 3

of the liver. These pre-erythrocytic stages are innocuous to the patient but serve, when mature and released into the circulation, as the initiators of the asexual erythrocytic cycle.

In the so-called relapsing malarias, caused by *Plamodium vivax*, *P. ovale* and *P. malariae*, some proportion of this mature population of pre-erythrocytic parasites invade healthy liver cells and initiate a persisting exo-erythrocytic cycle from which, on occasion, mature parasites may enter the circulation. The patient will then undergo a relapse, weeks, months or, exceptionally, years later. The importance of understanding these details which are sketched in Fig. 3, is that antimalarials differ in their ability to affect different stages of parasite development and hence have different clinical indications. In Table 1 are described the several points of clinical attack with indications where dihydrofolate reductase inhibitors play a prominent part.

C. Antimalarial Therapeutics

Very soon after the first laboratory demonstration of the antimalarial activity of substituted 2,4-diaminopyrimidines, large-scale screening and toxicity testing of promising compounds resulted in the selection of 2,4-diamino-5-p-chlorophenyl-6-ethylpyrimidine as the most clinically promising therapeutic agent. It is important to note that while the activity of this substance is the highest observed against *P. gallinaceum*, its activity against *P. berghei* was equalled or surpassed by other members of the series (HITCHINGS 1952; ROLLO 1952). Its final choice was based on consistent activity against all experimental malarias available at that time rather than the absolute level of activity reached. It is also important to note that all com-

Table 2. Data from first clinical trial of pyrimethamine given as a single oral dose to Nigerian schoolchildren. Comparison is made with single oral doses of established effective remedies (see ARCHIBALD 1951)

Treatment	*Plasmodium falciparum* trophozoite rate[a]					
	D[b]	D+2	D+4	D+7	D+14	D+30
Chloroguanide 300 mg	15/16	1/16	0/16			
Quinacrine 300 mg	12/14	0/12	0/12			
Pyrimethamine 25 mg	9/10	1/9	0/10			
Pyrimethamine 5 mg	45/48		0/28	1/44	0/40	0/27

[a] Number of individuals infected/total number of individuals in group
[b] "D" is on day of treatment just before dose given; "D+2" is day 3 of trial, and so on

parisons were carried out in vivo; at that time no reliable technique existed for the in vitro testing of antimalarial compounds. The activity quoted is, therefore, a function not only of intrinsic antimalarial activity but also of the various pharmacokinetic parameters which determine the fate of a substance in the body. These will, of course, differ appreciably from compound to compound and from host to host. A most interesting comparative study could now be carried out to determine the in vitro activity of individual compounds against different strains of plasmodia by utilizing a culture technique such as that described by JENSEN and TRAGER (1977).

I. Early Trials

Early trials of the therapeutic usefulness of pyrimethamine came shortly after the demonstration of its very high activity against the laboratory infections. The first report was published in 1951 in which ARCHIBALD described his field trials in Nigeria with single small doses administered to schoolchildren. The promptness of the report is remarkable in light of today's requirements for exhaustive pharmacological and toxicological data before a new drug may be given to humans; the substance was synthesized and received its first laboratory testing early in the year before the report. The reported data confirmed a high degree of activity and persistence of effect against *Plasmodium falciparum* and *P. malariae*, the species predominant in that part of West Africa. The smallest dosage tried, 5 mg in a single oral dose, caused disappearance of asexual parasites of both species. The effect persisted for 30 days but parasites reappeared within 60 days. The schizonticidal effect was equivalent to that of a much larger single dose, 300 mg, of either chloroguanide or quinacrine, although clearance of parasitaemia was slower than with the latter two. Gametocytes were apparently unaffected. In a parallel personal trial in Nigeria, GOODWIN (1952 a, b) was completely protected for several months by taking 5 mg daily. Protection was achieved not only against naturally acquired infection but also from several bites from laboratory-bred, infected *Anopheles gambiae*. Some of the data from ARCHIBALD's trial are shown in Table 2.

The early promise of these clinical trials led rapidly to more field testing in several parts of the world and to further evaluation of the proper place of pyrimeth-

Table 3. Data on early clinical trials with pyrimethamine (see GOODWIN 1952a)

Place	Plasmodium sp.	Dose[a]	Duration (days) Parasit-aemia	Fever	Cases	Failures
Gambia	P. falciparum	0.25–0.5	<3		29	1
	P. malariae	mg/kg	<4		3	0
Indochina	P. falciparum	(Various)	1.5	1.6	80	0
	P. vivax	(Various)	2.3	1.8	16	0
Tunisia	P. falciparum P. vivax	(Various)	1.7	1.6	36	1
Malaya	P. falciparum[b]	50	1.8	2.0	15	2
		50 × 2	2.3	2.1	39	4
		100 × 1 50 × 4	2.6	2.3	26	7
	P. vivax[b]	50 × 2	3.6	1.7	12	0
		50	3.1	2.1	10	0
Assam	P. falciparum	50	2.2	1.7	11	2
	P. vivax	50	2.0	3.0	1	0
Assam	P. falciparum	50	1.5	1.3	21	1
	P. malariae	50	1.5	1.5	1	0
	P. vivax	50	1.0	1.0	1	0
West Bengal	P. falciparum	50	2.3	1.8	6	0
	P. vivax	50	2.1	0.7	6	0

[a] Pyrimethamine, single dose of 50 mg unless stated otherwise
[b] Compared with chloroquine, single dose of 250 mg reduced fever more promptly

amine in antimalarial chemotherapy. An obvious test of antimalarial potential and one which enables rapid evaluation, is the treatment of overt malarial attacks, the ability of the compound to bring about clinical cure. Such trials were carried out in endemic areas of North and West Africa, India, and South-West Asia. These rapidly confirmed both the potency and the efficacy of the new antimalarial. A summary of these trials is shown in Table 3 (and see GOODWIN 1952a). From these and later trials (see THOMPSON and WERBEL 1972; HILL 1963) the schizonticidal potential of pyrimethamine became apparent. Its most outstanding property was its potency; single oral doses of 50 mg in the majority of cases produced a prompt response. In some trials even 25 mg as a single oral dose resulted in clinical cure.

II. Clinical Cure with Pyrimethamine

Despite this impressive demonstration of potency, however, the general usefulness of pyrimethamine in producing clinical cure was compromised by two undesirable properties. At the dosage used, and as shown in Table 3 and subsequent trials at higher dosage, the new antimalarial could not be relied upon to produce a cure in all cases, especially of falciparum malaria. For this species in particular, in which the clinicopathological picture includes the possibility of the lethal central nervous system involvement of cerebral malaria (BRUCE-CHWATT 1980), the lack of reliable response is a significant deterrent.

The second disadvantage was the relative slowness of its schizonticidal effects in all species of human malaria. This in itself is not a damning disadvantage, however when compared with chloroquine which produces a very rapid response, both in reducing parasitaemia and fever, and which had been the accepted therapeutic agent for many years, the comparison was not flattering. The debilitating and distressing effects of a malarial attack, particularly in the non-immune patient, demand as rapid as response to treatment as can possibly be achieved. In certain circumstances, however, especially when strains of falciparum malaria resistant to the action of chloroquine are involved, pyrimethamine does have a part to play. This situation is discussed in the following paragraphs.

The relative slowness of clinical response to pyrimethamine is associated directly with the stage of schizogony at which the drug has an obvious effect. Several observers have noted that pyrimethamine has little or no effect on trophozoites, the early stages of asexual development in the red cell. The most marked cytological effect is seen at the stage of schizont maturation when there is maximal synthesis of new nuclear material (see GOODWIN and ROLLO 1955). These observations are consistent with the action of pyrimethamine in inhibiting the biosynthesis of tetrahydrofolate. At the stage of trophozoite growth with relatively little demand for rapid nucleic acid biosynthesis, inhibition at a point both biochemically and temporally removed from these synthetic events would have little or no immediate effect. Moreover, HITCHINGS (1978) has proposed that subsequent to initial exposure to pyrimethamine, synthesis of DNA during the early stages of parasite growth could occur at the expense of existing pools of thymidylate and/or 5,10-methylenetetrahydrofolate. In contrast, chloroquine by its immediate intercalation with parasite DNA, its inhibition of both DNA and RNA polymerase, and possibly other interference with parasite metabolism, would be expected to affect the wellbeing of the parasite rapidly and disastrously (see ROLLO 1980). As a consequence, therefore, of the specificity of its action and of the nature of the metabolic inhibition it produces, pyrimethamine in most circumstances is not recommended as an agent of choice for the clinical cure, especially of falciparum malaria.

III. Causal Prophylaxis

Ideally, those persons living in or visiting malarious areas should be protected from acquiring malaria. Of the two measures possible to achieve this, elimination of the mosquito vector, and preventing parasite development in the human host, the former is by far the preferable and in many areas the more effective. Control programmes against mosquito larvae by drainage and by chemical or biological manipulation of breeding places have been highly successful in or near well-organized and advanced communities but less so under general rural conditions. Control of the adult mosquito by the use of persistent insecticides has also resulted in marked decreases in insect populations, however, the use of this method is limited by the development of resistant strains of mosquito, the costs involved, and potential health hazards from more recently introduced insecticides (see BRUCE-CHWATT 1980).

Chemotherapeutic control of early parasite development can be aimed at two stages of the plasmodium, the infective sporozoite and the pre-erythrocytic parasite. Of the two, the sporozoite is insensitive to all currently available antimalarial agents, at least to those concentrations present in the blood during conventional drug dosage. It is, therefore, impossible by chemotherapeutic means to prevent an individual, bitten by an infective mosquito, from becoming infected. Prophylactic chemotherapy must, therefore, be aimed at those early stages developing in the liver.

From the evidence available it appears that there are considerable differences in the sensitivity of the pre-erythrocytic stages of the different species of human malaria. In experiments with sporozoite-induced infections of the Chesson strain of *P. vivax* in volunteers, COATNEY et al. (1953) confirmed the effectiveness of pyrimethamine against frank attacks but were unable to demonstrate consistent causal prophylaxis. The volunteers were given 25 mg pyrimethamine once weekly, the recommended dosage for suppression. It was concluded that the drug did not appear to be a true causal prophylactic, although prolonged delays occurring before patent parasitaemia on cessation of treatment suggested some deleterious effects against early tissue stages of the parasite. Later trials by NEGULICI et al. (1960) also failed to demonstrate a consistent causal prophylactic effect.

Against the pre-erythrocytic stages of *P. falciparum*, however pyrimethamine has a much more consistent effect. Earlier work had demonstrated conclusively that chloroguanide, in adequate dosage, is an efficient causal prophylactic against many strains of this species (see PETERS 1970). Not surprisingly, COVELL et al. (1953a) were able to demonstrate a similar property for pyrimethamine. Volunteers infected with a West African strain of *P. falciparum* were treated weekly with 25 mg pyrimethamine. The times of infection relative to drug administration were distributed in such a manner as to cover all possible intervals between the individual doses. The treatment afforded complete protection against overt malarial attack in all individuals and the conclusion was drawn that pyrimethamine was an effective causal prophylactic. NEGULICI et al. (1960) confirmed this action against another strain of *P. falciparum*.

IV. Suppression and Mass Prophylaxis

In practical terms, however, the extremely high potency and efficacy of pyrimethamine as a suppressive agent, demonstrated from its earliest clinical trials, overcome any doubt of its effectiveness as a causal prophylactic. Many years of experience have confirmed the earlier results that pyrimethamine is an effective and safe antimalarial for individual suppression (COVELL et al. 1955). Its effectiveness as a suppressive agent given at weekly intervals is consistent with its pharmacokinetics. GOODWIN (1952a) and later SMITH and IHRIG (1959) were able to demonstrate long persistence of the drug following a high degree of absorption from the gastrointestinal tract. Data from the latter study showed that after single oral doses, pyrimethamine could be detected both chemically and microbiologically for 7 days in the serum and even longer in the urine. They compared their data with those of HERNANDEZ et al. (1953) who demonstrated successful suppression of *P. vivax* infection with doses as low as 0.25 mg/day. The rate of urinary excretion found by SMITH

Table 4. Data from mass prophylaxis trial by weekly self-administration of pyrimethamine in Ghana. The results of periodic malaria surveys at two villages (see CHARLES et al. 1962)

| | *Plasmodium falciparum* parasite rate (%) Week of treatment | | | | | | | | |
	0	4	6	16	22	26	37	38	49
Village 1	71[a]	6.5		5.5	3.2		25		59
Village 2	55[b]		7.4			28		57	

[a] 3 November 1958
[b] 14 January 1959

and IHRIG indicated that amounts in excess of this would be present in most individuals for at least 11 days after single oral doses, and for considerably longer in some subjects. More recent analysis of pyrimethamine kinetics has shown that its mean plasma half-life in humans is 85 h (CAVALLITO et al. 1978).

Despite its uniformly good record against initially sensitive strains of plasmodia, however, caution has had to be observed in those areas in which resistant strains have appeared. Such strains not only will not respond to pyrimethamine given in doses intended for clinical cure but are likely to fail with breakthrough parasitaemia and clinical attack despite continued weekly suppression. The problem of development of resistance has also bedevilled attempts at the rural control of malaria. Ideally such long-term control could be achieved by the regular self-administration of a long-lasting, potent, non-toxic antimalarial during that period of the year when transmission was significant. The exploratory trials of VINCKE and LIPS (1952) in which weekly doses of pyrimethamine brought malaria transmission virtually to a stand-still encouraged wider control in rural areas. Unfortunately experience has been disappointing as evidenced by mass prophylaxis trials against *P.falciparum* in Ghana (CHARLES et al. 1962). A dramatic fall in the parasite rates occurred in both of the villages selected for the trial for the first few weeks. By the 26th week in one village and the 37th week in the second, parasite rates were again increasing (Table 4).

The conclusions drawn from these trials and others were clear. Pyrimethamine has a very real part to play in suppression or chemoprophylaxis in compliant individuals visiting or working in malarious areas. In attempts at large scale suppression in less sophisticated rural communities, however, dependent upon unsupervised self-administration over long periods of time, initial success becomes tempered by the eventual selection or development of less responsive strains of the parasite. Use of pyrimethamine in such circumstances should be only a part of more general programme of prevention and control carried out by trained, highly motivated individuals.

V. Gametocyticidal Effects

Of considerable epidemiological importance are the effects of antimalarial drugs on the sexual stages of parasitaemia. Any effect of drugs on the gametocytes present in the bloodstream will have no observable effect on the clinical course of an infection, indeed gametocytes may persist for some time after an apparent clinical cure has been achieved. From the point of view of symptomatology, therefore, they are of no importance. However, from the point of view of transmission, any interference with the ability of the gametocytes to mature to male and female gametes in the midgut of the mosquito, to form the motile zygote, to form the oocyst and mature to infective sporozoite, will have immense benefit to the community. The treated individual will no longer become infective to mosquitos and hence will cease to be a reservoir of infection.

Early observations on the effect of pyrimethamine on the infectivity of gametocytes were made by FOY and KONDI (1952) who were unable to infect mosquitoes fed on a patient previously treated with the drug. Just prior to treatment, the mosquitos were readily infected and produced sporozoites in the salivary glands. Later, SHUTE and MARYON (1954) consolidating their earlier work with chloroguanide showed that in both *P. vivax* and *P. falciparum* infections, pyrimethamine in single doses of 50 and 25 mg, respectively, had no visible effect on circulating gametocytes but prevented the development of the oocyst in the mosquito, 5 mg had no effect on vivax gametocytes. This action might have been expected since, if pyrimethamine acts on the sexual stages just as it does on the asexual stages, then no effect will become obvious until there is substantial demand for the biosynthesis of nucleic acids. Subsequent to these observations many authors have confirmed the effectiveness of pyrimethamine in inhibiting the development of the parasite in the mosquito (see PETERS 1970).

The ideal antimalarial drug should possess properties such that it affects not only those stages of parasite development already discussed: the pre-erythrocytic tissue stage, the clinically important erythrocytic asexual schizonts, and the epidemiologically important gametocytes, but also those subsequent stages which in the case of the relapsing malarias persist as exo-erythrocytic parasites in the liver.

VI. Radical Cure

At the time of the introduction of pyrimethamine, only one drug could be relied upon to produce radical cure by eliminating the persisting parasites. The drug, primaquine, a derivative of 8-aminoquinoline, while undoubtedly effective in this function, had certain disadvantages. It has very limited activity against asexual parasitaemia and may have serious side effects in those individuals genetically deficient in glucose-6-phosphate dehydrogenase (see ROLLO 1980). The remarkably high schizonticidal activity and relative lack of toxicity of pyrimethamine, prompted its trial as an agent against the persisting tissue stage of *P. vivax*.

The trials, carried out by COVELL et al. (1953 b) involved infection by infective mosquito bite followed after parasitaemia became patent, by a 5-day course of treatment. The immediate clinical response was slow, confirming earlier reports involving nonimmune patients. All patients, however, subsequently relapsed, making it quite clear that treatment of the primary attack with pyrimethamine in full dosage was not effective in preventing relapse. Further treatment with a suppressive schedule of once weekly treatment for 2 months gave no indication of any effect on subsequent relapse rate. Despite this obvious lack of effect on persisting tissue forms, however, continuation of normal suppressive therapy for a period of up to 10 weeks after leaving a malarious area will provide suppressive cure with certain strains of *P. vivax*. The situation with these strains is analogous to that with falciparum malaria where the period of suppressive treatment is longer than the normal biological life span of the parasite in the host.

VII. Drug Resistance

Decreasing usefulness of an antimicrobial agent due to the development of drug-resistant strains is a common phenomenon in the treatment and control of infectious diseases. Antimalarials are no different in this respect. In one species or another or in one part of the world or another, resistance to the several agents is well documented (see PETERS 1970; ROLLO 1980). Inappropriate use or misuse of an initially useful agent is commonly involved, but whether or not this was the case with pyrimethamine is hard to tell. Nevertheless, as already shown, unsupervised long-term suppression in rural communities, while providing very promising early results, has often led to the development and dissemination of pyrimethamine-resistant strains. Such development should not have been unexpected. There seems to be a direct correlation between the readiness with which laboratory strains of plasmodia can develop resistance, and its development in the field. PETERS (1970) encyclopaedic work on drug resistance in malaria should be consulted for the vast coverage of the subject.

An early explanation of the development of pyrimethamine resistance in the avian plasmodium, *P. gallinaceum*, arose from a complex interrelationship of the action or lack of it of sulfonamide, chloroguanide or pyrimethamine in singly or multiply resistant strains (ROLLO 1955). The hypothesis involved a two-step action of pyrimethamine, resistance resulting from an impeding of access or uptake, the first of the two steps. This hypothesis lacked firm biochemical evidence.

A more rational explanation was provided by FERONE et al. (1969) when he showed marked differences between the dihydrofolate reductases of two strains of *P. berghei*, a rodent malaria, one originally sensitive, the other highly resistant to pyrimethamine. The enzyme extracted from the resistant strain was found to bind pyrimethamine 400–800 times less tightly than that extracted from the original sensitive strain. Furthermore, the concentration of pyrimethamine which, in vitro, was required to produce a 50% reduction in enyzme activity was increased 40-fold from 0.05 to 2.0×10^{-8} *M*.

VIII. Combination with Sulfonamides and Sulfones

1. Suppressive and Clinical Cure

The benefit of using combinations of dihydrofolate reductase inhibitors with either sulfonamides or sulfones is well established both experimentally in the laboratory and in clinical practice. What is now recognized as a very marked degree of antimicrobial potentiation was, in fact, first described between an antimalarial, chloroguanide, and sulfadiazine (GREENBERG et al. 1948). ROLLO (1955) extended this work later with pyrimethamine and showed by the construction of isobols that one-eighth the median effective dose (ED_{50}) of pyrimethamine plus one-seventh

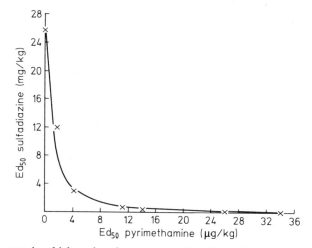

Fig. 4. Isobologram in which each point represents the ED_{50} of the drug or combination. ROLLO (1955)

the ED_{50} of sulfadiazine provided an optimal combination equivalent to one ED_{50} of either drug tested alone (Fig. 4). The action of chloroguanide and pyrimethamine given together was no greater than additive. HURLY (1959) was the first to test synergistic combinations in humans. He treated falciparum infections and found that less than one-tenth of an ED_{50} of pyrimethamine plus one-quarter of an ED_{50} of sulfadiazine was as effective in the treatment of acute infections as one ED_{50} of either drug alone. Subsequent trials have confirmed these original laboratory and field observations and have shown in addition that some sulfones can substitute for sulfonamides. These combinations act presumably by the same mechanism, that termed "sequential blockade" by HITCHINGS.

Such combinations offer tremendous potential advantages which can be itemized as follows:

a). In long-term suppression to prevent the development of pyrimethamine resistance particularly in those areas where such development has previously been shown to be a problem. The trial conducted by LUCAS et al. (1969) in Western Nigeria demonstrated the value of such use. In this it was found that when given alone at a usually effective suppressive dose, pyrimethamine produced a significant but incomplete suppression of asexual falciparum parasitaemia. The results confirmed and strengthened the evidence that pyrimethamine resistance in *P. falciparum* was present in that part of the African continent. In contrast, combinations of pyrimethamine at one-half the normal dose with either dapsone or sulformethoxine were clearly more effective. Parasitaemia was significantly and consistently lower than in those treated only with pyrimethamine. In addition, the drug combinations retained their effectiveness throughout 1 year of treatment with no indication at the end of the trial that strains resistant to the combinations had emerged.

b). The improved performance of combinations over pyrimethamine alone might be regarded as experimentally interesting but clinically of little account since over a very large part of the malarious world suppression has been effectively achieved by the 4-aminoquinoline antimalarial, chloroquine. This substance has been regarded in many areas as the ideal suppressive/clinically curative agent. It was effective as a suppressive agent in weekly, well-tolerated, doses, and as a highly effective rapidly acting schizonticide, producing clinical cure. In addition there was no evidence of the development of drug resistance. This position was maintained for 16 years of widespread use until, in 1961, the first report of chloroquine resistance in falciparum malaria was published. This first report, from Colombia, was soon followed by others in Central and South America and later in South-East Asia, the strains varying in degrees of resistance from very modest to almost completely insensitive to normal effective dosage. Currently such resistant strains have been reported from all parts of the world where falciparum malaria is endemic. It is in this situation that the combined use of pyrimethamine with either dapsone or a sulfonamide has proved so valuable. In areas where it is known that chloroquine suppression is inadequate and individuals are in danger of developing clinical attacks of the potentially life-threatening falciparum malaria, the choice of suppressive therapy should be such a combination. The pharmaceutical industry has risen to the occasion with preparations containing pyrimethamine and dapsone or sulfadoxine. In many parts of the world this has proven effective. Unfortunately, despite the benefits of pharmacological potentiation and the general usefulness of the combinations, in certain areas such as Cambodia where multiply resistant strains are already present, resistance to the combinations develops rapidly (VERDRAGER et al. 1968).

c). A further benefit from such combinations is in the therapy of chloroquine-resistant strains of *P. falciparum*. While pyrimethamine itself has proved to be slow in its action in the treatment of the acute clinical attack, the combinations have been found to have a speed of action comparable to that of chloroquine, in terms of both clearance of parasitaemia and clinical response (CHIN et al. 1966; HARINASUTA et al. 1967; HERRERO 1967). This has proved extremely valuable since, in some of the multiply resistant strains, the response to quinine which normally produces a very rapid response has been impaired. A combination of pyrimethamine with the long-acting sulfonamide, sulfadoxine, is available for this purpose and has already played a significant role in the management of patients infected with highly virulent strains.

2. Effect on Other Sporozoa

Potentiating combinations of dihyrofolate reductase inhibitors with sulfonamides have found clinical uses in the treatment of infections due to Sporozoa other than plasmodia. In these circumstances, the combination is required, not to prevent the development of resistance, but to provide as a combination, an efficacy which is lacking in the agents individually. The earliest such use was the treatment of toxoplasmosis. Pyrimethamine given concurrently with triple sulfonamides has been found useful in the treatment of this condition: (FELDMAN 1968). Unfortunately a course of treatment lasts 3–4 weeks. In order to obviate the haematological toxicity that may occur with such protracted daily administration of pyrimethamine, folinic acid should be given concurrently. This substance non-competitively antagonizes any block in folate metabolism produced by pyrimethamine in mammalian cells and hence inhibits any toxic potential. Folinic acid, however, has no effect in the parasitic cells since they lack the ability to actively take it up and are dependent on an exogenous supply of the precursor, p-aminobenzoate.

In the treatment of *Pneumocystis carinii* infection, a severe infection in impaired hosts, high dose therapy with trimethoprim and sulfamethoxazole has proved effective (LARTER et al. 1978). Similarly, low dose prophylaxis against this organism has also proved effective in neutropenic patients (see HUGHES et al. 1977).

Coccidiosis in poultry has often posed a problem, particularly under conditions of intensive husbandry. In these situations diaveridine, an analogue of pyrimethamine in combination with sulfaquinoxaline used prophylactically in the diet has proved beneficial. Similarly in human coccidiosis, caused by *Isospora belli*, trimethoprim/sulfamethoxozole has become a treatment of choice.

References

Archibald HM (1951) Preliminary field trials on a new schizonticide. Br Med J II:821–823

Bruce-Chwatt LJ (1980) Essential malariology. Heinemann, London

Carrington HC, Crowther AF, Davey DG, Levi AA, Rose FL (1951) A metabolite of "Paludrine" with high antimalarial activity. Nature 168:1080

Cavallito JC, Nichol CA, Brenckman WD, Deangelis RL, Stickney DR, Simmons WS, Sigal CW (1978) Lipid-soluble inhibitors of dihydrofolate reductase. 1. Kinetics, tissue distribution, and extent of metabolism of pyrimethamine, metoprine, and etoprine in the rat, dog, and man. Drug Metab Dispos 6:329–337

Charles LJ, Van der Kaay HJ, Vincke IH, Brady J (1962) The appearance of pyrimethamine resistance in *P. falciparum* following self-medication by a rural community in Ghana. Bull WHO 26:103–108

Chin W, Contacos PG, Coatney GR, King HK (1966) The evaluation of sufonamides, alone or in combination with pyrimethamine, in the treatment of multi-resistant falciparum malaria. Am J Trop Med Hyg 15:823–829

Coatney GR, Myatt AV, Hernandez T, Jeffery GM, Cooper WC (1953) Studies in human malaria. XXXII. The protective and therapeutic effects of pyrimethamine (Daraprim) against Chesson strain *vivax* malaria. Am J Trop Med Hyg 2:777–787

Covell G, Coatney GR, Field JW, Singh J (1955) Chemotherapy of malaria. WHO Monogr Ser 27

Covell G, Shute PG, Maryon M (1953a) Pyrimethamine ("daraprim") as a prophylactic agent against a West African strain of *P. falciparum*. Br Med J I:1081–1083

Covell G, Shute PG, Maryon M (1953b) Pyrimethamine ("daraprim") in the treatment of vivax malaria. Br Med J II:258–259

Falco EA, Hitchings GH, Russell PB, Vanderwerff H (1949) Antimalarials as antagonists of purines and pteroylglutamic acid. Nature 164:107–108

Feldman HA (1968) Toxoplasmosis. N Engl J Med 279:1370–1375, 1431–1437

Ferone R, Roland S (1980) Dihydrofolate reductase: thymidylate synthase, a bifunctional polypeptide from *Crithidia fasciculata*. Proc Natl Acad Sci USA 77:5802–5806

Ferone R, Burchall JJ, Hitchings GH (1969) *Plasmodium berghei* dihydrofolate reductase. Mol Pharmacol 5:49–59

Foy H, Kondi A (1952) Effect of daraprim on the gametocytes of *Plasmodium falciparum*. Trans R Soc Trop Med Hyg 46:370

Goodwin LG (1952a) Daraprim – Clinical trials and pharmacology. Trans R Soc Trop Med Hyg 46:485–495

Goodwin LG (1952b) Daraprim (B.W. 50–63) – a new antimalarial. Br Med J I:732–734

Goodwin LG, Rollo IM (1955) The chemotherapy of malaria, piroplasmosis, trypanosomiasis, and leishmaniasis. In: Hutner SH, Lwoff A (eds) Biochemistry and physiology of protozoa, vol II. Academic Press, New York, pp 225–276

Greenberg J, Boyd BL, Josephson ES (1948) Synergistic effect of chloroguanide and sulfadiazine against *Plasmodium gallinaceum* in the chick. J Pharmacol Exp Ther 94:60–64

Harinasuta T, Viravan C, Reid HA (1967) Sulphormethoxine in chloroquine-resistant falciparum malaria in Thailand. Lancet I:1117–1119

Hernandez T, Myatt AV, Coatney GR, Jeffery GM (1953) Studies in human malaria. XXXIV. Acquired resistance to pyrimethamine (Daraprim) by the Chesson strain of *Plasmodium vivax*. Am J Trop Med Hyg 2:797–804

Herrero J (1967) The use of long acting sulfonamides, alone or with pyrimethamine, in malaria (with special reference to sulformetoxine). Rev Soc Bras Med Trop 1:103–106

Hill J (1963) Chemotherapy of malaria. Part 2. The antimalarial drugs. In: Schnitzer RJ, Hawking F (eds) Experimental chemotherapy, vol 1. Academic Press, New York, pp 513–601

Hitchings GH (1952) Daraprim as an antagonist of folic and folinic acids. Trans R Soc Trop Med Hyg 46:467–473

Hitchings GH (1978) The metabolism of plasmodia and the chemotherapy of malarial infections. In: Wood C (ed) Tropical medicine: from romance to reality. Academic Press, London, pp 79–97

Hughes WT, Kuhn S, Chaudhary S, Feldman S, Verzosa M, Aur RJA, Pratt C, George SL (1977) Successful chemoprophylaxis for *Pneumocystis carinii* pneumonitis. N Engl J Med 297:1419–1426

Hurly MGD (1959) Potentiation of pyrimethamine by sulphadiazine in human malaria. Trans R Soc Trop Med Hyg 53:412–413

Jensen JB, Trager W (1977) *Plasmodium falciparum* in culture: Use of outdated erythrocytes and description of the candle jar method. J Parasitol 63:883–886

Larter WE, Sieber OF, Corrigan JJ (1978) Trimethoprim-sulfamethoxozole treatment of *Pneumocystis carinii* pneumonitis. J Pediatr 92:826–828

Lucas AO, Hendrickse RG, Okubadejo OA, Richards WHG, Neal RA, Kofie BAK (1969) The suppression of malarial parasitaemia by pyrimethamine in combination with dapsone or sulphormethoxine. Trans R Soc Trop Med Hyg 63:216–229

Negulici E, Constantinesco P, Teriteanu E, Cortez P, Cristesco A, Sandesco I (1960) L'action sporontocide et clino-prophylactique de la pyraméthamine simple ou associée à la chloroquine. Arch Roum Pathol Exp Microbiol 19:303–316

Peters W (1970) Chemotherapy and drug resistance in malaria. Academic Press, New York

Rollo IM (1952) Daraprim-experimental chemotherapy. Trans R Soc Trop Med Hyg 46:474–484

Rollo IM (1955) The mode of action of sulphonamides, proguanil and pyrimethamine on *Plasmodium gallinacium*. Br J Pharmacol 10:208–214

Rollo IM (1980) Drugs used in the chemotherapy of malaria. In: Gilman AG, Goodman LS, Gilman A (eds) The pharmacological basis of chemotherapy, 6th edn. Macmillan, New York, pp 1038–1060

Sherman IW (1979) Biochemistry of *Plasmodium* (malarial parasites). Microbiol Rev 43:453–495

Shute PG, Maryon M (1954) The effect of pyrimethamine (daraprim) on the gametocytes and oocysts of *Plasmodium falciparum* and *Plasmodium vivax*. Trans R Soc Trop Med Hyg 48:50–63

Smith CC, Ihrig J (1959) Persistent excretion of pyrimethamine following oral administration. Am J Trop Meg Hyg 8:60–62

Thompson PE, Werbel LM (1972) Antimalarial agents, chemistry and pharmacology. Medicinal chemistry, vol 12. Academic Press, New York

Verdrager J, Riche A, Chheang CM (1968) Action de l'association diaphenylsulfone-pyriméthamine sur le paludisme à *Plasmodium falciparum* au Cambodge. WHO/Mal/68.664

Vincke I, Lips M (1952) Note sur la prophylaxic médicamenteuse par daraprim en mileau rural. Ann Ist Med Trop 9:563–569

CHAPTER 14

Pediatric Uses of Sulfonamides, Trimethoprim, and the Combination

L.T. GUTMAN and C.M. WILFERT

A. Introduction

The subjects of this chapter include the major infectious diseases for which sulfon-amides, trimethoprim, or the combination have a major role in the treatment of children with infectious diseases. Although many of these topics will have been discussed in other chapters, their special uses in children are emphasized here.

B. Hemophilus influenzae Infections

Hemophilus influenzae represents a major pathogen which has a particular predilection for young children and infants. These organisms inhabit the respiratory tract which probably serves as the portal of entry for subsequent infection. In the vast majority of instances, invasive disease with bacteremia and secondary spread of infection to additional tissues is caused by strains which are encapsulated with type b polyribosephosphate, i.e., *H. influenzae* b (TODD and BRUHN 1975). Thus, almost all cases of bacteremia, meningitis, epiglottitis, pericarditis, cellulitis, arthritis, and pneumonia/empyema are caused by type b organisms. In contrast, many strains colonizing the respiratory tract are nonencapsulated and therefore nontypeable. These strains are frequently observed in otitis media.

Meningitis is the most common as well as the most severe consequence of *H. influenzae* b dissemination; the mortality rate has remained at 2%–10% in spite of currently optimal use of supportive measures and antimicrobial therapy. The peak incidence is in children who are between 3 months and 2 years of age (DAJANI et al. 1979), but a substantial proportion of cases occurs in infants ages 2–6 years; there is a 1 in 193 chance of contracting the disease by the age of 5 years (TARR and PETER 1978).

Ampicillin was the standard form of antimicrobial therapy for children with suspected systemic disease due to *H. influenzae* through the middle of the 1970s. Studies of the ampicillin sensitivity of *H. influenzae* b strains had demonstrated that the minimum inhibitory and minimum bactericidal concentrations (MIC and MBC) to ampicillin were usually less than 0.25 µg/ml. Ampicillin-resistant *H. influenzae* b meningitis was recognized in 1973 (W. THOMAS et al. 1974). Subsequent reports quickly established that this was occurring sporadically in many parts of the United States and other areas of the world (SCHIEFELE 1979). Subsequent studies have indicated a similar incidence of ampicillin resistance among type b and non-b *H. influenzae*. Similarly, resistance is comparable among those strains which are carried in the respiratory tract and those isolated from blood, spinal fluid, or other systemic sites (KIRVEN and THORNSBERRY 1978; PELTON et al. 1977).

Surveys in Alabama and Boston show a progressively increasing incidence of ampicillin resistance from 1970 to 1977. Ampicillin resistance of *H. influenzae* isolated from the middle ear increased from 1.4% to 13.6% in Alabama and from 5.3% to 15.6% in Boston in the years 1975–1977 (Syriopoulou et al. 1976, 1978). It is currently appreciated that there are substantial differences in reported rates of ampicillin resistance by geographic location within the United States. Infections due to *H. influenzae* in which there is a mixed population of ampicillin-sensitive and ampicillin-resistant strains have been reported (Albritton et al. 1977; Jubelirer and Yeager 1979). Ampicillin resistance is analogous to that of Enterobacteriaceae and has usually been conferred by a plasmid carrying the information for penicillinase production (Elwell et al. 1975). The problem of ampicillin resistance has stimulated a reassessment of appropriate therapy for the pediatric infections which are commonly caused by *Hemophilus* species. A role for TMP/SMX has emerged as current antimicrobial therapy for some of these infections.

I. Otitis Media

1. Acute

H. influenzae causes approximately 15%–25% of all cases of acute otitis media and is second only to *Streptococcus pneumoniae*. *H. influenzae* is more frequently isolated from younger, rather than older children. A minority (approximately 10%) of strains of *H. influenzae* isolated from middle ear aspirates are type b. Local disease due to nonencapsulated *H. influenzae* may lead to the familiar sequelae of relative or absolute deafness, chronic otitis media, serous otitis media, and mastoiditis. In addition, those children whose otitis media is due to encapsulated strains (type b) are at high risk for septicemia and/or meningitis.

Effective therapy for this infection must take into consideration the possibility of ampicillin-resistant *H. influenzae* strains as etiologic agents of acute otitis media. Laboratory studies of *H. influenzae* have indicated that most strains are sensitive to inhibition by trimethoprim/sulfamethoxazole (TMP/SMX), including type b organisms, nontypeable strains, penicillinase-producing strains, and non-penicillinase-producing strains. It has also been established that the distribution of both TMP and SMX to middle ear fluid is excellent (Klimek et al. 1980). TMP/SMX is equivalent to ampicillin in the therapy of acute otitis media due to *H. influenzae* (Shurin et al. 1976; Willner et al. 1977). Studies of penicillinase-producing *Hemophilus* infections of the middle ear have documented the failure of ampicillin therapy (Crosson et al. 1976; Shurin et al. 1976, 1980) and the efficacy of TMP/SMX (Schwartz et al. 1978, 1979; Rodriguez et al. 1978). Schwartz et al. (1980) reported the results of therapy with TMP/SMX of 16 children with acute otitis media due to ampicillin-resistant *H. influenzae*. Of the 16 children, 14 had failed a course of ampicillin therapy; 15 made a prompt recovery with TMP/SMX therapy, and there were no recurrences of otitis media within 1 month of therapy. TMP/SMX, therefore, should be one accepted approach to initial therapy of children with acute otitis media and may be preferred to ampicillin in areas where penicillinase-producing strains are common, or after a treatment failure has occurred. It is important to recognize that group A streptococcal pharyngitis is not successfully treated with TMP/SMX (Trickett et al. 1973). Therefore, children known or suspected to have group A streptococcal pharyngitis should receive another antimicrobial agent.

2. Serous and Chronic

Persistence of a middle ear effusion is a common sequel of acute otitis media. This is more frequently observed in infants less than 2 years of age. At the present time, it is not known whether the persistence of effusion relates to the frequency of viral respiratory tract infections, to the failure of the young infant to develop an appropriate immune response to the infecting pathogen, or to an abnormal function of the eustachian tube. The presence of effusion is not synonymous with failure to eradicate bacteria from the middle ear. Persistent effusions may relate to the subsequent high frequency of recurrent otitis media which affects some children (Shurin et al. 1979).

Studies of persistent middle ear effusions have demonstrated the presence of aerobic bacteria in as many as one-half of the children (Healy and Teele 1977). The presence of these organisms suggests they may be playing a role in the pathogenesis of serous and mucoid otitis media, which would provide a nidus for recolonization after the discontinuance of antimicrobial therapy for each acute episode. The organisms present in the middle ear are similar to those observed in acute otitis media. If chronic purulent otitis media is present or tympanic membrane perforation has occurred, a broader spectrum of microorganisms including staphylococcal species, *Neisseria catarrhalis*, and diphtheroids may be present.

These observations have stimulated initial studies of the prevention of recurrent otitis media by antimicrobial agents, and there are several studies indicating that antimicrobial prophylaxis may be effective. In 1974, Perrin et al. reported experience with a placebo-controlled crossover study of sulfisoxazole for 54 children who had had multiple episodes of otitis media during the previous year. The attack rate, in a 6-month period, was 1.05 for children in the placebo phase of the study, and 0.15 for children in the sulfisoxazole phase of the study. The results were most significant for the children in the younger age ranges. A subsequent study (Biedel 1978) described a similar decrease in incidence of otitis media in children who were treated with a sulfonamide, rather than a decongestant, when upper respiratory infections occurred after a previously documented episode of otitis media. Studies of the efficacy of TMP/SMX, of the influence of prior history of otitis media on response to preventive therapy, and of the influence of age on response to preventive therapy, are pending. The problems of treating persistent effusion and infection or recurrent/chronic otitis media in children are unresolved and require further evaluation.

II. Sinusitis

The diagnosis of sinusitis in childhood is especially imprecise. The sinuses may develop asymmetrically in normal children and roentgenographic evidence of opacification may represent mucosal thickening, purulent accumulation, or tears. Systemic findings, such as fever, bacteremia, leukocytosis, or elevated erythrocyte sedimentation rate, may or may not be present. The use of newer radiologic methods, such as radionucleotide scans or computerized assisted tomography have not yet been evaluated for their possible contribution in the diagnosis of sinus diseases in children.

The bacterial etiology of acute sinusitis in children seems to parallel that of other respiratory tract infections. Sinusitis or mastoiditis as an accompaniment to otitis media was frequent and the etiology was similar to that observed in acute otitis media (Hoshaw and Nickman 1974). A recent study of acute maxillary sinusitis in children (Wald et al. 1981) included maxillary sinus aspirate; bacteria in concentrations of greater than 10^4 organisms/ml were recovered from 77% of the children. The majority of the children had a single bacterial organism present and most of the bacterial species recovered were *Streptococcus* spp., *H. influenzae*, and *Neisseria* spp. There was very poor correlation between the organisms recovered from either the nasopharynx or throat culture and those present in the sinuses. In contrast to the findings in adult patients, no anaerobic bacteria were detected in the children with acute maxillary sinusitis.

These infections may have severe complications. One of the more commonly recognized is periorbital cellulitis or orbital cellulitis. Perinasal sinusitis, especially of the ethmoid, is the common setting in which this occurs (Watters et al. 1976). *H. influenzae* is the most prominent isolate, especially in children under the age of 3 years (Smith et al. 1978). Orbital cellulitis is usually a manifestation of sinus disease of children under 6 years of age (Gellady et al. 1978).

The efficacy of therapy with various antimicrobial agents has been difficult to evaluate because of the spectrum of responsible pathogens. A study of both adults and children has indicated that persistence of bacteria in sinus washings may correlate with poor healing or protracted illness (Nylen et al. 1972). Data derived from adults indicate overall equivalence of efficacy of ampicillin, amoxicillin, and TMP/SMX (Hamory et al. 1979).

It is the opinion of the authors that sinusitis in children under the age of 6 years should be treated with a regimen which is satisfactory for the eradication of *H. influenzae*. If the child is not apparently bacteremic, and does not have a major complication of sinusitis, TMP/SMX appears to be satisfactory. In instances of severe disease, chloramphenicol remains a part of the suggested regimen. Children with major complications of sinusitis may have osteomyelitis of the involved areas, and courses of therapy which are 2–3 weeks in duration may be necessary to prevent recurrence.

III. Prophylaxis to Prevent Secondary Infection

A subject of recent intense concern is the prevention of spread of bacteremic *H. influenzae* disease to intimate contacts within households or day-care centers. Tejani et al. (1977) reviewed 18 families in which multiple cases of systemic *H. influenzae* b infection had occurred. The majority of secondary cases occur within 5–7 days of recognition of the index case. Additional studies have further defined the high risk for the youngest household contacts; Filice et al. (1978) found that the rate of secondary disease in household contacts who were less than 4 years of age was 4.9%. It has also become apparent that other situations where intimate contact occurs among young children, for example, day-care centers, nursery schools, and chronic-care facilities, are settings in which multiple cases of systemic infection may occur. It is now appreciated that colonization of the nasopharynx with *H. influenzae* b is common in the members of a household in which a case has occurred, and is most prevalent in the youngest children (MICHAELIS and NORDEN 1977). Similarly, there is a relatively high rate of colonization of the nasopharynx in other children at day-care centers in which multiple cases have occurred (GRANOFF et al. 1979). This is in contrast to the colonization rates of normal populations of children, where the prevalence of *H. influenzae* b is quite low, possibly 2% (LERMAN et al. 1979).

There have been several approaches to attempts to eradicate nasopharyngeal colonization since high colonization rates and increased risk of systemic disease in young close contacts was first recognized to be a problem. The primary goal of antimicrobial prophylaxis is to prevent invasive infection, for which eradication of the carrier state must be reliably achieved in the majority of young children, and any drug selected for such prophylaxis must be safely administered with minimal side effects. Several clinical studies of totally different design have been independently reported in attempts to assess the efficacy of erythromycin and/or sulfonamide, cefaclor, ampicillin, TMP/SMX, and rifampin. Several studies indicate that approximately 25% of children will spontaneously cease carrying *H. influenzae* b organisms. There are too few data to form firm conclusions, but cefaclor, erythromycin/sulfonamide, and ampicillin would not appear to be reliably active in eradication of the carrier state.

Several different trials with TMP/SMX have been recorded in the day-care or chronic-care facility setting. Four cases of *H. influenzae* b disease were recognized over a 5-week period among 48 children in one day-care center. One-half of these children were colonized with *H. influenzae* b. A 4-day course of TMP/SMX was administered and subsequently all children were free of colonization (MELISH et al. 1976). No additional infection occurred in the next 2 months. The second trial, in a chronic care facility where 73%–100% of the patients were colonized with *H. influenzae* b, was reported by YOGEV in 1978. Treatment with TMP/SMX for 5 days resulted in 77% eradication of ampicillin-sensitive strains, but a failure of eradication of the eight persons who harbored ampicillin-resistant strains. Further study demonstrated that successful eradication of nasopharyngeal colonization by *H. influenzae* b with TMP/SMX was correlated with a sensitivity of the organism to TMP which was less than 0.5 µg/ml for bactericidal effect. This did not correlate with ampicillin sensitivity of the same strains (KIRVEN and THORNSBERRY 1978). One additional reported experience of a randomized crossover study comparing the efficacy of TMP/SMX with rifampin describes the results in 31 colonized children in a day-care setting. SUMAYA et al. (1980) reported that TMP/SMX successfully eradicated the carrier state in 12 of 14 children, whereas only 8 of 17 children were successfully treated with rifampin. It is probable that poor compliance and problems with dosing were responsible for the rifampin failures in the youngest children. Those youngsters who continued to be colonized were then treated with TMP/SMX and the carrier state was successfully eradicated.

Rifampin has been reported (GRANOFF et al. 1979) to eradicate carriage of *H. influenzae* b. Other reports indicate poor efficacy, especially in the young (GLO-

DE et al. 1981). It would appear that a dosage of 20 mg/kg more reliably achieves eradication of the carrier state than a dosage of 10 mg/kg/day. The Center for Disease Control is presently conducting a randomized placebo versus rifampin study to evaluate eradication of carriage and prevention of subsequent disease. The optimal form of chemoprophylaxis remains unknown at this time. Unfortunately, successful prophylaxis of all recognized contacts of systemic *Hemophilus* infection would prevent several hundred cases of disease each year, a relatively small fraction of the total number of cases of the disease occurring annually.

C. Meningitis

The most common agents of bacterial meningitis, *Streptococcus pneumoniae, Hemophilus influenzae*, and *Neisseria meningitidis*, all enjoy widely accepted regimens with which rapid sterilization of the infected sites is almost universally achieved. For this reason there has been marginal interest in developing experience with the use of other agents. Consequently, very little information exists concerning the use of TMP/SMX for the treatment of bacterial meningitis or the application of TMP/SMX in studies employing animal models of bacterial meningitis. In addition, TMP/SMX has only recently generally been generally available intravenously, and in the United States until this year was available for children only on study protocols. Nevertheless, it is worthwhile to discuss the potential use of this drug in meningitis.

Studies have indicated that both TMP and SMX achieve therapeutic levels in the cerebrospinal fluid (CSF) in the presence or absence of meningeal inflamation. After oral administration of drug, a peak CSF concentration of 13%–20% of the serum level of SMX is achieved after 6–8 h (BOGER and GAVIN 1960; SVEDHEM and IWARSON 1979). Parenteral administration of TMP at a dosage of 4 mg/kg demonstrated CSF concentrations that were 30%–40% of that of the corresponding serum concentration from 2–12 h after administration of the drug. One-half of the children receiving the drug had meningitis or encephalitis and one-half had no evidence of inflammatory process (FRIES et al. 1975).

Most preliminary clinical experiences with the use of TMP/SMX have been gained in three situations: infants with neonatal meningitis due to gram-negative enteric rods, children with infected ventricular shunts, and persons with *Salmonella* spp. meningitis. Results of therapy of the few patients with neonatal enteric meningitis appear to be comparable to those obtained with other forms of therapy. SABEL (1976) reported five children with *Escherichia coli*, one in combination with *Klebsiella*, meningitis. Several of the children had complicating factors such as myelomeningocele, infected shunt, renal failure, and primary immunologic deficiency. All had prompt sterilization of the CSF during therapy, although one had a recurrence. Another study of the use of intravenous TMP/SMX by ARDATI et al (1979) included two children with neonatal enteric meningitis with ventriculitis. Both children had a very delayed response to TMP/SMX as well as to other antimicrobial therapy, with persistently positive ventricular fluid or recurrent disease. Therefore, although therapy with TMP/SMX of neonatal enteric meningitis may be promptly efficacious (MORZARIA et al. 1969), delayed response and relapses are common, as is true with other therapeutic agents.

Staphylococcus epidermidis is the most frequentcause of infection in intraventricular shunts, and various forms of antimicrobial therapy with and without surgical removal of the shunt have been advocated. Two reports (ARDATI et al. 1979; SABEL 1976) have noted that TMP/SMX was efficacious in sterilizing the CSF in all of five instances. However, obstruction of the shunt and recurrent infections resulted in shunt removal in most instances. Thus, it is anticipated that TMP/SMX may be another antimicrobial agent which may be selected if the organism is sensitive in vitro, and will usually be used in conjunction with surgical removal of the shunt. Finally, *Salmonella* meningitis is a condition for which therapy is notoriously variable in efficacy, especially in the very young children who comprise the majority of cases (RABINOWITZ and MACLEON 1972). Reports of successful therapy with TMP/SMX following failures with other regimens suggest that this approach should receive increased attention (BRIGGS and ROBINSON 1975).

D. Urinary Tract Infections

I. Acute

TMP/SMX is an approved drug for the therapy of urinary tract infections (UTI) due to susceptible organisms. In the treatment of acute uncomplicated UTI of childhood, it has been shown to be as effective as ampicillin (ELLERSTEIN et al. 1977), and sulfamethoxazole (HOWARD and HOWARD 1978; FELDMAN et al. 1975). In the study of HOWARD et al., 61 children received TMP/SMX and 57 SMX alone. Cure, with all follow-up cultures negative, was achieved for 87% of both groups, and recurrence or reinfection were also similar for both treatment groups. *E. coli* were the predominant isolates, and in this study, recurrences were usually associated with the presence of anatomic or functional abnormalities. In the study of FELDMAN et al., recurrences within 3 months of therapy were significantly less common in children who had received TMP/SMX than in those who received SMX alone.

II. Structural Defects of the Urinary System

Several studies have substantiated the efficacy of TMP/SMX in children with structurally abnormal urinary tracts. BÖSE et al. (1974) reported the results of treatment with TMP/SMX compared with ampicillin. Of 20 such children treated with ampicillin, 9 had recurrences during therapy or within 4 days of the end of therapy compared with 3 of 36 children treated with TMP/SMX. Another study (M. THOMAS and HOPKINS 1972), which included 47 children with spina bifida cystica, found that TMP/SMX was more effective than cephalexin for a 2-week course of therapy.

III. Prevention

Efforts to prevent recurrences of UTI in children who have experienced frequent infections or who have structural defects which predispose to recurrent disease have included continuous medication for prolonged periods of time. Such an approach has been explored in adults, and experience with children has been accumulating since the early 1970s (Hobday 1971). Some studies have not included a comparative medication. For example, Zoethout (1973) reported the results of 42 children who received TMP/SMX for between 3 and 21 months. Of the 33 who had had an initially infected urine, 30 became sterile and remained so throughout the study. Smellie et al. (1976) reported the experience with 130 children treated continuously for 6 months to 6 years, and found 6 recurrences during this period. *Streptococcus faecalis (faecium)* was the predominant organism in the recurrences, an experience shared by others. Similarly, Forbes and Drummond (1973) reported on the results of prolonged therapy with TMP/SMX in 51 children with recurrent UTI. A sterile urine was maintained during therapy in 42 of these patients, but recurrences shortly after discontinuation of therapy were common.

Two studies have compared prophylaxis with TMP/SMX and another drug. Sher (1975) described ten children with recurrent UTI, five of whom received a variety of medications (ampicillin, nitrofurantoin, sulfisoxazole) and had had recurrences. Five additional children who received TMP/SMX were free of recurrences during therapy for 5–7 months. Second, Lines (1973) reported a double-blind study of SMX versus TMP/SMX for a 6-month course of prophylaxis of 36 patients with recurrent disease. Of the children receiving TMP/SMX, 63% were free of recurrences, as were 42% of children who received SMX, results which were not statistically significantly different.

IV. Therapy of Periurethral and Rectal Flora

Studies of the effect of TMP/SMX on periurethral and rectal flora have primarily involved adult women with recurrent UTI, in whom persistence of periurethral colonization is often associated with recurrent infections. A recent study by Sullivan et al. (1980) has demonstrated that therapy of female children with TMP/SMX leads to the eradication of periurethral colonization in most cases, which was not the case with ampicillin therapy. Rectal flora, similarly, show a dramatic decline in the density of aerobic organisms (Grüneberg et al. 1976), and the proportion of rectal organisms which were resistant to TMP or SMX did not rise. These results resemble those obtained in studies of adult patients. To the present time, the development of TMP/SMX-resistant enteric anaerobic flora, even during prolonged therapy, is a rare event. In summary, TMP/SMX is an effective antimicrobial agent in the therapy of urinary tract infections of children; its efficacy as a continuous prophylactic medication has been shown to be at least as good as ampicillin and cephalosporins.

V. Chlamydial Infections

Chlamydia are bacteria which are obligate intracellular parasites. They form cytoplasmic inclusions in affected cell cultures, and for many decades were erroneously thought to be viruses. Recent advances in diagnostic techniques have brought a rapid increase in understanding of the epidemiology, bacteriology, and clinical characteristics of these infections. There are two species of the genus *Chlamydia*,

C. trachomatis, and *C. psittaci*. *C. trachomatis* has been the subject of the majority of recent research on chlamydial infections. Newer laboratory methods have included tissue culture isolation techniques, typing of strains by microimmunofluorescent methods, and determination of antibody response to infection (SCHACHTER 1978).

The majority of children with recognized disease caused by *C. trachomatis* have inclusion conjunctivitis or pneumonitis. Inclusion conjunctivitis (IC) is an infection of the eye or other site of the newborn (SCHACHTER et al. 1979) which is usually acquired during passage through a birth canal which is infected with *C. trachomatis*. There is no evidence that silver nitrate drops prevent IC (SCHACHTER et al. 1979), and an infected infant will develop an acute unilateral or bilateral conjunctivitis. Strains of *C. trachomatis* which cause IC are strains which also cause genital disease in adults. IC resembles ocular trachoma in its acute phase. Although many children will eventually recover without compromise to their vision, the disease often runs a course which is weeks to months in length. Furthermore, severe disease with micropannus formation and conjunctival scarring may occur (MORDHORST 1967). Antimicrobial therapy of the disease, especially if instituted within the first 2 weeks of life, may prevent most of these sequelae (MORDHORST and DAWSON 1971). Systemic therapy is recommended, since infection may persist for long periods of time in children receiving only local antimicrobial agents to the eyes (ROWE et al. 1979). In addition, colonization of multiple anatomic sites is usual in children with conjunctival infections (SCHACHTER et al. 1979). Not only is the respiratory tract colonized (BEEM and SAXON 1977) but also the rectum and vagina.

The second major disease manifested by children and commonly caused by *C. trachomatis* is pneumonitis. It is primarily a disease of infancy, with the majority of affected babies being between 3 weeks and 4 months of age when they first come for medical attention. Distinguishing characteristics of infants with chlamydia pneumonia include roetgeongraphic findings of hyperinflation, prolonged cough and congestion, tachypnea, elevated serum IgG and IgA concentration, eosinophilia, lack of systemic response, the presence of conjunctivitis, and ear abnormalities (BEEM and SAXON 1977; HARRISON et al. 1978; TIPPLE et al. 1979). The infants characteristically have very high titers of specific antibody to the infecting strain of *C. trachomatis*. Approximately 50% of infants who are born to mothers who are genitally colonized by *C. trachomatis* acquire conjunctivitis or nasopharyngeal colonization, but not all of these children will develop pneumonitis (HAMMERSCHLAG et al. 1979). However, chlamydial pneumonia represents a very significant proportion of infants who are less than 3 months of age and are hospitalized for pneumonitis. HARRISON et al. (1978) found that in 13 of 21 (62%) infants with pneumonitis, chlamydia were implicated and BEEM et al. (1979) found that this infection accounted for 74% of infants admitted for afebrile pneumonia. The disease is responsible for significant morbidity, and deaths have occurred. In addition to the illnesses already mentioned, there is evidence that chlamydia may be associated with middle ear infection in infancy (TIPPLE et al. 1979), although not in older children (HAMMERSCHLAG et al. 1980). Gastrointestinal abnormalities of infants are also being studied for the possibility that chlamydia may play a role.

The susceptibility of *C. trachomatis* to TMP and SMX has been studied. Current data support the early observations that these organisms are inhibited by sulfonamides (BLACKMAN et al. 1977). A comparison of the efficacy of TMP, SMX, and TMP/SMX has shown that the large majority of the efficacy of TMP/SMX is attributable to SMX (JOHANNISSON et al. 1979). The MIC to TMP was > 100 µg/ml, to SMX was 50 µg/ml, and to TMP/SMX was 25 µg/ml. The authors concluded that synergism was not pronounced. Most studies of the treatment of *C. trachomatis* infections in children have been with a sulfonamide, rather than TMP/SMX in combination. The MIC of *C. trachomatis* to erythromycin is usually 1.0 µg/ml. The drug is well tolerated and usually safe in young children. Unfortunately, there has been a recent report of more resistant *C. trachomatis* isolates with MICs above 1 µg/ml (MOURAD et al. 1980).

Therapy of chlamydial pneumonia has utilized a sulfonamide or erythromycin, and a recent report enlarges this clinical experience. A total of 21 infants were treated with sulfisoxazole (150 mg/kg/d) and 11 infants were treated with erythromycin ethylsuccinate (40 mg/kg/d) for 10–21 days. Both regimens resulted in prompt cessation of shedding of organisms. The treatment regimens were equivalent when compared for the length of therapy before clinical improvement was apparent: 5–6 days, with a range of 2–10 days. Infants who had been ill longer did not respond more rapidly, indicating that spontaneous improvement was not a major factor. The authors concluded that the two regimens were equivalent, and that therapy had been beneficial (BEEM et al. 1979). There are other antimicrobial agents to which *C. trachomatis* isolates are sensitive. Tetracycline is effective, with an MIC of 1.0 µg/ml. However, tetracycline is usually avoided in the therapy of infections in young children. Rifampin has an MIC of 0.25 µg/ml (BLACKMAN et al. 1977). There has been, however, little clinical experience in the use of this drug for therapy of *C. trachomatis* infections.

E. Pneumocystis carinii Pneumonia

I. Therapy

Pneumocystis carinii is a protozoan which occurs as a common but largely asymptomatic infestation of humans as well as other animals. In humans, the disease first achieved clinical importance as an infection of the lungs of sickly or premature children in nurseries in Eastern Europe after World War II (GAJDUSEK 1957). It was then recognized to be a sporadic disease with a low incidence in various populations. In children, it was appreciated that frequently associated conditions were debilitation and protein/calorie malnutrition (HUGHES et al. 1974a). Most recently studies have identified *P. carinii* to be responsible for 14% of acute pneumonia which results in hospitalization of infants less than 3 months of age (STAGNO et al. 1980). The diagnosis was made by counter-immunoelectrophoresis (CIE) detection of circulating antigen. These immunocompetent infants have disease which clinically resembles *C. trachomatis* pneumonia of infancy.

Increased interest in *P. carinii* pneumonia has been the result of the recognition that the disease has become a major cause of illness and death in children and adults who are severely immunocompromized (HUGHES et al. 1973). Children with congenital syndromes which compromise the integrity of cell-mediated immunity, and children undergoing chemotherapy for malignancies, have suffered an increasing incidence of *P. carinii* pneumonia (PCP). PCP has occurred at the highest rates in children with most intensive courses of chemotherapy (CHUSID and HEYRMAN 1978). Rates of 3%–6% pertained for children with malignancies in 1970–1971 (HUGHES et al. 1973), but had increased to over 35% by 1975 in children with particularly intensive chemotherapy (HUGHES et al. 1975 b).

Diagnosis of *P. carinii* infection has undergone extensive evolution since effective therapy first became available. A definitive diagnosis may be made only by demonstration of the organisms from lung tissue or bronchial material. Open surgical biopsy has been recommended as most satisfactory. Other methods have included the endobronchial brush biopsy, transbronchial biopsy, and percutaneous lung biopsy. The organisms are then identified by methenamine–silver and/or toluidine blue stains. The organism has been propagated in the laboratory in several cell lines, including Vero cells and chick embryo epithelial lung cell cultures. These methods are not yet successful for isolation of organisms from clinical specimens and are not widely available.

Serologic methods of diagnosis are improving. It has recently been demonstrated that CIE and indirect immunofluorescence will detect *P. carinii* antigen and antibody to *P. carinii* cysts respectively (PIFER et al. 1978). By these methods, it has been shown that by the age of 4 years, the majority of children are antibody positive, indicating widespread subclinical infection. Antigenemia was found in 95% of children with tissue-proven PCP and in 15% of children with cancer without pneumonitis. Antigenemia was not detected in 120 normal children. Additional data are being developed with suggest that antigen detection will allow an adequate diagnosis without direct demonstration of organisms in tissue.

Therapy for PCP has been with three regimens: (a) pentamidine isothionate; (b) pyrimethamine/sulfadiazine; and (c) TMP/SMX. The toxicity of pentamidine isothionate has led to infrequent use of the drug. Steroid treatment of normal rats produces spontaneous infection and a model of PCP which has been widely used to study the efficacy of therapeutic regimens (HUGHES 1974 a). The rat model studies have indicated that both pyrimethamine/sulfadiazine and TMP/SMX regimens were equally or more effective than pentamidine (HUGHES et al. 1974 b).

Clinical studies have indicated that TMP/SMX is usually effective in the therapy of *P. carinii* of children (LARTER et al. 1978; HUGHES et al. 1975 a). The studies were extended when a crossover, randomized study of 50 patients with PCP was completed which compared TMP/SMX with pentamidine (HUGHES et al. 1978). The dose of TMP was 20 mg/kg/d and SMX was 200 mg/kg/d for 14 days; 17 of 25 TMP/SMX patients and 14 of 24 pentamidine-treated patients recovered without crossover therapy. Thus, it was demonstrated that TMP/SMX was at least as effective as pentamidine, and adverse reactions were minimal. Additional review of the therapy indicates that the response of children to therapy with TMP/SMX is as good as the response of adults (WINSTON et al. 1980).

II. Prevention

Successful therapy of PCP with a nontoxic drug, coupled with the rising incidence of this infection led directly to efforts to prevent the occurrence of symptomatic disease with this organism. Initial prophylactic regimens included short-term therapy with standard doses of TMP/SMX during the initial period of antitumor chemotherapy. Experience with this approach has shown the PCP may be delayed in onset, but later appears in a fully invasive form after the prophylactic therapy has been discontinued (WOLFF and BAEHNER 1978). Animal studies have also confirmed that TMP/SMX prevents development of disease in experimental studies of rats, but animals receiving steroids have emergence of disease following discontinuance of the antimicrobial therapy (HUGHES 1979). Accordingly, a randomized double-blind, placebo-controlled trial of 160 patients at high risk of PCP was reported in 1977. TMP/SMX was given in doses of 150 mg/day TMP + 750 mg/day with a maximum of 320 mg day/TMP. Children received continuous therapy for as long as 2 years (HUGHES et al. 1977). Results of the study showed that 21% of the 80 patients in a placebo-treated group developed PCP, whereas none of the 80 patients in the TMP/SMX-treated group developed PCP ($P < 0.01$). Of unexpected, but equal importance was the observed decrease in acute bacterial infections in the TMP/SMX-treated group, especially bacterial sepsis, otitis media, pneumonia, sinusitis, and cellulitis. However, the TMP/SMX-treated group had a greater incidence of oral candidiasis and the possibility of a higher rate of systemic candidiasis. Two additional published reports have recorded the use of TMP/SMX for prophylaxis of PCP. A review of the results of the use of TMP/SMX in 229 children deemed to be at high risk of developing PCP showed that none of these children developed the disease, while 5 of 10 high risk children not on preventive therapy contracted PCP (HARRIS et al. 1980). The second report, covering a 3-year study period, observed 786 patients who were assessed by the attending oncologist to be at risk of PCP. None of the 786 patients receiving TMP/SMX developed PCP, but 43 (5.5%) developed an adverse reaction (WILBER et al. 1980). In summary, TMP/SMX has been demonstrated to be efficacious in the therapy of PCP and to serve as the best available prophylactic measure to prevent this infection in immunocompromised children. (See also Chap. 20.)

F. Enteric Diseases

I. Salmonellosis

The vast majority of infections due to *Salmonella* species in the United States are non-typhoidal enteric infections. Resolution of clinical symptoms of this condition is not enhanced by therapy with ampicillin or chloramphenicol and prolongation of fecal excretion of *Salmonella* occurs following therapy as compared with untreated patients (KAZEMI et al. 1973). Uncomplicated *Salmonella* enteritis, therefore, is best treated symptomatically and without antimicrobial therapy. Treatment of complicated or systemic non-typhoidal *Salmonella* infections of children has not received extensive clinical study. The clinical settings where these are more likely to occur include infancy, old age, patients with malignancy, sickle cell disease, or chronic granulomatous disease. In these circumstances, the extensive clinical experiences in the treatment of *Salmonella typhi* have been extrapolated and applied.

Until approximately 1970, chloramphenicol was almost universally recognized to be the drug of choice for therapy of typhoid fever. During the early 1970 s, chloramphenicol-resistant strains of *S. typhi* emerged in several areas of the world, especially in Mexico and the Far East. During the Mexican epidemic of 1972–1973 occasional strains were also ampicillin resistant, creating an impetus for the development of alternative therapy. For reasons that are not understood, there has been a marked subsequent decline in the prevalence of these strains, and currently most Mexican strains are again chloramphenicol sensitive. In the United States, chloramphenicol-resistant *Salmonella* strains were rare between 1968 and 1975, with a rate of approximately 0.001% (CHERUBIN et al. 1977). Between 1975 and 1976 there were 209 cases of typhoid fever in the United States reported to the Center for Disease Control. The majority were acquired within the United States, and were not associated with outbreaks. Of these strains, 95% were sensitive to ampicillin and chloramphenicol, 3% were ampicillin resistant, and 2% were chloramphenicol resistant (RYDER and BLAKE 1979). Resistance to TMP/SMX continues to be very rare (BARROS et al. 1977; SNYDER et al. 1973) in other *Salmonella* spp. as well as *S. typhi*.

Numerous studies have described the clinical response, relapse rate, and carrier rate of children and adults who are treated for typhoid fever with TMP/SMX. Although some studies indicate that a significant proportion of patients have a slow response to therapy (SCRAGG and RUBIDGE 1971) or that relapses are common (GEDDES et al. 1971; PORTNOY and SEAH 1979), other studies indicated that defervescence in patients receiving TMP/SMX was as rapid as in those receiving chloramphenicol (JONSSON 1974) and relapses were very rare (UWAYDAH et al. 1975). In addition, JONSSON (1974) demonstrated that fecal excretion was more prolonged for patients receiving chloramphenicol compared with those who received TMP/SMX. Specific studies by GILMAN et al. (1975) on the efficacy of ampicillin or TMP/SMX for therapy of patients with chloramphenicol-sensitive or chloramphenicol-resistant strains of *S. typhi* indicated that the clinical responses to either drug were comparable, regardless of the chloramphenicol sensitivity of the strain.

Medical therapy of chronic *Salmonella* carriers has a low rate of success (MUSHER and RUBENSTEIN 1973). Relapses following attempts at therapy with TMP/SMX are as common as these following other antimicrobial regimens (PICKLER et al. 1973). In summary, uncomplicated *Salmonella* infections limited to the gastrointestinal tract should receive no antimicrobial therapy. In patients requiring hospitalization, with recognized complications of infection, or in high risk situations, e.g., newborns, antimicrobial therapy is indicated. Ampicillin or TMP/SMX are the drugs of choice. In *S. typhi* infections, chloramphenicol or TMP/SMX appear to be similarly efficacious.

II. Shigellosis

In contrast to salmonellosis patients, those with shigellosis derive benefit symptomatically from treatment, and prolongation of the carrier state has not been a complication of therapy (WEISSMAN et al. 1974). Therefore, most patients have been treated when the disease is recognized and ampicillin has constituted standard therapy. However, in the past decade, ampicillin resistance has emerged as a common characteristic of all species of *Shigella* (ROSS et al. 1972; RUDOY et al. 1974).

Since virtually all strains of *Shigella* have been sensitive in vitro to TMP/SMX, experience with the use of this therapy has been generated. Patients with ampicillin-resistant and ampicillin-sensitive strains respond promptly to the use of TMP/SMX, and patients with ampicillin-sensitive strains had a response to ampicillin equivalent to TMP/SMX. Currently (NELSON et al. 1976; CHANG et al. 1977), TMP/SMX is the therapy of choice for treatment of shigellosis in areas in which ampicillin resistance occurs. Successful therapy of *Shigella* infections, clinical improvement and eradication of the organisms, has been accomplished by ampicillin and by TMP/SMX. (See also Chap. 17.)

III. Yersinia Infections

In the United States most *Yersinia* infections are due to *Yersinia enterocolitica*. This is a common pathogen, and in some areas is more common than *Shigella*. The disease is primarily sporadic, but more than one member of a family may be affected (GUTMAN et al. 1973a). The organism is moderately virulent; in a single human volunteer experiment, 3.5×10^9 organisms were required to cause intestinal disease. The organism, therefore, seldom spreads widely through a community, although large outbreaks have been reported (ASAKAWA et al. 1973).

Y. enterocolitica infection is a zoonotic disease and has been demonstrated in a rather wide variety of wildlife. The animal species with which disease is most consistently associated are pigs and dogs (WILSON et al. 1976). Both of these animals suffer disease from strains which resemble those isolated from humans, and should be considered to be possible foci during the investigation of an outbreak. Fecal-oral spread appears to be the primary method of transmission, with contamination of food a common vehicle. An increasingly common source of large outbreaks has been the contamination of milk products, with contamination during processing of containers, of chocolate additives, and of a milk separator.

In some large epidemics, the source has never been identified. In a large Japanese school epidemic, over 500 pupils were probably infected and ill, all cases occurred within a few days, and no secondary cases in family members were discovered. In contrast, person-to-person transmission in families, between visiting relatives, and within hospitals has been documented. Surveys of stool cultures of healthy adults seldom yield *Y. enterocolitica*. Infections with *Y. enterocolitica* are most commonly recognized in the younger child; a recent report from Montreal showed that of 64 cases in children under 17 years of age, 37 (58%) were 3 years of age or less (LAFLEUR et al. 1972). These 64 children had the following presentations

Acute gastroenteritis; symptoms for 7 days or less: 53%

Chronic gastroenteritis; symptoms for greater than 7 days: 33%

Abdominal pain; appendicitis: 8%

Miscellaneous; other: 6%

These data are notably different from the initial reports of the disease spectrum of this organism, which had reflected the difficulties in isolating the agent from contaminated sites, such as the feces, and therefore favored recognition of septicemic disease.

1. Acute Enteritis

Acute enteritis is the most common presentation of *Y. enterocolitica* disease in children. Most of the children with this presentation are otherwise normal, and underlying defects in host defense are rarely diagnosed. The onset of symptoms is usually rapid, with development of abdominal pain, fever, diarrhea, headache, weakness, and nausea within 1 day. Differentiation from other causes of dysentery cannot be made on clinical grounds. If there are other young children in the household, a family history will often reveal that other members are experiencing abdominal pain with or without diarrhea.

2. Chronic Enteritis

Subacute presentations with very prolonged symptoms of diarrhea are usually increasingly commonly recognized features of *Y. enterocolitica* enteritis (SCHIEVEN and RANDALL 1974). These children may be afebrile, and may not have had an acute febrile onset. The diarrhea is often mucoid, several stools a day, and abdominal pain may be intermittent, or may not occur. Mild weight loss or failure to thrive are common. The disease may present as protein-losing enteropathy with low serum albumin and peripheral edema.

3. Mesenteric Adenitis

The most commonly recognized syndrome caused by *Y. enterocolitica* in the earlier literature was acute mesenteric adenitis. This presentation includes acute abdominal pain, often localized to the right lower quadrant, fever, leukocytosis, and peritoneal irritation. Diarrhea was variable. Understandably, children were commonly believed to have acute appendicitis; at exploration, enlarged mesenteric nodes were found. There have been a number of fatalities due to *Y. enterocolitica*, and there appear to be three settings in which this occurs. Several children who were less than 2 years of age have died. At autopsy, acute peritonitis with rupture of extensive conglomerated mesenteric nodes and extensive involvement of the intestines in the region of the ileum and proximal colon have been described (BRADFORD et al. 1974). Second, children and adults with hemolytic processes or with primary diseases of the liver appear to be at greater risk of septicemia with rapid progression, secondary localization, and fatalities (RABSON et al. 1975). Finally, there is an occasional fatality in a person who is experiencing a complication of the basic enteric disease. For example, a young teenager recently died of complications of the exploratory surgery which he underwent for his acute abdominal pain.

Controlled studies of the therapy of *Y. enterocolitica* diseases have not been accomplished and so the approaches to therapy are derived from in vitro assessment of antimicrobial susceptibility and the numerous reports of results in groups of patients. As demonstrated by the frequency of chronic diarrhea as a presentation, the disease does not appear to be rapidly self-limited. Antimicrobial therapy does not appear to lengthen a carrier status, and most patients cease to harbor the organism in their stools after therapy. For these reasons, treatment of symptomatic persons is recommended. Studies by GUTMAN et al. (1973b), MAKI et al. (1980),

Hammerberg et al. (1977) have shown that all of 78 strains tested were sensitive to TMP/SMX. Individual case reports have suggested a prompt symptomatic response to TMP/SMX therapy.

G. Miscellaneous Conditions

I. Chronic Granulomatous Disease

Chronic granulomatous disease of childhood is a disease in which there is defective leukocyte-killing capability, involving infections with a group of microorganisms which are characterized by the production of peroxidase (Lazarus and Neu 1975). The exact nature of the deficit is not certain. The disease is characterized by recurrent abscess of the skin, liver, lungs, and lymph nodes. The condition, untreated, is frequently fatal during infancy and early childhood. Serendipitous experiences with the care of patients with this condition have indicated that continuous therapy with a sulfonamide appears to modify the severity of the illness. In vitro studies of the function of leukocytes from children with chronic granulomatous disease have shown that leukocyte bactericidal capacity is enhanced in the presence of a sulfonamide, even if the challenge bacterium is sulfonamide resistant (Johnston et al. 1975). Clinical research on this subject is progressing, but the mechanism of the sulfonamide enhancement of polymorphonuclear cell function is not known. At the present time, continuous therapy of children with this disease with a sulfonamide is standard practice in many medical centers.

II. Osteomyelitis

Osteomyelitis of children is usually acute, hematogenous disease due to *Staphylococcus aureus*. Occasional instances of chronic disease due to other organisms also occur, however. The therapy of chronic osteomyelitis, especially when due to enteric organisms, is difficult and usually involves meticulous debridement of dead tissue together with a prolonged course of antimicrobial therapy. Bone levels of TMP have been found to be in a therapeutic range (Hansen 1975). Although clinical trials of children with osteomyelitis due to enteric organisms and treated with TMP/SMX have not been reported, individual experiences have been favorable and indicate that this approach to these difficult problems may be considered in some instances.

III. Ascending Cholangitis

Ascending infection of the liver via the biliary system is a rare disease in children. However, there are instances in which it is recognized to occur. In children with biliary atresia, an enterohepatic anastomosis may be employed, which allows direct drainage of the hepatic bed into the duodenum. Subsequent infections of the liver are common occurrences, and often refractory to antimicrobial therapy. Experience with children who receive TMP/SMX for therapy indicates that an excellent response may be hoped for (H. Filston 1981, personal communication).

References

Albritton WL, Hammond G, Hoban S et al. (1977) Ampicillin-resistant *H. influenzae* subdural empyema following successful treatment of apparently ampicillin-sensitive *H. influenzae* meningitis. J Pediatr 90:320–321

Ardati KO, Thirumoorthi MC, Dajani A (1979) Intravenous trimethoprim-sulfamethoxazole in the treatment of serious infections in children. J Pediatr 95:801–806

Asakawa Y, Akahane S, Kagata N, Noguchi M, Sakazaki R, Tamura K (1973) Two community outbreaks of human infection with *Yersinia enterocolitica*. J Hyg (Lond) 71:715–723

Barros F, Korzeniowski OM, Sande MA et al. (1977) Invitro antibiotic susceptibility of Salmonellae. Antimicrob Agents Chemother 11:1071–1073

Beem MO, Saxon EM (1977) Respiratory-tract colonization and a distinctive pneumonia syndrome in infants infected with *Chlamydia* trachomatis. N Engl J Med 296:306–310

Beem MO, Saxon EM, Tipple MA (1979) Treatment of chlamydial pneumonia of infancy. Pediatrics 63:198–203

Biedel CW (1978) Modification of recurrent otitis media by short-term sulfonamide therapy. Am J Dis Child 132:681–683

Blackman HJ, Yoneda C, Dawson CR, Schachter J (1977) Antibiotic susceptibility of *Chlamydia trachomatis*. Antimicrob Agents Chemother 12:673–677

Böse W, Linzenmeier G, Karama A, Olbing H, Wellman P (1974) Controlled trial of cotrimoxazole in children with urinary tract infection. Bacteriological and haematological toxicity. Lancet 2:614–616

Boger WP, Gavin JJ (1960) Sulfamethoxazole: Comparison with sulfisoxazole and sulfaethiodole and cerebrospinal fluid diffusion. Antibiot Chemother 10:572–580

Bradford WD, Noce PS, Gutman LT (1974) Pathologic features of enteric infection with *Yersinia enterocolitica*. Arch Pathol 98:17–22

Briggs AE, Robinson ME (1975) Salmonella meningitis treatment with intravenous trimethoprim. Aust NZJ Med 5:364–366

Chang MJ, Dunkle LM, VanReben D, Anderson D, Wong ML, Feigin RD (1977) Trimethoprim-sulfamethoxazole compared with ampicillin in the treatment of shigellosis. Pediatrics 59:726–729

Cherubin CE, Neu HC, Rahal JJ, Sabath LD (1977) Emergence of resistance to chloramphenicol in *Salmonella*. J Infect Dis 135:807–812

Chusid MJ, Heyrman KA (1978) An outbreak of *Pneumocystis carinii* pneumonia at a pediatric hospital. Pediatrics 62:1031–1035

Crosson JF, Watson C, Bailey DW, MacLowry JD (1976) Acute otitis media caused by ampicillin-resistant *Haemophilus influenzae* type B. JAMA 236:2778–2779

Dajani AS, Asmar BI, Thirumoorthi MC (1979) Systemic *Haemophilus influenzae* disease: an overview. J Pediatr 94:355–364

Ellerstein NS, Sullivan TD, Baliah T, Neter (1977) Trimethoprim-sulfamethoxazole and ampicillin in the treatment of acute urinary tract infections in children: a double-blind study. Pediatrics 60:245–247

Elwell LP, Graaff J de, Seibert D et al. (1975) Plasmid-linked ampicillin resistance in *Haemophilus influenzae* type b. Infect Immun 12:404–410

Feldman W, Johnson DM, Newberry P, Weldon A, Naidoo S (1975) Comparison of trimethoprim-sulfamethoxazole with sulfamethoxazole in urinary tract infections of children. Can Med Assoc J 112:19 S–21 S

Filice GA, Andrews J-S, Hudgins MF, Fraser DW (1978) Spread of *Haemophilus influenzae*. Am J Dis Child 132:757–759

Forbes PA, Drummond KN (1973) Trimethoprim-sulfamethoxazole in recurrent urinary tract infection in children. J Infect Dis [Suppl] 128:S 626–S 628

Fries VN, Keuth U, Braun JS (1975) Investigations of cerebrospinal fluid diffusion of trimethoprim in infants and children. Fortschr Med 93:1178–1183

Gajdusek C (1957) *Pneumocystis carinii*: etiologic agent of interstitial plasma cell pneumonia of premature and young infants. Pediatrics 19:543

Geddes AM, Fothergill R, Goodall JAD, Dorken PR (1971) Evaluation of trimethoprim-sulfamethoxazole compound in treatment of salmonella infections. Br Med J 3:451–454

Gellady AM, Shulman ST, Ayoub EM (1978) Periorbital and orbital cellulitis in children. Pediatrics 61:272–277

Gilman RH, Terminel N, Levine MM et al. (1975) Comparison of trimethoprim-sulfamethoxazole and amoxicillin in therapy of chloramphenicol-resistant and chloramphenicol-sensitive typhoid fever. J Infect Dis 132:630–635

Glode M, Daum R, Goldman D et al. (1981) Chemoprophylaxis for contacts of children with invasive *Hemophilus influenzae* type B (HIB) disease. Pediatr Res 14:611

Granoff DM, Gilsdorf J, Gessert C, Basden M (1979) *Haemophilus influenzae* type B disease in a day care center: erradication of carrier state by rifampin. Pediatrics 63:397–401

Grüneberg RN, Smellie J, Leakey A, Atkin W (1976) Long-term low-dose co-trimoxazole in prophylaxis of childhood urinary tract infection: bacteriological aspects. Br Med J 2:206–208

Gutman LT, Ottesen EA, Quan TJ et al. (1973a) An inter-familial outbreak of *Yersinia enterocolitica* enteritis. N Engl J Med 288:1372–1377

Gutman LT, Wilfert CM, Quan TJ (1973b) Susceptibility of *Yersinia enterocolitica* to trimethoprim-sulfamethoxazole. J Infect Dis 128:S 538

Hammerberg S, Sorger S, Marks MI (1977) Antimicrobial susceptibilities of *Yersinia enterocolitica* Biotype 4, serotype 0: 3. Antimicrob Agents Chemother 11:566–568

Hammerschlag MR, Andorka M, Semine DZ, McComb D, McCormack WM (1979) Prospective study of maternal and infantile infection with *Chlamydia trachomatis*. Pediatrics 64:142–148

Hammerschlag MR, Hammerschlag PE, Alexander ER (1980) The role of *Chlamydia trachomatis* in middle ear effusions in children. Pediatrics 63:628–632

Hamory BH, Sande MA, Sydnor A et al. (1979) Etiology and antimicrobial therapy of acute maxillary sinusitis. J Infect Dis 139:197–202

Hansen I (1975) A new method for homoginization of bone exemplified by measurement of trimethoprim in human bone tissue. Acta Pharmacol Toxicol 37:33–42

Harris RE, McCallister JA, Allen SA, Barton AS, Baehner RL (1980) Prevention of pneumocystis pneumonia. Am J Dis Child 134:35–38

Harrison HR, English MG, Lee CK, Alexander ER (1978) *Chlamydia trachomatis* infant pneumonitis. N Engl J Med 298:702–708

Healy GB, Teele DW (1977) The microbiology of chronic middle ear effusions in children. Laryngoscope 98:1472–1478

Hobday JD (1971) The prophylactic treatment of recurrent urinary tract infections with sulphamethoxazole-trimethoprim. Aust Paediatr J 7:199–202

Hoshaw TC, Nickman NJ (1974) Sinusitis and otitis in children. Arch Otolaryngol 100:194–195

Howard JB, Howard JE (1978) Trimethoprim-sulfamethoxazole vs sulfamethoxazole for acute urinary tract infections in children. Am J Dis Child 132:1085–1087

Hughes WT (1979) Limited effect of trimethoprim-sulfamethoxazole prophylaxis on *Pneumocystis carinii*. Antimicrob Agents Chemother 16:333–335

Hughes WT, Price RA, Kim H-K, Coburn TP, Grigsby D, Feldman S (1973) *Pneumocystis carinii* pneumonitis in children with malignancies. J Pediatr 82:404–415

Hughes WT, Price RA, Sisko F, Havron WS, Kafatos AG, Schonland M, Smythe PM (1974a) Protein calorie malnutrition a host determinant for *Pneumocystis carinii* infection. Am J Dis Child 128:44–52

Hughes WT, McNabb PC, Makres TD (1974b) Efficacy of trimethoprim and sulfamethoxazole in the prevention and treatment of *Pneumocystis carinii* pneumonitis. Antimicrob Agents Chemother 5:289–293

Hughes WT, Feldman S, Sanyal SR (1975a) Treatment of *Pneumocystis carinii* pneumonia with trimethoprim-sulfamethoxazole. Can Med Assoc J 14:47S–50S

Hughes WT, Feldman S, Aur RJA, Verzosa MS, Hustu HO, Simone TV (1975b) Intensity of immuno suppressive therapy and the incidence of *Pneumocystis carinii* pneumonia. Cancer 6:2004–2009

Hughes WT, Kuhn S, Chaudhary S et al. (1977) Successful chemoprophylaxis for *Pneumocystis carinii* pneumonia. N Engl J Med 297:1419–1426

Hughes WT, Feldman S, Chaudhary SC, Ossi MJ, Cox F, Sanyal SK (1978) Comparison of pentamidine isethionate and trimethoprim-sulfamethoxazole in the treatment of *Pneumocystis carinii*. J Pediatr 92:285–291

Johannisson G, Sernyrd A, Lycke E (1979) Susceptibility of *Chlamydia trachomatis* to antibiotics in vitro and in vivo. Sex Transm Dis 6:50–57

Jonsson N (1974) The treatment of typhoid and parathyroid fevers with co-trimoxazole in a comparative triad with chloramphenicol. Scand J Infect Dis [Suppl] 8:81–83

Johnston RB, Wilfert CM, Buckley RH, Webb LS, De Chatelet LR, McCall CE (1975) Enchanged bactericidal activity of phagocytes from patients with chronic granulomatous disease in the presence of sulphisoxazole. Lancet 1:824–827

Jubelirer DP, Yeager AS (1979) Simultaneous recovery of ampicillin-sensitive and ampicillin-resistant organisms in *Haemophilus influenzae* type B meningitis. J Pediatr 95:415–416

Kazemi M, Gumpert TG, Marks MI (1973) A controlled trial comparing sulfamethoxazole-trimethoprim, ampicillin, and no therapy in the treatment of salmonella gastroenteritis in children. J Pediatr 83:646–650

Kirven LA, Thornsberry C (1978) Minimum bactericidal concentration of Sulfamethoxazole-trimethoprim for *Haemophilus influenzae*: correlation with prophylaxis. Antimicrob Agents Chemother 14:731–736

Klimek JJ, Bates TR, Nightingale C, Lehmann WB, Ziemniak JA, Quintiliani R (1980) Penetration characteristics of trimethoprim-sulfamethoxazole in middle ear fluid of patients with chronic serous otitis media. J Pediatr 96:1087–1089

LaFleur L, Martineau B, Chicoine L (1972) Yersinia enterocolitica. Union Med Can 101:2407–2413

Larter WE, John TJ, Sieber OF, Johnson H, Corrigan JJ, Fuginiti VA (1978) Trimethoprim sulfamethoxazole treatment of *Pneumocystis carinii* pneumonitis. J Pediatr 92:826–828

Lazarus GM, Neu HC (1975) Agents responsible for infection in chronic granulomatous disease of childhood. J Pediatr 86:415–417

Lerman SJ, Kucera JC, Brunken JM (1979) Nasopharyngeal carriage of antibiotic-resistant *Haemophilus influenzae* in healthy children. Pediatrics 64:287–291

Lines DR (1973) The effectiveness and safety of sulfamethoxazole-trimethoprim compound in childhood urinary tract infections. Aust Paediatr J 9:205–207

Maki M, Vesikari T, Rantala I, Gronroos P (1980) Yersinia in children. Arch Dis Child 44:861–865

Melish ME, Nelson AJ, Martin TE, Norden CW (1976) Epidemic spread of *H. influenzae* type B (HIB) among children in a day care center. Clin Res 24:184 A

Michaels RH, Norden CW (1977) Pharyngeal colonization with *Haemophilus influenzae* type b: a longitudinal study of families with a child with meningitis or epiglottitis due to *H. influenzae* type B. J Infect Dis 136:222–228

Morzaria RN, Walton IG, Pickering D (1969) Neonatal meningitis treated with trimethoprim and sulfamethoxazole. Br Med J 2:511–512

Mordhorst CH (1967) Studies on occulogenital TRIC agents isolated in Denmark. Am J Ophthalmol 63:1282–1288

Mordhorst CH, Dawson C (1971) Sequelae of neonatal inclusion conjunctivitis and associated disease in parents. Am J Ophthalmol 71:861–867

Mourad A, Sweet RL, Sugg N, Schachter J (1980) Relative resistance to erythromycin in *Chlamydia trachomatis*. Antimicrob Agents Chemother 18:696–698

Musher DM, Rubenstein AD (1973) Permanent carriers of nontyphosa salmonellae. Arch Intern Med 132:869–872

Nelson JD, Kusmiesz H, Jackson LH (1976) Comparison of trimethoprim-sulfamethoxazole and ampicillin therapy for shigellosis in ambulatory patients. J Pediatr 89:491–493

Nylén O, Jeppson PH, Branefors-Helander P (1972) Acute sinusitis. Scand J Infect Dis 4:43–48

Pelton SI, Shurin PA, Klein JO, Finland M (1977) Quantitative inhibition of *Haemophilus influenzae* by trimethoprim-sulfamethoxazole. Antimicrob Agents Chemother 12:649–654

Perrin JM, Charney E, MacWhitney JB, Miller RL, Nazarian RF (1974) Sulfisoxazole chemoprophylaxis for recurrent otitis media. A double-blind crossover study in pediatric practice. N Engl J Med 291:664–667

Pifer LL, Hughes WT, Stagno S, Woods D (1978) *Pneumocystis carinii* infection: evidence for high prevalence in normal and immunosuppressed children. Pediatrics 61:35–41

Pickler H, Knothe H, Spitzy KH, Vielkind G (1973) Treatment of chronic carriers of *Salmonella typhi* and *Salmonella paratyphi B* with trimethoprim-sulfamethoxazole. J Infect Dis 128:S 743–S 744

Porotnoy D, Seah S (1979) Typhoid fever: treatment failure and multiple relapses with trimethoprim-sulfamethoxazole and chloramphenicol therapy. Can Med Assoc J 120:1264–1265

Rabinowitz SG, MacLeon NR (1972) Salmonella meningitis. A report of three cases and a review of the literature. Am J Dis Child 123:259–262

Rabson AR, Hallett AF, Koornhof HJ (1975) Generalized *Yersinia enterocolitica* infection. J Infect Dis 131:447–451

Rodriguez WJ, Schwartz R, Barsanti R, Mann R, Khan W, Ross S (1978) Trimethoprim-sulfamethoxazole (TMP/SMX) in the treatment of otitis media (O.M.) secondary to ampicillin-resistant strains of H. influenzae (H. flu^R). 18 th Intersci Conf Antimicrob Agents Chemother, Atlanta, Georgia

Ross S, Controni G, Khan W (1972) Resistance of Shigellae to ampicillin and other antibiotics. JAMA 221:45–47

Rowe DS, Aicardi BZ, Dawson CR, Schachter J (1979) Purulent ocular discharge in neonates: significance of *Chlamydia trachomatis*. Pediatrics 63:628–632

Rudoy RC, Nelson JD, Haltalin KC (1974) In vitro susceptibility of *Shigella* strains to trimethoprim and sulfamethoxazole. Antimicrob Agents Chemother 5:439–443

Ryder RW, Blake PA (1979) Typhoid fever in the Unites States, 1975 and 1976. J Infect Dis 139:124–126

Sabel K-G (1976) Treatment of meningitis in infants with co-trimoxazole administered parenterally. Scand J Infect Dis [Suppl] 8:86–89

Schachter J (1979) Chlamydial infections. N Engl J Med 298:428–435, 490–495, 540–549

Schachter J, Grossman M, Holt J, Sweet R, Spector S (1979) Infection with *Chlamydia trachomatis*: involvement of multiple anatomic sites in neonates. J Infect Dis 139:231–234

Schiefele DW (1979) Ampicillin-resistant *Hemophilus influenzae* in Canada: nationwide survey of hospital laboratories. Can Med Assoc J 21:198–221

Schieven BC, Randall C (1974) Enteritis due to *Yersinia enterocolitica*. J Pediatr 84:402–404

Schwartz R, Rodriguez W, Khan W et al. (1978) The increasing incidence of ampicillin-resistant *Haemophilus influenzae*. A cause of otitis media. JAMA 239:320–323

Schwartz R, Rodriguez WJ, Ross S et al. (1979) Treatment of otitis media with trimethoprim-sulfamethoxazole. J Pediatr 95:666–667

Schwartz R, Rodrigruez WJ, Khan W, Mann R, Barsanti RG, Ross S (1980) Trimethoprim-sulfamethoxazole in the treatment of otitis media secondary to ampicillin-resistant strains of *Haemophilus influenzae*. Ann Otol Rhinol Laryngol 89:281–284

Scragg JN, Rubdige CJ (1971) Trimethoprim and sulfamethoxazole in typhoid fever in children. Br Med J 3:738–741

Sher N (1975) Prophylactic chemotherapy with low-dose TMP/SMX following acute urinary tract infections in children. Can Med Assoc J 112:16S–18S

Shurin PA, Pelton SI, Scheifele D, Klein JO (1976) Otitis media caused by non-typable ampicillin-resistant strains of *Haemophilus influenzae*. J Pediatr 88:646–649

Shurin PA, Pelton SI, Donner A, Klein JO (1979) Persistence of middle-ear effusion after acute otitis media in children. N Engl J Med 300:1121–1123

Shurin PA, Pelton SI, Donner A, Finkelstein J, Klein JO (1980) Trimethoprim-sulfamethoxazole compared with ampicillin in the treatment of acute otitis media. J Pediatr 96:1081–1087

Smellie JM, Grüneberg RN, Leakey A, Atkin WS (1976) Long-term low-dose co-trimoxazole infection: clinical aspects. Br Med J 2:203–206

Smith TF, O'Day D, Wright PF (1978) Clinical implications of septal (periorbital) cellulitis in childhood. Pediatrics 62:1006–1009

Snyder MJ, Perroni J, Gonzalez O et al. (1973) Trimethoprim-sulfamethoxazole in the treatment of typhoid and paratyphoid fevers. J Infect Dis 128:S 734–S 737

Stagno S, Pifer LL, Hughes WT, Bradfield DM, Tiller RE (1980) *Pneumocystis carinii* pneumonitis in young immunocompetent infants. Pediatrics 66:56–62

Sullivan TD, Ellerstein NS, Neter E (1980) The effects of ampicillin and trimethoprim-sulphamethoxazole on the periurethral flora of children with urinary tract infection. Infection 8:S 339–S 341

Sumaya CV, Jorgensen JH, Townsend S, Littlefield LC (1980) Comparison of trimethoprim-sulfa and rifampin in eradication of *Haemophilus influenzae* type B (HIB) infections in a day care center. Pediatr Res 14:565

Svedhem A, Iwarson S (1979) Cerebrospinal fluid concentrations of trimethoprim during oral and parenteral treatment. Antimicrob Agents Chemother 5:717–720

Syriopoulou V, Scheifele D, Howie V et al. (1976) Incidence of ampicillin-resistant *Hemophilus influenzae* in otitis media. J Pediatr 89:839–841

Syriopoulou V, Schiefele D, Smith AL et al. (1978) Increasing incidence of ampicillin resistance to *Haemophilus influenzae*. J Pediatr 92:889–892

Tarr PI, Peter G (1978) Demographic factors in the epidemiology of *Hemophilus influenzae* meningitis in young children. J Pediatr 92:884–888

Tejani A, Dobias B, Nangia BS, Velkuru H (1977) Intrafamily spread of *Haemophilus influenzae*. Am J Dis Child 131:778–781

Thomas M, Hopkins JM (1972) Co-trimoxazole and cephalexin. A clinical trial in urinary tract infections in children with spina bifida cystica. Dev Med Child Neurol 14:342–349

Thomas WJ, McReynolds JW, Mock CR et al. (1974) Ampicillin-resistant *Haemophilus influenzae* meningitis. Lancet 1:313

Tipple MA, Been MO, Saxon EM (1979) Clinical characteristics of the afebrile pneumonia associated with Chlamydia trachomatis in infants less than 6 months of age. Pediatrics 63:192–197

Todd JK, Bruhn IW (1975) Severe *Haemophilus influenzae* infections. Am J Dis Child 129:607–611

Trickett PC, Dineen P, Mogabgab W (1973) Trimethoprim-sulfamethoxazole versus penicillin G in the treatment of group A beta-hemolytic streptococcal pharyngitis and tonsillitis. J Infect Dis 128:S 693–695

Uwaydah M, Marossian R, Balabanian M (1975) Cotrimoxazole compared with chloramphenicol in the treatment of enteric fever. Scand J Infected Dis 7:123–126

Wald ER, Milmore GJ, Bowen AD, Ledesma-Medina J, Salamon N, Bluestone CD (1981) Acute maxillary sinusitis in children. N Engl J Med 304:749–754

Watters E, Wallar PH, Hiles DA et al. (1976) Acute orbital cellulitis. Arch Otolaryngol 94:785–788

Weissman JB, Gangarosa EJ, Dupont HL, Nelson JD, Haltalin KC (1974) Shigellosis. JAMA 229:1215–1216

Wilber RB, Feldman S, Malone WS, Ryan M, Aur RJA, Hughes WI (1980) Chemoprophylaxis for *Pneumocystis carinii* pneumonitis. Outcome of unstructured delivery. Am J Dis Child 134:643–684

Willner M, Dull T, MacDonald H (1977) Comparison of TMP-SMX and ampicillin in the treatment of acute bacterial otitis media in children. In: Current chemotherapy. Proc 10 th Int Congr Chemother, vol 1, pp 125–127

Wilson HD, McCormick JB, Feeley JC (1976) Yersinia enterocolitica infection in a 4-month old infant associated with infection in household dogs. J Pediatr 89:767–769

Winston DS, Lau WK, Gale RP, Young LS (1980) Trimethoprim-sulfamethoxazole for the treatment of *Pneumocystis carinii* pneumonia. Ann Intern Med 92:762–769

Wolff LJ, Baehner RL (1978) Delayed development of Pneumocystis pneumonia following short-term high-dosage trimethoprim-sulfamethoxazole. AM J Dis Child 132:525–526

Yogev R, Lander HB, Davis AT (1978) Effect of TMP/SMX on nasopharyngeal carriage of ampicillin-sensitive and ampicillin-resistant *Haemophilus influenzae* type B. J Pediatr 93:394–397

Zoethout HE (1973) Long-term treatment of urinary tract infection with trimethoprim/sulphamethoxazole in children. In: Bernstein L, Salter AT (eds) Trimethoprim-sulphamethoxazole in bacterial infections. Churchill-Livingstone, Edinburgh, p 175

CHAPTER 15

Use of Co-trimoxazole in Urinary Tract Infection

F. O'GRADY

A. Introduction

Infections of the urinary tract are commonly caused by organisms which are sensitive to a large number of antimicrobial agents and the choice of agents for treatment is consequently wide. There is, moreover, ample evidence to show that acute urinary tract infection responds equally well to almost any agent to which the infecting organism is sensitive. Many clinical trials with an assortment of agents show that about 80%–90% of patients respond despite marked differences between the agents in activity, antibacterial range, and pharmacokinetics.

It is against this background that we have to judge whether a special place can be defined for co-trimoxazole in the treatment of urinary infection and the question is more complicated than it would be for other agents because until recently trimethoprim was available only in combination with sulfonamide and we have therefore to assess to what extent any special place defined for co-trimoxazole can be ascribed to the properties of the individual components or to interaction between them.

B. Co-trimoxazole in Acute Urinary Tract Infection

The results of trials of co-trimoxazole in acute urinary infection have followed the general pattern in that response rates around 80%–95% have been obtained (BRUMFITT et al. 1969; BRUMFITT and PURSELL 1972; GOWER and TASKER 1976; GRÜNEBERG and KOLBE 1969; KOCH et al. 1973; REEVES et al. 1969; SYMPOSIUM 1973 a, b). These results – on the high side of general experience – require the prevalence of resistance to the drug to be very low. Overall, because of the relative frequency with which different species cause urinary infection and the proportions of strains of those species resistant to the agents commonly used for treatment, there is little to choose among them, except that the position of co-trimoxazole is favourable or unfavourable depending on whether the judgement of sensitivity is based on the trimethoprim component alone (to which resistance is currently relatively uncommon) or on the sum of resistances to trimethoprim and sulfonamide (to which resistance is relatively wide-spread). On the basis of the argument (see Sect. D) that the effect of co-trimoxazole on urinary infection is dominated by the trimethoprim component, the low prevalence of resistance makes its position particularly favourable. How long it will remain so depends on the future rate and extent to which resistant strains come to prevail.

I. Epidemiology of Resistance

Undoubtedly the most striking feature of the resistance of urinary tract pathogens over a considerable number of years has been its stability (Grüneberg 1976) and this has been general experience with trimethoprim (Correspondence 1977; Grey et al. 1979; Towner et al. 1980). Nevertheless, history repeatedly teaches us that stability of resistance patterns over many years is far from being a guarantee that upturn will not at some time occur. Moreover, there may be little warning of change in the shape of a modest but progressive increase: the emergence of tetracycline-resistant *Streptococcus pyogenes* and sulfonamide-resistant meningococci, amongst others, showed that long periods of stable sensitivity can give way rapidly to a predominance of resistant strains. There has consequently been considerable interest in monitoring the situation with co-trimoxazole and our own experience is based on studies of patients treated for long periods (Pearson et al. 1979) and on surveys of the prevalence of resistance in organisms recovered from urinary infection in successive years (Towner et al. 1980). These findings extended other experience that the absolute prevalence of trimethoprim resistance was low and stable, but recently there have been indications of a systematic increase and before that, within the stable overall level, some striking shifts in the nature of resistance (Towner 1982).

1. Types of Resistance

Of the mechanisms by which organisms become resistant to trimethoprim: decreased permeability to the drug, over-production or modification of the target enzyme and loss of ability to synthesise thymine, we have not encountered thymine dependency in our strains and such mutants have been rare in the experience of others (Amyes et al. 1978; Grey et al. 1979; Jobanputra and Datta 1974). However, one of the most important aspects of resistance in relation to choice of therapy is its patchy geographical distribution and Maskell et al. (1978) continue to report isolation of thymine-requiring strains. (See Chaps. 1, 4 for discussion of the availability of thymidine in body fluids.)

Our own and general experience up to 1978 was that about 10% or less of resistance was plasmid borne (Amyes et al. 1978; Grey et al. 1979; Towner et al. 1980). Modest increases were then noted in hospital (Amyes et al. 1978, Grüneberg and Bendall 1979) and in our study of strains derived from both domiciliary and hospital practice over a year, although the absolute prevalence remained low, the proportion of resistance attributed to R plasmids almost trebled (Towner et al. 1980). Amyes et al. (1978) noted a change in the nature of sulfonamide resistance in their strains and from one annual survey to the next we observed a sharp increase in non-transferable high level resistance compatible with spread of the Tn 7 transposon. Subsequently an increase in the overall prevalence of resistance has been observed (Towner 1982).

There cannot, therefore, be any doubt about the variety and efficacy of means for generating and spreading trimethoprim resistance amongst wild strains, yet until recently therapy has not been in any measure threatened by resistance despite the large scale on which the drug (as combinations) has been prescribed. As long as changes in the nature of resistance occurred without affecting its overall prevalence, co-trimoxazole continued to enjoy a particularly favourable place amongst rival agents in terms of the proportion of urinary strains susceptible to it. There is, unfortunately, no way of predicting how long this desirable state of affairs will now continue, but a partial explanation for it may be sought in some unusual and striking features of the drug's behaviour.

II. Effects on Carriage Sites

It is generally conceded that urinary infection arises from the colonisation of the anterior urethra by organisms resident in the patient's own bowel which are transferred to the bladder during or at the end of micturition where, in some cases, they multiply. In a minority of patients, the bladder organisms ascend the ureter and invade the kidney. Elegant evidence of this sequence of events is provided by STAMEY's (1973) serial studies over prolonged periods. In this sequential process, cycles of urethral colonisation and bladder invasion occur by different serotypes and account for the fact that relapse (failure to eradicate the infecting organism) is a relatively uncommon cause of recurrent urinary infection and most patients suffer serial reinfections with different strains (KUNIN 1962). It follows that elimination of the common urinary pathogens from the bowel or prevention of their establishment in the anterior urethra could play a major part in the control of recurrent urinary infection; in achieving both these ends, trimethoprim is unusually effective.

1. Effect on Gut Flora

By and large, antibiotics are incompletely absorbed and residual active agent reaching the colonised sites of the lower bowel inhibits the propagation of susceptible species and provides room for their replacement by resistant relatives. The ability of ampicillin and especially tetracycline to effect such changes is well known (DATTA et al. 1971) and its recognition as an undesirable effect remote from the treated lesion is well exemplified by the experience of VALTONEN et al. (1976) who noted the frequency with which enterobacteria carrying tetracycline R plasmids were recovered from the faeces of patients treated with tetracycline for acne.

By comparison, the position of co-trimoxazole is remarkable. It was established very early in its history that conventional doses exert a dramatic effect in reducing the numbers of enterobacteria in the gut (KNOTHE 1973; SPELLER and BRUTEN 1972; MOORHOUSE and FARRELL 1973) yet the extent to which the vacated microbial niche was occupied by trimethoprim-resistant organisms was very limited (TOIVANEN et al. 1976). Moreover, on cessation of treatment, even the few resistant organisms that intruded promptly withdrew and the antecedent susceptible flora was restored (GRÜNEBERG et al. 1976). This remarkable freedom from overgrowth of resistant strains has been seen even in our patients treated for years with low doses of the combination (PEARSON et al. 1979).

2. Effect on Urethral Colonisation

The persistent suppressant effect of trimethoprim on the faecal *Escherichia* could go a long way to explain the success of co-trimoxazole in the control of recurrent urinary tract infection, but there is another important feature. In co-trimoxazole-treated patients, the anterior urethra, the launch site for enterobacteria poised to enter the bladder, is sterile. All agents used to treat urinary tract infection are ex-creted in the urine in high concentrations and this no doubt plays an important part in eliminating bacteria colonising the anterior urethra, but nitrofurantoin, for ex-ample, is a good deal less effective than co-trimoxazole in eliminating vaginal en-terobacteria (STAMEY et al. 1977). The difference can be accounted for by the phar-macokinetics of the agents (STAMEY and CONDY 1975). Unlike other drugs custom-arily used in the treatment of urinary infection, trimethoprim is a lipid-soluble weak base, un-ionised at the pH of the vaginal fluid and therefore concentrated in the vaginal secretion. The resulting exceptional levels of an agent active against the great majority of *Escherichia* virtually precludes urethral colonisation, thereby blocking the essential first step in the genesis of urinary infection.

Why this extraordinary capacity of trimethoprim to abolish natural carriage at both faecal and urethral sites has not already been overtaken by the incursion of appropriately adapted resistant strains has not been explained and, if experience is anything to go by, will not continue indefinitely unless exposure to the drug is curtailed. If we add to this the potential benefits of reducing cost and the probabil-ity of toxicity it plainly behoves us to define, if we can, the minimum effective dose.

III. Overtreatment

Many years ago, GOULD et al. (1953) showed that bacteria commonly disappear from infected urine within hours of initiating therapy and by following the bacteri-al counts in serially voided specimens we showed (CATTELL et al. 1968) that in many patients a single dose of an agent to which the organism was sensitive rendered the urine "sterile" on conventional testing for several days (Fig. 1). The obvious impli-cation that patients who customarily receive several doses of antibacterial agents a day for 1 week or more are being vastly overtreated has taken time to reach clini-cal practice, but several recent studies have shown that the great majority of patients will respond to a few doses or even a single dose of an appropriate agent. CHARLTON et al. (1976) showed that the effects of treatment with co-trimoxazole for 3 or 10 days were indistinguishable and it is now clear that even briefer treat-ment is just as effective. In general, the single doses given of various agents have been large but certainly effective: BAILEY and ABBOTT (1978) achieved 90% success rate with a single dose of 0.4 g trimethoprim + 2.4 g sulfamethoxazole.

We have argued that there is little advantage to be gained by raising the dosage to very high levels (GREENWOOD et al. 1980) and in a later study, BAILEY and BLAKE (1980) showed a single conventional dose (two tablets) to be effective, but recom-mended that the dose should be at least four tablets – the dose successfully used by HARBORD and GRÜNEBERG (1981). In these circumstances it is not surprising that the success of a large dose can be matched by giving a conventional dose night-

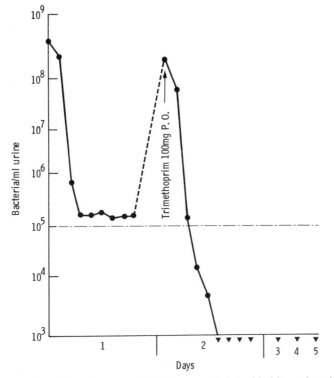

Fig. 1. When a patient with urinary tract infection emptied the bladder at hourly intervals the bacterial concentration in the voided samples fell precipitantly over 4 h and then remained approximately constant at about 10^5 organisms/ml until the patient retired to bed. On the following day frequent regular micturition was resumed after taking one oral dose of 100 mg trimethoprim. The counts fell rapidly below the minimum detectable level (10^3 organisms/ml) and were still uncountable after 5 days. (After CATTELL et al. 1968)

ly for 3 nights (RAPOPORT et al. 1981), or conventional therapy for 1 day (RUSS et al. 1980). Which of several possible effective regimens will gain the greatest patient acceptance remains to be shown.

C. Control of Recurrent Infection

In view of the prolonged levels of trimethoprim produced in the urine by conventional dosage, it is doubtful whether the extra-urinary effects on the faecal enterobacteria and urethral colonisation play an important part in the elimination of acute urinary infection, but they probably make a major contribution to the success of co-trimoxazole in the control of recurrent infection.

In 1929, the Royal Society of Medicine held a discussion on urinary antiseptics (BROWN 1929) in the course of which SWIFT JOLLY said "any infection of the kidney which persisted for longer than a few months would continue indefinitely" and LANGDON BROWN admitted that the subject was a disappointing one, saying "there was very little satisfactory evidence pathologically as to the efficacy of drugs in common use". Thirty years later, despite the introduction of a number of agents effective in the management of acute urinary infection, the expectation that the outcome of therapy in chronic urinary infection would be disappointing was still prevalent. At that time at St. Bartholomew's Hospital, our attempts to control infections which had been pronounced by others as "incurable" were not encouraging.

It is fair to say that the advent of trimethoprim changed all that and we were able to report (O'GRADY et al. 1969) that of 31 patients with intractable infection, 25 had been controlled. Perhaps the most remarkable feature of this study was that patients who had suffered for years refused to stop taking the drug and we were driven to weaning them from it by progressively reducing the dose. We thereby established that control can be maintained by a single dose given at night two or three times a week (CATTELL et al. 1971).

It had been argued for years that failure to control persistently relapsing patients was the result of using too short a course of therapy. Several well-designed studies quickly disposed of the belief that 6 or 8 weeks treatment would succeed where 2 weeks treatment failed, though treatment of infection in the male with co-trimoxazole may be an exception to this (GLECKMAN et al. 1979), and an important result of the use of diminishing doses of co-trimoxazole for long periods (designed essentially for symptomatic control) was that after 6 or 9 months in about one-half the patients persistent relapse or frequent reinfection no longer occurred (O'GRADY et al. 1973). Several other groups have since reported similar success in the control of intractable infection both in children (FORBES and DRUMMOND 1973; SMELLIE et al. 1976, 1978) and in adults (GLECKMAN 1973; HARDING and RONALD 1974). Even in patients with calculus disease who are particularly difficult to control, co-trimoxazole has been described as the drug of choice (CHINN et al. 1976). Except in patients harbouring multiply resistant organisms, infection can now almost always be brought under control and it is very likely that the long-term suppressive effects of co-trimoxazole on the bowel and urethral flora are important elements in this efficacy. However, other agents which do not share these properties can be equally effective and there has been much experience of alternatives, particularly nitrofurantoin (BAILEY et al. 1971).

In protracted antimicrobial therapy, there are two obvious foreseeable hazards: cumulative toxicity and superinfection with resistant strains or species. HARDING and RONALD (1974) noted an increased frequency of infection with enterococci in their patients and warned, very properly, that this might portend future trouble. In our 10 years experience of long-term, low dose co-trimoxazole, breakthrough infections with resistant organisms have been uncommon and very rarely led to therapeutic difficulties. In a particularly intensively studied group (PEARSON et al. 1979), we found that more than half the breakthrough infections were due to trimethoprim-sensitive organisms and therefore concluded "not only that breakthrough infections were uncommon but other reasons for failure (including, presumably, non-compliance) were more important numerically than was the emergence of resistance." The antibacterial activity and range of co-trimoxazole, its peculiarly favourable pharmacokinetics, its effect on the bowel and vaginal flora and (for the time being at least) the low prevalence of resistance to it, both de novo and in the course of long-term therapy, must make it close to a tailor-made agent for the control of intractable urinary infection.

D. Role of the Combination

If co-trimoxazole is held to have particularly favourable properties in relation to chronic urinary infection, to what extent do these properties depend on the mixture and to what extent on the components? In the laboratory, substantial bacteristatic synergy between trimethoprim and sulfonamide can be readily demonstrated against many organisms and bactericidal synergy can be demonstrated in appropriate conditions. The magnitude and the regularity of synergy between the agents in vitro is so striking that it was natural to assume that this would be projected into clinical benefit, providing a sulfonamide with reasonably matching pharmacokinetics could be found. Over the years, the validity of the belief that clinical benefit and in vitro synergy are intimately linked has been increasingly questioned. The substance of these doubts is well known: that many organisms are sulfonamide resistant and therefore not accessible to a synergic contribution by the sulfonamide component; that the distribution of the components of the mixture differs so much that many sites where synergy might be valuable are reached in appropriate concentrations only by the trimethoprim and that in other situations, notably in the urine, trimethoprim is present in such concentrations for such prolonged periods that it alone is sufficient to eliminate infection. Bacteriostatic synergy is demonstrable only where each agent is present in subinhibitory concentrations; if either is present in an inhibitory concentration there is nothing for the other agent to do.

I. Contrasting Effects of Trimethoprim and Sulfonamide in the Urine

The significance of this in urinary tract infection can be seen in Fig. 2 which shows the elimination of bacteria from a mechanical model of bladder infection by trimethoprim and sulfonamide alone and together (GREENWOOD and O'GRADY 1976). The bacterial concentration in the urine is high when "the patient rises in the morning" and falls to a state of fluctuating equilibrium in response to dilution by the day-time rate of flow of ureteric urine and hourly micturition. The concentration of bacteria does not fall further unless an antibacterial agent is exhibited.

When the infection is treated with sulfonamide, several intermicturition cycles are required for the drug to take effect because the folate possessed by the organism must be depleted by sharing amongst the progeny before the effect of folate starvation induced by the sulfonamide is felt. In contrast, when trimethoprim is used there is a very rapid effect as the recycling of tetrahydrofolate is halted. It follows that trimethoprim, excreted in urine after a normal dose in concentrations which remain superinhibitory for days, affects the organisms before an effect of sulfonamide is even within sight: the sulfonamide is superfluous. It can even be held (GREENWOOD 1979) that since the trimethoprim "hare" deprives the sulfonamide "tortoise" of the chance of acting it can be regarded as a sulfonamide antagonist! It may be argued that within the kidney the position of trimethoprim is not so dominant, but there is no reason to believe that it is not effective alone and at other sites, notably the prostate, differential access to the tissue ensures that all the work is done by trimethoprim. For the same reason the clearance of organisms from the urethral colonisation sites is wholly attributed to trimethoprim. This also almost certainly applies to the elimination of enterobacteria from the faeces.

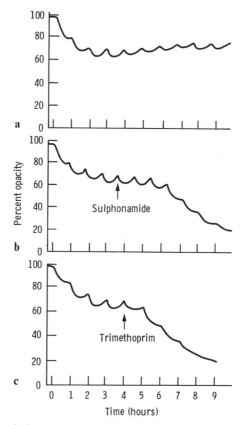

Fig. 2a-c. In a mechanical model simulating the growth conditions of the infected bladder **a** hourly micturition caused the bacterial concentration (measured by opacity) to fall over 3 h from the "overnight" value and then to remain approximately constant; **b** treatment with sulfonamide produced little effect for 3 h; **c** the effect of trimethoprim by contrast was visible within 1 h. (After GREENWOOD and O'GRADY 1976)

In the face of such arguments the reputation of the combination has been upheld, partly by claims that even in the treatment of sulfonamide-resistant organisms, the combination is superior (GRÜNEBERG 1975; SOURANDER et al. 1972) but principally by the belief that the presence of sulfonamide plays a significant role in controlling the emergence of trimethoprim resistance. Some have seriously doubted that this could be so because many organisms are already sulfonamide resistant, and in R factor resistance both sulfonamide and trimethoprim are commonly conferred together. Evidence on this crucial point has not come either freely or convincingly. Our own very limited experience of the use of trimethoprim alone for the control of intractable urinary infection (in patients intolerant of sulfonamide) has shown no excess of resistance by comparison with patients treated with co-trimoxazole (TOWNER et al. 1980) and this is in keeping with claims from Finland (HUOVINEN and TOIVANEN 1980) based on very large numbers of patients. It must be said, however, that the overall prevalence of resistance in the Finnish studies is extremely high compared with experience in the United Kingdom.

II. Toxicity

One effect of separation of the mixture is not in doubt: the frequency of side effects can be expected to fall. There has been disagreement about the relative contribution to toxic manifestations made by each of the components, but the prevalence of reaction to two drugs must be greater than that to one unless there are no patients who react to only one component – a very unlikely event. Long-term therapy is not to be entered on lightly. Patients with impairment of their renal function or folate status, or those requiring admission to hospital or instrumentation must be particularly carefully appraised and all must be observed regularly for the possible emergence of chronic toxicity or infection with resistant species or strains. Using the sequential system of treatment described several times (O'GRADY et al. 1973) in regularly monitored patients over many years we have had very little trouble with either. It is very much to be hoped that this state of affairs will continue because co-trimoxazole has unquestionably made a major contribution to the control of otherwise intractable urinary tract infection.

References

Amyes SGB, Emmerson AM, Smith JT (1978) R-factor mediated trimethoprim resistance: result of two three-month clinical surveys. J Clin Pathol 31:850–854

Bailey RR, Abbott GD (1978) Treatment of urinary tract infection with a single dose of trimethoprim-sulfamethoxazole. Can Med Assoc J 118:551–552

Bailey RR, Blake E (1980) Treatment of uncomplicated urinary-tract infections with a single dose of co-trimoxazole. NZ Med J 92:285–286

Bailey RR, Roberts AP, Gower PE et al. (1971) Prevention of urinary tract infection with low-dose nitrofurantoin. Lancet 2:1112–1114

Brown WL (1929) Discussion on urinary antiseptics. Proc R Soc Med 22:1127–1150

Brumfitt W, Pursell R (1972) Double blind trial to compare ampicillin, cephalexin, co-trimoxazole and trimethoprim in treatment of urinary infection. Br Med J 2:673–676

Brumfitt W, Faiers MC, Pursell RE et al. (1969) Bacteriological pharmacological and clinical studies with trimethoprim-sulphonamide combinations. Postgrad Med J [Suppl] 45:56–65

Cattell WR, Sardeson JM, Sutcliffe MB, O'Grady F (1968) Kinetics of urinary bacterial response to antibacterial agents. In: O'Grady F, Brumfitt W (eds) Urinary tract infection. Oxford University Press, London, p 212

Cattell WR, Chamberlain DA, Fry JK et al. (1971) Long-term control of bacteriuria with trimethoprim-sulphonamide. Br Med J 1:377–379

Charlton CAC, Crowther A, Davies JG et al. (1976) Three-day and ten-day chemotherapy for urinary tract infections in general practice. Br Med J 1:124–126

Chinn RH, Maskell R, Mead JA, Polak A (1976) Renal stones and urinary infection: A study of antibiotic treatment. Br Med J 2:1411–1413

Correspondence (1977) Trimethoprim-resistant coliforms. Lancet 2:774, 926

Datta N, Faiers MC, Reeves DS et al. (1971) R factors in Escherichia coli in faeces after oral chemotherapy in general practice. Lancet 1:312–315

Forbes PA, Drummond KN (1973) Trimethoprim-sulphamethoxazole in recurrent urinary tract infection in children. J Infect Dis [Suppl] 128:S 626–S 628

Gleckman RA (1973) A co-operative controlled study of the use of trimethoprim-sulphamethoxazole in chronic urinary tract infections. J Infect Dis [Suppl] 128:S 647–S 651

Gleckman R, Crowley M, Natsius GA (1979) Therapy of recurrent invasive urinary-tract infections of men. N Engl J med 301:878–880

Gould JC, Bowie JH, Cameron JDS (1953) Dosage of antibiotics: Relation between the in vitro and in vivo concentrations effective in urinary tract infections. Lancet 1:361–364

Gower PE, Tasker PRW (1976) Comparative double-blind study of cephalexin and co-trimoxazole in urinary tract infections. Br Med J 1:684–686

Greenwood D (1979) Laboratory methods for the evaluation of synergy. In: Williams JD (ed) Antibiotic interactions. Academic Press, London, p 53

Greenwood D, O'Grady F (1976) Activity and interaction of trimethoprim and sulphamethoxazole against Escherichia coli. J Clin Pathol 28:162–166

Greenwood D, Kawada Y, O'Grady F (1980) An in vitro model for assessing optimum antibiotic dosage in urinary tract infection. Infection [Suppl 1] 8:S 35–S 38

Grey D, Hamilton-Miller JMT, Brumfitt W (1979) Incidence and mechanism of resistance to trimethoprim in clinically isolated Gram negative bacteria. Chemotherapy 25:147–156

Grüneberg RN (1975) The use of co-trimoxazole in sulphonamide-resistant Escherichia coli urinary tract infection. J Antimicrob Chemother 1:305–310

Grüneberg RN (1976) Susceptibility of urinary pathogens to various antimicrobial substances: a four year study. J Clin Pathol 29:292–295

Grüneberg RN, Bendall MJ (1979) Hospital outbreak of trimethoprim resistance in pathogenic coliform bacteria. Br Med J 2:7–9

Grüneberg RN, Kolbe R (1969) Trimethoprim in the treatment of urinary infections in hospital. Br Med J 1:545–547

Grüneberg RN, Smellie JM, Leakey A, Atkin WS (1976) Long-term low-dose co-trimoxazole in prophylaxis of childhood urinary tract infection: Bacteriological aspects. Br Med J 2:206–208

Harbord RB, Grüneberg RN (1981) Treatment of urinary tract infection with a single dose of amoxycillin, co-trimoxazole, or trimethoprim. Brit Med J 283:1301–1302

Harding GKM, Ronald AR (1974) A controlled study of antimicrobial prophylaxis of recurrent urinary infection in women. N Engl J Med 291:597–601

Huovinen P, Tiovanen P (1980) Trimethoprim resistance in Finland after five years of use of plain trimethoprim. Br Med J 1:72–74

Jobanputra RS, Datta N (1974) Trimethoprim R factors in enterobacteria from clinical specimens. J Med Microbiol 8:169–177

Knothe H (1973) The effect of a combined preparation of trimethoprim and sulphamethoxazole following short-term and long-term administration on the flora of the human gut. Chemotherapy 18:285–296

Koch UJ, Schumann KP, Küchler R, Kewitz H (1973) Efficacy of trimethoprim, sulphamethoxazole and the combination of both in acute urinary tract infection. Chemotherapy 19:314–321

Kunin CM (1962) Microbial persistence versus reinfection in recurrent urinary tract infections. Antimicrob Agents Chemother 3:21–25

Maskell R, Okubadejo OA, Payne RH, Pead L (1978) Human infections with thymine-requiring bacteria. J Med Microbiol 11:33–45

Moorhouse EC, Farrell W (1973) Effect of co-trimoxazole on faecal enterobacteria: no emergence of resistant strains. J Med Microbiol 6:249–252

O'Grady F, Chamberlain DA, Stark JE et al. (1969) Long-term, low-dosage, trimethoprim-sulphonamide in the control of chronic bacteriuria. Postgrad Med J [Suppl Nov] 45:61–64

O'Grady F, Fry JK, McSherry A, Cattell WR (1973) Long-term treatment of persistent or recurrent urinary tract infection with trimethoprim-sulfamethoxazole. J Infect Dis [Suppl Nov] 128:S 652–S 656

Pearson NJ, Towner KJ, McSherry AM et al. (1979) Emergence of trimethoprim-resistant enterobacteria in patients receiving long-term co-trimoxazole for the control of intractable urinary-tract infection. Lancet 2:1205–1208

Rapoport J, Rees GA, Willmott NJ et al. (1981) Treatment of acute urinary tract infection with three doses of co-trimoxazole. Brit Med J 283:1302–1303

Reeves DS, Faiers MC, Pursell RE, Brumfitt W (1969) Trimethoprim-sulphamethoxazole: comparative study in urinary infection in hospital. Br Med J 1:541–544

Russ GR, Mathew TH, Caon A (1980) Single day or single dose treatment of urinary tract infection with co-trimoxazole. Aust NZ J Med 10:604–607

Smellie JM, Grüneberg RN, Leakey A, Atkin WS (1976) Long-term low-dose co-trimoxazole in prophylaxis of childhood urinary tract infection: clinical aspects. Br Med J 2:203–206

Smellie JM, Katz G, Grüneberg RN (1978) Controlled trial of prophylactic treatment in childhood urinary-tract infection. Lancet 2:175–178

Sourander L, Saarimaa H, Arvilommi H (1972) Treatment of sulphonamide-resistant urinary tract infections with a combination of sulphonamide and trimethoprim. Acta Med Scand 191:1–3

Speller DCE, Bruten DM (1972) Faecal flora after prolonged co-trimoxazole treatment. Br Med J 3:416

Stamey TA (1973) The role of introital enterobacteria in recurrent urinary infections. J Urol 109:467–472

Stamey TA, Condy M (1975) The diffusion and concentration of trimethoprim in human vaginal fluid. J Infect Dis 131:261–266

Stamey TA, Condy M, Mihara G (1977) Nitrofurantoin and trimethoprim-sulfamethoxazole prophylaxis of urinary tract infection. N Engl J Med 296:780–783

Symposium (1973 a) Session V clinical experiences: genitourinary infections. A. Infections of the urinary tract. J Infect Dis [Suppl] 128:S 641–S 665

Symposium (1973 b) Septrim symposia. Med J Aust [Suppl June] I:1–76

Toivanen A, Kasanen A, Sundquist H, Toivanen P (1976) Effect of trimethoprim on the occurrence of drug-resistant coliform bacteria in the faecal flora. Chemotherapy 22:97–103

Towner KJ (1982) Resistance to trimethoprim among urinary tract isolates in the United Kingdom. Rev Infect Dis 4: in the press

Towner KJ, Pearson NJ, Pinn PA, O'Grady F (1980) Increasing importance of plasmid-mediated trimethoprim resistance in enterobacteria: two six-month clinical surveys. Br Med J 280:517–579

Valtonen MV, Valtonen VV, Salo OP, Mäkelä PH (1976) The effect of long-term tetracycline treatment for acne vulgaris on the occurrence of R factors in the intestinal flora of man. Br J Dermatol 95:311–316

Treatment of Genital Infections with Trimethoprim, Sulfonamides, and Combinations

W.E. STAMM

A. Introduction

Shortly after their introduction into clinical medicine in the late 1930s, sulfonamides were found to be effective treatment for several sexually transmitted diseases, specifically gonorrhea, chancroid, and lymphogranuloma venereum. Early studies showed that 80%–90% of gonococcal isolates were sensitive in vitro to sulfonamides, but by 1942 rapid emergence of resistance occurred and the majority of isolates from patients with uncomplicated gonorrhea were resistant to sulfonamides in vitro. Penicillin replaced sulfonamides as the preferred treatment for gonorrhea. Interestingly, by 1954 and continuing to the present, most gonococci again show in vitro sensitivity to sulfonamide. Unlike gonorrhea, chancroid, and lymphogranuloma venereum have been treated successfully with sulfonamides consistently since 1938.

The advent of the combination drug trimethoprim sulfamethoxazole has reawakened interest in sulfonamide-containing regimens for treatment of genital infections (CARROLL and NICOL 1970; WORMSER 1978). Used alone, trimethoprim in vitro has little activity against *Neisseria gonorrhoeae*, *Chlamydia trachomatis*, or *Hemophilus ducreyi*, but the combination of these two drugs exhibits excellent in vitro activity against these agents. Further impetus for studying trimethoprim/sulfonamides in treatment of genital infections stems from other considerations. Effective forms of treatment for gonorrhea other than penicillins have become increasingly important owing to the spread of β-lactamase-producing *N. gonorrhoeae* and the recognition of frequent coinfection with *C. trachomatis* (against which penicillin is ineffective) and *N. gonorrhoeae*. The increasing number and types of genital infections due to *C. trachomatis*, while usually successfully treated by tetracycline, may require alternate forms of therapy in some cases and trimethoprim/sulfonamides may be useful in this regard. In this chapter, the current role of trimethoprim/sulfamethoxazole in the treatment of genital infections will be examined.

B. Treatment of Gonorrhea with Trimethoprim/Sulfamethoxazole

I. Uncomplicated Anogenital Infection

Despite the ineffectiveness of either trimethoprim or sulfamethoxazole alone in the treatment of uncomplicated gonococcal infections, the combination trimethoprim/sulfamethoxazole or trimethoprim with other sulfonamide preparations has been shown to be efficacious for uncomplicated anogenital gonorrhea. However, widely disparate results have been reported by various groups. Several factors underlie these differences in the reported efficacy of trimethoprim/sulfamethoxazole in the treatment of gonorrhea, including: (1) true differences among the drug regimens utilized; (2) differences in the populations studied in terms of sex, sexual preference, sexual activity, or compliance; (3) regional variations in susceptibility of gonococci to trimethoprim, sulfonamides, or the combination; and (4) differences in study design and data analysis. Unfortunately, most studies have not reported the in vitro sensitivities of their gonococcal isolates and thus differences attributable to this factor can be assessed in selected studies only. To facilitate comparison of the efficacy of trimethoprim/sulfamethoxazole combinations in the treatment of gonococcal infections, Tables 1–4 show the efficacy of various dose–duration combinations in the treatment of uncomplicated gonococcal urethritis in men and uncomplicated anogenital gonorrhea in women. Studies included in this analysis all provided evidence of gonococcal infection and eradication based upon appropriate cultures; included a minimum of 20 patients in each dose–duration trial; and stated clearly in their results numbers of patients enrolled, defaulters, patients felt to be reinfected, and patients representing treatment failures. To facilitate comparison of studies, efficacy for each study was recalculated using the formula

$$\text{Efficacy} = \frac{\text{Patients cured} - (\text{patients reinfected} + \text{patients failed})}{\text{Patients successfully completing follow-up}}.$$

Thus, efficacy in these tables does not differentiate reinfection from failure and doubtlessly provides minimal estimates of efficacy for this reason. However, since reinfection cannot realistically be distinguished from therapeutic failure in all instances and since reinfection was variously defined by different investigators, this formula provides for a more meaningful comparison of studies. Defaulters were excluded from the analysis by using as the denominator patients successfully completing follow-up.

The majority of therapeutic data have been accumulated in studies of males with gonococcal urethritis. Since single-dose or at least single-day therapy has always proven preferable to multiple-day regimens for the treatment of sexually transmitted diseases, early trials with trimethoprim/sulfamethoxazole focused upon single-dose schedules in which 6–12 tablets containing 80–400 mg trimethoprim/sulfamethoxazole were given at a single session. Unfortunately, single-day regimens given in this manner resulted in unacceptably low efficacy. WIGFIELD et al. (1973) gave six tablets at a single session and achieved a 70% success rate; five separate studies utilizing 8 tablets given at a single session achieved efficacies of 83%, 78%, 84%, 85%, and 90%, respectively (Table 1). In a study done at the Center for Disease Control in the United States, 9 tablets at a single sitting resulted in a 77% cure rate (ELIOTT et al. 1977). In earlier studies of tolerance and pharmacokinetics, 12 tablets given simultaneously resulted in unacceptable rates of nausea and vomiting (ELLIOTT et al. 1977). For this reason, studies administering more than 9 tablets simultaneously have not been undertaken.

As it became evident that single-dose therapy was not sufficiently effective, other regimens utilizing a single dose upon diagnosis and a subsequent dose 6–8 h later were proposed. In general, these regimens appear to have resulted in slightly

Table 1. Single-dose or single-day regimens for treatment of gonococcal urethritis

Reference	Regimen	Efficacy[a]	Postgonococcal urethritis[b]
Lawrence et al. (1973)	8 tablets single dose	159/176 (90)	NS
Wigfield et al. (1973)	6 tablets single dose	16/23 (70)	6/23 (26)
Meheus et al. (1974)	8 tablets single dose	50/64 (78)	6/14 (43)
Rahim (1975)	8 tablets single dose	765/918 (83)	46/794 (6)
Brathwaite (1975)	8 tablets single dose	43/51 (84)	NS
Brathwaite (1975)	8 tablets single dose (trimethoprim/ sulfadiazine)	41/48 (85)	NS
Elliott et al. (1977)	9 tablets single dose	51/66 (77)	NS
Arya et al. (1970)	4 tablets given twice, 8 h apart	14/23 (61)	6/23 (26)
Ullman et al. (1971)	5 tablets given twice, 8 h apart	62/64 (97)	NS
Nelson et al. (1975)	6 tablets given twice, 6 h apart	22/25 (88)	1/25 (4)
Kristensen and From (1975)	5 tablets given twice, 8 h apart	214/232 (92)	8/232 (3.4)
Elliott et al. (1977)	6 tablets given twice, 6 h apart	60/74 (81)	NS

[a] $Efficacy = \dfrac{Patients\ cured - (patients\ reinfected + patients\ failed)}{Patients\ successfully\ completing\ follow-up}$. Numbers in parentheses are percentages

[b] NS = not stated

higher overall cure rates than did single-dose therapy. Kristensen and From (1975), for example, cured 214 of 232 men treated with five tablets of trimethoprim/sulfamethoxazole given upon diagnosis and 8 h later. Ullman et al. (1971) also used this regimen and cured 62 (97%) of 64 patients. Nelson et al. (1975) used six tablets given twice on the day of diagnosis at a 6-h interval and cured 88% of males with gonococcal urethritis. However, Eliott et al. (1977) at the Center for Disease Control cured only 81% of patients by means of this same regimen. Arya et al. (1970) used four tablets given twice on the day of diagnosis, separated by an 8-h interval, and cured only 61% of patients.

Table 2 exhibits 20 different multiple-day dosage regimens that have been used for treatment of gonococcal urethritis in men. In general, multiple-day regimens appear more successful than the single-dose or single-day regimens. With the 12 single-day regimens reported in Table 1, the median efficacy was 83.5%, with the range being 61%–97%. With the multiple-dose regimens, the median efficacy was 93%, with a range of 80%–97%. If one uses either the Mann–Whitney test or the rank sum test, these two distributions are clearly different, efficacy being significantly greater in the multiple-day regimens.

Within the various dose–duration schedules used for multiple-day regimens, the most effective appear to be those giving a single daily dose of trimethoprim/sulfamethoxazole rather than spreading the tablets over the day in twice-daily or four-times-daily regimens. In a direct comparison of the same number of tablets given in different schedules, Robin and Seth (1972) gave one tablet four times a

Table 2. Multiple-day regimens for treatment of gonococcal urethritis

Reference	Regimen[a]	Efficacy[b]	Postgono-coccal urethritis[c]
CSONKA and KNIGHT (1967)	Trimethoprim/sulfatrid (400/4000) ×4 days	33/37 (89)	3/37 (8)
CSONKA and KNIGHT (1967)	Trimethoprim (400 mg) + sulfamethoxazole (2,000 mg) × 4 days	39/42 (93)	4/42 (10)
ARYA et al. (1970)	4 tablets × 3 doses over 1–5 days	23/24 (96)	1/23 (4)
ARYA et al. (1970)	4 tablets × 4 doses	27/28 (96)	1/27 (4)
EVANS et al. (1972)	4 tablets b.i.d. × 1 day, followed by 2 b.i.d. to 22 tablets total	47/59 (80)	8/111 (7)
AUSTIN et al. (1973)	6 tablets q.d. × 3 days	74/80 (93)	4/80 (5)
AUSTIN et al. (1973)	3 tablets b.i.d. × 3 days	68/85 (80)	10/85 (12)
SVINDLAND (1973)	2 tablets b.i.d. × 5 days	105/123 (85)	NS
SVINDLAND (1973)	3 tablets b.i.d. × 5 days + 2 at end	100/112 (89)	NS
SVINDLAND (1973)	4 tablets b.i.d. × 2 days	95/103 (92)	NS
MAHONEY et al. (1973)	4 tablets + 2 tablets on day 1, then 2 b.i.d. × 4 days	105/118 (89)	7/118 (6)
LAWRENCE et al. (1973)	4 tablets q.d. × 5 days	97/102 (97)	NS
LAWRENCE et al. (1973)	1 tablet q.i.d. × 5 days	85/103 (83)	NS
LAWRENCE et al. (1973)	4 tablets b.i.d. × 2 days	669/687 (97)	NS
LAWRENCE et al. (1973)	5 tablets b.i.d. × 1 day, then 5 tablets q.d. × 1 day	589/610 (96)	NS
MEHEUS et al. (1974)	2 tablets a.m. + 3 tablets p.m. × 4 days	45/56 (80)	3/12 (25)
BRATHWAITE (1975)	8 tablets q.d. × 2 days	46/48 (96)	NS
BRATHWAITE (1975)	8 tablets q.d. × 2 days (trimethoprim/sulphadiazine)	35/41 (85)	NS
DUNCAN et al. (1975)	6 tablets q.d. × 3 days	50/54 (93)	0/50 (0)
SATTLER and RUSKIN (1978)	4 tablets b.i.d. × 2 days	41/43 (95)	1/43 (2)

[a] Abbreviations: a.m. in the morning; b.i.d. twice a day; p.m. in the afternoon; q.d. once a day; q.i.d. four times a day

[b] Efficacy = $\dfrac{\text{Patients cured} - (\text{patients reinfected} + \text{patients failed})}{\text{Patients successfully completing follow-up}}$. Numbers in parentheses are percentages

[c] NS = not stated

day, two tablets twice a day, or four tablets once a day for 5 days, in men with gonococcal urethritis and found that 100% (43 of 43) were cured with the third regimen, while 92% and 88%, respectively, were cured with the first and second regimens. Similarly, LAWRENCE et al. (1973) achieved a 97% cure rate, giving four tablets daily for 5 days, but only an 83% cure rate, giving one tablet four times a day for 5 days. AUSTIN et al. (1973) cured 74 of 80 patients with six tablets given daily for 3 days, but only 80% of patients given three tablets twice daily for 3 days. It would thus appear that a single peak concentration of antimicrobial once a day has greater efficacy than sustained lower levels of antimicrobial activity. The exact explanation for this phenomenon is not clear.

Fewer studies of treatment of uncomplicated anogenital gonorrhea in women have been published. However, of five studies using single-dose or single-day regi-

Table 3. Treatment of uncomplicated gonorrhea in women; single-dose or single-day regimens

Reference	Regimen	Efficacy[a]
LAWRENCE et al. (1973)	8 tablets single dose	38/38 (100)
RAHIM (1975)	8 tablets single dose	258/275 (94)
NELSON et al. (1975)	6 tablets given twice, 6 h apart	77/86 (90)
ULLMAN et al. (1971)	5 tablets given twice, 8 h apart	36/36 (100)
KRISTENSEN and FROM (1975)	5 tablets given twice, 8 h apart	176/182 (97)

[a] $\text{Efficacy} = \dfrac{\text{Patients cured} - (\text{patients reinfected} + \text{patients failed})}{\text{Patients successfully completing follow-up}}$. Numbers in parentheses are percentages

Table 4. Treatment of uncomplicated gonorrhea in women; multiple-day regimens

Reference	Regimen[a]	Efficacy[b]
SVINDLAND (1973)	2 tablets b.i.d. × 5 days	100/111 (90)
SVINDLAND (1973)	3 tablets b.i.d. × 5 days + 2 tablets at end	74/85 (87)
SVINDLAND (1973)	4 tablets b.i.d. × 2 days	87/95 (92)
MAHONEY et al. (1973)	4 tablets on day 1, then 2 b.i.d. × 4 days	47/48 (98)
NELSON et al. (1975)	6 tablets q.d. × 3 days	66/82 (80)
LAWRENCE et al. (1973)	4 tablets b.i.d. × 2 days	164/169 (97)
LAWRENCE et al. (1973)	5 tablets b.i.d. × 7 days	409/416 (98)

[a] Abbreviations: b.i.d. twice a day; q.d. once a day

[b] $\text{Efficacy} = \dfrac{\text{Patients cured} - (\text{patients reinfected} + \text{patients failed})}{\text{Patients successfully completing follow-up}}$. Numbers in parentheses are percentages

mens in women with gonorrhea, cure rates of between 90% and 100% were achieved (Table 3). It is of interest that the cure rates achieved with single-dose or single-day therapy in women seem higher than those achieved with comparable regimens in men. As shown in Table 1, use of these regimens in men resulted in cures ranging from 61% to 97%, with a median of 83.5%. Comparison of these numbers with the efficacy figures in Table 3 suggests that single-dose or single-day therapies may be more successful in women. LAWRENCE et al. (1973) cured 38 of 38 women given eight tablets daily for gonorrhea, but only 90% of men treated with the same regimen. Using the same regimen, RAHIM (1975) cured 258 (94%) of 275 women, but only 765 (83%) of 918 men. It is thus possible that single-dose therapy may be more efficacious in women than men, although further data would be necessary to confirm this hypothesis. The explanation for this phenomenon is unclear, but might be that women achieve higher levels of drug on a mg/kg basis, or excrete the drug into urogenital tissues in higher concentrations than men. Table 3 also lists three studies in which single-day regimens were utilized in both males and females. In these studies, there appeared to be little difference between the efficacy noted in each sex.

Most multiple-day regimens were highly effective in treatment of uncomplicated gonorrhea in women as well as men. Of the studies listed in Table 4, only that of NELSON et al. (1975) resulted in a relatively low cure rate. These investigators used six tablets daily for 3 days and cured only 80% of women. In contrast, LAWRENCE et al. (1973) cured 97% of women given four tablets twice a day for 2 days or five tablets twice a day for 2 days. Not enough studies have been published to assess accurately which of the multiple-day regimens used to date is most effective in women. However, it appears that single-day therapy might well work in many women and should perhaps be given further consideration.

II. Rectal Infection

Few studies have specifically addressed the question of treating rectal gonorrhea with trimethoprim/sulfamethoxazole. KRISTENSEN and FROM (1975), using five tablets given twice on the day of diagnosis, 8 h apart, cured 53 of 53 women with anal infection. To date, few studies on the efficacy of trimethoprim/sulfamethoxazole in male homosexuals with asymptomatic gonorrhea or proctitis have been published. With increasing appreciation of the spectrum and frequency of gonococcal proctitis, further data in this regard would be useful. Men with gonococcal proctitis may have coinfection with other organisms, including *C. trachomatis*, and hence studies on the effectiveness of relatively broad spectrum agents like trimethoprim/sulfamethoxazole for this condition would be useful. SATTLER and RUSKIN (1978) reported cure of anal gonococcal infection in two male homosexuals.

III. Pharyngeal Infection

As with anal infection, little data exists on the use of TMP/SMX treatment of pharyngeal gonococcal infection. KRISTENSEN and FROM (1975) cured nine of nine patients with gonococcal pharyngeal infection. BRO-JORGENSEN and JENSEN (1973) studied 29 patients who had gonococcal pharyngeal infection and were given trimethoprim/sulfamethoxazole, two tablets three times a day for 1 week. Of the 29 patients, 28 were cured, and the one who was still infected at follow-up admitted reexposure. The available data thus suggest that trimethoprim/sulfamethoxazole successfully treats gonococcal pharyngitis.

IV. In Vitro Studies and Treatment of Gonorrhea with Trimethoprim/Sulfamethoxazole

In vitro studies of resistance to trimethoprim, sulfamethoxazole, or trimethoprim/sulfamethoxazole in isolates obtained from clinical studies have raised several important questions. First, is therapeutic failure associated with in vitro resistance to either of these drugs singly, or to the combination, or both? Second, will increasing use of trimethoprim/sulfamethoxazole result in increasing resistance of gonococci to sulfonamides, as occurred when sulfonamides were introduced in the late 1930 s? And, third, is resistance to penicillin linked to resistance to sulfamethoxazole, to trimethoprim, or to the combination? The latter question has particular importance if trimethoprim/sulfamethoxazole is to be considered a drug for treatment of penicillin failures or for treatment of penicillinase-producing gonococcal infections.

Several studies clearly indicate that failure to cure gonococcal infection with trimethoprim/sulfamethoxazole occurs more frequently in patients whose infections are caused by organisms which show in vitro resistance to trimethoprim/sulfamethoxazole. In a study done by the Center for Disease Control, ELLIOTT et al. (1977) nicely demonstrated that increasing in vitro resistance to either sulfamethoxazole or trimethoprim/sulfamethoxazole correlated with an increasing clinical failure rate. In their study, increasing resistance to trimethoprim alone was not related to clinical failure. RAHIM (1975) also showed that cases failing therapy had increased in vitro resistance to trimethoprim/sulfamethoxazole. On the other hand, SVINDLAND (1973) showed that many strains resistant or relatively resistant to sulfonamides were successfully treated with trimethoprim/sulfamethoxazole and none of the treatment failures had sulfonamide-resistant strains. AUSTIN and HOLMES (1975) showed that the minimum inhibitory concentrations (MICs) against sulfamethoxazole for isolates from seven clinical failures were significantly higher than the MICs of successfully treated strains. This was also true for MICs against trimethoprim/sulfamethoxazole, but not for MICs against trimethoprim alone.

These results agreed with those of ELLIOTT et al. (1977) at the Center for Disease Control in suggesting that resistance to trimethoprim/sulfamethoxazole seemed most associated with in vitro resistance to sulfamethoxazole rather than trimethoprim. LAWRENCE et al. (1973), on the other hand, found that the reverse was true. In their study, there was a significant correlation between clinical failure and high level resistance to trimethoprim (MIC $\geq$ 50 µg/ml), but little relationship between clinical failure and in vitro resistance to sulfamethoxazole. They, like other investigators, found that an MIC of >4 µg/ml against the combination was associated with an elevated failure rate. WIGFIELD et al. (1973) also found that when many strains demonstrated in vitro resistance to trimethoprim, failure rates with trimethoprim/sulfamethoxazole were high. Most likely, these differences in outcome are explained by the small numbers of study organisms tested. In all likelihood, when larger numbers of organisms are tested, increased in vitro resistance to either trimethoprim or to sulfamethoxazole would probably correlate with clinical failure when treatment with the combination was used. AUSTIN and HOLMES (1975) also showed that geographic variation in sensitivity to trimethoprim and/or sulfamethoxazole occurs.

ELLIOTT et al. (1977) showed that increasing resistance to trimethoprim/sulfamethoxazole was perhaps associated with increasing resistance to penicillin. LAWRENCE et al. (1973) also found a correlation between increasing MICs of penicillin and trimethoprim/sulfamethoxazole. However, SATTLER and RUSKIN (1978) found no correlation between MICs to ampicillin and those to trimethoprim/sulfamethoxazole. These results correspond to clinical results recently described by WATKO et al. (1977), who studied gonorrhea in the Philippines, where 40% of strains are penicillinase producers. In this setting, trimethoprim/sulfamethoxazole gives cure rates exceeding 90% for gonococcal urethritis in men, suggesting that little cross-resistance between trimethoprim/sulfamethoxazole and penicillin exists and that, at least at the present time, trimethoprim/sulfamethoxazole does not share the cross-resistance that is found between tetracycline, erythromycin, and penicillin.

SATTLER and RUSKIN (1978) found that 97.6% of 490 strains of *N. gonorrhoeae* were sensitive to <2 µg/ml of a 1:19 ratio of trimethoprim:sulfamethoxazole and that there was no correlation of increased MICs to trimethoprim/sulfamethoxazole with elevated MICs against ampicillin. EVANS et al. (1972) reported that clinical failures occurred in 17 of 43 patients given trimethoprim/sulfamethoxazole whose isolates exhibited sensitivity to penicillin of >0.1 µg/ml, as opposed to one of 58 clinical failures in patients whose strains were sensitive to <0.1 µg/ml penicillin. Thus, at this point controversy remains regarding the potential cross-resistance between trimethoprim/sulfamethoxazole and penicillin, and further studies are needed.

At present, little data regarding changes in susceptibility of *N. gonorrhoeae* to trimethoprim/sulfamethoxazole is available. LAWRENCE et al. (1973) did report that in their clinic, where the drug was being used for studies over a period of 3 years, the fraction of organisms resistant to 12.5 µg/ml sulfamethoxazole did not increase between 1970 and 1972. However, the percentage of strains resistant to 50 µg/ml trimethoprim rose from 22% to 44%. It is thus of concern that, with widespread use of trimethoprim/sulfamethoxazole, either increased resistance to trimethoprim, as appears to have occurred in England (LAWRENCE et al. 1973), or increased resistance to sulfonamides might render the combination ineffective. For *N. gonorrhoeae*, trimethoprim becomes effective only when a minimum concentration of sulfonamides is achieved (see Chap. 4).

C. Infections Due to Chlamydia trachomatis

I. Postgonococcal Urethritis

Many of the studies assessing the efficacy of trimethoprim/sulfamethoxazole in the treatment of gonorrhea have also reported numbers of cases of postgonococcal urethritis occurring in their study patients. Unfortunately, most studies have had inadequate follow-up for optimal evaluation of postgonococcal urethritis since often only a single follow-up 7–10 days after therapy or immediately after therapy and 1–2 weeks later were performed. In addition, none of the published studies to date have obtained chlamydial cultures before treatment for gonorrhea, and thus the specific effect of trimethoprim/sulfamethoxazole upon chlamydial infection and its relationship to postgonococcal urethritis have been inadequately assessed. Finally, in most studies the number of cases of postgonococcal urethritis occurring has been small and not truly adequate to assess therapeutic differences between trimethoprim/sulfamethoxazole and other drugs. Despite these deficiencies, several studies suggest that trimethoprim/sulfamethoxazole, when used for treatment of gonorrhea, is followed by fewer cases of postgonococcal urethritis than penicillin drugs. KRISTENSEN and FROM (1975) found that trimethoprim/sulfamethoxazole given as two doses of five tablets separated by 8 h resulted in 3.4% of cases subsequently incurring postgonococcal urethritis. By comparison, patients given pivampicillin and probenecid had a 7.7% rate of postgonococcal urethritis. Similarly, EVANS et al. (1972) found that when trimethoprim/sulfamethoxazole was given as four tablets initially, then two tablets twice a day for a total of 22 tablets, 8 of 111 patients given this regimen developed postgonococcal urethritis compared with 18 of 111 patients treated with the standard penicillin regimen of 4.8×10^6 IU intramuscularly with 1 g probenecid orally. SATTLER and RUSKIN (1978) detected postgonococcal urethritis in 2% of cases treated with four tablets of trimethoprim/ sulfamethoxazole twice daily for 2 days compared with 9.5% of cases given 3.5 g ampicillin plus 1.1 g probenecid in a single dose. AUSTIN et al. (1973) compared occurrence of postgonococcal urethritis after four different regimens for the treatment of gonococcal urethritis. Trimethoprim/sulfamethoxazole given as six tablets daily for 3 days was followed by postgonococcal urethritis in 5% of patients, while trimethoprim/sulfamethoxazole given as three tablets twice a day for 3 days resulted in postgonococcal urethritis occurring in 12% of patients. Comparative drugs used in this study were tetracycline (500 mg orally four times a day for 7 days) which was followed by postgonococcal urethritis in 4% of cases and the standard penicillin regimen of 4.8×10^6 IU intramuscularly together with 1 g probenecid which resulted in 10% of cases developing postgonococcal urethritis. In other studies involving small numbers of patients, MAHONEY et al. (1974) and LEE (1975) also felt that trimethoprim/sulfamethoxazole aborted postgonococcal urethritis.

In summary, it appears that trimethoprim/sulfamethoxazole may well be more effective in preventing postgonococcal urethritis than penicillin regimens used for treatment of gonorrhea. This would be expected based on trimethoprim/sulfamethoxazole's known in vitro activity against C. trachomatis. However, studies to date have not documented the effects of trimethoprim/sulfamethoxazole on concomitant chlamydial and gonococcal infection, and the optimal dose and duration for preventing postgonococcal urethritis have not been studied. One might anticipate that single-day regimens would be less effective than regimens given over several days, based on previous studies with use of tetracyclines or erythromycins for treatment of chlamydial infections which had caused nongonococcal urethritis or postgonococcal urethritis. However, further studies must be done to assess the effects of trimethoprim/sulfamethoxazole on postgonococcal morbidity. To date, no studies have assessed the effects of trimethoprim/sulfamethoxazole on the comorbidity of chlamydial and gonococcal infections in women.

II. Nongonococcal Urethritis

In vitro studies have shown that most genital strains of C. trachomatis are susceptible to sulfamethoxazole, while trimethoprim alone appears ineffective. Since chlamydiae probably cause 40%–50% of cases of nongonococcal urethritis, one might anticipate that sulfonamides alone or trimethoprim/sulfamethoxazole would be effective agents for treatment of this disease. However, Ureaplasma urealyticum, another probable etiologic agent in this syndrome, is not susceptible to trimethoprim/sulfamethoxazole in vitro. BOWIE et al. (1976) treated men who had nongonococcal urethritis with sulphafurazole, 500 mg orally four times a day for 10 days, and showed that 7 of 7 men whose pretreatment cultures grew C. trachomatis but not U. urealyticum were cured, while only 2 of 6 whose pretreatment cultures were positive for both chlamydia and ureaplasma, and only 5 of 19 whose pretreatment cultures were positive for ureaplasma alone were cured. DANIELSSON and WIRKSTRÖM (1975) cured 68% of 78 men given trimethoprim/sulfamethoxazole for nongonococcal urethritis, and showed partial response in another 17%. However, chlamydia cultures were not obtained and sex partners were not treated.

In a recent study by Paavonen et al. (1980), men with nongonococcal urethritis were treated with trimethoprim/sulfadiazine or placebo. Cultures for *C. trachomatis* were obtained before therapy and sex partners were examined and treated as well. The therapeutic regimen used was one tablet twice a day, containing trimethoprim (160 mg) and sulfadiazine (500 mg), daily for 2 weeks. A sample of 34 men was randomized to receive the trimethoprim/sulfadiazine regimen and 19 of these men had *C. trachomatis* isolated before therapy was given. At reexamination 4 weeks after the beginning of treatment, only 1 of the 34 men receiving trimethoprim/sulfadiazine had not responded to treatment. In the placebo-treated group, 21 of 41 patients failed to improve and 16 of 21 continued to be chlamydia positive. Of 33 women who were chlamydia positive prior to therapy, 32 were cured using the trimethoprim/sulfadiazine regimen, while 12 of 15 women given placebo continued to excrete chlamydia after their initial visit. These results suggest that trimethoprim/sulfamethoxazole has promise as a drug for the treatment of chlamydial infections in both men with nongonococcal urethritis and women with genital chlamydial infection. Further studies are necessary to assess its effect upon chlamydia-negative urethritis in men, a more difficult therapeutic problem.

III. Lymphogranuloma Venereum

Shortly after sulfonamides became available, Levaditi (1938) showed that sulfonamide administered orally to mice prevented the meningoencephalitis ordinarily induced by intracerebral injection of what was then thought to be the lymphogranuloma virus. This work was subsequently substantiated by MacCallum and Findlay (1938). Later, numerous studies demonstrated that orally administered sulfonamides were highly successful in the treatment of early lymphogranuloma venereum. These studies have been nicely summarized by Koteen (1945), who recommended sulfathiazole or sulfadiazine, 1 g orally four times daily for 2 weeks for lymphogranuloma venereum. Current recommendations for treatment of lymphogranuloma venereum have changed little. Most authors recommend sulfisoxazole, 1 g orally four times a day for 21 days, or triple sulfonamide, $60-75 \text{ mg kg}^{-1} \text{ day}^{-1}$ given as four divided doses every 6 h. Studies of the in vitro susceptibility of *C. trachomatis* lymphogranuloma venereum immunotype strains to sulfonamides has indicated consistent sensitivity. To date, trimethoprim/sulfamethoxazole has not been extensively tested in the treatment of lymphogranuloma venereum.

D. Chancroid

In 1938, sulfanilamide was shown to be effective for treating chancroidal ulcers, and sulfonamides have remained an effective therapeutic regimen for treatment of chancroid since then (Wilcox 1963). Most authorities have recommended sulfisoxazole, 1 g orally every 6 h for 7–14 days. With this regimen, therapeutic improvement is usually rapid, often occurring on the second or third day. Other sulfonamides useful in the treatment of chancroid include sulfadiazine, also given 1 g orally every 6 h for 7–14 days, and sulfamethoxytyridazine, given as a 1.5 g loading dose followed by 500 mg orally each day for 7–14 days. CAERASQUES (1966) felt the once-daily regimen using sulfamethoxytyridazine resulted in better patient compliance.

Unfortunately, few therapeutic trials involving chancroid have required isolation of *Hemophilus ducreyi* for confirmation of cases. In nearly all studies published to date, either a compatible clinical syndrome in and of itself, or a compatible clinical syndrome and a Gram's stain of the lesion showing small gram-negative rods was considered sufficient for diagnosis. In some studies, the Ito–Reenstierna skin test was used for confirmation of cases. Given our present knowledge of the inaccuracy of both the Gram's stain for *H. ducreyi* and of the Ito–Reenstierna skin test, it is difficult to interpret many of the previous therapeutic studies. Further, since isolates are not available in most studies, little is known about the in vitro antimicrobial spectrum of *H. ducreyi* strains causing illness. Most in vitro data, however, have consistently demonstrated susceptibility of *H. ducreyi* to sulfonamides. HAMMOND et al. (1978), reporting work done on strains from a recent outbreak of chancroidal illness in Winnipeg, found that all 19 outbreak strains and four reference strains they tested were highly susceptible to ≤ 8 µg/ml sulfisoxazole. All strains were also susceptible to tetracycline, but three strains demonstrated high level resistance to penicillin and produced β-lactamase.

Recent experience regarding the treatment of chancroid has come primarily from American servicemen in South-East Asia and Korea. KERBER et al. (1969) reported that 24 of 27 men with chancroid responded readily to sulfisoxazole, but only 7 of 23 treated initially with tetracycline responded adequately. They found that both drugs given together were 100% successful when used as initial therapy or for follow-up of cases that failed to respond to either drug given individually. The authors recommended that sulfisoxazole remains the drug of choice for treatment of chancroid and suggested that tetracycline-resistant strains may be prevalent in South-East Asia, where there is widespread use of tetracycline by prostitutes. However, isolation attempts were unsuccessful in all of the study patients and hence none of the cases were confirmed microbiologically and no isolates were available for testing in vitro antimicrobial susceptibility. MARMAR (1972) reported on management of chancroidal ulcers in American servicemen returning from Vietnam. He found most cases responded initially to sulfisoxazole. However, some cases did not and in cases termed "resistant" (defined as patients failing long-term therapy with sulfasoxazole, tetracycline, and other drugs), the author reported that 67 of 67 patients responded to kanamycin, 500 mg intramuscularly twice a day for 10–14 days. The author also recommended that cephalothin, 3 g intravenously daily for 10–14 days, could be used for management of these cases. Again, no microbiologic confirmation of cases was carried out.

Although chancroid is susceptible to trimethoprim/sulfamethoxazole in vitro, few data exist on the clinical use of trimethoprim/sulfamethoxazole for its treatment. STAMPS (1974) commented that the use of a single dose of trimethoprim/sulfamethoxazole (eight tablets) gave promising results, but no specific numbers were provided. He also reported that single-dose sulfonamides, given as eight tablets or 4 g triple sulfonamide on one occasion, caused frequent nausea and vomiting, posed a potential renal hazard, and caused 50% treatment failure. In view of the possibility of plasmid-mediated β-lactamase in strains of *H. ducreyi*, as demonstrated by HAMMOND et al. (1978), and in view of increasing tetracycline resistance in South-East Asia, sulfonamides may become the mainstay of therapy for chancroidal ulcers. In order to forestall emergence of resistance to sulfonamides, the use of trimethoprim/sulfamethoxazole may prove valuable in this situation. Further studies with this drug are warranted.

E. Syphilis

Trimethoprim/sulfamethoxazole in the doses and durations used for treatment of gonorrhea does not appear to provide adequate therapy for incubating or early syphilis. RAHIM (1975) reported two cases of syphilitic chancre developing on trimethoprim/sulfamethoxazole therapy and LAWRENCE et al. (1973) reported that three patients with chancres remained dark-field positive during therapy with trimethoprim/sulfamethoxazole. While no studies of syphilis treated by this combination have been published, it seems safe to conclude that the combination is not effective therapy for all cases of syphilis. Whether the combination does cure some cases of incubating syphilis is unknown. Patients given trimethoprim/sulfamethoxazole for treatment of gonorrhea should have serologic tests for syphilis done following therapy to rule out syphilis.

References

Arya OP, Pearson CH, Rao SJ, Blowers R (1970) Treatment of gonorrhea with trimethoprim-sulfamethoxazole in Uganda. Br J Vener Dis 46:214–216

Asin J (1952) Chancroid – a report of 1,402 cases. Am J Syphilis Gonorrhea Vener Dis 36:483–487

Austin TW, Holmes KK (1975) The use of trimethoprim-sulfamethoxazole in gonococcal infections. Can Med Assoc J 112:37S–39S

Austin TW, Brooks GF, Bethel M, Roberts FL, Turck M, Holmes KK (1973) Trimethoprim-sulfamethoxazole in the treatment of gonococcal urethritis: clinical and laboratory correlates. J Infect Dis 128:S666–S672

Bowie WR, Alexander ER, Floyd JF, Holmes J, Miller Y, Holmes KK (1976) Differential response of chlamydial and ureaplasma-associated urethritis to sulphafurazole (sulfisoxazole) and aminocyclitols. Lancet 2:1276–1278

Brathwaite AR (1975) Treatment of gonorrhea in the male with trimethoprim-sulfamethoxazole using a one- or two-dose regimen. Can Med Assoc J 112:43S–46S

Bro-Jorgensen A, Jensen T (1973) Gonococcal pharyngeal infections: report of 110 cases. Br J Vener Dis 49:491–499

Caerasques LG (1966) Chancroid treatment with sulfamethoxytyridazine. Dermatologica [Venezolana] 5:86–87

Carroll BRT, Nicol CS (1970) Trimethoprim-sulfamethoxazole in NGU and gonorrhea. Br J Vener Dis 46:31–33

Csonka TW, Knight GJ (1967) Therapeutic trial of trimethoprim as a potentiator of sulfonamides in gonorrhea. Br J Vener Dis 43:161–165

Danielsson D, Wikström KJ (1975) Diagnostic aspects of gonococcal and nongonococcal urethritis. Results of treatment with trimethoprim-sulfamethoxazole. In: Danielsson D, Juhlin L, Mårdh PA (eds) Genital infections and their complications. Almqvist and Viksel, Stockholm, pp 299–307

Duncan WC, Knox JM, Jackson TH (1975) Trimethoprim-sulfamethoxazole in the treatment of gonorrhea. South Med J 68:1147–1151

Elliott WC, Reynolds G, Thornsberry C et al. (1977) Treatment of gonorrhea with trimethoprim-sulfamethoxazole. J Infect Dis 135:939–943

Evans AJ, Churcher TM, Human RP (1972) Trimethoprim-sulfamethoxazole in the treatment of gonorrhea. Br J Vener Dis 48:179–181

Hammond GW, Lian CJ, Wilt JC, Ronald AR (1978) Antimicrobial susceptibility of *Hemophilus ducreyi*. Antimicrob Agents Chemother 13:608–612

Kerber RE, Row CE, Gilbert KR (1969) Treatment of chancroid. Arch Dermatol 100:604–607

Koteen H (1945) Lymphogranuloma venereum. Medicine 24:1–69

Kristensen JK, From E (1975) Trimethoprim-sulfamethoxazole in gonorrhea: a comparison with pivampicillin combined with probenecid. Br J Vener Dis 51:31–33

Lawrence A, Phillips I, Nicol C (1973) Various regimens of trimethoprim-sulfamethoxazole used in the treatment of gonorrhea. J Infect Dis 128:S 673–S 678

Lee VS (1975) Therapie-Erfahrung mit Trimethoprim-Sulfamethoxazole bei der post-gonorrhoischen Urethritis. Z Allg Med 27:1207–1209

Levaditi C (1938) Chemotherapie de la lymphogranulomatose inguinale experimentale. C R Soc Biol (Paris) 128:138–142

MacCallum FO, Findlay GM (1938) Chemotherapeutic experiments on the virus of lymphogranuloma inguinale in the mouse. Lancet 2:136–138

Mahoney JDH, McCann JS, Harris JRW (1973) Comparison of trimethoprim-sulfamethoxazole and penicillin in the treatment of gonorrhea. Br J Vener Dis 49:517–520

Mahoney JDH, McCann JS, Harris JRW, Howe JG, Dougan HJ (1974) Oxytetracycline compared with single-dose therapy with sulfamethopyrazine/streptomycin sulfate in NGU in males. Br J Clin Pract 28:179–181

Marmar JL (1972) The management of resistant chancroid in Vietnam. J Urol 107:807–808

Meheus AZ, Ngamige E, Freyens P (1974) Treatment of gonorrhea with trimethoprim-sulfamethoxazole and probenecid plus procaine penicillin in Rwanda. Br J Vener Dis 50:447–449

Nelson M, Bresher JT, Duncan WC, Eakins W, Knox JM (1975) Comparison of trimethoprim-sulfamethoxazole with penicillin and tetracycline in the treatment of uncomplicated gonorrhea in women. Can Med Assoc J 112:43 S–46 S

Paavonen J, Kousa M, Saikku T, Vartiainen E, Kanerva L, Lassus A (1980) Treatment of nongonococcal urethritis with trimethoprim-sulfadiazine and with placebo: a double-blind, partner-controlled study. Br J Vener Dis 56:101–104

Rahim G (1975) Single-dose treatment of gonorrhea with cotrimoxazole – a report of 1,023 cases. Br J Vener Dis 51:179–182

Rodin T, Seth AD (1972) Treatment of gonorrhea with cotrimoxazole, procaine penicillin alone, and procaine penicillin plus probenecid. Br J Vener Dis 48:517–521

Sattler FR, Ruskin J (1978) Therapy of gonorrhea: comparison of trimethoprim-sulfamethoxazole and ampicillin. JAMA 240:2267–2270

Stamps TJ (1974) Experience with doxycycline in the treatment of chancroid. J Trop Med Hyg 77:55–60

Svindland HB (1973) Treatment of gonorrhea with trimethoprim-sulfamethoxazole: Lack of effect on concomitant syphilis. Br J Vener Dis 49:50–53

Ullman S, Niordson AM, Zachariae H (1971) Trimethoprim-sulfamethoxazole in gonorrhea. Acta Derm Venereol (Stockh) 51:394–395

Watko LP, Kilpatrick ME, Hooper RR, Harrison WO (1977) Evaluation of cotrimoxazole in the treatment of penicillin-resistant gonorrhea. Program Abstr 17th Intersci Conf Antimicrob Agents Chemother, Abstr 262. American Society for Microbiology, Washington, DC

Wigfield AS, Selkon JB, Rich GE (1973) Single-session treatment of uncomplicated gonorrhea in men using penicillin combined with cotrimoxazole. Br J Vener Dis 49:277–290

Wilcox RR (1963) The treatment of chancroid. Br J Clin Pract 17:455–460

Wormser GP (1978) Trimethoprim-sulfamethoxazole in the treatment of genital infections. NY State J Med 78:2058–2067

CHAPTER 17

Treatment of Enteric Infections and Combinations

M.L. Clements, R.E. Black, and M.M. Levine

A. Escherichia coli Diarrhea

I. Introduction

Escherichia coli are gram-negative facultative bacilli that are part of the normal colonic flora in humans, but can also be important causes of diarrhea. *E. coli* are known to cause diarrhea by a variety of pathogenic mechanisms, including the ability of the bacteria to produce toxins (enterotoxigenic) or to penetrate the colonic mucosa (enteroinvasive). Some specific *E. coli* serotypes (designated by letter and number based on three separate antigenic groups: O, K, and H) that were associated with outbreaks of diarrhea in hospital nurseries in the 1950s and 1960s, are referred to as enteropathogenic.

Enterotoxigenic *E. coli* are known to produce two plasmid-mediated enterotoxins: one heat labile and the other heat stable. These toxins cause loss of fluid and electrolytes from the intestine as a result of stimulation of adenylate cyclase or guanylate cyclase, respectively, and the resulting illness is characterized by watery stools without inflammatory exudate. These organisms are now recognized as the most frequent cause of diarrhea in children in developing countries and in travelers to these countries (BLACK et al. 1981; MERSON et al. 1976).

The so-called enteropathogenic *E. coli* also produce a watery diarrhea compatible with enterotoxin mediation. Such toxins have been demonstrated in laboratory studies, but remain poorly characterized. Thus, these organisms are still identified solely on the basis of their serotype. In recent years, nursery epidemics associated with enteropathogenic serotypes appear to have decreased in the United States, but continue in the United Kingdom and some other countries.

Enteroinvasive *E. coli* and *Shigella*-like organisms that produce diarrhea, usually accompanied by abdominal pain, fever, and inflammatory exudate in the stool, appear to be infrequently identified pathogens in the areas of the world in which they have been sought. As in the treatment of cholera, fluid and electrolyte replacement is the mainstay of therapy of *E. coli* diarrhea. Antibiotic administration may be useful in some cases to reduce the volume and duration of diarrhea and therefore the requirements for fluid replacement.

II. Trimethoprim/Sulfamethoxazole Treatment of E. coli Diarrhea

1. In Vitro Studies

Although in many areas of the world enterotoxigenic and enteropathogenic *E. coli* are resistant to tetracycline and/or sulfa drugs, susceptibility to trimethoprim

(TMP) exceeds 90% (Echeverria et al. 1978; Thóren 1980). It is likely that the increasing use of trimethoprim for a variety of indications and the emergence of *E. coli* with plasmid-borne trimethoprim resistance will result in a greater prevalence of trimethoprim resistance in the future (Smith 1980).

2. Clinical Studies

In a double-blind study of the treatment of enterotoxigenic *E. coli* by Black et al. (1982), diarrhea was induced in volunteers using a trimethoprim/sulfamethoxazole(TMP/SMX)-susceptible strain of *E. coli* that produces both heat-stable and heat-labile toxin. Persons with diarrhea were then treated with TMP, TMP/SMX, or placebo. Compared with the placebo-treated group, ill volunteers in the antibiotic treatment groups had diarrhea for half as long and had a corresponding reduction in the number of stools and in the volume of diarrhea. The antibiotic-treated volunteers also had a reduction in the duration of abdominal cramps and anorexia. In five of ten TMP-treated volunteers, but not in ten TMP/SMX-treated persons, TMP-resistant enterotoxigenic *E. coli* emerged within 48 h after treatment was initiated, and in two persons the appearance of the resistant organisms was associated with a clinical relapse.

A study by Thóren et al. (1980) demonstrated that children with diarrhea associated with an enteropathogenic *E. coli* who were treated with TMP/SMX or mecillinam had a shorter duration of illness and a more rapid eradication of the *E. coli* from the stool than children who were not treated with an antibiotic.

III. Summary

The combination TMP/SMX may be a useful addition to oral and intravenous fluid therapy in some persons with diarrhea due to enterotoxigenic or enteropathogenic *E. coli*. Since antibiotic therapy appears to reduce the volume and duration of diarrhea substantially, and therefore the requirements for fluid replacement, it may be particularly important for travelers with cardiac or renal disease, in whom management of fluid and electrolyte balance is difficult. Such therapy may also be indicated for persons with severe diarrhea who are far from medical facilities. On the other hand, preliminary information suggests that treatment of enteric infections with TMP alone may be less efficacious owing to the rapid development of TMP resistance during therapy and the possibility that these resistant strains will become predominant in the fecal flora and cause prolongation of the illness or clinical relapse.

B. Isospora belli Infections

I. Introduction

Coccidiosis caused by *Isospora belli* is usually a self-limited illness of acute onset with fever, diarrhea, and colicky abdominal pain lasting several weeks. Occasionally chronic diarrhea may persist for many years. Stool examinations unfortunately are usually negative; thus, small bowel biopsy is important in making the diagnosis. Many antibiotics and other agents have been used to treat the illnesses, but none have been uniformly successful.

II. Trimethoprim/Sulfamethoxazole Treatment of an Isospora belli Infection

WESTERMAN and CHRISTENSEN (1979) reported one case of severe, chronic diarrhea associated with chronic *Isospora belli* infection which had been unresponsive to many treatments, including metronidazole and tetracycline. This patient received 160 mg TMP + 800 mg SMX every 6 h for the first 10 days, then twice daily for 3 weeks. Within 48 h after treatment with TMP/SMX, the diarrhea subsided; subsequently, the infection resolved. Further evaluation of TMP/SMX in therapeutic trials is needed before any definitive conclusions can be made regarding its role in the treatment of *Isospora belli* infections.

C. Salmonella Infections

I. Introduction

Salmonellae, gram-negative, motile bacilli of the family *Enterobacteriaceae*, belong, strictly speaking, to one of three species, *Salmonella typhi* (1 serotype), *S. choleraesuis* (1 serotype), and *S. enteritidis* (more than 1,700 serotypes). In this discussion, however, the more conventional nomenclature, referring to the genus *Salmonella* and serotype, will be used. *Salmonella* can cause a variety of clinical syndromes, including gastroenteritis, enteric fever, bacteremia, and focal metastatic infections (such as abscesses and osteomyelitis). The enteric infections are discussed in the rest of this section. Most patients continue to excrete *Salmonella* organism in stool or urine for a few weeks after the enteric infection. Those persons who excrete the organism for a year or longer after the illness or the initial discovery of the pathogen are designated as chronic carriers. The incidence of the chronic carrier state after typhoid fever is 1%–3%, whereas it is far less common (less than 1%) after non-typhoidal salmonellosis. Chronic carriers are asymptomatic. They tend to be older (often in the sixth decade) and to have a higher incidence of gallbladder disease than the general population.

1. Typhoidal and Paratyphoidal Salmonella Infections

S. typhi and *S. paratyphi* are responsible for typhoid and paratyphoid fever, also known as enteric fever. The clinical features of typhoid fever and paratyphoid fever are similar, although the latter tends to be a milder illness. A full-blown case of typhoid fever is characterized by a spiking fever which progresses in stepwise fashion, abdominal cramps, headache, severe malaise, and toxemia. When they appear (usually on the abdomen) rose spots which are maculopapular erythematous lesions are very helpful to diagnosis. In older children and adults, typhoid and paratyphoid fever may be accompanied by constipation; whereas in young children enteric fever may be accompanied by diarrhea (see Chap. 14, sect. F.I). In mild cases and relapses, enteric fever is mainly manifested by fever and malaise. The diagnosis can be made bacteriologically by isolation of *S. typhi* or *S. paratyphi* from blood, stool, or bone marrow. The strain should be examined for its sensitivity to antibiotics.

Since humans are the only known natural reservoir of *S. typhi*, infections with *S. typhi* can be transmitted only by direct or indirect exposure to a human source. Paratyphoid and typhoid fever usually are acquired by ingestion of fecally contaminated food (or water). Since 1948, chloramphenicol has been the drug of choice for paratyphoid and typhoid fever. Clinical responses to treatment with chloramphenicol are usually gradual with defervescence within 2–5 days. Because of its high relapse rate and risk of bone marrow toxicity, chloramphenicol has not been an ideal drug. Since the widespread emergence of *S. typhi* strains with R factor-mediated chloramphenicol resistance, other antimicrobial agents have been sought as alternatives.

While many other antibiotics have been active in vitro against *S. typhi*, only ampicillin and TMP/SMX have been used successfully to treat patients with chloramphenicol-resistant *S. typhi*. In Mexico, however, some strains of chloramphenicol-resistant *S. typhi* have also developed resistance against ampicillin (OLARTE and GALINDO 1973). Although the R-factor coding for chloramphenicol resistance also codes for sulfonamide resistance, the trimethoprim portion of the combination remained active against multiply resistant strains. In view of its efficacy in *S. typhi* infections, even in those which are multiply drug resistant, and its low toxicity, TMP/SMX now appears to be a preferred therapeutic agent for use in acute typhoid fever.

The dose of TMP/SMX recommended for adults with acute typhoid fever is 160–320 mg TMP and 800–1,600 mg SMX. The dose in children is 8–10 mg kg^{-1} day^{-1} TMP and 40–50 mg kg^{-1} day^{-1} SMX in two divided doses for 2 weeks (see Chap. 14, sect. F. I). Chronic typhoid carriers are usually treated with intravenous ampicillin or oral amoxicillin. Those who have gallbladder disease sometimes require a cholecystectomy to eradicate *S. typhi* excretion. At present, there is insufficient data to evaluate the value of TMP/SMX therapy in eliminating chronic typhoid carriage.

2. Non-Typhoidal Salmonella Infections

S. typhimurium, *S. enteritidis*, and *S. heidelberg* (and many others, depending on the geographic area) commonly cause gastroenteritis characterized by a sudden onset of abdominal pain, watery stools (occasionally mixed with blood or mucus), fever, nausea, and vomiting. These symptoms, usually self-limited, subside within 2 or 3 days. On the other hand, the disease may be more severe in infants, in the elderly, in the immunosuppressed host, in gastric surgical patients, and in persons with achlorhydria, ulcerative colitis, sickle cell anemia, or other debilitating disease.

Diagnosis is usually made by stool cultures; blood cultures are negative in the vast majority of cases. Since animals harbor most non-typhoidal *Salmonella*, most infections with non-typhoidal *Salmonella* in humans can be traced to ingestion of inadequately cooked poultry or poultry products, meats, dairy products, or occasionally, food contaminated by a chronic carrier or to exposure to infected pets or domestic animals.

The use of oral fluids containing glucose and electrolytes has been the mainstay of treatment for diarrheal dehydration due to *Salmonella*. Although most *Salmonella* are sensitive in vitro to many antibiotics, at least five prospective randomized trials of *Salmonella* gastroenteritis have shown no significant effect of orally administered antibiotics on the duration of diarrhea or of *Salmonella* excretion (MacDonald et al. 1954; Pettersson et al. 1964; Kazemi et al. 1973; Garcia de Olarte et al. 1974; Nelson et al. 1980). These antibiotics include TMP/SMX, as well as, chloramphenicol, ampicillin, amoxicillin, and neomycin. Nelson et al. (1980) also found that treatment with ampicillin substantially increased the risk of bacteriologic and symptomatic relapse. There are certain patients with *Salmonella* infections, however, who may benefit from antibiotic therapy. They include the immunosuppressed host, those with ulcerative colitis, and those with chronic, failure-to-thrive syndrome.

II. Trimethoprim/Sulfamethoxazole in the Treatment of Salmonella typhi Infections

1. Therapeutic Studies in Antibiotic-Sensitive S. typhi Infections

The combination TMP/SMX has emerged as a preferred treatment in typhoid fever. Between 1968 and 1975, more than 1,000 documented cases of typhoid fever were successfully treated with TMP/SMX. In an analysis of the results of 15 open and 3 double-blind comparative trials, involving a total of 1,255 cases, Herzog (1976) found little differences overall between the TMP/SMX and chloramphenicol treatment groups in term of mean duration of fever (4.84 and 4.78 days, respectively), treatment failure (up to 12.6% and 10%), or relapse rates (up to 12.9% and 12.6%).

We reviewed further those controlled trials in which TMP/SMX was compared with chloramphenicol or other antimicrobial agents in the treatment of acute typhoid fever. Reports of three controlled studies in India and Sudan have claimed that TMP/SMX was superior to chloramphenicol in relieving toxemia in typhoid fever (Kamat 1970; Sardesai et al. 1973; Omer 1975). In each study, however, the criteria of toxemia varied and included features, such as headache, apathy, and confusion, that would seem to be difficult to evaluate objectively. Therefore, in this discussion objective parameters, such as duration of fever and stool excretion, will be relied upon to evaluate therapeutic responses of different agents.

The results of six trials with a total of 568 patients conducted in Nigeria, South Africa, Egypt, Sri Lanka, and India demonstrated that response to treatment with TMP/SMX was as good as with chloramphenicol in terms of duration of fever. In these studies, cure rates were similar, ranging from 89.1% to 100% in the TMP/SMX-treated group and 76.3% to 100% in those treated with chloramphenicol (Akinkugbe et al. 1968; Kamat 1970; Cardoso 1972; Sardesai et al. 1973; Hassan et al. 1975; Ramachandran et al. 1978).

In two separate trials reported by Mahapatra et al. (1979) from India and Omer (1975) from Sudan, defervescence was more rapid in the groups treated with TMP/SMX (87 cases) than in those (99 cases) who received chloramphenicol.

Since patients in these two studies were assigned to treatment groups in an alternate or rotational manner rather than at random, it is possible that the better outcome in the TMP/SMX treatment group was due in part to other characteristics of the subjects, not accounted for in the assignment.

In contrast, one controlled trial showed that chloramphenicol was more effective than either TMP/SMX or ampicillin in reducing the duration of fever and fecal excretion of *Salmonella*. In this randomized clinical study in Chile, SNYDER et al. (1976) compared simultaneously the efficacy of oral TMP/SMX, oral and parenteral chloramphenicol, and parenteral ampicillin in 92 patients with culture-positive typhoid or paratyphoid fever. Within 2 days of therapy, blood cultures of all patients became negative. Although most patients responded well to TMP/SMX treatment, two had fever persisting for 14 days and four more patients had unremitting fever that necessitated a change to chloramphenicol therapy between days 11 and 13. A separate report (SNYDER et al. 1973) presented the data of the TMP/SMX and chloramphenicol treatment groups in more detail. The mean time required for defervescence in chloramphenicol-treated patients was about 4.75 days compared with approximately 7 days in the group that received the combination. However, when the slow responders in the latter group were excluded, there were no significant differences between the two groups. They noted a tendency for mean levels of SMX to increase and TMP to decrease with time during therapy, but concluded that neither the levels of drugs in serum nor the in vitro sensitivities of *Salmonella* isolates could account for the slow response to TMP/SMX. This experience suggested that, while TMP/SMX is a good drug in the majority of patients, a small fraction of patients may respond slowly or not at all to the combination. Other factors pertaining to the host or the organism, as well as the in vitro resistance to the combination, may be responsible for other therapeutic failures with TMP/SMX.

RAMACHANDRAN et al. (1978) and MAHAPATRA et al. (1979) also reported persistence of fever in approximately 10% and 15%, respectively, of the typhoid patients treated with TMP/SMX in their studies. In four studies (SARDESAI et al. 1973; HASSAN et al. 1975; RAMACHANDRAN et al. 1978; MAHAPATRA et al. 1979), fewer relapses were noted following TMP/SMX treatment than after chloramphenicol treatment: 0 versus 4%, 5% versus 12.5%, 0 versus 8.1%, and 5.7% versus 12.5%, respectively. In three studies by KAMAT (1970), SARDESAI et al. (1973), and MAHAPATRA et al. (1979), toxic crises (i.e., drug-induced exacerbation of toxemia) occurred in approximately 4%–8% of the patients who received chloramphenicol.

Two nonrandomized studies reported higher failure rates with TMP/SMX than with chloramphenicol treatment of patients with typhoid fever. These conclusions were based on bacteriologic results of stool cultures in the study by SCRAGG and RUBIDGE (1971) and on relapses and slow or no response to therapy in the study by JAQUES and VAN DER HYDE (1972). In the former study, the doses of TMP/SMX used to treat the children may have been inadequate. In both studies, the comparison groups may have been dissimilar before treatment, since the assignment was not made at random. Because of this flaw in these study designs, it is possible that other factors in addition to the antimicrobial agents may have influenced the results.

2. Studies in Infections Due to Chloramphenicol-Resistant S. typhi Strains

Despite the widespread use of chloramphenicol in areas where typhoid was endemic, until 1971 resistance of *S. typhi* to this antibiotic was sporadic. In 1971, however, antimicrobial-resistant typhoid fever emerged in South Vietnam (BUTLER et al. 1973) and spread rapidly (ANDERSON 1975). At about the same time, during 1972, epidemic typhoid fever caused by *S. typhi* resistant to chloramphenicol (ANDERSON and SMITH 1972) and sporadically resistant to ampicillin appeared in Mexico (OLARTE and GALINDO 1973). In searching for antibiotics to replace chloramphenicol (and ampicillin), several studies were carried out to evaluate the efficacy of TMP/SMX in treatment of typhoid fever due to multiply resistant strains.

a) In Vitro Studies

One of the main concerns with the widespread use of TMP/SMX is the possible emergence of organisms resistant to trimethoprim. PINNEY and SMITH (1973) showed that *S. typhi*, *S. enteritidis*, and two strains of *E. coli* (including one enteropathogenic serotype 0111) can mutate in vitro to TMP resistance. They showed that strains resistant to a combination of TMP and SMX may arise spontaneously, provided the bacteria harbor an R factor that mediates SMX resistance. They found that all trimethoprim-resistant mutants isolated in vitro required thymidine. These findings suggested that the frequency of isolation of organisms resistant to TMP might be increased if the medium employed is supplemented with thymidine.

From 1973 to 1975, BUTLER et al. (1977) examined in vitro the microbial susceptibilities of 87 *S. typhi* strains isolated from Vietnamese patients and found 65 (75%) to be resistant to chloramphenicol, streptomycin, sulfonamide, and tetracycline. This multiple drug resistance was transferable to *E. coli* and was found in 11 different Vi ("virulence") phage types, in contrast to a single Vi phage type in chloramphenicol-resistant strains isolated during the epidemic in Mexico (ANDERSON and SMITH 1972). All isolates were susceptible to TMP/SMX and to ampicillin. Agar dilution studies of TMP/SMX showed synergistic inhibition of growth in all nonresistant isolates and 12 of 48 resistant strains tested.

In 1981, DATTA et al. reported a case in which an antibiotic-sensitive strain of *S. typhi* in the bowel of a patient with enteric fever treated with chloramphenicol and later TMP/SMX became resistant to both drugs. The original sensitive *S. typhi* had no detectable plasmids, however, the resistant *S. typhi* at the end of treatment had acquired two plasmids. Chloramphenicol and sulfonamide resistances were carried by a plasmid of incompatibility group H. Trimethoprim resistance was determined by transposon 7 carried in another plasmid of incompatibility group I. Presumably *S. typhi* clones in the patient's intestine acquired resistant plasmids by transfer from an antibiotic-resistant *Klebsiella aerogenes* present in the patient's urine before treatment, and the resistant clones replaced the original sensitive *S. typhi* as a result of antibiotic treatment. Although this is only one instance of *S. typhi* acquiring a TMP-resistant plasmid, two factors suggest that it will happen again: (1) the capacity of the TMP-resistance transposon 7 to spread between plasmids (RICHARDS and DATTA 1981; RICHARDS et al. 1978); and (2) the selection exerted by TMP treatment of enteric fever (MCKENDRICK et al. 1981).

b) Clinical Studies

LINH (1974) reported that 72% of 56 S. typhi isolated during 1973 from hospitalized patients in South Vietnam were resistant to chloramphenicol. On an alternate admission basis, 26 of these patients received TMP/SMX intramuscularly and 27 took chloramphenicol orally. Of the TMP/SMX-treated patients, 93% became afebrile after 5 days while only 45% of the chloramphenicol-treated group had a similarly good response. Of the non-responders in the latter group, 12 recovered subsequently with TMP/SMX treatment. LINH concluded that TMP/SMX was a useful drug in the treatment of chloramphenicol-resistant typhoid fever. Since LINH did not specify the antibiotic resistance of the strains in the TMP/SMX-treated patients, we cannot be certain that his conclusion was correct.

During 1975, BUTLER et al. (1977) compared ampicillin with TMP/SMX treatment of typhoid fever in South Vietnam where antimicrobial (chloramphenicol, streptomycin, sulfonamides, and tetracycline) resistance was endemic. In this study, 20 patients with laboratory-proven typhoid fever were randomly assigned to receive either TMP/SMX or ampicillin intravenously for 3–5 days, then orally. Their results indicated that ampicillin and TMP/SMX were equally effective against typhoid infections, in defervescence (5.5 and 5.0 days, respectively). In both treatment groups, patients with antibiotic-sensitive S. typhi strains had poorer clinical responses (two deaths and two with persistent fever) than in those with resistant strains (one with persistent fever), suggesting that chloramphenicol treatment might be preferable in antibiotic-sensitive typhoid fever.

During an epidemic of chloramphenicol-resistant typhoid in Mexico, GILMAN et al. (1975) conducted a clinical trial in which 64 patients with proven typhoid were randomly assigned to receive TMP/SMX or amoxicillin administered orally for 10 days. Their results showed that both drug regimens were equally effective in chloramphenicol-resistant infections, as evidenced by duration of fever and bacteremia. Therapy with TMP/SMX caused more rapid lysis of fever in chloramphenicol-sensitive typhoid infections than amoxicillin therapy. In vitro studies conducted with these R factor-containing (chloramphenicol-resistant) strains revealed very high levels of resistance to SMX and lack of synergy when SMX was added to TMP.

3. Trimethoprim/Sulfamethoxazole Treatment of Typhoid Carriers

An analysis of the literature has revealed that there are no conclusive studies on the therapeutic efficacy of TMP/SMX in chronic excreters (or carriers) of S. typhi or S. paratyphi. In published case reports or in treatment studies, most authors cite good results from treatment with the combination, but thus far none has reported studies with thorough follow-up. Therefore, the actual incidence of the carrier state following treatment remains unknown. A few reports are mentioned briefly.

BRODIE et al. (1970) from Aberdeen, Scotland, reported that treatment with 160 mg TMP + 800 mg SMX twice a day for about 1 month resulted in successful clearance of Salmonella pathogens from stools in four male patients: one chronic (6-year) typhoid carrier, one short-term convalescent typhoid excreter, and two chronic non-typhoidal Salmonella carriers. Treatment failures were observed in three female typhoid carriers, all with radiologic abnormalities of the gallbladder.

PICHLER et al. (1973) reported preliminary results of 46 chronic carriers with *S. typhi* or *S. paratyphi* B who were treated with TMP/SMX twice daily for 3 months; 34 of these patients had negative coprocultures throughout a follow-up period of one year; 12 patients relapsed, within 5 weeks of discontinuation of therapy in 11 patients and by 9 months in 1 patient. The *Salmonella* strains of the relapsed carriers showed the same antibiotic sensitivity before and after treatment.

Based on experience obtained in a clinical study in Borstel, FREERKSEN et al. (1977) reported that 35 of 40 *S. typhi* excreters, 7 of 19 *S. paratyphi* excreters, and 8 of 28 *S. enteritidis* excreters were cured of their chronic carrier state by treatment with both TMP/SMX and rifampicin. In a report by SARKIS-KECHICHE (1980), 11 female *Salmonella* carriers (3 with *S. typhi*, 4 with *S. typhimurium*, and the remainder with other Salmonella serotypes) were successfully treated with TMP/SMX without side effects. The average period of treatment was 19.8 weeks. No relapses occurred during the follow-up period of up to 29 months after termination of therapy.

4. Adverse Effects

Adverse effects, such as urticarial skin rashes, hemolysis, and other hematologic changes, have been associated with TMP/SMX in a few instances during treatment for typhoid fever. A few reports are mentioned. In 1972, OWUSU et al. suggested that TMP/SMX triggered an episode of acute hemolysis in a typhoid patient with glucose-6-phosphate dehydrogenase (G6PD) deficiency. Others disagreed with this observation (CHAN 1972; MEYER 1973). LEXOMBOON and UNKURAPIANA (1978) determined the efficacy and hazards of TMP/SMX treatment in children with G6PD deficiencies before treatment and with laboratory-proven typhoid fever (see Chap. 14, Sect. F.I). One of the 37 G6PD deficient children developed acute hemolysis on the second day of medication, but the hemolysis subsided during 14 days with the continuation of TMP/SMX therapy. All patients responded satisfactorily to treatment, with the mean period of defervescence about 8 days. The authors concluded that TMP/SMX, in doses of 6–10 mg/kg TMP and 30–50 mg/kg SMX, twice daily for 14 days, can be used successfully in the treatment of typhoid fever in G6PD-deficient children with little risk of serious adverse reactions.

GEDDES et al. (1971) and others have mentioned occasional occurrences of maculopapular rashes of varying severity and development of macrocytic anemia in their series of typhoid patients treated with the combination. SCRAGG and RUBIDGE (1971) and others reported instances of neutropenia, thrombocytopenia, and hypoplastic anemia during treatment. Recognizing these possible toxicities of TMP/SMX, it is necessary, as with chloramphenicol, to monitor blood counts and to check renal and liver function tests during therapy.

5. Summary

Most controlled clinical trials have demonstrated that, in terms of efficacy and low toxicity TMP/SMX, is equal to or better than chloramphenicol in the treatment of enteric fever. A few patients may not respond as well to TMP/SMX as to chloramphenicol. The variations in different study results may be attributed in part to different doses administered, variations in strains of *S. typhi*, and inherent host and immunologic differences in persons living in different geographic areas. TMP/SMX is the drug of choice for enteric fever due to chloramphenicol-resistant strains of *S. typhi*. The role of TMP/SMX in eradicating chronic carriage of *S. typhi* is not clear.

III. Trimethoprim Alone in Treatment of Enteric Fever

Since side effects of TMP/SMX treatment, mainly rash, are usually due to the sulfonamide portion and since increasing numbers of *S. typhi* strains are resistant to sulfonamides, it was suggested that patients with typhoid fever might be treated with TMP alone. McKENDRICK et al. (1981) treated seven patients with typhoid fever and one with enteric fever caused by *S. paratyphi* A with trimethoprim 100–300 mg twice daily for 14 days. In all eight patients, treatment was effective and well tolerated. All patients were cured by a single course of TMP except for one 14-year-old boy who had a clinical and microbiologic relapse 13 days after stopping treatment. He was successfully retreated with a further 12 days TMP at 300 mg twice daily. Trimethoprim MICs for the eight strains isolated ranged from 0.05 mg/l to 0.2 mg/l. The results of this clinical study are limited, but suggest that TMP alone might be useful against enteric fever. Additional treatment studies with TMP alone are needed. It is likely, however, that widespread TMP treatment of enteric fever may result in the increased incidence of plasmid-encoded TMP resistance in *S. typhi* strains.

IV. Trimethoprim/Sulfamethoxazole Therapy in Non-Typhoidal Salmonellosis

1. In Vitro Studies

Although culture methods, strains tested, and drug concentrations have varied, numerous studies have revealed that most strains of *Salmonella* are susceptible in vitro to TMP/SMX in combination. Two reports of susceptibility testing and three reports of TMP/SMX resistance are mentioned.

BUSHBY (1973) consolidated 28 reports from different geographic areas of studies in which sensitivities of 594 strains of *Salmonella* were measured by disc diffusion. The sensitvity discs containing 1.25 mg TMP and 23.75 mg SMX were used in each study, but the media varied. From these data, BUSHBY reported that 98.6% of 594 strains of *Salmonella* spp. were susceptible to the TMP/SMX combination. MARKS et al. (1973b) from Montreal tested 115 clinical isolates of non-typhoidal *Salmonella* species and found 91% of the strains to be sensitive in vitro to TMP/SMX in a 1:10 ratio.

McCARTHY et al. (1977) identified a thymidine-dependent mutant from a clinical isolate of *Salmonella* spp. Their in vitro testing revealed that the first isolate from a patient with *S. oslo* infection was sensitive to TMP/SMX before therapy with the combination. A second strain of *S. oslo* isolated from the patient's stool after 10 days TMP/SMX therapy was resistant in vitro to TMP/SMX combination and was characterized as thymidine dependent. After several passages on nutritionally complex media, this strain reverted to thymidine independence. The frequency of developing resistance to TMP/SMX via dependence on exogenous thymine or thymidine has not been established, but is probably low.

Between 1977 and 1979, ANDERSON (1980) examined 16 ampicillin-resistant strains of *S. typhimurum* phage 179 (the most common phage type isolated in Australia) which had been isolated from human feces in New Zealand. Of 8 ampicillin-resistant strains isolated during 1978, 7 were found to be also resistant to trimethoprim, sulfafurazole, and tetracycline. All resistances could be transferred to *E. coli* K_{12}. Characterization of the plasmids contained in these strains revealed that the resistance to sulfafurazole and trimethoprim was carried on a plasmid with a molecular weight of 5.2×10^6 daltons, whereas resistance to ampicillin and tetracycline was carried on a plasmid with a molecular weight of approximately 60×10^6 daltons.

In 1978, plasmid-encoded TMP resistance appeared in multiply resistant epidemic *S. typhimurium* strains (type 204) that were isolated during outbreaks of salmonellosis in Britain in cattle and later in one human infection (THRELFALL et al. 1978). In 1979, a similar, but not identical TMP-resistant strain of multiply resistant *S. typhimurium* (type 204c) caused outbreaks among calves on at least 56 farms and was identified in 20 human infections (THRELFALL et al. 1980). Cattle appeared to be the main source of the human infections. Trimethoprim had been used to prevent and treat bovine salmonellosis, and this usage probably resulted in the increased incidence of TMP-resistant *S. typhimurium* in cattle.

2. Clinical Studies

One controlled trial and other nonrandomized treatment studies have demonstrated that TMP/SMX therapy is no more effective than other antibiotics or no therapy. KAZEMI et al. (1973) in a controlled trial in Montreal to evaluate the role of TMP/SMX and other antibiotics in the therapy of *Salmonella* gastroenteritis, randomly assigned 78 children, aged between 10 months and 15 years, to one of three groups, TMP/SMX $(20+100 \text{ mg kg}^{-1} \text{ day}^{-1}$, respectively), ampicillin $(100 \text{ mg kg}^{-1} \text{ day}^{-1})$, or no therapy. The antibiotics were given orally for 7 days. A total of 42 children were excluded from long-term follow-up. Of the 36 patients followed for 6 months, there were no significant differences in the duration of diarrhea or fever, bacteriologic cure rates (63%–72% at one week), or carrier states (none at 8 weeks) among the three groups. All isolates remained sensitive in vitro to TMP/SMX and ampicillin. Pharmacokinetic studies in 13 of 14 patients receiving TMP/SMX (MARKS et al. 1973a) showed prompt absorption and optimal drug concentrations and ratios in serum and urine. KAZEMI et al. (1973) concluded that in spite of its adequate absorption in vivo and high activity in vitro the combination of TMP/SMX was no more effective than ampicillin. Neither of the antibiotics offered any benefit over no antibiotics in the therapy of *Salmonella* gastroenteritis in children. The high exclusion rate (54%) in this study could have biased their observations, however, these findings correspond with those of previous studies that demonstrated no therapeutic effect with antibiotics on the acute symptoms or in eradicating *Salmonella* in convalescent carriers (MACDONALD et al. 1954; PETTERSSON et al. 1964).

Other nonrandomized studies have reported similar findings. In a clinical trial comparing TMP/SMX and ampicillin treatment of *S. typhimurium* gastroenteritis in 113 adults in Halifax, Nova Scotia, SMITH and BRADLEY (1971) demonstrated no superiority of the combination to ampicillin or no therapy during the acute part of illness. Their follow-up period (4 weeks) was too short and number of carriers (5 cases) too few to make any meaningful conclusions about efficacy of TMP/SMX in shortening fecal excretion of *Salmonella*. In another study reported by BAILEY et al. (1972), 76 British bacon factory workers and others excreting *S. panama* were treated with 80 mg TMP + 400 mg SMX four times daily for 10 days; 21 persons were not treated. Treatment with TMP/SMX appeared to prolong the carrier state, but the differences between the two groups were not statistically significant.

In contrast, CLEMENTI (1975) reported that a 2-week course of TMP/SMX eradicated *S. enteritidis* fecal excretion in the majority of patients over 2 years of age, including those who had received prior antibiotic treatment. These conclusions may not be valid and are certainly difficult to accept for the following reasons: the patients were not randomly assigned to receive treatment; the comparison groups (TMP/SMX and no therapy) were not matched for age, by serotype of *Salmonella*, or by duration of carriage; coprocultures were not carried out at regular or sufficient intervals (before, during, and after treatment); and the patients previously treated with other antibiotics were combined with those who received TMP/SMX alone for comparison with the group not treated.

3. Summary

Treatment with TMP/SMX offers no benefit over no therapy in acute non-typhoidal *Salmonella* gastroenteritis. Studies on its usefulness in non-typhoidal *Salmonella* carriers are inconclusive.

D. Shigella

I. Introduction

Shigellosis is an acute human enteric infection caused by aerobic, gram-negative bacilli belonging to the species *Shigella boydii*, *S. dysenteriae*, *S. flexneri*, or *S. sonnei*. Shigella organisms are responsible for a range of clinical illness from asymptomatic infection, through diarrhea without fever to severe dysentery characterized by high fever, chills, toxemia, convulsions (in children), tenesmus, and bloody mucoid stools (see Chap. 14, Sect. F.II). *S. dysenteriae* 1, Shiga's bacillus, is known for its virulence and for causing pandemics. *Shigella*, for which humans are the natural host and reservoir, is spread usually by contact with infected hands and less commonly by contaminated food and water. Wherever personal hygiene is suboptimal, as in day-care facilities, institutions for the mentally handicapped, and those for the emotionally disturbed, the risks of transmission and infection may be great.

Treatment with appropriate antibiotics shortens the duration of diarrhea, fever, and the excretion of *Shigella* in the stools. However, despite the fact that many antibiotics are effective in vitro, only a few antibiotics (ampicillin, oxolinic acid, nalidixic acid, tetracycline, and TMP/SMX) have been shown to be clinically effective. Treatment with antibiotics is advocated mainly for serious illnesses, particularly in debilitated patients or when the likelihood of secondary transmission is great. When indicated, TMP/SMX is the therapeutic choice for *Shigella* infections since antimicrobial resistance to ampicillin and tetracycline is common. The dose of TMP/SMX recommended in adults is 160 mg TMP + 800 mg SMX twice a day for 5 days; in children, 10 mg kg^{-1} day^{-1} and 50 mg kg^{-1} day^{-1} SMX in two equal doses twice daily for 5 days (see Chap. 14, Sect. F.II).

II. Trimethoprim/Sulfamethoxazole Treatment in Shigellosis

1. In Vitro Studies

Although culture media and techniques, drug concentrations, and strains tested varied from study to study, several in vitro studies in England, Germany, Thailand, and the United States generally revealed that all of 1,046 *Shigella* strains tested were highly susceptible to the combination TMP/SMX (JARVIS and SCRIMGEOUR 1970; TITZE 1971; LEXOMBLOON et al. 1972; RUDOY et al. 1974; GORDON et al. 1975; BYERS et al. 1976). BUSHBY (1973) confirmed these individual claims after reviewing 28 reports from different geographic areas in which the sensitivities of *Shigella* strains were measured by disc diffusion. He found overall that 8 (67%) of 12 *S. dysenteriae* strains and 222 (98%) of 226 other *Shigella* strains were sensitive to TMP/SMX.

Most strains in these studies were susceptible to TMP alone, but many were resistant to SMX. LEXOMBOON et al. (1972) found that some *Shigella* isolates were not sensitive to TMP alone; nevertheless, when SMX was added to it, the bacterial activity of TMP was potentiated by the SMX. RUDOY et al. (1974) reported that the addition of SMX slightly reduced the MIC of TMP, especially of *S. flexneri* strains susceptible to SMX. On the other hand, JARVIS and SCRIMGEOUR noted potentiation of inhibition against SMX-susceptible *S. sonnei*, but not against SMX-resistant strains.

Recent reports announced the emergence of TMP-resistant and TMP/SMX-resistant strains of *Shigella*. In the first reports by BANNATYNE et al. (1980a, b), approximately 3% of 482 human isolates of *Shigella* strains (four *S. sonnei* and four *S. flexneri* 2a) surveyed in Ontario during 1977–1978 were found to be resistant in vitro to TMP. These *S. sonnei* strains were also resistant to sulfamethoxazole and tetracycline, but were susceptible to ampicillin and chloramphenicol, whereas the *S. flexneri* 2a isolates were resistant to sulfamethoxazole, tetracycline, ampicillin, and chloramphenicol. The TMP-resistant *S. sonnei* cases were temporally and geographically unrelated and belonged to different bacteriocine types. The TMP-resistant *S. flexneri* 2a isolates, on the other hand, were collected from patients who had shared a meal at the same house around the time of the outbreak of TMP-resistant *S. flexneri* 2a infection.

During 1980, FINLAYSON (1980) also isolated TMP/SMX-resistant strains of *S. sonnei* from 18 patients from Alberta, Canada. There were two dominant strains: one from northwestern Alberta that was resistant to ampicillin, sulfonamides, and tetracycline; and the other from eastern Alberta that was sensitive to ampicillin, but resistant to sulfonamides and tetracycline. The minimum inhibitory concentrations of trimethoprim were lower (ranging between 50 and 100 μg/ml) than those reported (MICs $\geq$ 128 μg/ml) by BANNATYNE et al. (1980b).

TAYLOR et al. (1980) from Ontario reported a case of shigellosis acquired in Brazil in which treatment with the combination for two 14-day courses was unsuccessful. The strain of S. sonnei was found by agar plate dilution method to be resistant to both TMP and SMX as well as to ampicillin, chloramphenicol, streptomycin, and tetracycline. Resistance to all these antibiotics was transferred in vitro to a strain of E. coli K_{12}, indicating that the trimethoprim resistance of this TMP-resistant strain of Shigella was located on a transmissible plasmid. Further analysis revealed that resistance to TMP, SMX, and streptomycin was carried simultaneously on an R plasmid, whereas resistance to ampicillin, chloramphenicol, tetracycline, streptomycin, and SMX was encoded by another unrelated plasmid in the same isolate of S. sonnei.

2. Clinical Studies

Five randomized, prospective clinical trials described in this section have demonstrated that TMP/SMX therapy in patients with shigellosis is effective in reducing the duration of symptoms and fecal excretion of Shigella organisms. The combination appears to be superior to furazolidone and sulfadimidine. TMP/SMX is as effective as ampicillin in the treatment of illnesses due to ampicillin-sensitive strains, and superior in those cases with ampicillin-resistant shigellosis.

LEXOMBOON et al. (1972) in Bangkok, compared TMP/SMX with furazolidone in two groups of 33 and 30 randomly assigned outpatients, respectively. By 4 days of treatment all of the TMP/SMX group had improved clinically and their coprocultures were negative for Shigella; whereas even after 7 days furazolidone therapy, approximately one-quarter failed to respond clinically or bacteriologically.

In another randomized trial MABADEJE (1974) in Nigeria, compared the therapeutic effects of TMP/SMX in adults with Shigella dysentery; patients treated with sulfadimidine served as the control group. The treatment response achieved with TMP/SMX was definitely superior to that with the control drug by day 3 of treatment, all 50 TMP/SMX-treated patients were asymptomatic, whereas 8 of the 50 controls continued to have diarrhea beyond the 5-day treatment period. All six types of Shigella isolates (including S. dysenteriae and S. boydii) were sensitive to TMP/SMX, while 88.3% were resistant to sulfadimidine.

In an inpatient study, NELSON et al. (1976a) in Dallas, Texas, randomly assigned 28 infants hospitalized with severe shigellosis to receive 5 days of treatment with either oral ampicillin or the combination TMP/SMX. The same dose and treatment schedules were employed in a second randomized study (NELSON et al. 1976b), comparing both antibiotic therapies for shigellosis in 65 ambulatory patients. In both studies, similar, prompt bacteriologic and clinical responses were observed in the patients treated with TMP/SMX and in those with susceptible Shigella treated with ampicillin. By the completion of therapy, most of the patients in both groups had negative coprocultures for Shigella and formed stools. In both studies, four patients with ampicillin-resistant Shigella failed to respond to ampicillin therapy and continued to have diarrhea and positive coprocultures; subsequently, they responded favorably to treatment with TMP/SMX.

In a small study in 20 hospitalized children with shigellosis, CHANG et al. (1977) in St. Louis, evaluated TMP/SMX therapy in shigellosis and confirmed the findings of the two studies by NELSON and co-workers. In addition their data suggest that in comparison with ampicillin therapy, TMP/SMX treatment results in significantly fewer stools per day and may eliminate *Shigella* excretion in stools more rapidly. One of the ampicillin-resistant patients treated with ampicillin remained symptomatic until his therapy was changed to TMP/SMX. Other nonrandomized studies (FRANZEN et al. 1972; GEDDES et al. 1975; FREIBERG 1971) showed similar good responses to TMP/SMX treatment of *Shigella* dysentery.

3. Summary

Numerous in vitro studies have almost uniformly indicated that TMP and SMX in combination are effective in inhibiting growth of most strains of *Shigella*. Results from two controlled studies showed that TMP/SMX and ampicillin have similar efficacies in the treatment of most patients with shigellosis (*S. flexneri* or *S. sonnei*); and TMP/SMX treatment was clearly superior in those cases with ampicillin-resistant *Shigella*. It appears, therefore, that TMP/SMX is currently a very effective antibiotic for treatment of shigellosis. A word of caution is warranted, however, since emerging resistance to TMP/SMX in *Shigella* organisms and its associated resistance to other preferred antimicrobial agents, as evidenced in a few strains in Canada, could prove to be a major therapeutic problem. Therefore, in vitro susceptibility testing is important for proper selection of antimicrobial therapy.

E. Vibrio cholerae Infections

I. Introduction

Vibrio cholerae, a noninvasive enteropathogen that causes cholera in humans, is an aerobic, gram-negative bacillus with a polar flagellum. *V. cholerae* belong to either the classical biotype, the cause of two previous pandemics, or El Tor biotype, responsible for the current pandemic. The serotypes include Inaba, Ogawa, and Hikojima. Cholera, an acute, self-limited gastrointestinal illness is characterized by the sudden onset of vomiting and mild or occasionally severe watery diarrhea (cholera gravis). When copious losses of gastrointestinal fluids and electrolytes are not replaced, dehydration and metabolic acidosis ensue; such losses may be so severe as to cause hypovolemic shock, renal failure, and death.

Cholera remains endemic in the Ganges Delta of eastern India and Bangladesh. Since 1961, cholera epidemics have occurred in Asia, the Middle East, Africa, and in certain European countries. Persons with asymptomatic or mild infections may contribute to the transmission of cholera when they travel to other areas since the vibrios are excreted in stools for a brief period (usually 5–9 days). A few convalescent patients (often with underlying gallbladder disease) may sporadically excrete the vibrios for a year or longer. Such carriers may occasionally serve as reservoirs of *V. cholerae* between epidemics.

Replacement of fluids and electrolyte losses and maintenance of hydration are the mainstays of treatment in cholera. Antibiotics are useful adjuncts to fluid therapy since they reduce the duration and volume of diarrheal fluid losses (and thus, diminish the volume of replacement fluids required) and shorten the excretion time of the vibrios from the stool. Tetracycline is the drug of choice in the treatment of illness and eradication of vibrio excretion in stools. The combination TMP/SMX, a practical alternative to tetracycline, is particularly useful in tetracycline-resistant cholera cases and in the treatment of children. Chloramphenicol and furazolidone are also effective in the treatment of cholera. The doses of TMP/SMX used successfully in adults have ranged from 160 to 320 mg TMP and from 800 to 1,600 mg SMX daily in divided doses for 3–5 days. Children have usually received 6–10 mg TMP and 30–50 mg SMX daily in divided doses for the same duration. In the following section, in vitro studies and clinical controlled trials to evaluate the effectiveness of treatment with TMP/SMX in cholera will be discussed.

II. Trimethoprim/Sulfamethoxazole Treatment in Cholera

1. In Vitro Studies

Both El Tor and classical biotypes of *V. cholerae* were highly susceptible in vitro to TMP and SMX in combination. The MICs of TMP/SMX against the cholera strains tested were about the same as those of tetracycline. NORTHRUP et al. (1972) studied in vitro susceptibilities by an agar dilution method of six El Tor and five classical *V. cholerae* strains to TMP and SMX alone and in combination. Their results indicated that TMP was equally active against both strains, while SMX alone was much less active against the classical than the El Tor biotypes. The combination of these agents in a 1:5 ratio was clearly synergistic against both biotypes of *V. cholerae*. The MICs for the TMP/SMX reported in this study were consistent with those reported by CASH et al. (1973). Their sensitivity studies by tube dilution showed similar MICs of the TMP/SMX combination and tetracycline for 18 El Tor and 14 classical *V. cholerae* strains.

2. Clinical Studies

In three studies of patients with cholera, compared with tetracycline therapy, the results of treatment with TMP/SMX were similar in volume of stools (CASH et al. 1973), duration of diarrhea (CASH et al. 1973; FRANCIS et al. 1971), and period of vibrio excretion (CASH et al. 1973; GHARAGOZLOO et al. 1970). The results of studies by FRANCIS et al. (1971) and DUTTA et al. (1978) conflicted: in the former study, tetracycline eliminated the vibrios from stools more rapidly than TMP/SMX; in the latter study the opposite results were found.

The only treatment study in patients with *V. cholerae* of the classical biotype (serotype Inaba) was conducted by CASH et al. (1973) in Bangladesh (formerly East Pakistan). A total of 96 patients, divided according to fluid treatment received (intravenous only or intravenous and oral therapy) and subdivided according to pediatric (3–10 years) or adult (older than 10 years) age groups were alternatively allocated to receive TMP/SMX or tetracycline. The results indicated that stool volume, duration of diarrhea, and duration of excretion of vibrios were slightly, but not significantly, greater in the groups treated with TMP/SMX than with tetracycline.

In a randomized treatment study in Iran, GHARAGOZLOO et al. (1970) compared the combination TMP/SMX with tetracycline, chloramphenicol, or placebo (dextrose) treatment in 42 patients hospitalized with cholera. Treatment for 4 days with TMP/SMX or tetracycline was adequate to eradicate the *V. cholerae* (El Tor Inaba) from stools of patients, whereas 4–7 days were required with chloramphenicol. In another randomized study, FRANCIS et al. (1971) allocated 65 dehydrated Nigerian patients with cholera (El Tor Ogawa) to receive treatment with TMP/SMX, tetracycline, sulfamethoxine, or no treatment. The latter two groups were dropped early from the study because 20 patients in these groups fared worse clinically than those in the other treatment groups. Their results showed that TMP/SMX and tetracycline were both more effective in shortening the duration of diarrhea (mean values 3.4 and 3.3 days, respectively) in comparison with the placebo group (5.3 days) Tetracycline treatment on the average eliminated vibrio excretion (1.7 days) from stools more rapidly than the combination (2.8 days).

DUTTA et al. (1978) from New Delhi in a randomized trial in 175 patients with bacteriologically confirmed *V. cholerae* (El Tor Ogawa), showed that treatment with TMP/SMX for 3 days resulted in earlier vibrio clearance (2.3 days) from stools than with chloramphenicol (2.8 days), tetracycline (3.2 days), or placebo (8.6 days). These data also supported the contention that TMP/SMX treatment shortens the duration of diarrhea in cholera illness as effectively as tetracycline therapy (mean values 2.2 and 2.4 days, respectively).

In a nonrandomized trial with 67 adult cholera patients in southern Italy, PASTORE et al. (1977) compared TMP/SMX, tetracycline, or chloramphenicol in the treatment of El Tor Ogawa infections. With the exception of one case which had negative coprocultures after 4 days of TMP/SMX treatment, all three antimicrobial agents eliminated vibrio excretion within 3 days. On the basis of this experience they concluded that treatment with TMP/SMX should be continued for at least 4 days. They reported that bacteriologic relapses occurred in two patients 10 and 12 days after completing chloramphenicol treatment, suggesting that chloramphenicol treatment was not as effective in eradication of vibrio excretion.

3. Summary

The combination TMP/SMX compares favorably with tetracycline bacteriologically and clinically in the treatment of cholera. Both antimicrobial agents are effective in reducing the duration and volume of diarrhea and clearance of vibrio excretion in stools. Both drugs are superior to chloramphenicol. Sulfamethoxine is not an effective treatment. These studies indicate that TMP/SMX is a practical alternative to tetracycline and might be very useful in areas where cholera is tetracycline resistant, or in the treatment of children.

F. Yersinia enterocolitica Infections

I. Introduction

Yersinia enterocolitica, a gram-negative coccobacillary, facultative anaerobe, causes a spectrum of clinical illnesses that vary with the age and physical state of the host. Young children usually experience a self-limited illness with diarrhea (sometimes with blood and mucus), fever, and occasionally erythematous rashes (see Chap. 14, Sect. F.III). Older children often develop self-limited acute mesenteric adenitis or terminal ileitis that may mimic appendicitis. In adults, the acute febrile diarrhea is occasionally associated with extraintestinal manifestations, including seronegative nonpurulent arthritis, a Reiter-like syndrome, or an erythematous skin rash. Protein-losing enteropathy may be associated with more severe cases of diarrhea. Patients with septicemia (many with underlying diseases) may develop a typhoid-like syndrome of headache, malaise, abdominal pain, and vomiting, but with an early onset of diarrhea and hepatomegaly, and without rose spots or leukopenia.

The infection is probably transmitted by fecally contaminated food vehicles. The diagnosis can be made by culturing blood, abscess fluid, mesenteric nodes, or stool specimens. *Y. enterocolitica* is usually sensitive in vitro to several antibiotics, including TMP/SMX. The value of antimicrobial therapy in cases of mesenteric adenitis and gastroenteritis or dysentery is unclear since these infections are usually self-limited. Patients with *Y. enterocolitica* septicemia, which has high mortality rate, and severe infections should receive antibiotic therapy. At present, there are insufficient clinical data to substantiate whether treatment with TMP/SMX or the antibiotics usually recommended (chloramphenicol or aminoglycosides) is beneficial.

II. Trimethoprim/Sulfamethoxazole and Yersinia enterocolitica

Published experience with TMP/SMX is currently limited to the in vitro studies and one case report mentioned in Sect. F.II.2.

1. In Vitro Studies

GUTMAN et al. (1973) reported the agar dilution drug susceptibilities of 23 human isolates of *Y. enterocolitica* (11 strains) to TMP and SMX, alone and in combination. All strains were inhibited by clinically achievable levels of each antimicrobial agent when used alone: the MIC to TMP was between 0.15 and 1.5 μg/ml and the MIC to SMX between 2.45 and 24.5 μg/ml. All strains demonstrated greater susceptibility to each drug when used in combination: the MIC to TMP ranged from 0.015 μg/ml to 0.15 μg/ml; and for SMX, from 0.285 μg/ml to 2.85 μg/ml.

HAMMERBERG et al. (1977) performed disc diffusion tests on 23 isolates from stool or appendiceal specimens of 22 ill children. All isolates were *Y. enterocolitica* biotype 4, serotype 3, the predominant serotype associated with clinical infection in Canadian patients. When TMP and SMX were combined in a 1:20 ratio, marked synergism resulted, reducing the MIC of the former at least eight-fold and the latter at least four-fold. These isolates were slightly more susceptible to SMX alone (MIC 3.1–6.3 μg/ml) than reported by GUTMAN et al., but slightly more resistant to TMP alone (MIC 0.16–1.25 μg/ml). Their results demonstrated that the most active antimicrobials in vitro against these strains were the aminoglycosides and the combination TMP/SMX. They found that the isolates were less susceptible to chloramphenicol, tetracycline, and rifampin and that they were resistant to ampicillin, carbenicillin, cloxacillin, erythromycin, and cephalothin. These results suggested that TMP/SMX (or aminoglycosides) might be clinically useful in the therapy of *Y. enterocolitica*.

2. Clinical Report

ERIKSSON and OLCÉN (1975) reported one case of *Y. enterocolitica* (biotype 4, serotype 3) septicemia that failed to respond to intravenous TMP/SMX treatment in spite of complete inhibitory, bactericidal, and synergistic effects in vitro. After the treatment was changed to tetracycline, the patient completely recovered.

3. Summary

While in vitro sensitivities of *Y. enterocolitica* suggest that TMP/SMX may be useful in the therapy of the illness; the role of TMP/SMX in *Y. enterocolitica* infections is unclear. Clinical trials are needed to evaluate its effectiveness in vivo.

References

Akinkugbe OO, Lewis EA, Montefiore D, Okubadejo OA (1968) Trimethoprim and sulphamethoxazole in typhoid. Br Med J 3:721–722

Anderson DM (1980) Plasmid studies of Salmonella typhimurium phage type 179 resistant to ampicillin, tetracycline, sulphonamides, and trimethoprim. J Hyg (Lond) 85:293–300

Anderson ES (1975) The problem and implications of chloramphenicol resistance in the typhoid bacillus. J Hyg (Camb) 74:289–299

Anderson ES, Smith HR (1972) Chloramphenicol resistance in the typhoid bacillus. Br Med J III:329–331

Bailey GK, Fraser PK, Ward CP, Bouttell G, Kinnear E (1972) Enteritis due to *Salmonella panama* from infected ham. J Hyg (Lond) 70:113–119

Bannatyne RM, Toma S, Cheung R, Hu G (1980a) Resistance to trimethoprim and other antibiotics in Ontario *Shigellae* (letter). Lancet 1:425–426

Bannatyne RM, Toma S, Cheung R, Hu G (1980b) Resistance to trimethoprim and other antibiotics in shigellae isolated in the Province of Ontario. Can J Microbiol 26:1256–1258

Black RE, Hug I, Merson MH, Alim ARMA (1981) Incidence and severity of rotavirus and *Escherichia coli* diarrhoea in rural Bangladesh. Lancet 2:141–143

Black RE, Levine MM, Clements ML, Cisneros L, Daya V (1982) Treatment of experimentally induced enterotoxigenic *Escherichia coli* diarrhea with trimethoprim, trimethoprim/sulfamethoxazole, or placebo. Rev Infect Dis 4:540–545

Brodie J, Macqueen IA, Livingstone D (1970) Effect of trimethoprim-sulphamethoxazole on typhoid and salmonella carriers. Br Med J 3:318–319

Bushby SRM (1973) Sensitivity testing with trimethoprim/sulphamethoxazole. Med J Aust [Suppl] 1:10–18

Butler T, Linh NN, Arnold K, Pollack M (1973) Chloramphenicol-resistant typhoid fever in Vietnam associated with R factor. Lancet 2:983–985

Butler T, Lingh NN, Arnold K, Adickman MD, Chau DM, Muoi MM (1977) Therapy of antimicrobial-resistant typhoid fever. Antimicrob Agents Chemother 11:645–650

Byers PA, DuPont HL, Goldschmidt MC (1976) Antimicrobial susceptibilities of shigellae isolated in Houston, Texas, in 1974. Antimicrob Agents Chemother 9:288–291

Cardoso N (1972) Double-blind trial with chloramphenicol and the combination trimethoprim/sulphamethoxazole (Bactrim) in typhoid. S Afr Med J 46:1286–1287

Cash RA, Northrup RS, Rahman ASMM (1973) Trimethoprim and sulfamethoxazole in clinical cholera: comparison with tetracycline. J Infect Dis [Suppl] 128:S 749–S 753

Chan TK (1972) G.-6P.D. deficiency, typhoid, and co-trimoxazole (letter). Lancet 2:1258

Chang MJ, Dunkle LM, Van Reken D, Anderson D, Wong ML, Feigin RD (1977) Trimethoprim-sulfamethoxazole compared to ampicillin in the treatment of shigellosis. Pediatrics 59:726–729

Clementi KJ (1975) Treatment of Salmonella carriers with trimethoprim-sulfamethoxazole. Can Med Assoc J 112:S 28–S 32

Datta N, Richards H, Datta C (1981) *Salmonella typhi* in vivo acquires resistance to both chloramphenicol and co-trimoxazole. Lancet I:1181–1183

Dutta JK, Santhanam S, Misra BS, Ray SN (1978) Effect of trimethoprim-sulphamethoxazole in vibrio clearance in cholera (El Tor): a comparative study. Trans R Soc Trop Med Hyg 72:40–42

Eriksson M, Olcen P (1975) Septicaemia due to *Yersinia enterocolitica* in a non-compromised host. Scand J Infect Dis 7:78–80

Echeverria P, Ulyangco CV, Ho MT, Verhaert L, Komalarini S, Ørskov F (1978) Antimicrobial resistance and enterotoxin production among isolates of *Escherichia coli* in the Far East. Lancet 2:589–592

Finlayson M (1980) *Shigella sonnei* resistant to cotrimoxazole. Can Med Assoc J 123:718–719

Francis TI, Lewis EA, Oyediran ABOO et al. (1971) Effect of chemotherapy on the duration of diarrhoea, and on vibrio excretion by cholera patients. J Trop Med Hyg 74:172–176

Franzen C, Lindin-Janson G, Nygren B (1972) Trimethoprim-sulphamethoxazole in enteric infections. Scand J Infect Dis 4:231–240

Freerksen E, Rosenfeld M, Freerkson R, Krüger-Thiemer M (1977) Treatment of chronic salmonella carriers. Chemotherapy 23:192–210

Freiberg T (1971) Erfahrungen mit der Kombination Sulfamethoxazole + Trimethoprim bei der Behandlung von *Shigella-Flexner*-Erkrankungen. Arneim Forsch 21:599–600

Garcia de Olarte D, Trujillo SH, Agudelo ON, Nelson JD, Haltalin KC (1974) Treatment of diarrhea in malnourished infants and children: a double-blind study comparing ampicillin and placebo. Am J Dis Child 127:379–388

Geddes AM, Fothergill R, Goodall JAD, Dorken PR (1971) Evaluation of trimethoprim-sulphamethoxazole compound in treatment of salmonella infections. Br Med J 3:451–454

Geddes AM, Pugh RNH, Nye FJ (1975) Treatment and follow-up studies with co-trimoxazole in enteric fever and in typhoid carriers. J Antimicrob Chemother 1:51–54

Gharagozloo RA, Naficy K, Mouin M, Nassirzadeh MH, Yalda R (1970) Comparative trial of tetracycline, chloramphenicol, and trimethoprim/sulphamethoxazole in eradication of *Vibrio cholerae* El Tor. Br Med J 4:281–282

Gilman RH, Terminel M, Levine MM et al. (1975) Comparison of trimethoprim-sulfamethoxazole and amoxicillin in therapy of chloramphenicol-resistant and chloramphenicol-sensitive typhoid fever. J Infect Dis 132:630–636

Gordon RC, Thompson TR, Carlson W, Dyke JW, Stevens LI (1975) Antimicrobial resistance of shigellae isolated in Michigan. JAMA 231:1159–1161

Gutman LT, Wilfert MC, Quan T (1973) Susceptibility of Yersinia enterocolitica to trimethoprim-sulfamethoxazole. J Infect Dis [Suppl] 128:S 538

Hammerberg S, Sorger S, Marks MI (1977) Antimicrobial susceptibilities of *Yersinia enterocolitica* biotype 4, serotype 0:3. Antimicrob Agents Chemother 11:566–568

Hassan A, Hathout S, Safwat Y et al. (1975) A comparative evaluation of the treatment of typhoid fevers with co-trimoxazole and chloramphenicol in Egypt. J Trop Med Hyg 78:50–53

Herzog C (1976) Chemotherapy of typhoid fever: a review of literature. Infection 4:166–173

Jarvis KJ, Scrimgeour G (1970) In-vitro sensitivity of *Shigella sonnei* to trimethoprim and sulphamethoxazole. J Med Microbiol 3:554–557

Jacques PH, Van der Heyde H (1972) Combination of trimethoprim and sulphamethoxazole in typhoid fever. S Afr Med J 46:281–284

Kamat SA (1970) Evaluation of therapeutic efficacy of trimethoprim-sulphamethoxazole and chloramphenicol in enteric fever. Br Med J 3:320–322

Kazemi M, Gumpert TG, Marks MI (1973) A controlled trial comparing sulfamethoxazole-trimethoprim, ampicillin, and no therapy in the treatment of salmonella gastroenteritis in children. J Pediatr 83:646–650

Lexomboon J, Mansuwan P, Duangmani C, Benjadol P, McMinn MT (1972) Clinical evaluation of co-trimoxazole and furazolidone in treatment of shigellosis in children. Br Med J 3:23–26

Lexomboon U, Unkurapiana N (1978) Co-trimoxazole in the treatment of typhoid fever in children with glucose-6-phosphate dehydrogenase deficiency. Southeast Asian J Trop Med Public Health 9:576–580

Linh NN (1974) Typhoid fever treated with chloramphenicol and co-trimoxazole (letter). Lancet 2:1222

Mabadeje BAF (1974) A controlled clinical trial of trimethoprim-sulphamethoxazole in shigella dysentery. J Trop Med Hyg 77:50–54

MacDonald WB, Friday F, McEacharn M (1954) The effect of chloramphenicol in salmonella enteritis of infancy. Arch Dis Child 29:238–241

Mahapatra GB, Broacha ER, Toprani HT (1979) Enteric fevers in children – a prospective study on comparative evaluation of three drugs chloramphenicol, furazolidone and co-trimethoxazole. Indians Pediatr 16:259–265

Marks MI, Kazemi M, Hales B, Neims AH (1973 a) Pharmacokinetic studies of trimethoprim-sulfamethoxazole in children with gastroenteritis. J Infect Dis [Suppl] 128:S 622–S 625

Marks MI, Kazemi M, MacKay E (1973 b) In vitro sensitivity of Salmonella to ten antimicrobial agents including sulfamethoxazole and trimethoprim, alone and in combination. Antimicrob Agents Chemother 4:555–559

McCarthy LR, Chmel H, Bell G, Armstrong D (1977) Thymidine-dependent strain of Salmonella oslo selected by trimethoprim-sulfamethoxazole therapy. Am J Clin Path 68:307–310

McKendrick MW, Geddes AM, Farrell ID (1981) Trimethoprim in enteric fever. Br Med J 282:364

Merson MH, Morris GK, Sack DA et al. (1976) Travelers' diarrhea in Mexico, a prospective study of physicians and family members attending a congress. N Engl J Med 294:1299–1305

Meyer HA (1973) Acute haemolysis associated with typhoid fever and G.-6-P.D. deficiency (letter). Lancet 2:729–730

Nelson JD, Kusmiesz H, Jackson LH (1976 a) Comparison of trimethoprim-sulfamethoxazole and ampicillin therapy for shigellosis in ambulatory patients. J Pediatr 89:491–493

Nelson JD, Kusmiesz H, Jackson LH, Woodman E (1976 b) Trimethoprim-sulfamethoxazole therapy for shigellosis. JAMA 235:1239–1243

Nelson JD, Kusmiesz H, Jackson LH, Woodman E (1980) Treatment of salmonella gastroenteritis with ampicillin, amoxicillin, or placebo. Pediatrics 65:1125–1130

Northrup RS, Doyle MA, Feeley JC (1972) In vitro susceptibility of El Tor and classical Vibrio cholerae strains to trimethoprim and sulfamethoxazole. Antimicrob Agents Chemother 1:310–314

Olarte J, Galindo E (1973) Salmonella typhi resistant to chloramphenicol, ampicillin and other antimicrobial agents: strains isolated during an extensive typhoid fever epidemic in Mexico. Antimicrob Agents Chemother 4:596–601

Omer AMI (1975) Trimethoprim-sulphamethoxazole in the treatment of enteric fever. J Trop Med Hyg 78:162–166

Owusu SK (1972) Acute haemolysis complicating co-trimoxazole therapy for typhoid fever in a patient with G.-6-P.D. deficiency (letter). Lancet 2:819

Pastore G, Rizzo G, Fera G, Schiraldi O (1977) Trimethoprim-sulphamethoxazole in the treatment of cholera. Chemotherapy 23:121–128

Pettersson T, Klemola E, Wagner O (1964) Treatment of acute cases of salmonella infection and salmonella carriers with ampicillin and neomycin. Acta Med Scand 175:185–190

Pichler H, Knothe H, Spitzy KH, Vielkind G (1973) Treatment of chronic carriers of Salmonella typhi and Salmonella paratyphi B with trimethoprim-sulfamethoxazole. J Infect Dis [Suppl] 128:S 743–S 744

Pinney RJ, Smith JT (1973) Joint trimethoprim and sulphamethoxazole resistance in bacteria infected with R factors. J Med Microbiol 6:13–19

Ramachandran S, Godfrey JJ, Lionel NDW (1978) A comparative trial of co-trimoxazole and chloramphenicol in typhoid and paratyphoid fever. J Trop Med Hyg 81:36–39

Richards H, Datta N (1981) Transposons and trimethoprim-resistance. Br Med J 282:1118–1119

Richards H, Datta N, Sojka WJ, Wray C (1978) Trimethoprim-resistance plasmids and transposons in salmonellae. Lancet II:1194–1195

Rudoy RE, Nelson JD, Haltalin KC (1974) In vitro susceptibility of shigella strains to trimethoprim and sulfamethoxazole. Antimicrob Agents Chemother 5:439–443

Sardesai HV, Karandikar RS, Harkshe RG (1973) Comparative trial of Co-trimoxazole and chloramphenicol in typhoid fever. Br Med J I:82–83

Sarkis-Kechiche VJ (1980) Bericht über die erfolgreiche Behandlung von elf weiblichen Salmonellenausscheidern mit Co-soltrim. Wien Med Wochensch 130:489–491

Scragg JN, Rubidge CJ (1971) Trimethoprim and sulphamethoxazole in typhoid fever in children. Br Med J 3:738–741

Smith ER, Bradley BWD (1971) Treatment of Salmonella enteritis and its effect on the carrier state. Can Med Assoc J 104:1004–1006

Smith HW (1980) Antibiotic-resistant *Escherichia coli* in market pigs in 1956–1979: the emergence of organisms with plasmid-borne trimethoprim resistance. J Hyg (Lond) 84:467–477

Snyder MJ, Perroni J, Gonzalez O et al. (1973) Trimethoprim-sulfamethoxazole in the treatment of typhoid and paratyphoid fevers. J Infect Dis [Suppl] 128:S 734–S 737

Snyder MJ, Perroni J, Gonzalez O et al. (1976) Comparative efficacy of chloramphenicol, ampicillin, and co-trimoxazole in the treatment of typhoid fever. Lancet 2:1155–1157

Taylor DE, Keystone JS, Devlin HR (1980) Resistance to trimethoprim and other antibiotics in Ontario Shigellae (letter). Lancet 1:426

Thóren A (1980) Antibiotic sensitivity of enteropathogenic *Escherichia coli* to mecillinam, trimethoprim-sulfamethoxazole and other antibiotics. Acta Pathol Microbiol Scand [B] 88:265–268

Thóren A, Wolde-Mariam T, Stintzing G, Wadström T, Habte D (1980) Antibiotic in the treatment of gastroenteritis caused by enteropathogenic *Escherichia coli*. J Infect Dis 141:27–31

Threlfall EJ, Ward LR, Ashley AS, Rowe B (1980) Plasmid-encoded trimethoprim resistance in multi-resistant epidemic *Salmonella typhimurium* phage types 204 and 193 in Britain. Br Med J I:1210–1211

Threfall EJ, Ward LR, Rowe B (1978) Spread of multiresistant strains of *Salmonella typhimurium* phage types 204 and 193 in Britain. Br Med J II:997

Titze W (1971) Resistenzbestimmungen bei Erregern der Bakterienruhr unter Berücksichtigung von Sulfamethoxazole-Trimethoprim. Arzneim Forsch 21:597–598

Westerman EL, Christensen RP (1979) Chronic *Isospora belli* infection treated with co-trimoxazole. Ann Intern Med 91:413–414

CHAPTER 18

Prostatitis

T.A. STAMEY

A. Introduction

Prostatitis is a common and frustrating problem for the patient, the general practitioner, and the urologist. It is a difficult subject to review because much of the literature is so imprecise as to definition of the disease and acceptable diagnostic techniques that most of the available data are impossible to interpret. In truth, the term prostatitis has been a "wastebasket" diagnosis for any patient with unexplained pelvic, genitourinary, or ejaculatory symptoms whose prostate appears tender on examination. There is no generally accepted definition, no clearly established criteria for making the diagnosis, and no definite pathophysiology. The incidence of prostatitis is unclear. One of the greatest problems confronted in reviewing the literature is the multiplicity of patient types which are considered as having prostatitis by various authors without any objective criteria for making the diagnosis. Moreover, the findings used to diagnose prostatitis, even in the most thoughtful studies, are so nonspecific that refutation of these studies is easy because it can be shown that selected patients are in most ways no different from some healthy adult men among the general population. Because very few authors have defined prostatitis, and almost no two works used the same criteria for inclusion of patients within a study, few direct comparisons can be made of the findings of one author with those of another. Indeed, except for true bacterial prostatitis due to Enterobacteriaceae, pseudomonas, and enterococci, which is invariably associated with recurrent bacteriuria and which most of this review will concentrate upon, it is fair to comment that little more is known about prostatitis than was presented by HUGH H. YOUNG in 1906 (YOUNG et al. 1906).

B. Classification and Description of Patient Categories

Precisely because of the difficulties discussed in Sect. A, DRACH, MEARES, FAIR, and STAMEY proposed a classification of prostatitis in 1978 which is presented in Table 1 (DRACH et al. 1978). As can be seen in this table, the distinguishing features of this classification are that acute and chronic bacterial prostatitis are always characterized by recurrent bacteriuria, and the responsible organism can be recovered from the prostate once the bacteriuria has cleared, while nonbacterial prostatitis is never associated with urinary tract infection (bacteriuria) nor can any etiologic agent be identified as the cause of the inflammatory reaction in the prostate. Prostatodynia is a term applied to a subset of patients with symptoms identical to those with nonbacterial prostatitis, but who have no evidence of inflammatory disease in their prostatic fluid.

In acute bacterial prostatitis, the infection often begins with malaise, fever, and myalgias several days before local prostatic inflammation produces symptoms of urinary frequency, urgency, dysuria, and ultimately obstructive voiding often requiring catheterization for acute retention. On rectal examination, the prostate is often irregular, hard, and even suggestive of prostatic cancer, rectal findings which gradually return to normal with subsidence of the inflammation. The bladder urine is infected almost invariably within 24 h of the lower tract symptoms. BRUCE and FOX (1960) reviewed 78 cases of acute prostatitis and 13 cases of prostatic abscess treated over a 5-year period at St. Peter's and St. Paul's Hospitals in London in 1960. Except for a handful of cases preceded by urologic instrumentation or injection of hemorrhoids, no etiologic factor could be demonstrated in 86 of the patients who, in fact, enjoyed excellent health prior to the onset of their infection (BRUCE and FOX 1960). The status of the prostate is not described in this paper, but those with prostatic abscess were found to have a "softened" area in the prostate. The mean age of these patients was 45 years, the predominant infecting strain was *Escherichia coli*, and the length of illness as well as the incidence of prostatic recurrences was proportional to the type of antimicrobial therapy, with sulfonamides alone yielding the worst results.

In chronic bacterial prostatitis, by contrast, symptoms are limited to those associated with the bladder or renal infection, the prostate is always normal to palpation, and appears normal upon cystoscopic examination. While the symptoms are usually limited to the acute onset of dysuria and frequency, recurrent bacteriuria in these patients can be asymptomatic. The prostate is not tender to palpation; the diagnosis can only be made by bacteriologically proving the site of bacterial persistence to be the prostate at a time when the urine is sterile. Bacterial persistence in the prostate, after sterilizing the urine and stopping antimicrobial therapy, is characterized by bacteriuric recurrences with the same pathogen at time intervals varying between 48 h and 6 months after stopping antimicrobial therapy (STAMEY 1980). While the infecting bacteria in both acute and chronic bacterial prostatitis are usually members of the Enterobacteriaceae family, pseudomonas as well enterococci are also responsible for prostatic infections (STAMEY 1980). The incidence of acute and chronic bacterial prostatitis is unknown, but since they represent the major cause of recurrent bacteriuria in males (STAMEY 1980), the prevalence rate probably approaches that of bacteriuria in males which is less than 1% of males below the age of 50 years, but 1%–3% above 60 years (FREEDMAN et al. 1965).

"Nonbacterial" prostatitis ("abacterial" prostatitis) and prostatodynia (Table 1) are characterized by a variety of pelvic symptoms which in general may be characterized as urinary, ejaculatory, or referred pain. The pain may be suprapubic, infrapubic, perineal, inguinal, scrotal, or low back discomfort. These patients never have bacteriuria. The cause of the inflammatory reaction in the expressed prostatic secretion (EPS) of patients with nonbacterial prostatitis is unknown.

Prostatodynia is a term of exclusion reserved for those patients who have pelvic symptomatology similar to patients with nonbacterial prostatitis, but who have no

Table 1. Clinical classification of prostatitis (STAMEY 1980)

	Evidence of inflammation (EPS)	Culture positive (EPS)	Culture positive (bladder)	Common etiologic bacteria	Rectal examination (prostata)
Acute bacterical prostatitis	+	+	+[a]	Entero-bacteriaceae	Abnormal
Chronic bacterial prostatitis	+	+	+[b]	Entero-bacteriaceae	Normal
Nonbacterical prostatitis	+	0	0	?	Normal
Prostatodynia	0	0	0	0	Normal

[a] Acute bacterial prostatitis is nearly always accompanied by bladder infection
[b] Characterized by reccurrent bacteriuria, at varying intervals up to several months, after stopping antimicrobial therapy

evidence of inflammatory reaction in their EPS. According to NILSSON et al. (1975), many of these patients with prostatodynia have serious personality disturbances and problems with sex identification, but it is not known whether psychiatric counseling is beneficial or not.

Because the distinction between nonbacterial prostatitis and prostatodynia rests exclusively with the number of inflammatory leukocytes in the EPS, the number of leukocytes characteristic of normal EPS in healthy males free of urinary tract disease is important. The observations reported by BLACKLOCK (1969), PFAU et al. (1978), and ANDERSON and WELLER (1979) have led me to estimate that 12 white blood cells (WBC) per high power field of the microscope in a cover slip examination of EPS should include 95% of all normal controls (STAMEY 1980). Using a Fuchs-Rosenthal counting chamber, ANDERSON and WELLER (1979) reported that 1,165 WBC/mm^3 includes 2.5 standard deviations of a carefully selected, control group of healthy men; in this detailed and quantitative study, 40 men with nonbacterial prostatitis had a five-fold increase in the number of leukocytes in their EPS in comparison with 20 healthy controls; histiocytes (oval fat macrophages), also characteristic of inflammation in the EPS, were increased eight-fold in these patients. JAMESON (1967) reported that EPS from healthy men obtained within 48 h of ejaculation contained between 10 and 20 WBC per high power field in the cover slip examination (JAMESON 1967); these observations remain to be confirmed and could be due to the confusion of unseparated spermatids from the seminal fluid with polymorphonuclear leukocytes as well as the confusion of early spermatids from the ejaculate with lymphocytes (COUTURE et al. 1976).

While general or family practice studies on the incidence of males with nonbacterial prostatitis and prostatodynia are needed to establish the prevalence of this syndrome, the clinical impression is that it exceeds by many times the incidence of males with recurrent bacteriuria, which represents the maximal incidence of true bacterial prostatitis. Because of these substantial differences in prevalence, most of the literature on "prostatitis" relates mainly to either nonbacterial prostatitis or to prostatodynia. Unfortunately, however, even in the more careful studies such as those carried out by the University of Lund group in Sweden (COLLEEN and

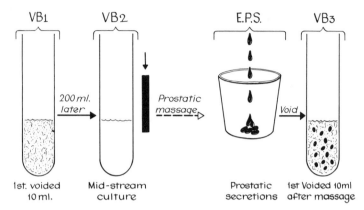

Fig. 1. Illustration of the technique for obtaining segmented cultures of the lower urinary tract in the male. With this technique, bacterial persistence in the prostate can be distinguished from persistence in the urethra as foci of recurrent urinary tract infections (MEARES and STAMEY 1968)

MÅRDH 1975), their term "nonacute prostatitis" also included some patients who probably had chronic bacterial prostatitis. It is this failure to separate true bacterial prostatitis from nonbacterial prostatitis and prostatodynia (Table 1), of which the latter conditions constitute the vast majority of cases, that makes a review of the literature very difficult. Despite these limitations, there are a number of contributions which have added significantly to our knowledge.

C. Acute and Chronic Bacterial Prostatitis

I. Diagnosis

STAMEY et al. (1965) called attention to the value of segmenting the voided urinary stream into urethral (VB$_1$ for "voided bladder one"), midstream (VB$_2$), and post prostatic massage (VB$_3$) urine aliquots in the presence of a sterile, midstream urine in order to separate urethral from prostatic infection. MEARES and STAMEY (1968), however, documented the importance of a direct culture of the EPS when the VB$_1$ and VB$_3$ urine aliquots were equivalent in bacterial numbers, and further emphasized the usefulness of antibacterial therapy – especially nitrofurantoin and oral penicillin G – as diagnostic tools in clearing the urethra of prostatic organisms; they further demonstrated the reproducibility of these culture techniques in longitudinal studies on patients with recurrent bacteriuria who had bacterial persistence in the prostate. Figure 1, taken from their 1968 paper, illustrates the culture technique while Table 2 shows several diagnostic examples, both on and off antimicrobial therapy. The critical observation rests with the demonstration that the numbers of bacteria recovered in the EPS or VB$_3$ must not be accounted for by similar bacteria added to these prostatic aliquots from the urethral mucosa. The most indisputable localization studies show that bacteria are absent from the VB$_1$ and VB$_2$, but present in the EPS or VB$_3$; antimicrobial agents like nitrofurantoin or oral penicillin G, which will not affect the organisms in the prostate, are often

Table 2. Examples of bacteriologic localization cultures to the prostate in several men on and off antimicrobial therapy

Patient	Antibiotic	VB$_1$	VB$_2$	EPS	VB$_3$	Organism
1	Yes	0	0	5,000	100	*Escherichia coli*
1	Yes	50	10	10,000	1,500	*Escherichia coli*
2	Yes	120	0	3,600	370	*Escherichia coli*
2	No	2,000	200	100,000	4,000	*Escherichia coli*
3	No	60	20	2,000	40	*Escherichia coli*
3	Yes	20	0	10,000	180	*Escherichia coli*
3	Yes	100	0	1,000	10	*Escherichia coli*
4	Yes	670	0	100,000	1,200	*Escherichia coli*
4	Yes	10	0	1,900	30	*Escherichia coli*
5	Yes	250	20	5,000	330	*Klebsiella* sp.
5	No	0	0	50	0	*Klebsiella* sp.
5	No	20	0	10,000	2,000	*Klebsiella* sp.
6	Yes	90	0	800	20	*Escherichia coli*
6	No	10	0	1,000	20	*Escherichia coli*
7	Yes	0	0	1,000	0	*enterococci*
7	Yes	20	0	4,000	10	*enterococci*
8	Yes	0	0	660	190	*Escherichia coli*
		10	0	400	40	*Aerobacter aerogenes*
		0	0	500	20	*Proteus mirabilis*
		0	0	200	0	*Proteus morgani*
8	Yes	50	0	165	150	*Escherichia coli*
		0	0	50	20	*Escherichia aerogenes*
		0	0	560	50	*Proteus mirabilis*
		0	0	140	0	*Proteus morgani*
9	Yes	20	0	5,000	50	*Klebsiella* sp.
9	Yes	50	0	100,000	1,000	*Klebsiella* sp.
10	No	60	0	1,000	20	*Escherichia coli*
10	No	640	40	100,000	220	*Escherichia coli*

required for this demonstration. Long-term follow-up studies of 10 years or more on many of these patients with chronic bacterial prostatitis have been published (STAMEY 1980).

All of the reports from Stanford, including the therapeutic trials of MEARES (1973a, 1979) have been on patients with recurrent bacteriuria due to strains of Enterobacteriaceae, pseudomonas, or enterococci. DRACH (1974), however, using the same collection technique as in the figure, reported a very high proportion of gram-positive organisms (37% *Staphylococcus epidermidis*, 21% α-hemolytic streptococci, and 12% diphtheroids) in 153 localizations in 85 patients, organisms considered by the Stanford group to be urethral contaminants. For example, data are not available to show that therapy with urinary antimicrobial agents like nitrofurantoin or oral penicillin G sterilizes the urethra while demonstrating positive EPS or VB$_3$ cultures. There is also the possibility that the more viscous EPS, as it traverses the urethra and the fossa navicularis, with its high concentration of normal urethral flora, adsorbs greater numbers of normal, indigenous urethral flora, thereby giving a falsely positive EPS culture (STAMEY 1980).

For those few patients from whom one cannot obtain either EPS or a cloudy VB_3 containing EPS, cultures of the seminal fluid can be obtained by ejaculation (MOBLEY 1975). With this technique, however, a sterile VB_1 must be demonstrated prior to ejaculation because massage of the distal urethra which accompanies masturbation produces far more urethral bacteria onto the urethral lumen to contaminate the seminal fluid than are present in the normal voiding of a VB_1 aliquot.

II. Pathology

In 1937, MOORE studied 581 unselected prostates at autopsy from men between 20 and 90 years of age; each prostate was studied microscopically in 4 mm step sections for the presence of inflammation. It was found that 36 (6.3%) showed typical histologic changes of acute or chronic inflammation, 26 of which were considered clear examples of ascending ductal inflammation. The incidence of inflammation was related to increasing age, being 16.3% in patients 81–90 years old (MOORE 1937). MOORE also called attention to several noninfectious causes of cellular infiltrate, including sclerotic atrophy and ductal obstruction.

The classic studies of MCNEAL (1968, 1972), who divided the true prostate (as opposed to the periurethral elements of benign hyperplasia) into the central and peripheral zones, showed a substantially greater frequency of inflammation in the peripheral zone. The anatomic and functional factors which theoretically might allow greater involvement of the peripheral zone in an ascending infection have been pointed out (BLACKLOCK 1974).

While the pathologic entity of granulomatous prostatitis can be caused by tuberculosis and fungi, a much more common cause is resolving acute bacterial prostatitis, where the prostate is grossly distorted by the inflammatory reaction (STAMEY 1980); the granulomatous reaction is possibly from the extravasated prostatic secretions (possibly lipids) as suggested by KELALIS et al. (1965) in the Mayo Clinic series of patients with granulomatous prostatitis.

III. Prostatic Immunoglobulins

Immunoglobulins IgG and IgA in noninfected prostatic fluid were first reported by CHODIRKER and TOMASI (1963); in 17 samples of EPS, they observed a mean concentration for IgA of 26 mg/100 ml and 157 mg/100 ml for IgG. GRAY et al. (1974), using radial immunodiffusion agar plates, quantitated the total amount of IgG, IgA, and IgM in EPS from 33 controls and 48 patients with prostatitis; it is estimated that about one-half of these patients had true bacterial prostatitis while the other half had nonbacterial prostatitis (N.J. BLACKLOCK, 10 January 1979, personal communication). Although IgA was measured with antiserum raised against human serum, immunoelectrophoretic analysis suggested that only secretory IgA was present in their normal reference group as well as in the "chronic cases." In the normal group, these authors reported a mean of 38 mg/100 ml for IgG, 12 mg/100 ml for IgA, and 14 mg/100 ml for IgM. Their patients with "unresolved" prostatitis, most of whom were probably chronic bacterial prostatitis, showed a three-fold increase in IgG above the normal reference group, a seven-fold increase in IgA (85 mg/100 ml) and a 2.5-fold rise in IgM. In those patients whose prostatitis was thought to have resolved, IgG returned to normal levels, while both IgA and IgM remained at concentrations twice normal. These authors felt that the large increase of IgA over the normal level expected in EPS was a sensitive indicator of challenge by a foreign bacterial antigen (GRAY et al. 1974).

Using direct immunofluorescence of normal human prostatic tissue, ABLIN et al. (1971) observed IgG and IgA in secretory granules lying within the ductular lumen; surprisingly, IgG was observed in the basal portion of the cytoplasm of secretory epithelial cells, but the authors were unable to show IgA in epithelial cells, even though it was noted occasionally in plasma cells within the stroma. MEARES (1977) has reported bacterial agglutination titers in the serum of patients with chronic bacterial prostatitis and compared these titers with both normal controls and patients whose urethra was colonized with Enterobacteriaceae; he later reported longitudinal studies on serum antibody titers in the treatment of chronic bacterial prostatitis with trimethoprim/sulfamethoxazole (MEARES 1978). A few patients failed to show significant titers, probably because bacterial agglutination primarily measures IgM rather than IgG or IgA. Serum and prostatic fluid agglutinins have also been reported in 60 patients against strains of staphylococci considered to be prostatic in origin (MAGED and KHAFAGA 1965); bacteriologic documentation that these staphylococci were prostatic rather than urethral in origin did not accompany this report.

At Stanford, we have modified the solid phase radioimmunoassay developed by ZOLLINGER et al. (1976) and his associates to measure antigen-specific antibodies against a purified meningococcal antigen. Using formalin-fixed whole bacterial antigen isolated from the prostate, we have followed patients longitudinally with acute and chronic bacterial prostatitis, measuring antigen-specific secretory IgA and IgG antibodies in both their EPS and serum (SHORTLIFFE et al. 1981a and b). We have shown that antigen-specific secretory IgA in EPS is several hundred times greater than that in the serum, leaving little doubt that the source of the IgA is a local immune response. The immunologic response in the serum is mainly IgG, but it so exceeds the antigen-specific antibodies in normal serum from healthy control volunteers that these IgG-specific antibodies against Enterobacteriaceae antigen represent a sensitive diagnostic indicator of true bacterial prostatitis. EPS from normal volunteers has virtually no detectable antigen-specific antibody against E. coli; we have shown that patients with chronic bacterial prostatitis have 10,000 times more antigen-specific IgA in their EPS than we can measure in control volunteers.

IV. The Antibacterial Factor in Prostatic Fluid

During the course of experimental studies at Stanford on the diffusion of antimicrobial agents from plasma to prostatic fluid in the dog in the mid-1960s, we observed that canine prostatic fluid appeared remarkably sterile, despite casual laboratory handling at room temperature. Because of this observation, we added E. coli and other Entrobacteriaceae to canine prostatic fluid which showed substantial bactericidal activity (STAMEY et al. 1968). When we added E. coli to VB_2

and VB_3 urines obtained from normal human males, we observed a similar bactericidal activity in the VB_3 urine (which contained human prostatic fluid) as had occurred in the canine prostatic secretion; the VB_2 aliquot (the midstream urine without prostatic fluid) supported growth of bacteria (STAMEY et al. 1968). We were unaware until much later that YOUMANS et al. (1938), also investigating the bactericidal action of urinary antiseptics in dogs, had also observed and studied canine prostatic fluid for its antibacterial activity. FAIR et al. (1976), in a laborious effort to identify the antimicrobial substance, have shown it to be zinc; of equal importance, they have demonstrated that men with chronic bacterial prostatitis average only 50 µg/ml zinc in their EPS compared with control levels in healthy volunteers of about 450 µg/ml. They have further observed that serum levels of zinc were normal in patients with chronic bacterial prostatitis and, what is often ignored in clinical practice, that oral exogenous zinc did not change the markedly depressed levels of zinc in the EPS of patients with chronic bacterial prostatitis (FAIR et al. 1976). In an experimental extension of these data, LEVY and FAIR (1973) localized a similar activity in the EPS from the dorsolateral lobe of the rat's prostate. FRIEDLANDER et al. (1972) observed that experimental pyelonephritis in the male rat was sustained by bacterial prostatitis which spared the dorsolateral lobe of the prostate and mainly involved the ventral lobe where LEVY and FAIR (1973) found minimal antimicrobial activity. EPS has also been shown to be inhibitory to *Candida albicans* (GIP and MOLIN 1970). Human semen has also been shown to have antibacterial activity against several bacterial species (TALLGREN et al. 1968).

V. Treatment

Clinical observations in the 1960s clearly showed that sensitive strains of Enterobacteriaceae were persisting in the prostatic fluid, despite serum levels of bactericidal antimicrobial agents which exceeded the minimal inhibitory concentration of the infecting bacteria by severalfold (MEARES and STAMEY 1968; STAMEY 1972). We suspected that antimicrobial drugs were not penetrating into the prostatic fluid. While we did not know then, nor now, whether the site of bacterial persistence involved the interstitial tissue of the prostate, we were certain that some of the bacteria were in the secretory fluid, because of the culture methodology (Table 2). We turned to a simple model in the dog, where the diffusion characteristics of antimicrobial agents from the plasma across noninflamed glandular epithelium of the canine prostate could be investigated. The ureters were separated from the bladder to prevent urinary contamination of prostatic secretions, the vas deferens was ligated from each testis to exclude secretions from that source, and the bladder neck was ligated to seal off bladder secretions. After establishing plasma levels by intravenous infusion of antimicrobial agents, secretion of prostatic fluid was stimulated by intravenous pilocarpine, which usually resulted in rapid prostatic fluid flow rates. The concentrations of nine antimicrobial agents in plasma, urine and prostatic fluid, studied in 16 dogs was first reported in 1968 (WINNINGHAM et al. 1968). The diffusion of sulfonamides (WINNINGHAM and STAMEY 1970), tetracyclines (HESSL and STAMEY 1971), and, when it became available later, trimethoprim (GRANATO et al. 1973) were studied in succession. These results are summarized in Table 3.

Table 3. Diffusion gradients between plasma and prostatic fluid in the dog and the physico-chemical characteristics that determine diffusion (STAMEY 1980)

Antimicrobial drug	Plasma (μg/ml)	Prostatic fluid (μg/ml)	Acid or Base	Lipid soluble at at pH 7.4	pK$_a$	Unchanged in Plasma (%)
Penicillin G	62	< 0.2[a]	Acid	No	2.7	0.001
Ampicillin	54	< 0.2[a]	Acid	No	2.5	0.001
Cephalothin	63	< 0.4[a]	Acid	No	2.5	0.001
Nitrofurantoin	15	3.2	Acid	Sligthly	7.2	39.0
Nalidixic acid	53	< 5.0[a]	Acid	Yes	6.0	4.0
Sulfisoxazole	15	0.3	Acid	Yes	5.0	0.4
Sulfamethoxazole	12.6	1.3	Acid	Yes	6.0	4.0
Sulfadimidine	8.5	4.6	Acid	Yes	7.7	67.0
Oxytetracylcine	10	< 2.0[a]	Amphoteric	No	3.5, 7.6, 9.2	
Tetracycline	19	4.0	Amphoteric	Partially	3.3, 7.7, 9.7	
Polymyxin B	14	< 0.5[a]	Base	No	8.9	8.0
Kanamycin	41	< 2.0[a]	Base	No	7.2	39.0
Erythromycin	16	38.0	Base	Yes	8.8	4.0
Oleandomycin	12	39.0	Base	Yes	8.5	8.0
Trimethoprim	4	7.0	Base	Yes	7.3	56.0

[a] Indicates the lower limits of sensitivity of the bioassay

As can be seen, most of the useful antimicrobial agents against gram-negative bacteria which cause urinary infections were either undetectable in prostatic fluid or present in subinhibitory concentrations, even in the presence of pathologic plasma levels from the intravenous infusion. The surprising diffusion and concentration of the basic macrolides, erythromycin, and oleandomycin, represented the key to recognizing the importance of lipid solubility, pK$_a$, and whether the antimicrobial agent was an acid or a base in terms of ion trapping in the more acidic prostatic fluid (WINNINGHAM et al. 1968). The sulfonamides, for example, diffused from the plasma into prostatic fluid in direct proportion to their pK$_a$, suggesting that their lipid solubility differences were insignificant in terms of diffusion (WINNINGHAM and STAMEY 1970). In the early studies with the basic macrolides, erythromycin and oleandomycin, the ion trapping of these bases in prostatic fluid could not be maintained at rapid rates of prostatic secretion (WINNINGHAM et al. 1968). Trimethoprim, on the other hand, always showed concentrations in prostatic fluid which exceeded the plasma level, regardless of prostatic fluid flow rates; indeed, when trimethoprim and pilocarpine were injected intravenously in the same syringe, the first prostatic fluid to appear moments later always showed ion trapping of trimethoprim which substantially exceeded the plasma levels (GRANTO et al. 1973); for example, with the simultaneous administration of pilocarpine and trimethoprim, the prostatic fluid obtained during the first 15 min after injection showed prostatic fluid: serum ratios of trimethoprim as high as 8.3:1. Moreover, without further trimethoprim administration, these diffusion gradients were maintained even after 3 h continuous prostatic fluid secretion.

So impressed were we with these gradients of trimethoprim concentration in prostatic fluid over serum levels, that we designed experiments to exclude an active transport system by the prostatic glandular epithelium for pumping trimethoprim from plasma into prostatic fluid (STAMEY et al. 1973). In these latter experiments, enormous intravenous doses of trimethoprim were given to the dog without demonstrating saturation of an active transport system. In addition, with careful arterial and prostatic fluid pH measurements, the established diffusion gradient between plasma and prostatic fluid was always less than the theoretical, expected diffusion. The differences in diffusion gradients between the basic macrolides and trimethoprim is probably related to the small fraction of uncharged molecules of the basic macrolides available for diffusion.

REEVES and GHILCHIK (1970), on the basis of the earlier studies by WINNINGHAM et al. (1968), were the first to study the diffusion of trimethoprim. Further studies by REEVES et al. (1973) showed that 7-chlorolincomycin was concentrated in prostatic fluid, in comparison with serum, and that lincomycin and chloramphenicol achieved concentrations in prostatic fluid equal to that of serum. BAUMUELLER and MADSEN (1977) compared the diffusion of trimethoprim, sulfamethoxazole, erythromycin, doxycycline, and ampicillin before and after the induction of bacterial prostatitis in dogs with an *E. coli* 06 injected into a branch of the prostatic artery; erythromycin appeared to concentrate better in prostatic fluid after inducing prostatitis, while trimethoprim also showed an increased concentration which was not statistically significant. Prostatic fluid pH in these animals appeared to be reduced after prostatic infection. When trimethoprim and sulfamethoxazole concentrations were measured in homogenized prostatic tissue obtained at the time of prostatectomy in humans, trimethoprim averaged 8.2 µg/g in prostatic tissue compared with a simultaneous plasma level of 4.0 µg/ml; sulfamethoxazole achieved one-third the concentration of biologically active drug in the prostate of that which occurred in the plasma (DABHOIWALA et al. 1976). In our canine studies (STAMEY et al. 1973), prostatic tissue concentrations exceeded the serum levels by about four-fold at a time when the prostatic fluid levels were nine times greater than the serum concentration. While one might assume that the four-fold increase in tissue concentration was due to ion trapping in the prostatic fluid, it is interesting that the levels in the canine lung tissue also exceeded the serum by four-fold, just as much as the prostatic tissue (STAMEY et al. 1973). The mechanism of trimethoprim concentration in lung tissue is unknown, but presumably the bronchial secretions in these experiments must have been more acidic than plasma.

Because of these substantial concentrations of trimethoprim in prostatic fluid produced by ion trapping, trimethoprim appeared to be the ideal antimicrobial drug for the treatment of chronic bacterial prostatitis. Using trimethoprim/sulfamethoxazole (TMP/SMX) at a dosage of 160 mg TMP and 800 mg SMX twice a day for 14 days, two of 13 patients were cured with sterile monthly cultures for 6 months after therapy; an additional nine patients had EPS cultures which were sterile while on therapy (MEARES 1973a). Because of the apparent sterilization of the EPS during therapy in these 9 patients, 19 patients then received full dosage therapy for 12 weeks: 6 were cured (32%) and 8 had sterile EPS during therapy but the infection recurred after treatment (MEARES 1979). If 4 of the failures from these 19 patients are excluded because they also failed the initial 14-day course, the cure rate was 40% (STAMEY 1980). SMITH et al. (1979) randomized 30 male patients, all of whom had antibody-coated bacteria in their urine and one-half of whom were proven to have prostatic infection, to either 10 days or 12 weeks of TMP/SMX therapy: 9 of 15 were cured on the 12-week course (60%) while 3 of 15 were cured on the 10-day course ($P = 0.06$). These data suggest that a prolonged course of full-dosage TMP/SMX for 12 weeks will cure about one-half of the patients with chronic bacterial prostatitis, provided the infecting organism is sensitive to TMP. If the infecting organism is recovered from EPS during the first weeks of therapy, it is pointless to continue treatment (MEARES 1979). When TMP/SMX fails, a 10–14 day course of kanamycin is worthwhile; we reported one documented cure (STAMEY 1972) while PFAU and SACHS (1976) have added two others.

The question arises as to why 50% of patients fail TMP/SMX therapy, even though this success rate far exceeded previous experience with other antimicrobial agents. In the presence of prostatic calcifications, the bacteria could persist inside prostatic stones just as they do in renal struvite calculi (STAMEY and NEMOY 1971). Others have presented evidence that prostatic calculi can become secondarily infected (MEARS 1974; EYKYN et al. 1974), but even in such cases, the prostatic tissue per se is usually infected as well. Nonetheless, it is possible that secondary infection of these prostatic stones may prevent antimicrobial cure of the prostatic infection. Since most patients with bacterial prostatitis do not have radiologically detectable calcifications, it is possible that the mucoprotein matrix of corpora amylacea, present in every prostate (SMITH 1966), could serve as a nidus of bacterial persistence in some of these patients.

Failure is clearly not due to development of bacterial resistance. Dr. S.R.M. BUSHBY at the Wellcome Laboratories, Research Triangle Park, North Carolina, determined the minimal inhibitory concentrations for each of the infecting strains causing chronic bacterial prostatitis in the 15 patients from Stanford who received TMP/SMX for 12 weeks (MEARES 1979; STAMEY 1980). These data show that neither the cures, the improved cases (those whose EPS was sterile during therapy), nor the bacteriologic failures could be explained by in vitro sensitivities. Except for a single naturally resistant *Pseudomonas aeruginosa*, all of the infecting strains were sensitive to 0.5 µg/ml TMP or less, regardless of the bacteriologic result; SMX resistance occurred in three of the six cures and in none of the four failures (STAMEY 1980). Moreover, there was no significant change in the sensitivity of the strains during or after therapy with TMP/SMX.

YOUNG (1906), LUDWIK (1964), BLACKLOCK and BEAVIS (1974), ANDERSON and FAIR (1976), and PFAU et al. (1978) have all shown that the pH of prostatic fluid is alkaline in the presence of inflammatory leukocytes in the EPS. With resolution of the inflammatory reaction, BLACKLOCK and BEAVIS (1974) and PFAU et al. (1978) showed a fall in the alkaline pH to more acidic levels. BLACKLOCK and BEAVIS (1974) and PFAU et al. (1978) believe that EPS from normal, healthy men is acid (the mean pH was 6.4 in BLACKLOCK and BEAVIS' study) but ANDERSON and FAIR (1976), collecting EPS from men who had not voided for several hours to avoid contamination with urine, reported a pH of 7.6 in older men (mean age 50 years). FAIR et al. (1979) argue that an alkaline pH of the EPS in patients with chronic bacterial prostatitis might explain the clinical failure of therapy with TMP/SMX, which I have already shown is 40%–60%. It is true that since TMP is a base, ion trapping of TMP cannot occur in an alkaline EPS, but since 50% of the TMP molecules are uncharged in plasma, these un-ionized molecules should diffuse into the EPS and approximate the plasma level at equilibrium. Since plasma concentrations of TMP are by no means insignificant (about 1.7 µg/ml TMP 2 h after 160 mg/ 800 mg SMX with a serum half-life of 10 h for TMP), the concentration of uncharged TMP, even in alkaline EPS should be at least 0.5 µg/ml. It should be noted that the MIC of TMP to all the 15 infecting organisms treated for 12 weeks at Stanford (MEARES 1979; STAMEY 1980) was 0.5 µg/ml or less except for the one strain of *P. aeruginosa*, which should not have been included in the study; in fact, 10 of the 15 organisms had an MIC to TMP of 0.15 µg/ml (STAMEY 1980). A close examination of the MICs in relation to cures, improved group, and failures shows no relationship as to whether the MIC was 0.15 or 0.5 µg/ml TMP, all of which makes one doubt that the failures of TMP/SMX therapy were related to diffusion difficulties of TMP into an alkaline EPS.

It is clear from the theoretical determinants of antimicrobial diffusion from plasma to prostatic fluid (STAMEY et al. 1970) that an alkaline EPS in chronic bacterial prostatitis does mean that a lipid-soluble, antimicrobial acid with a favorable pK_a might be ion trapped in prostatic fluid when it is highly alkaline at the height of the inflammatory response (a pH of 8.32 ± 0.07 in the studies by FAIR et al. 1979). We believe that factors other than diffusion of TMP into prostatic fluid are responsible for the 40%–60% failure rate with the 12-week course of therapy; my guess is that since sterilization of the prostatic fluid occurs in 75% of patients during therapy, bacteria are probably persisting in some focus within the prostate, perhaps the mucoprotein of the corpora amylacea, which the TMP cannot penetrate.

Transurethral resection of the prostate, which is the only operation short of total prostatectomy which has a chance to remove the nonhyperplastic tissue of the true outer prostate, has about a 33% chance of cure in our experience (STAMEY 1980). In 1968 we documented, with multiple localizing cultures, the first reported cure of chronic bacterial prostatitis by transurethral resection, as well as the first documented cure by radical prostatectomy in the same report (MEARES and STAMEY 1968). SMART and JENKINS (1973) reported that 72% of patients were "rendered asymptomatic" after transurethral resection, but there is no documentation that their patients had true chronic bacterial prostatitis; in a later paper this same group reported that 50% of their patients were asymptomatic at follow-up, but they relied on unquantitated, tissue-positive broth cultures at the time of resection for evidence of chronic bacterial prostatitis (SMART et al. 1976), many of which may have represented urethral or even urine contaminants. Without documenting data similar to that presented in Table 2, it is impossible to know whether the prostate was infected or not.

One reason bacteriologic cures from transurethral resection of the prostate, as opposed to total prostatectomy, are unlikely to be much better than 33% is the fact that MCNEAL's (1968) studies show that most of the infection is in the peripheral zone of the prostate, and as emphasized by BLACKLOCK (1974), all of the ducts from the peripheral zone empty into the urethra distal to the verumontanum; a radical transurethral resection in this area carries a high risk of urinary incontinence.

D. Nonbacterial Prostatitis

The inflammatory reaction in the EPS of patients with nonbacterial prostatitis is indistinguishable, with the light microscope, from that of patients with chronic bacterial prostatitis (Table 1). It is a clinical fact that patients with nonbacterial prostatitis do not respond to antimicrobial agents and that all efforts to prove the etiology of the inflammatory reaction have been unsuccessful so far.

Our attempts at Stanford to prove the presence of *Neisseria* spp., *Ureaplasma urealyticum*, aerobic and anaerobic bacteria were without success (MEARES 1973 b). MÅRDH and COLLEEN (1975), recognizing the difficulty of accurate diagnosis because of urethral contamination of EPS, wisely compared their bacteriologic findings with those in 20 healthy, normal volunteers; in their search for aerobes, strict anaerobes, mycoplasmas, fungi, trichomonads, and viruses, they found no greater incidence in their patients than their control subjects. These authors concluded that "the cultures of the expressed prostatic fluids and the samples of semen gave no information of the occurrence of bacteria over and above that obtainable from examination of the urethral specimens." Although complement-fixing antibodies to *Chlamydia* were found in 33% of the patients in comparison with 5% of the control subjects (MÅRDH and COLLEEN 1975), in a later publication MÅRDH et al. (1978) appear to have excluded *Chlamydia trachomatis* as an etiologic agent in nonbacterial prostatitis. GORDON et al. (1972) and NIELSEN and VESTERGAARD (1973) were unable to isolate viruses as etiologic agents, either from urine, EPS, or prostatic biopsies in patients with prostatitis. NIELSEN and JUSTESEN (1974) confirmed the absence of obligate anaerobes in the urine, EPS, and in prostatic biopsies; they showed the importance of culturing the perineal skin in order to control for the contamination of the perineal needle biopsy of the prostate. NIELSEN et al. (1973) performed transperineal needle biopsies of the prostate in 18 patients with nonbacterial prostatitis as well as 18 with chronic urethritis; interestingly, there was as much prostatic inflammation in the urethritis group as in the patients with "prostatitis."

C-reactive protein in the serum was found in only 6 of 78 patients with predominantly nonbacterial prostatitis (COLLEEN and MÅRDH 1975); these authors' also reported that seminal fluid spermiograms were similar in control subjects and patients with prostatitis, an important observation for those who believe that prostatitis affects male fertility. Although COLLEEN and MÅRDH (1975) showed no difference between patients and control subjects with respect to the concentration of zinc and magnesium in their EPS, FAIR et al. (1976) have clearly shown that zinc is substantially reduced in patients who have chronic bacterial prostatitis. Thus, it would appear that zinc is reduced in patients with chronic bacterial prostatitis, but not in those with nonbacterial prostatitis.

Since *C. trachomatis* is recognized as the cause of non-gonococcal urethritis in 40% of men (HOLMES et al. 1975) as well as the major cause of acute epididymitis in men under 35 years of age (BERGER et al. 1978), this intracellular agent remains an excellent candidate for the causative organism in nonbacterial prostatitis, despite the evidence of MARDH et al. (1978) which appears to exclude *C. trachomatis* as a major cause of nonbacterial prostatitis. It is of interest that BALLARD et al. (1979) have suggested, on the basis of single but detailed case study, that nonbacterial prostatitis may be a manifestation of delayed hypersensitivity to *C. trachomatis*. More recently, WISHNOW et al. (1982), using the solid phase radioimmunoassay of SHORTLIFFE et al. (1981 a), have shown that patients with nonbacterial prostatitis have no antigen specific antibodies to Enterobacteriaceae or pseudomonas in their prostatic fluid; indeed, their immunologic reactivity is similar to the prostatic fluid of normal healthy controls who have never had prostatic inflammation. These observations mean that if a microbial agent is the cause of nonbacterial prostatitis, it has no shared antigens with *E. coli* or other members of the Enterobacterioceae family. Even the total immunoglobulins A and G are minimally elevated, if at all, in comparison to the Ig response in bacterial prostatitis (WISHNOW et al. 1982), suggesting that the inflammatory agent in nonbacterial prostatitis is non-immunogenic.

It is possible that nonbacterial prostatitis is caused by a chemical rather than an infectious agent. I have always been intrigued at how asymptomatic men who have true chronic bacterial prostatitis can be, as long as their bladder infections are prevented by low-dosage, antimicrobial prophylaxis. For example, despite years of demonstrating bacterial persistence of *E. coli*, *Pseudomonas aeruginosa*, or *Proteus mirabilis* in the EPS, these men have no urinary, ejaculatory, or pelvic pain as long as their bladder urine remains uninfected. Thus, if thousands and sometimes tens of thousands of *Pseudomonas aeruginosa* can persist in the prostate without symptoms, it is hard to imagine what kind of infectious agent must be present in patients with nonbacterial prostatitis to produce such devastating pelvic symptomatology.

Whatever the cause of nonbacterial prostatitis, treatment is largely unsatisfactory. Our best results have occurred when the patient is informed that no one knows the cause of his inflammatory reaction, that it is unlikely to be an infectious agent, that antimicrobial agents are a waste of money, and that his symptoms will ultimately improve. It is important for the physician to recognize nonbacterial prostatitis and to refrain from prescribing antimicrobial agents for what is probably a nonexistent infection. Such prescribing simply creates more anxiety for the patient, prolongs his misery, and strengthens his concern that there must be a mysterious underlying infection which his physicians are unable to cure.

References

Ablin RJ, Soanes WA, Gonder MJ (1971) Localization of immunoglobulins in human prostatic tissue. J Immunol 107:603–604

Anderson RU, Fair WR (1976) Physical and chemical determinations of prostatic secretion in benign hyperplasia, prostatitis, and adenocarcinoma. Invest Urol 14:137–140

Anderson RJ, Weller C (1979) Prostatic secretion leukocyte studies in non-bacterial prostatitis (prostatosis). J Urol 121:292–294

Ballard RC, Block C, Koornhof HJ, Haitas B (1979) Delayed hypersensitivity to Chlamydia trachomatis: cause of chronic prostatitis? Lancet 2:1305–1306

Baumueller A, Madsen PO (1977) Secretion of various antimicrobial substances in dogs with experimental bacterial prostatitis. Urol Res 5:215–218

Berger RE, Holmes KK, Alexander ER, Monda GD, Ansell J, McCormick G (1978) Chlamydia trachomatis as a cause of acute "idiopathic" epididymitis. N Eng J Med 298:301–304

Blacklock NJ (1969) Some observations on prostatitis. In: Williams DC, Briggs MN, Staniford M (eds) Advances in the study of the prostate. Heinemann, London, pp 37–61

Blacklock NJ (1974) Anatomical factors in prostatitis. Br J Urol 46:47–54

Blacklock NJ, Beavis JP (1974) The response of prostatic fluid pH in inflammation. Br J Urol 46:537–542

Bruce AW, Fox M (1960) Acute infections of the prostate gland. Br J Urol 32:302–305

Chodirker WB, Tomasi TB (1963) Gamma-globulins: quantitative relationships in human serum and nonvascular fluids. Science 142:1080–1081

Colleen S, Mardh P-A (1975) Studies on non-acute prostatis: clinical and laboratory findings in patients with symptoms of non-acute prostatitis. In: Danielsson D, Juhlin L, Mardh P-A (eds) Genital infections and their complications. Alqvist and Wiksell, Stockholm, pp 121–131

Couture M, Ulstein M, Leonard J (1976) Improved staining method for differentiating immature germ cells from white blood cells in human seminal fluid. Andrologia 8:61–66

Dabhoiwala NF, Bye A, Claridge M (1976) A study of concentrations of trimethoprim-sulphamethoxazole in the human prostate gland. Br J Urol 48:77–81

Drach GW (1974) Problems in diagnosis of bacterial prostatitis: gram-negative, gram-positive, and mixed infections. J Urol 111:630–636

Drach GW, Meares EM, Stamey TA (1978) Classification of benign diseases associated with prostatic pain: prostatitis or prostatodynia (letter to the editor)? J Urol 120:266

Eykyn S, Bultitude M, Mavo ME (1974) Prostatic calculi as a source of recurrent bacteriuria in the male. Br J Urol 46:527–532

Fair WR, Couch J, Wehner N (1976) Prostatic antibacterial factor-identity and significance. Urology 7:169–177

Fair WR, Crane DB, Schiller N, Heston WDW (1979) A re-appraisal of treatment in chronic bacterial prostatitis. J Urol 121:437–441

Freedman LR, Phair JP, Seki M, Hamilton HB, Nefzger MD (1965) The epidemiology of urinary tract infections in Hiroshima. Yale J Biol Med 37:262–282

Friedlander AM, Braude AI, Singler R, Kornfield P (1972) Experimental prostatitis: relationship to pyelonephritis. J Infect Dis 126:645–651

Gip L, Molin L (1970) On the inhibitory activity of human prostatic fluid on Candida albicans. Mykosen (1) 13:61–63

Gordon HL, Miller DH, Rawls WE (1972) Viral studies in patients with nonspecific prostatourethritis. J Urol 108:299–300

Granato JJ, Gross DM, Stamey TA (1973) Trimethoprim diffusion into prostatic and salivary secretions of the dog. Invest Urol 11:205–210

Gray SP, Billings J, Blacklock NJ (1974) Distribution of the immunoglobulins G, A and M in the prostatic fluid of patients with prostatitis. Clin Chim Acta 57:163–169

Hessl JM, Stamey TA (1971) The passage of tetracyclines across epithelial membranes with special reference to prostatic epithelium. J Urol 106:253–256

Holmes KK, Handsfield HH, Wang SP, Wentworth BB, Turck M, Anderson JB, Alexander ER (1975) Etiology of nongonococcal urethritis. N Eng J Med 292:1199–1205

Jameson RM (1967) Sexual activity and the variations of the white cell content of the prostatic secretion. Invest Urol 5:297–302

Kelalis PP, Greene LF, Harrison EG (1965) Granulomatous prostatitis – a mimic of carcinoma of the prostrate. JAMA 191:111–113

Levy BJ, Fair WR (1973) The location of antibacterial activity in the rat prostatic secretions. Invest Urol 11:173–177

Ludvik W (1964) Zur Diagnostik der chronischen Prostatitis. Deutsche Med Wochenschr 89:2366–2369

Maged Z, Khafaga H (1965) Bacteriological and serological study of chronic prostatis patients. Br J Vener Dis 41:202–207

Mårdh P-A, Colleen S (1975) Search for uro-genital tract infections in patients with symptoms of prostatitis. Scand J Urol Nephrol 9:8–16

Mårdh P-A, Darougar S, Ripa KT, Colleen S, Treharne JD (1978) Role of Chlamydia trachomatis in non-acute prostatitis. Br J Vener Dis 54:330–334

McNeal JE (1968) Regional morphology and pathology of the prostate. Am J Clin Pathol 49:347–357

McNeal JE (1972) The prostate and prostatic urethra: a morphologic synthesis. J Urol 107:1008–1016

Meares EM Jr (1973a) Observations on activity of trimethoprim-sulfamethoxazole in the prostate. J Infect Dis [Suppl] 128:S679–S685

Meares EM Jr (1973b) Bacterial prostatitis vs "prostatosis" – a clinical and bacteriological study. JAMA 224:1372–1375

Meares EM Jr (1974) Infection stones of prostate gland-laboratory diagnosis and clinical management. Urology 4:560–566

Meares EM Jr (1977) Serum antibody titers in urethritis and chronic bacterial prostatitis. Urology 10:305–309

Meares EM Jr (1978) Serum antibody titers in treatment with trimethoprim-sulfamethoxazole for chronic prostatitis. Urology 11:142–146

Meares EM Jr (1979) Long-term therapy of chronic bacterial prostatitis with trimethoprim-sulfamethoxazole. Can Med Assoc J 112:22S–25S

Meares EM Jr, Stamey TA (1968) Bacteriologic localization patterns in bacterial prostatitis and urethritis. Invest Urol 5:492–518

Mobley DF (1975) Serum cultures in the diagnosis of bacterial prostatitis. J Urol 114:83–85

Moore RA (1937) Inflammation of the prostate gland. J Urol 38:173–182

Nielsen ML, Justesen T (1974) Studies on the pathology of prostatitis – a search for prostatic infections with obligate anaerobes in patients with chronic prostatitis and chronic urethritis. Scand J Urol Nephrol 8:1–6

Nielsen ML, Vestergaard BF (1973) Virological investigations in chronic prostatitis. J Urol 109:1023–1025

Nielsen ML, Asnaes S, Hattel T (1973) Inflammatory changes in the non-infected prostate gland. A clinical, microbiological and histological investigation. J Urol 110:423–426

Nilsson I-K, Colleen S, Mårdh P-A (1975) Relationship between psychological and laboratory findings in patients with symptoms of non-acute prostatitis. In: Danielsson D, Juhlin L, Mårdh P-A (eds) Genital infections and their complications. Almqvist and Wiksell, Uppsala, pp 133–144

Pfau A, Sacks T (1976) Chronic bacterial prostatitis: new therapeutic aspects. Br J Urol 48:245–253

Pfau A, Perlberg S, Shapira A (1978) The pH of the prostatic fluid in health and disease: implications of treatment in chronic bacterial prostatitis. J Urol 119:384–387

Reeves DS, Ghilchick MB (1970) Secretion of the antibacterial substance trimethoprim in the prostatic fluid of dogs. Br J Urol 42:66–72

Reeves DS, Rowe RCG, Snell ME, Thomas ABW (1973) Further studies on the secretion of antibiotics in the prostatid fluid of the dog. In: Brumfitt W, Asscher AW (eds) Urinary Proceedings of the Second National Symposium. University Press, London, pp 197–205

Shortliffe LMD, Wehner N, Stamey TA (1981) The use of a solid phase radioimmunoassay and formalin-fixed whole bacterial antigen in the detection of antigen-specific immunoglobulin in human prostatic fluid. J Clin Invest 67:790–799

Shortliffe LMD, Wehner N, Stamey TA (1981 b) The detection of a local prostatic immunologic responese to bacterial prostatitis. J. Urol 125:509–515

Smart CJ, Jenkins JD (1973) The role of transurethral prostatectomy in chronic prostatitis. Br J Urol 45:654–662

Smart CJ, Jenkins JD, Lloyd RS (1976) The painful prostate. Br J Urol 47:861–869

Smith JW, Jones JR, Reed WP, Tice AD, Deupree RH, Kaijser B (1979) Recurrent urinary tract infections in men: characteristics and response to therapy. Ann Intern Med 91:544–548

Smith MJV (1966) Prostatic corpora amylacea. Monogr Surg Sci 3:209–265

Stamey TA (1972) Urinary infections. Williams and Wilkins, Baltimore

Stamey TA (1980) Pathogenesis and treatment of Urinary Tract Infections. Williams and Wilkins, Baltimore

Stamey TA, Nemoy NJ (1971) Surgical bacteriological and biochemical management of: "infection stones". JAMA 215:1470–1476

Stamey TA, Govan DE, Palmer JM (1965) The localization and treatment of urinary tract infections: the role of bactericidal urine levels as opposed to serum levels. Medicine 44:1–36

Stamey TA, Fair WR, Timothy MM, Chung HK (1968) Antibacterial nature of prostatic fluid. Nature 218:444–447

Stamey TA, Meares EM, Winningham DG (1970) Chronic bacterial prostatitis and the diffusion of drugs into prostatic fluid. J Urol 103:187–194

Stamey TA, Bushby SRM, Bragonje J (1973) The concentration of trimethoprim in prostatic fluid: nonionic diffusion or active transport? J Infect Dis [Suppl] 128:S 686–S 690

Tallgren LG, Rusk J, Alfthan DS (1968) Antibacterial activity in semen and its relation to semen quality. Ann Chir Gynaecol Fenn 57:540–543

Winningham DG, Stamey TA (1970) Diffusion of sulfonamides from plasma into prostatic fluid. J Urol 104:559–563

Winningham DG, Nemoy NJ, Stamey TA (1968) Diffusion of antibiotics from plasma into prostatic fluid. Nature 219:139–143

Wishnow KI, Wehner N, Stamey TA (1982) The diagnostic value of the immunologic response in bacterial and nonbacterial prostatitis. J Urol 127:689–694

Youmans GP, Liebling J, Lyman RY (1938) The bactericidal action of prostatic fluid in dogs. J Infect Dis 63:117–121

Young HH, Geraghty JJT, Stevens AR (1906) Chronic prostatitis – an experimental and clinical study with an analysis of 358 cases. Johns Hopkins Hospital Reports 13:272–341

Zollinger WD, Dalrymple JM, Artenstein MS (1976) Analysis of parameters affecting the solid phase radioimmunoassay quantitation of antibody to meningococcal antigens. J Immunol 117:1788–1798

CHAPTER 19

Co-trimoxazole in Chest Infections Including its Long-Term Use in Chest Disease

D.T.D. Hughes

A. Introduction

The development of combinations of a diaminopyrimidine and a sulfonamide as a potent antibacterial combination has already been described earlier in this volume. The degree of synergy was pointed out by Bushby and Hitchings (1968) and emphasized by Darrell et al. (1968), who also gave some striking examples of the clinical efficacy of the combination. Synergy between the two components of co-trimoxazole could be demonstrated in vitro over quite a wide range of ratios of one drug to another. Furthermore, the pharmacokinetics were such (see Chap. 10) that although the trimethoprim and sulfonamide might be administered in one particular ratio by mouth, the ultimate levels in the various tissues might be different. In addition, the infecting organisms differed between tissues. Thus, it was at least theoretically possible that whilst a ratio of 1 part trimethoprim to 5 parts sulfamethoxazole might be most appropriate for treating infections of one organ, a ratio of 1:20 might be better elsewhere.

B. Exacerbations of Chronic Bronchitis

The initial studies in chest disease were carried out using a combination of trimethoprim (TMP) and sulfamethoxazole (SMX) in a ratio of 1:2, administering 500 mg/day TMP and 1 g/day SMX in divided doses given 12 h apart. Drew et al. (1967a) treated 50 cases of chronic bronchitis with this combination using a 5- to 7-day course. Some patients had additional bronchiectasis; all had purulent sputum before treatment which was rendered mucoid in every case. Recognised bacterial pathogens were isolated from the sputum before treatment in 33 cases, the commonest being *Hemophilus influenzae* and *Streptococcus pneumoniae*. These pathogens were eradicated and in only two cases was the same organism isolated after therapy and both of these had responded well clinically. There were no significant side effects or effects on the blood count in this early trial.

This initial promising success led on to a trial to attempt to see what ratio of TMP:SMX appeared to be the best in treating exacerbations of chronic bronchitis. Two additional groups of 50 patients with exacerbations of their chronic bronchitis were treated during the next year and the results were compared (D. Hughes et al. 1969). As shown in Table 1, it appeared that the *lower* ratio of SMX:TMP and the higher daily dosage of TMP gave the best results. In practice, there was little difference between the 1:5 and 1:2 ratios of TMP:SMX and the comparison was a relatively crude one, being carried out as a sequential study. It therefore seemed

Table 1. Clinical and bacteriological cures in three successive groups of 50 patients with exacerbations of chronic bronchitis each treated with combinations of TMP and SMX (D. Hughes et al. 1969, adapted)

Group	1	2	3
Ratio TMP:SMX	1:10	1:5	1:2
Daily TMP (mg)	200	320	500
Daily SMX (mg)	2,000	1,600	1,000
Clinical failures[a]	10 (20)	3 (6)	1 (2)
Bacteriological failures[a]	12 (24)	8 (16)	5 (10)

[a] Figures in parentheses are percentages

Table 2. Isolation of pathogens, particularly *Hemophilus influenzae*, from the sputum of patients with exacerbations of chronic bronchitis

Reference	No. of patients	No. with pathogens[a]	No. whose sputum grew H. influenzae[a]
Drew et al. (1967)	50	33 (66)	17 (34)
D. Hughes et al. (1969)	50	27 (54)	13 (26)
D. Hughes (1969)	50	35 (70)	15 (30)
D. Hughes (1970 unpublished work)	30	24 (80)	18 (60)

[a] Figures in parentheses are percentages

quite appropriate for treating chronic bronchitis when the 1:5 ratio was finally adopted (following pharmacokinetic studies and clinical trials of infections in other organs) as the universally recommended dosage giving a daily total of 320 mg TMP and 1,600 mg SMX. Meanwhile, Pines et al. (1969) had shown that, in patients with very purulent heavily infected sputum when the 1:5 ratio combination was used, a total daily dose of 480 mg TMP and 2,400 mg SMX was even more effective than the recommended standard dose. Consideration of these clinical results leads to the suggestion that perhaps greater efficacy in treating exacerbations of chronic bronchitis might be achieved with larger daily doses of TMP (i.e. 500 mg as suggested by Hughes et al. and 480 mg as suggested by Pines et al.).

Carrying out clinical trials in such exacerbations is not straightforward, however (D. Hughes 1979 a). Sputum bacteriology is often unsatisfactory and, apparently purulent sputum is often reported to contain no pathogens, and conversely, a pathogen may be cultured from apparently mucoid sputum. There are several reasons for this. First, *H. influenzae* (the commonest pathogen) is quite a delicate organism with rather fastidious requirements when grown in culture media, needing both factor X and factor Y. If sputum is sent to the laboratory fresh, and cultured with care, a higher rate of positive cultures is obtained. This is illustrated in Table 2, which shows the proportion of pathogenic organisms cultured from sputum samples over a series of winters (Drew et al. 1967 a; D. Hughes et al. 1969; D. Hughes 1969). Certain organisms such as *Proteus* and *Pseudomonas* spp. may

Table 3. Pathogenic organisms cultured from the sputum of 161 consecutive patients with exacerbations of chronic bronchitis (mostly treated as hospital in-patients)

1. *Hemophilus influenzae*	29
2. *Streptococcus pneumoniae*	17
3. *H. influenzae* plus *S. pneumoniae*	14
4. *Escherichia coli*	17
5. *Proteus* spp.	13
6. *Staphylococcus pyogenes*	5
7. *Klebsiella pneumoniae*	4
8. *Pseudomonas* spp.	3
Total number of organisms[a]	102
	5
Total no. of patients whose sputum grew pathogens	97
No. of patients growing no pathogens	64
Total	161

[a] Neglecting cases (other than 3) in which two organisms were isolated

grow very readily on artifical culture media and swamp a more sparse growth of *H. influenzae*. Such organisms may also be cultured from mucoid uninfected sputum. Table 3 shows the organisms cultured from 161 consecutive patients with exacerbations of chronic bronchitis studied during three winters. *H. influenzae* and *S. pneumoniae*, either singly or in combination, were by far the commonest organisms grown, but some other organisms were isolated. It is often difficult to determine the role of such additional pathogens in exacerbations of chronic bronchitis. Furthermore, *clinical* improvement seems to correlate best with conversion of purulent to mucoid sputum rather than eradication of a pathogen.

It is also necessary to define chronic bronchitis as precisely as possible. In Britain, the MEDICAL RESEARCH COUNCIL (1965) has designed a questionnaire to detect its presence and has also produced a classification of sputum purulence. In some of the early studies the patients might not have conformed precisely to the MRC criteria, but these were adhered to in some of the subsequent studies.

I. Levels of Two Components in Sputum

Since chronic bronchitis is characterised by the excessive production of sputum, and during exacerbations this becomes infected and purulent, it seemed appropriate to study the levels of TMP and SMX in the sputum after oral administration. Several such studies have been carried out. D. HUGHES et al. (1972) studied the levels of both drugs in the serum and sputum of ten patients with exacerbations of chronic bronchitis who received the combination for a period of 5 days. Blood samples were withdrawn at 9 a.m. (just before the morning dose), 12 noon and 4. p.m. and sputum collected from 9 a.m. to 4 p.m.. The sputum was fully homogenised with an ultrasonic probe. The results are shown in Tables 4 and 5. From these it will be seen that TMP is concentrated in sputum so that the level exceeds that in the blood; whereas SMX was only found in much smaller amounts. Other

Table 4. Levels of trimethoprim in serum and sputum (µg/ml)

Time (h)	Serum		Standard error of mean	Sputum		Standard error of mean
	Mean	Range[b]		Mean	Range	
09.00	2.15	0.50–3.45	0.4088			
12.00	2.89	0.75–4.30	0.4870			
16.00	2.71	0.50–5.10	0.5337			
Mean[a]	2.587			4.51	2.05–6.85	0.6964

[a] Ratio of sputum TMP:serum TMP = 1.75:1
[b] Values of < 1 µg/ml were observed on four occasions only

Table 5. Levels of sulfamethoxazole in serum and sputum (6 patients); standard error of mean given in parentheses

Time (h)	Serum		Sputum	
	Before hydrolysis	After hydrolysis	Before hydrolysis	After hydrolysis
09.00	42.40 (±4.65)	79.58 (±11.10)		
12.00	70.27 (±5.31)	113.20 (± 9.31)		
16.00	61.64 (±5.03)	116.80 (± 9.46)		
Mean[a]	58.10 (±6.73)	103.19 (± 9.68)	12.40 (3.89)	19.35 (10.44)

[a] Sputum: serum ratios – before hydrolysis 0.213:1, after hydrolysis 0.284:1

studies gave similar results so that it appears that in sputum the ratio of TMP:SMX is greater than 1:5. The sputum TMP levels certainly exceed the minimum inhibitory concentrations (MICs) needed to kill *H. influenzae* and *S. pneumoniae* (whether SMX is present or not), whereas those of sulfamethoxazole probably do not, though there may be sufficient SMX to have an effect on some other chest pathogens, such as *Klebsiella pneumoniae*.

II. Comparative Trials

A number of trials comparing the effects of co-trimoxazole with that of other antibacterials in treating exacerbations of chronic bronchitis have been carried out. The most important of these are summarised in Table 6. From this table it will be seen that in all the trials carried out, combinations of trimethoprim and sulfamethoxazole had an equal or better effect than the antibiotics with which they were compared. These included ampicillin, tetracycline, dimethylchlortetracycline, doxycycline, ampiclox, amoxycillin, and cephalexin. These trials were carried out both on hospital patients and patients treated in general practice, and in a number of different countries. The overall conclusion must undoubtedly be that co-trimoxazole is an effective treatment for exacerbations of chronic bronchitis. There are several points to be made from all these studies, however, whilst some of them are worth mentioning in a little more detail. All the studies suffered from the difficulties inherent in testing the effects of antibacterial substances in chronic bronchitis

Table 6. Comparative trials in chronic bronchitis

Reference	Dose and regimen of co-trimoxazole[a]		Agent compared, dose and regimen	Practice type	Result
D. Hughes (1969)	S	7 days	Ampicillin, 2 g	Hospital	TMP/SMX better
Lal and Bhalla (1969)	S	7 days	Tetracycline, 1 g	Hospital	TMP/SMX better
Beumer (1972)	S	14 days	Dimethylchlortetracycline (Ledermycin), 600 mg	Hospital	TMP/SMX better
General Practitioner Group (1972)	S	7 days	Doxycycline, 100 mg	General practice	TMP/SMX better
Kaplan and Stegman (1972)	6×5 / 4×5	10 days	Ampiclox $2 \times 4 \times 2$ / $1 \times 4 \times 8$ } 10 days	Hospital	Equal effect
Carroll et al. (1977)	S	5 days	Amoxycillin, 750 mg	General practice	Equal effect
Tandon (1977)	6	7 days	Amoxycillin, 1500 mg	Hospital	Equal effect
Pines et al. (1977)	6	10 days	Amoxycillin, 1500 mg	Hospital	Equal effect
Cooper and McGillion (1978)	S	7 days	Cephalexin, 2 g	General practice	TMP/SMX better

[a] S = standard dose of co-trimoxazole. Numbers indicate numbers of tablets a day in other instances, e.g. several trials used six tablets a day. In the trial by Kaplan and Stegman (1972), six tablets a day were given for 5 days and four tablets a day for 5 days.

that have already been referred to. In addition, the patient population would not have been identical in each. For example, in the study of Pines et al. (1977) shown in Table 6 and in other trials carried out by this group, all are very long-standing chronic patients producing highly infected purulent sputum. At the other end of the spectrum are likely to be some of the patients who were studied in general practice. The trials varied in their strictness of criteria for admission; for example, the study of D. Hughes (1969) took only patients who conformed 100% to the criteria set down by the Medical Research Council for a diagnosis of chronic bronchitis. He judged the effect of TMP/SMX and ampicillin by the effect on sputum volume, sputum purulence and eradication of pathogenic organisms. In that particular study there was a significantly greater reduction in sputum purulence after treatment with co-trimoxazole than there was after treatment with ampicillin. There was also a significant difference in the proportion of cases whose sputum was rendered mucoid. Though more pathogens were eradicated with the TMP/SMX combinations, this was not significantly greater than when ampicillin was used. Pathogenic organisms were isolated from only 29 of 50 patients, the commonest being *H. influenzae* and *S. pneumoniae*.

A rather similar pattern was found in the other trials, though some of those, particularly those carried out in general practice, had an even lower rate of isolation of pathogenic organisms. From Table 6 it will be evident that some of the trials were carried out with rather higher doses of antibacterial substances. Following the early suggestion of Pines, various authors tried using a bigger dose of the combination, namely 480 mg trimethoprim and 2,400 mg sulfamethoxazole. The trial carried out by Pines et al. (1977) is of particular interest since, although they found that this higher dose regimen of the combination gave a comparable effect to the amoxycillin at rather higher dosage, namely 1,500 mg/day, this was only true when one considered the immediate treatment period of 10 days. If these patients were followed up for longer, during the next month a much higher proportion of those patients who had received the combination relapsed and had purulent sputum (growing pathogens again) than those who had received amoxycillin, implying that perhaps amoxycillin has a much more lasting effect in sterilising the bacterial flora of the sputum in such patients. Nevertheless, the total evidence in support of the combination in treating acute exacerbations of bronchitis remains impressive. It is also interesting that in most of these trials side effects were minimal. Occasional nausea occurred, blood counts when monitored did not alter significantly. Thus, the use of the combination in treating exacerbations of chronic bronchitis seems established.

C. Other Acute Conditions

Of these most important is pneumonia. D. Hughes (1973) has reported the results of treating 15 cases of lobar pneumonia with the combination of trimethoprim/sulfamethoxazole in conventional dosage, treatment being carried out for periods of 7–14 days (Table 7). All 15 patients responded well and some dramatically, as is shown by the illustrative case history. Interestingly enough, a further six patients were treated by the combination, but at a different ratio. Three patients with pneumonia responded well to 500 mg/day trimethoprim and 1,000 mg/day sulfameth-

Table 7. Details of cases of pneumonia treated with 320 mg TMP + 1600 mg SMX

Patient	Sex	Age (years)	Site[a]	Organism	Result
1	M	44	LLL	*Escherichia coli*	Cured
2	M	39	RUL	*Hemophilus influenzae*	Cured
3	M	65	LLL	*Streptococcus pneumoniae*	Cured
4	M	61	BLL	*Proteus* sp.	Cured
5	M	50	RLL	No pathogens	Cured
6	F	65	RLL	*Escherichia coli*	Cured
7	M	62	BLL	*Escherichia coli*	Cured
8	M	33	RUL	*Proteus* sp.	Cured
9	M	65	LUL	*Streptococcus pneumoniae*	Cured
10	M	70	BLL	*Escherichia coli*	Cured
11	F	63	RLL	*Stapholococcus pyogenes*	Cured
12	M	50	RLL	*Staphylococcus pyogenes*	Cured
13	F	71	BLL	*Proteus*	Cured
14	M	45	LLL	*Proteus*	Cured
15	M	50	RLL	*Streptococcus pneumoniae*	Cured

[a] Abbreviations: BLL both lower lobes; LLL left lower lobe; LUL left upper lobe; RLL right lower lobe; RUL right upper lobe

oxazole, but of the three patients treated with 200 mg trimethoprim and 2,000 mg sulfamethoxazole, only one responded to treatment. This again implies that a larger dose of trimethoprim may be needed.

Case History
A 65-year-old man was admitted to hospital acutely ill. He was delirious and cyanosed and had a temperature of 39.5 °C. He was producing purulent sputum which was occasionally bloodstained and from which *S. pneumoniae* was cultured. The chest radiograph showed consolidation of the left upper lobe. Within 48 h of oral administration of co-trimoxazole his condition was much improved. His temperature returned to normal and his sputum was mucoid and free of pathogens by the sixth day of treatment. Complete radiological resolution also occurred.

D. HUGHES (1973) in the same paper described the successful treatment of three cases of lung abscess due to *Staphylococcus pyogenes*, one of which was penicillin resitant. In addition a number of patients with exacerbations of infection associated with bronchiectasis were also treated successfully with the combination. Trimethoprim/sulphamethoxazole is bactericidal against *Bordetella pertussis*. A trial in patients infected with this organism, most of whom had typical "whooping cough," was therefore carried out by ADCOCK et al. (1972) Two groups of 44 children were treated with either TMP/SMX or tetracycline. The results were difficult to interpret although it appeared that there might have been a slight advantage for TMP/SMX over tetracycline, but only in children with a history of less than 10 days cough.

I. Pneumocystis carinii Pneumonia

This is a severe and often fatal form of pneumonia caused by the protozoan, *Pneumocystis carinii*. It usually occurs in debilitated children or else in patients (children and adults) receiving treatment with cytotoxic, immunosuppressive or steroid drugs. Until the introduction of co-trimoxazole, treatment had been with penta-midine which, although effective, gave rise to many unwanted side effects. The ef-ficacy of TMP/SMX was first demonstrated in children by W. Hughes et al. (1975) and in adults by Lau and Young (1976). Both groups used the drug given orally to treat established *Pneumocystis* infections and with favourable results and mini-mal toxicity. They found that high dosage was needed, however. Hughes' group, from this initial and other studies, recommended a total daily oral dosage of 20 mg kg^{-1} day^{-1} TMP and 100 mg kg^{-1} day^{-1} SMX whilst Lau and Young (1976) in adults used comparable doses of the order of 960–1,200 mg TMP and 480–6,000 mg SMX. Occasional treatment failures occurred, some of which were as-sociated with a failure to reach the high serum level needed following oral dosage owing to inadequate absorption in some instances. For this reason Winston et al. (1980) employed *intravenous* TMP/SMX using a daily dose of 10–15 mg/kg TMP and 50–75 mg/kg SMX. They obtained excellent results in 11 patients, only one of whom failed to respond. They also reviewed previous experience with TMP/SMX combinations in this condition, including its prophylactic use in patients known to be at risk. The use of such chemoprophylaxis seems justified in selected high risk cases, especially in children with certain types of leukaemia who are receiving treat-ment with multiple drugs (W. Hughes et al. 1977) (cf. Chap. 14).

D. Long-Term Treatment

The main long-term use of the combination in chest disease has been in the prophy-laxis of chronic bronchitis. There is a considerable amount of literature on the pos-sible value of chemoprophylaxis in the management of chronic bronchitis and this has been reviewed by D. Hughes (1976). It would be true to say that there is no complete agreement on the subject, but that many authorities would agree that some of the patients with more severe chronic bronchitis, in whom an exacerbation could lead to a possibly fatal episode of respiratory failure, may well be usefully protected by long-term treatment with an antibacterial substance.

Most of the earlier work on long-term chemoprophylaxis had been with tetra-cycline; for example that study carried out in Britain by the Medical Research Council Working Party (1966). However, it seemed worthwhile to see if TMP/SMX would prove a useful agent. Most of the work on long-term prophylaxis has been carried out by The London Hospital group and, indeed, the initial clinical re-ports on the usefulness of the combination included a study of ten patients with bronchitis or bronchiectasis who had received the combination in a 1:2 ratio, that is to say 500 mg/day trimethoprim and 1 g/day sulfamethoxazole (Drew et al. 1967b; Jenkins et al. 1970). The patients received treatment for a period of about 3 months, the duration of therapy being in the range 45–113 days. This treatment not only eradicated any pathogens that were present in the sputum, but kept these patients well and out of hospital. This represented a significant clinical improve-ment since eight of the ten had had repeated hospital admissions during the preced-ing winters. Toxicity was slight, though one patient did have a fall in his platelet count which had to be reversed by the administration of calcium folinate.

A more pertinent and definitive study was reported by D. Hughes et al. (1975). In this study, nine patients with bronchitis and one with bronchiectasis received co-trimoxazole at the standard dosage and 1:5 ratio for long periods of time ranging from 3 to 30 months with a mean of 10.6 months. Sputum was taken for bacteriological culture before treatment was started and at approximately monthly intervals throughout. From the sputum of the nine patients with chronic bronchitis, *H. influenzae* was isolated on a total of eight occasions, *Streptococcus pneumoniae* six times and *Staphylococcus aureus* once. All these isolates whenever taken were sensitive to co-trimoxazole. Pathogens were completely eradicated in seven cases, though it was interesting that *H. influenzae* was isolated once *during* therapy. Sputum was also cultured on a monthly basis in several patients after therapy had stopped; one patient grew no pathogens until 3 months after therapy, when *S. pneumoniae* and *H. influenzae* were isolated, whilst another grew *H. influenzae* 4 months after treatment was stopped. During therapy, *Candida albicans* was isolated from the sputum of two patients, neither of whom, however, had any symptoms of fungal infection. The haematological changes were all very minor and a full discussion of them is beyond the scope of this chapter. The study showed again how effective the combination could be in selected patients in preventing further exacerbations of chronic bronchitis. Combinations of TMP/SMX have also been used in bronchiectasis and cystis fibrosis and it is worth reporting the experience of D. Hughes and RUSSELL (1982) in cystic fibrosis.

Eight subjects with cystic fibrosis from 15 to 21 years old have now been followed for a number of years. Four of them had already been receiving long-term treatment with trimethoprim/sulfamethoxazole which had been previously initiated by the paediatricians. For various reasons, two remained on this long-term therapy and have by and large remained well, whilst the two who had to discontinue it have had repeated chest infections. The number is too small to draw any conclusions from, but it was thought that inclusion of an illustrative case history would be helpful. In such young patients one does not seem to run into trouble with toxicity, nor have any organisms resistant to trimethoprim or sulfamethoxazole been isolated.

Case History
A 15-year-old schoolboy came under our care in August 1975. He had been missing a lot of schooling on account of recurrent episodes of purulent chest infection. A number of pathogenic organisms had been isolated from the sputum in the preceeding 6 months, including *Pseudomonas* spp., *Staphylococcus aureus*, *H. influenzae*, and *Streptococcus pneumoniae*. The last three were sensitive to co-trimoxazole. Because of these frequent infections the paediatrician had started him on long-term co-trimoxazole (at the standard adult dosage) in February. Following this he had missed no more time from school up to the time of seeing us. He remained on this regime continuously until January 1980 (4.5 years) during which time he remained well and was not absent from his studies. He was so successful in these as to be able to go to University in the Autumn of 1978. Repeated cultures of his always somewhat purulent sputum grew no pathogens, or else *S. pneumoniae* sensitive to co-trimoxazole. In January 1980 he had to be admitted to hospital with weight loss and a particularly severe chest infection. This was found to be due to *Pseudomonas* for which he received a course of gentamicin. His weight loss was due to his developing diabetes which had almost certainly also been a factor in the development of this severe episode of infection. His blood count had remained normal throughout.

PINES et al. (1972) carried out a useful trial of the effects of TMP/SMX in the *prophylaxis* of chronic bronchitis as well as in its treatment. They took 30 patients and treated them with one tablet twice a day (that is to say 160 mg trimethoprim and 800 mg sulfamethoxazole), until a purulent exacerbation occurred or treatment had lasted for 3 months. Of the 30 patients, 26 deteriorated and it was concluded that in this group of patients the dosage was inadequate; 21 patients, therefore, were given the standard dosage and under the same conditions, only 4 deteriorated. This served to confirm the usefulness of the combination in the prophylaxis of chronic bronchitis and also that the prophylactic dose is probably the same as the therapeutic one. Again, toxicity was almost non-existent though skin rashes were encountered.

E. Parenteral TMP/SMX

An intramuscular form of the combination has been introduced which has been tested in chest infections (IGLAUER et al. 1978); 79 patients aged 21–90 years were treated. The preparation consists of ampoules of 3 ml, each corresponding to 160 mg TMP and 800 mg SMX and the usual dosage was one ampoule every 12 h, corresponding exactly to the oral dosage. A few cases received three ampoules in 24 h. Approximately equal numbers of patients had bronchopneumonia (29), purlent bronchitis (26), and obstructive purulent bronchitis (20). Details of bacteriology are not given in any detail, but the clinical response appears to have been excellent in all three groups. It is certainly useful to have a parenteral preparation available and it may even be that the absence of one in the past rather inhibited some clinicians from using the combination in gravely ill patients with pneumonia. IGLAUER et al. (1978) point out that in many cases a patient can be started on the parenteral preparation and then be transferred to the oral one.

F. Alternative Drugs

Alternative sulfonamides to SMX have been tried in combination with trimethoprim in treating chest infections. KNOTHE and WETTENGEL (1978) have used sulfamoxole and this combination, called co-trifamol or Supristol, was compared with co-trimoxazole. In a double-blind study involving 163 patients, 320 mg TMP and 1,600 SMX were compared with 320 mg TMP and 1,600 mg sulfamoxazole. Patients with exacerbations of their bronchitis received a 14-day course of either treatment. Only patients from whose sputum pathogenic bacteria sensitive to trimethoprim and sulfonamide were isolated, were included in the trial. This meant that of an initial 163 patients, only 61 were left for study. Of these, 28 received Supristol and 33 co-trimoxazole. The sputum cultures grew *Streptococcus pneumoniae* in 28 cases and *H. influenzae* in 5, whilst other organisms, such as *Staphylococcus* and *Klebsiella* spp. were grown from some other cases. Taking the bacteriological results from the whole 61 patients, the causative agent was eliminated by Supristol in 95.3% of cases and by co-trimoxazole in 93.2%. This result was interpreted by the authors as showing no significant difference between the treatments. There was also no difference between the treatments as regards clinical improvement and side effects, which were few.

It has also been questioned whether SDZ might penetrate better into the sputum. In a small study D. HUGHES et al. (1979) compared levels of SMX and sulfadiazine in bronchial secretions obtained by suction through a fibre optic bronchoscope. There was little difference in levels of the two sulfonamides, both of which were found in much lower concentrations than in the blood. Sulfadiazine (SDZ) has also been suggested as a logical partner for TMP. A recent clinical study by J. ROBERTSON et al. (1982, unpublished work) suggested that such a combination may indeed be effective in treating chronic bronchitis, though no comparison was made directly with TMP/SMX. They used tablets, each containing 125 mg TMP and 375 mg SDZ (1:3 ratio) giving two tablets every 12 h (a daily dosage of 500 mg TMP and 1,500 mg SDZ) for 7 days.

Other diaminopyrimidines had been considered by HITCHING's group in the 1950s and 1960s (see BUSHBY and HITCHINGS 1968), but more recently another member of this series has been investigated bacteriologically and clinically (see Antibacterial Folate Inhibitors, 1979, WISE R. and REEVES DS, eds., J Antimicrob Chemother [Suppl] 5). This is tetroxoprim, which chemically is 2,4-diamino-5(3,5-dimethoxy-4(2-methoxyethoxy)benzylpyrimidine, which is also a selective blocker of the bacterial, but not the human, enzyme, dihydrofolate reductase. Two clinical studies of the use of tetroxoprim combined with sulfadiazine in chest infections have been reported. The first of these was by PINES and RAAFAT (1979). In this, tetroxoprim 100 mg and sulfadiazine 250 mg was given as two doses 12 h apart daily for 10 days to treat patients with purulent bronchial infections. This gave a daily dose of 200 mg tetroxoprim and 500 mg SDZ. A comparison with ampicillin (2 g/day) was made in 60 patients, 30 patients receiving each treatment in a single-blind trial. In both groups, purulent sputum was rendered mucoid in 24/30 patients. The mean time to achieve such mucoid sputum was 5 days with both treatments. The clinical success rate was the same for both groups. No side effects were found in the tetroxoprim/sulfadiazine group, whereas three patients receiving ampicillin had gastrointestinal upsets, necessitating withdrawal of treatment in two cases. The authors concluded that this novel combination was at least as effective as ampicillin at 2 g/day and possibly less toxic. They also pointed out (see Chap. 4) that four species of *H. influenzae* isolated from sputum were resistant as graded by sensitivity discs of tetroxoprim and sulfadiazine which contained 50 µg of the combination in a 1:9 ratio. The relevance of such apparent resistance to TMP and sulfonamides to true resistance in vivo remains uncertain.

In a second study, FERBER and AHRENS (1979) used tetroxoprim/SDZ to treat both chest and urinary infections. Rather scant details of the patients are given, but some 213 patients with "acute bronchitis" were treated with favourable results. Insufficient data were presented to allow any critical assessment of the efficacy of the combination in their hands.

G. Trimethoprim Alone

Because of the high urinary levels that can be achieved, trimethoprim alone has been used extensively and successfully in the treatment of both acute and chronic urinary infections. It has not, so far, found such extensive use in treating chest infections, though there is evidence to suggest that it would be quite logical to use the agent *alone* in this situation. The fact that it is concentrated whilst SMX is diluted in the sputum has already been referred to. Several workers have pointed out that the low concentrations of sulfonamide in the sputum may contribute but little to any antibacterial effect of the combination and that it is the sulfonamide component that produces most of the toxicity.

WILKINSON and REEVES (1979) conclude a useful review as to which sulfonamide should be combined with TMP, with the statement "Since sulphonamides alone are not active at low concentrations and a ratio with low sulphonamide content (as in sputum) is unsatisfactory for obtaining synergy against the majority of bacteria, even in antagonistic-free media, the exact role of sulphonamides in general therapy with co-trimoxazole is still open to debate". Many would agree with this view. LACEY has long been sceptical of the relevance of in vitro synergy of TMP and sulfonamides to the in vivo efficacy of the combination. He has pointed out that in several situations in the body – either due to the pharmacokinetics of the two components or the nature of the infecting organism – the sulfonamide component may be having little effect. So far he is the only author to have *published* results of any study comparing the effect of TMP alone and combined with sulfonamide in *chest* infections.

In a recent paper (LACEY et al. 1980), he describes results in some 279 patients treated in general practice and in hospital geriatric wards. The nature of the patients and their infections is not enlarged upon, but the main respiratory diagnoses appear to have been exacerbations of chronic bronchitis and pneumonia. Patients had to be excluded for various reasons so that he was finally left with 216 patients with chest infections suitable for study. Of these, 107 received TMP 200 mg twice daily for 5 days and 109 two co-trimoxazole tablets twice daily (320 mg TMP and 1,600 mg SMX in 24 h). The tablets were made to resemble each other and the trial was randomised and double-blind. Both regimes produced a good response and after 7 days, purulent sputum had become non-purulent and most pathogenic organisms, which had been present before treatment, had been eradicated. There was no difference between the two treatments. In none of the sputum samples taken, either at the beginning of the trial or after treatment, was any strain of *H. influenzae* or *S. pneumoniae* resistant to TMP or sulfonamide cultured. This is too short a period for any resistance to be expected to develop, but one of the reasons put forward initially to justify the combination of TMP with sulfonamide was to prevent the emergence of a resistant organism.

The whole question of the possible emergence of resistant organisms following the use of TMP alone is a complex one that is considered in Chap. 2. LACEY et al. (1980) make a strong case for using TMP alone in chest as well as in urinary tract infections. Their conclusions may need to be taken with caution, however. In a preliminary trial (D. HUGHES, 1979 b), rather disappointing results were obtained with TMP alone at 250 mg twice a day. Further work with TMP alone in chest infections, and in defined diagnostic categories, is needed to assess its possible value.

H. Future Developments

In spite of all the comparisons and criticisms as to whether a sulfonamide, and if so, which, should be combined with TMP, there can be no doubt that for all its theoretical disadvantages a 1:5 ratio combination of TMP and SMX as formulated in co-trimoxazole in a daily dosage of 320 mg TMP and 1,600 mg SMX, has proved effective in treating many types of chest infection. It will be interesting to see if, for all the controversy, either TMP alone (at *any* dosage) or TMP combined with another sulfonamide, will prove any more effective. It will certainly be difficult to prove any such increased efficacy in clinical terms, though were TMP alone to be of comparable efficacy it might be preferred on grounds of both toxicity and cost.

References

Adcock KJ, Reddy S, Okubadejo OA, Montefiore D (1972) TMP/SMX in pertussis: comparison with tetracycline. Arch Dis Child 47:311–313

Beumer HM (1972) Double-blind trial with sulfamethoxazole plus trimethoprim (Bactrim) versus demethyl-chlortetracycline (Ledermycin) in chronic respiratory tract infections. Respiration 29:257–269

Bushby SRM, Hitchings GH (1968) Trimethoprim, a sulphonamide potentiator. Br J Pharmacol Chemother 33:72–90

Carroll PG, Krejci SP, Mitchell J, Puranik V, Thomas R, Wilson B (1977) A comparative study of co-trimoxazole and amoxycillin in the treatment of acute bronchitis in General Practice. Med J Aust 2:286–287

Cooper J, McGillion FB (1978) Treatment of acute exacerbations of chronic bronchitis. A double-blind trial of co-trimoxazole and cephalexin. Practitioner 221:428–432

Darrell JH, Garrod LP, Waterworth PM (1968) Trimethoprim: laboratory and clinical studies. J Clin Pathol 21:202–209

Drew CDM, Hughes DTD, Fowle ASE, Cassell M (1967a) Effective treatment of chronic bronchitis with short-term trimethoprim and sulphamethoxazole. Proc 5th Int Cong Chemother [Suppl] Al-5a/3:293–296. Verlag der Wien med Akad

Drew CDM, Hughes DTD, Jenkins CG (1967b) Long-term treatment of chronic bronchitis with trimethoprim and sulphamethoxazole. Proc 5th Int Congr Chemother [Suppl] Al-5a/3:107–109. Verlag der Wien med Akad

Ferber H, Ahrens KH (1979) A short-term study of tetroxoprim/sulphadiazine in the treatment of acute bronchitis and urinary tract infections. J Antimicrob Chemother [Suppl B] 5:231–235

General Practitioner Group (1972) A further comparative trial of co-trimoxazole in chronic bronchitis. Practitioner 209:838–840

Hughes DTD (1969) Single-blind comparative trial of trimethoprim-sulphamethoxazole and ampicillin in the treatment of exacerbations of chronic bronchitis. Br Med J 4:470–473

Hughes DTD (1973) Use of combinations of trimethoprim and sulfamethoxazole in the treatment of chest infections. J Infect Dis [Suppl] 128:S701–S705

Hughes DTD (1976) Chemoprophylaxis in chronic bronchitis. J Antimicrob Chemother 2:320–322

Hughes DTD (1979a) Antibiotic treatment of chronic bronchitis. J R Coll Physicians Lond 13:26–28

Hughes DTD (1979b) Trials of TMP alone in the treatment of exacerbations, of chronic bronchitis. Internal Report filed with Wellcome Research Laboratories, Beckenham

Hughes DTD, Drew CDM, Johnson TBW, Jarvis JD (1969) Trimethoprim and sulphamethoxazole in the treatment of chronic chest infections. Chemotherapy 14:151–157

Hughes DTD, Bye A, Hodder P (1972) Levels of trimethoprim and sulphamethoxazole in blood and sputum in relation to treatment of chest infections. Adv Antimicrob Antineoplast Chemother 1/2:1105–1106

Hughes DTD, Jenkins GC, Gurney JD (1975) The clinical, haematological and bacteriological effects of long-term treatment with co-trimoxazole. J Antimicrob Chemother 1:55–65

Hughes DTD, Land G, McDonnell KA (1979) Study of the comparative levels of sulphadiazine and sulphamethoxazole in plasma, saliva and bronchial secretions. Internal Report field with Wellcome Research Laboratories, Beckenham

Hughes DTD, Russell NJ (1982) The use of co-trimoxazole in treating chest infections. Rev Infect Dis. 4, 528–532

Hughes WT, Feldman S, Sanyal SK (1975) Treatment of Pneumocystis carinii pneumonia with TMP-SMX. Can Med Assoc J [Suppl] 112:475–505

Hughes WT, Kuhn S, Chaudhary S (1977) Successful chemoprophylaxis for Pneumocystis carinii pneumonitis. N Eng J Med 297:1419–1426

Iglauer E, Wieser O, Zechner E (1978) Trial of the clinical tolerance of a new form of co-trimoxazole for intramuscular injection in patients with bronchopulmonary infections. Wien Med Wochenschr 128:400–402

Jenkins GC, Hughes DTD, Hall PC (1970) A haematological study of patients receiving long-term treatment with trimethoprim and sulphonamide. J Clin Pathol 23:392–396

Kaplan L, Stegman TM (1972) Single-blind comparative trial of trimethoprim-sulphamethoxazole and ampiclox. S Afr Med J 46:318–321

Knothe H, Wettengel R (1978) Treatment of chronic bronchitis with supristol and a co-trimoxazole preparation. Comparative bacteriological and clinical findings, results of a double-blind study. Med Klin 73:1780–1784

Lacey RW, Lord VL, Gunasekera HKW, Leiberman PJ, Luxton DEA (1980) Comparison of trimethoprim alone with trimethoprim sulphamethoxazole in the treatment of respiratory and urinary infections with particular reference to selection of trimethoprim resistance. Lancet 1:1270–1273

Lal S, Bhalla KK (1969) Comparison of tetracycline and TMP-SMX in acute episodes in chronic chest infections. Postgrad Med J [Suppl] 45:91–93

Lau WK, Young LS (1976) Trimethoprim-sulfamethoxazole treatment of Pneumocystis carinii pneumonia in adults. N Engl J Med 295:716–718

Medical Research Council (1965) Comittee on aetiology of chronic bronchitis: Definition and classification of chronic bronchitis for clinical and epidemiological purposes. Lancet 1:775–779

Medical Research Council Working Party (1966) Value of chemoprophylaxis and chemotherapy in early chronic bronchitis. Br Med J 1:117–122

Pines A, Raafat H (1979) A comparative clinical trial of tetroxoprim/sulphadiazine and ampicillin in the treatment of purulent bronchial infections. J Antimicrob Chemother [Suppl B] 5:201–205

Pines A, Greenfield JSB, Raafat H, Rahman M, Siddiqui AM (1969) Preliminary experience with trimethoprim and sulphamethoxazole in the treatment of purulent chronic bronchitis. Postgrad Med J [Suppl] 45:89–90

Pines A, Raafat H, Greenfield JSB, Siddiqui G, Lennox-Smith I, Linsell WD (1972) The management of purulent exacerbations of chronic bronchitis – a comparison of co-trimoxazole and tetracycline. Practitioner 208:265–270

Pines A, Nandi AR, Raafat H, Rahman M (1977) Amoxycillin and co-trimoxazole in acute purulent exacerbations of chronic bronchitis. Chemotherapy 23:58–64

Tandon MK (1977) A comparative trial of co-trimoxazole and amoxycillin in the treatment of acute exacerbations of chronic bronchitis. Med J Aust 2:281–284

Wilkinson PJ, Reeves DS (1979) Tissue penetration of trimethoprim and sulphonamides. J Antimicrob Chemother [Suppl B] 5:159–168

Winston DJ, Lau WK, Gale RP, Young S (1980) TMP-SMX for the treatment of Pneumocystis carinii pneumonia. Ann Intern Med 92:762–769

Treatment of Miscellaneous and Unusual Infections with Trimethoprim and Trimethoprim/Sulfonamide Combinations

R.E. DESJARDINS

A. Introduction

The broad spectrum of in vitro antimicrobial activity and frequent observations of synergy with the combination of trimethoprim and sulfamethoxazole (co-trimoxazole) have lead to its evaluation clinically in a large variety of infectious diseases. Many of these are discussed in other chapters. However, a few notable exceptions remain. The present chapter is a summary of data from studies in a variety of diseases in which the combination has been evaluated in some detail, though well-controlled clinical studies have not been reported in most cases. These include brucellosis, toxoplasmosis, nocardiosis, the "atypical" mycobacterioses, histoplasmosis, paracoccidioidomycosis, phycomycosis, and chromomycosis. A few additional examples are included because of their inherent interest, despite the paucity of available information; i.e., bubonic plaque, Q fever, *Isospora belli* infections, pneumonitis due to the "Pittsburgh pneumonia agent," malakoplakia, and pediculosis capitis.

Most of these diseases are relatively uncommon in any one location. The opportunity, therefore, for well controlled clinical studies is remote. In such cases, judgments as to the relative merit of one or another mode of therapy are extremely dependent on the reliability of observations recorded by the physicians directly involved in the care of these patients. For the many such observations reported in the world medical literature upon which this review is based, I am deeply grateful. In some cases, the data reviewed and results presented suggest at least a tentative conclusion regarding the efficacy of the combination in the condition being considered. Where such conclusions are stated they represent the opinion only of the present author.

B. Brucellosis

This zoonotic infection has its natural reservoir in a variety of domestic animals such as cattle, pigs, goats, and sheep. It is, therefore, often seen in agricultural workers or following the ingestion of unpasteurized milk. The most common species infecting humans are *Brucella melitensis* (of goats), *Brucella suis* (of pigs), and *Brucella abortus* (of cattle).

In humans, the affliction resulting from infection with any of these species of *Brucella* is highly variable. Its designation, "undulant fever," is an apt description of the most common symptom of the disease; a remitting and relapsing fever. In its usual course, permanent remission of fever and associated symptoms such as anorexia, malaise, headache, weakness, insomnia, and mental depression, occurs within 3–6 months. It may relapse following apparent recovery with or without treatment, and a chronic form of the disease is seen in some patients in whom symptoms may persist for up to 2 years. It is often difficult, though, to rule out the possibility of reinfection in individuals with continuing occupational exposure. Treatment with tetracycline for 3–4 weeks may bring about a more rapid recovery. Patients with unusually severe undulant fever may, in addition, be treated with streptomycin. The use of trimethoprim/sulfamethoxazole (TMP/SMX) in the treatment of this disease has also been described.

Several investigators have demonstrated convincingly the synergistic activity of TMP and SMX against various species of *Brucella*. Barnett and Bushby (1970) first reported assessment of in vitro activity of the combination using Wellcome Nutrient Agar supplemented with 5% lysed horse blood, against 18 isolates of *B. abortus*. The minimum inhibitory concentration of TMP alone was 15 µg/ml, of SMX alone, 3 µg/ml and of a 1:20 ratio, of the combination, 0.05 µg/ml TMP + 1.0 µg/ml SMX. Identical results were reported by Lal et al. (1970) with two clinical isolates of *B. abortus*. Additional confirmation of the synergistic effect of the combination against *B. abortus* has been reported by many investigators (Colonnello et al. 1970; Calongi et al. 1973; Robertson et al. 1973; Roux et al. 1974). Activity of TMP/SMX has also been demonstrated in vitro against *B. melitensis* (Ktenidou et al. 1974) and other species of *Brucella* (Pilet and Monteil 1972).

Philippon et al. (1972) described the use of a murine model to evaluate various antimicrobial drugs against infection with *B. melitensis*. Fifteen days after intraperitoneal inoculation with 3×10^5 organisms, the animals were given the test drug once daily for 19 days by gastric lavage. Tetracycline was the most potent agent evaluated, resulting in a 1,000-fold reduction in the number of organisms found in the spleen at the end of therapy. TMP/SMX showed only slight activity in this model. However, as noted by Grossman and Remington (1979) in their evaluation of this combination against toxoplasmosis, the laboratory mouse may be unsuitable for the evaluation of TMP because of the exceedingly short half-life of the drug in this species (24 min) compared with humans (10 h).

Clinical reports of the use of co-trimoxazole to treat brucellosis have appeared frequently since the introduction of the drug in 1969. Alberola et al. (1969) first reported successful therapy in two patients with Malta fever, but did not include any details regarding the clinical status of their patients or the regimen used to treat them. A more complete report by Lal et al. (1970) included in vitro assessment of the sensitivity of the isolates from two of their four patients to TMP/SMX. These four patients were treated with four tablets daily (80 mg TMP + 400 mg SMX in each tablet) for periods varying from 18 days to 8 weeks. All of these patients responded well to treatment, but one had a subsequent rise in antibrucella antibody titer 4 months after treatment, suggesting a possible relapse of the infection. Lal et al. (1970) suggested that some of their patients may have been treated longer than was necessary, and the one patient who apparently relapsed was treated for only 18 days. Eight patients of Hassan et al. (1971) with infection due to *B. melitensis* responded rapidly to treatment with TMP/SMX, 2–4 tablets daily for 3 weeks, but three of these relapsed within 3 weeks of ending therapy. This prompted Hassan et al. (1971) to suggest that therapy be continued for at least 6 weeks. Giunchi

Table 1. Reported cases of human brucellosis treated with TMP/SMX

Reference	Country	No. of patients		
		Treated	Cured	Relapsed or poor response
ALBEROLA et al. (1969)	Spain	2	2	
LAL et al. (1970)	England	4	3	1
GIUNCHI et al. (1971)	Italy	9	8	1
BILLI and FRONGILLO (1971)	Italy	3	3	
HASSAN et al. (1971)	Egypt	8	8	
BARBA and MERLO (1972)	Italy	8	8	
CANTALAMESSA et al. (1972)	Italy	14	13	1
GIUNCHI et al. (1972)	Italy	27	25	2
PASCHETTA (1972)	Italy	14	14	
SUERI (1972)	Italy	35	24	11
SUERI (1973)	Italy	14	10	4
DAIKOS et al. (1973)	Greece	86	78	8
PORTO et al. (1974)	Italy	25	18	7
SUERI and IELASI (1974)	Italy	20	19	1
D'ALESSANDRO et al. (1974)	Italy	20	18	2
MINOPRIO (1974)	Argentina	56	54	2
KERI and TELEGOY (1975)	Hungary	6	4	2
ARROYO and NORIEGA (1976)	Spain	4	4	
BERTAGGIA (1975)	Italy	2	2	
TELEGDY and KERI (1976)	Hungary	19	9	10
RIGATOS et al. (1975)	Greece	30	24	6
OOMEN (1976)	Kenya	10	5	5
LOPEZ et al. (1976)	Spain	19	14	5
ARIZA et al. (1977)	Spain	31	21	10
FIORI et al. (1978)	Italy	47	45	2
SUERI et al. (1978)	Italy	24	20	4

et al. (1971) described treatment of nine patients with daily doses of 4–6 tablets of co-trimoxazole for periods ranging from 12 to 43 days. One patient relapsed following 16 days treatment and was subsequently cured by a second course of co-trimoxazole for an additional 12 days. The remaining eight patients had remission of fever after only 2–4 days treatment and no evidence of relapse during a follow-up period of 1–5 months. GIUNCHI et al. (1971) concluded that TMP/SMX was a good alternative to tetracycline for the treatment of acute brucellosis in humans. A similar conclusion was reached by ARIZA et al. (1977) based on their experience with the use of the combination in the treatment of 33 patients with acute brucellosis. All patients were treated uniformly with six tablets daily for 15 days followed by four tablets daily for an additional 30 days. This regimen was completed and well tolerated by 31 of the 33 patients. All but one patient (who had brucellar spondylitis) responded well initially, though serologic or bacteriologic evidence of relapse occurred in eight.

Since 1969, over 500 cases of brucellosis treated with TMP/SMX have been reported in the medical literature from many different countries. These are summarized in Table 1. Represented in this summary are a variety of clinical presentations treated with an even greater variety of dosage regimens. In some cases a combination of several drugs was used, though the majority report treatment with co-trimoxazole alone. With very few exceptions, the results reported have been excellent. Of the total of 535 cases in the table, 449 (84%) were reported as cured or significantly improved. In those cases in which rapidity of response was noted, the patients generally became afebrile after 2–8 days therapy.

The experience of two groups of investigators (DAIKOS et al. 1973; SUERI 1972, 1973; SUERI and IELASI 1974; SUERI et al. 1978) has been quite extensive. DAIKOS et al. (1973) reported the results of treatment with co-trimoxazole of 86 patients with brucellosis. These patients were treated with doses ranging from four tablets a day for 15 days to six tablets a day for as long as 2 months, depending on the clinical presentation and severity of the illness. A few cases (patients with endocarditis or osteomyelitis) were given as many as eight tablets a day for an initial period of 1 week or longer. In 39 cases, the diagnosis was made by culture of the organism from blood. In the remainder, serologic tests confirmed the diagnosis. The response to treatment was reported as "very good" in 78 of the 86 patients; 8 patients did not respond initially and 3 others relapsed during a follow-up period of 2 months.

SUERI (1972, 1973), SUERI and IELASI (1974), and SUERI et al. (1978) reported a series of patients with brucellosis treated with co-trimoxazole over several years. In the earlier reports, results of treatment with TMP/SMX were compared with results of treatment with tetracycline. The first report (SUERI 1972) described treatment of 35 patients with 4 tablets of co-trimoxazole a day or 2 g/day tetracycline for 15–25 days. While most of these patients responded favorably, the rate of relapse was 37% with co-trimoxazole and 18% with tetracycline during a follow-up period of 3–4 months. Subsequently (SUERI 1973) a group of 14 patients was treated with 640 mg/day TMP + 3,200 mg/day SMX (one-half of the dose was given intravenously) for 15 days, and a control group of 15 patients was treated with 3–4 g/day tetracycline for 15 days. Again, the response to treatment was excellent in both groups and the relapse rates were 10% following co-trimoxazole and 11% following tetracycline therapy.

In a review of the use of TMP/SMX for the treatment of human brucellosis, CHALHOUB (1976) concluded that this combination appears to be quite effective. The dose requirement is probably higher than the standard dose of two tablets twice daily, recommended for most bacterial infections, and for a period longer than the usual 10–15 days. This conclusion appears reasonable at the present time, though it is likely that a small proportion of patients will relapse despite such a regimen. The relapse rate with tetracycline or chloramphenicol, the standard treatment for brucellosis, is also considerable. TMP/SMX may, therefore, be recommended as acceptable therapy for brucellosis.

C. Toxoplasmosis

This protean disease, due to infection with the coccidian parasite *Toxoplasma gondii*, has become recognized as one of the most widespread and common human infections with a prevalence in the world of approximately 500 million cases (KEAN

1972). Fortunately, most of these are asymptomatic infections recognized retrospectively by various serologic tests. The disease in its more active forms is recognized as occurring in four distinct clinical presentations
1. Acquired acute lymphadenopathic toxoplasmosis
2. Congenital toxoplasmosis
3. Toxoplasmic retinochoroiditis
4. Toxoplasmosis in the immune deficient host.
The first of these exhibits a highly variable but usually self-limited course without therapy. It most often presents as a febrile lymphadenopathy with frequent involvement of the spleen, skeletal muscle, myocardium, brain and, less often, liver and skin. The remaining presentations, however, are either life-threatening or involve serious sequelae, and therefore always require appropriate chemotherapy. Therapeutic intervention is effective only during the proliferative phase, and therefore requires early recognition of active disease. There is no effective therapy for the dormant or cyst stage of the infection. Effective therapy with the synergistic combination of pyrimethamine and sulfadiazine was first described by EYLES and COLEMAN (1953), and has changed little since that time. Because of the frequent bone marrow suppression associated with this combination when used in the doses required for the treatment of toxoplasmosis, folinic acid is often given concurrently.

Interest in the use of trimethoprim rather than pyrimethamine, in the hope of achieving reasonable efficacy with less hematologic toxicity, led to evaluation of this drug in combination with a sulfonamide in experimental models of the disease. FELDMAN (1973) reported the use of a combination of TMP and sulfasoxazole in a murine model with dissappointing results. In that study, the drugs were administered in a dose of approximately 5 mg kg^{-1} day^{-1} TMP $+ 20$ mg kg^{-1} day^{-1} sulfasoxazole added to the animals' drinking water. Failure of this combination to affect the course of the infection was attributed by FELDMAN to the possible use of an unsuitable sulfonamide and the need for further studies of TMP with a different sulfonamide was suggested.

Using a higher dose of TMP/SMX in a similar model, SANDER and MIDTVEDT (1970) reported definite evidence of synergy with this combination, whereas SMX alone had been reported to be ineffective (MACHADO et al. 1967). Subsequent reports presented variable results, but generally supported the impression of a synergistic effect of this combination in rodents (STADTSBAEDER and CALVIN-PREVAL 1973; TERRAGNA et al. 1973; LAFRENZ et al. 1973; CELLESI et al. 1973; SZAFLARSKI et al. 1974; TERRAGNA et al. 1974a, b; WERNER and EGGER 1975; MAIER and PIEKARSKI 1976; FREZZOTTI et al. 1978; THIERMANN et al. 1978). With intraperitoneal administration of the drugs at a dose of 2 mg/day TMP $+ 10$ mg/day SMX for 20 days, TERRAGNA et al. (1973) reported 91.3% survival of treated mice in two separate experiments in which all control mice died. SEAH (1975) demonstrated the efficacy of TMP/SMX added to the food of mice infected by intraperitoneal inoculation of 10^4 trophozoites of T. gondii. However, in that study, SMX alone was only slightly less effective than an identical dose of TMP/SMX, which was in turn less effective than pyrimethamine/sulfadiazine (PMA/SDZ), all administered for 7 days. Mean survival times of mice treated with SMX alone, TMP/SMX, and PMA/SDZ were 13.76 ± 1.95, 18.73 ± 3.03, and 21.26 ± 2.25 days respectively.

SEAH concluded that TMP/SMX was synergistic, but less effective than PMA/SDZ in this murine model.

The synergistic activity of TMP/SMX on the multiplication of *T. gondii* trophozoites in mouse peritoneal macrophages in vitro was demonstrated by NGUYEN and STADTSBAEDER (1975). Inhibition of replication was 19.6% ± 4.6% with TMP alone at 2 μg/ml, 17.0% ± 3.9% with SMX alone at 70 μg/ml and 96.3% ± 2.7% with the two drugs combined at 2 μg/ml TMP + 70 μg/ml SMX in tissue culture medium. These investigators later called attention to the apparent discrepancy between these in vitro results with TMP and failure of this drug alone in an experimental murine infection with the same parasite (NGUYEN et al. 1977). They furthermore confirmed earlier reports of the superiority of PMA/sulfonamide over TMP/sulfonamide in the mouse model.

REMINGTON (1976) first reported that TMP was ineffective alone and did not add to the activity of sulfamethoxazole in mice infected with the RH strain of *T. gondii*. These early experiments were conducted by adding the drugs to the animals' food. Later experiments, in which the drug was administered by gavage were reported by GROSSMAN et al. (1978) as showing evidence of a synergistic effect of TMP/SMX. They also reported that the combination was highly effective in vitro against multiplication of *T. gondii* in mouse bladder tumor cells. These observations were later extended to show a marked effect of TMP in vitro, as indicated by suppression of uptake of uracil ³H by *T. gondii* cultured in mouse peritoneal macrophages (GROSSMAN and REMINGTON 1979). In a series of elegant experiments, synergism was clearly demonstrated in vitro with TMP/SMX. Additional experiments in mice further confirmed the activity of the combination in vivo at concentrations that were ineffective when each agent was used alone. A significant aspect of these in vivo experiments was the frequent measurement of TMP concentrations in the serum of these animals by which it was shown that the half-life of this drug in the mouse was 24 min. Noting that the half-life of PMA in this animal is 6.5 h, a plausible explanation for the discrepancies in various comparative studies was offered, based on the differing metabolism of the drugs in mice. Knowing also that the half-life of trimethoprim in humans is between 10 and 14 h, GROSSMAN and REMINGTON (1979) concluded that the in vivo mouse model may not reflect the potential efficacy of TMP/SMX for the treatment of toxoplasmosis in humans. They further pointed out that the in vitro results "demonstrate remarkable synergism against intracellular *T. gondii* with drug levels easily achievable in man."

Several reports of the use of co-trimoxazole clinically in the treatment of toxoplasmosis have appeared during the past 10 years. MÖSSNER (1970) reported the results of treatment of 9 patients with TMP alone and 11 patients with TMP/SMX. All of these patients were adults with acquired lymphadenopathic toxoplasmosis. TMP alone was inadequate, but the therapeutic activity of the combination was considered equivalent to that of standard therapy with PMA/SDZ. LAFRENZ et al. (1973) reported similar results in 12 patients with toxoplasmosis treated with a dose of 160 mg TMP + 800 mg SMX twice daily for ten days. Several additional cases of acquired toxoplasmosis treated successfully with TMP/sulfonamide have appeared in the literature (DOMART et al. 1973; KUSCHNAROFF et al. 1973; GEDDES et al. 1973; PARADISI et al. 1976; KOUBA et al. 1978; GAMBARELLA et al. 1978;

CALONGHI et al. 1978). NORRBY (1975) reported good results with TMP/SMX in five of six patients with acquired lymphadenopathic toxoplasmosis and in one 22-month-old child with severe toxoplasmic retinochoroiditis. The most extensive experience with the use of the combination in the treatment of ocular toxoplasmosis is that of FREZZOTTI et al. (1978). These authors evaluated a regimen of TMP/SMX administered for 21 days of each month with total treatment durations of 2–36 months in 57 patients with a variety of ocular manifestations of toxoplasmosis. Among these patients, 40 had chorioretinitis, 33 with macular involvement. Their results were described as excellent (rapid cure, with complete recovery) in 10 cases, good (rapid cure, with residual traces) in 33 cases, moderate (slow cure, with serious sequelae) in 11 cases, and poor (no therapeutic response) in 3 cases. The treatment regimen was well tolerated in most cases with only four patients having to discontinue the medication owing to gastrointestinal intolerance or cutaneous allergy.

It must be acknowledged that, with the exception of FREZZOTTI et al. (1978), most of the clinical reports of successful therapy with co-trimoxazole have described treatment of patients with acquired lymphadenopathic toxoplasmosis, a self-limited disease with a highly variable course, and none has been a controlled study. However, bone marrow suppression is not at all uncommon with PMA/SDZ at the recommended doses, and a safer effective therapy would be greatly appreciated by physicians and their patients. This is especially true for women who manifest the disease during pregnancy (FUCHS et al. 1974), and infants (WILLIAMS 1977). If the disease is recognized in the first trimester, termination of pregnancy by induced abortion is commonly recommended because of concern about the possible teratogenic risk associated with the use of PMA in the first trimester, based on laboratory data in mice.

In patients with life-threatening toxoplasmosis and toxoplasmic retinochoroiditis, the paucity of clinical data regarding use of TMP and the established efficacy of PMA combined with a long-acting sulfonamide support the continued use of the latter regimen, despite the problems associated with hematopoietic toxicity. However, recent in vitro data discussed previously, and the recognition of the unsuitability of the murine model for evaluation of TMP, indicate the desirability of addition experimental data in a more suitable animal such as the dog or nonhuman primates. If studies in these species provide good evidence of efficacy, controlled clinical trials with TMP/SMX compared with PMA/SDZ would be justifiable. More frequent use of antidotal leucovorin is also indicated, see Chap. 1.

D. Nocardiosis

This relatively uncommon but widespread disease is caused by infection with *Nocardia asteroides* (the most prevalent organism causing systemic nocardiosis), *N. brasiliensis*, and *N. caviae*. Though the disease caused by infection with *N. asteroides* most often presents as a bronchopulmonary infection, it has a distressing tendency to spread, with involvement of the brain and other organs. Infections with *N. brasiliensis* typically cause mycetoma or lymphocutaneous disease.

Pulmonary nocardiosis may occur in otherwise healthy individuals, but patients with impaired immunity are particularly susceptible. Treatment usually requires prolonged administration of appropriate antimicrobial drugs. LYONS et al. (1943) first reported successful therapy with SDZ. Though other agents have been advocated, including chloramphenicol (RIVERA and PEREZ 1957), tetracycline (PEABODY and SEABURY 1960), and erythromycin/ampicillin (BACH et al. 1973 a), long- or intermediate-acting sulfonamides are still most commonly employed.

Early reports of successful therapy of mycetoma due to infection with *N. brasiliensis* with TMP/SMX suggested the possibility of synergistic activity of these two agents against *Nocardia* spp. (OCHOA and TAMAYO 1969; ESCALONA 1969; PENICHE et al. 1969; EVANS and BENSON 1971; MAHGOUB 1972). A more recent review of these early reports (LOPES 1976 a) concluded that treatment with this combination had been effective in 44 of 46 reported cases of infection with *N. brasiliensis*, and recommended two tablets (160 mg TMP + 800 mg SMX) twice daily until all lesions were healed, followed by prolonged "maintenance therapy" with one tablet twice daily – the latter because of the considerable tendency to relapse. Additional cases of successful therapy of nocardial mycetoma due to *N. brasiliensis* and *N. asteroides* with co-trimoxazole have been reported (MAIBACH and GORHAM 1975; NITIDANDHAPRABHAS and SITTAPAIROCHANA 1975; MAHGOUB 1977).

The relative inhibitory activity of TMP against the dihydrofolate reductase derived from *N. brasiliensis* and mammalian cells (rat liver) was shown by JAFFE et al. (1972) to be 40:1; only a moderate therapeutic ratio compared with *Plasmodium berghei*, where the ratio was 4,000:1. Several investigators have evaluated the potential synergy of TMP/SMX in vitro against various species of *Nocardia* with varying results. W. BLACK and MCNELLIS (1970) first reported the results of their in vitro evaluation of this combination with nine isolates of *N. asteroides*, two of *N. caviae*, and one of *N. blackwellii*. The minimum inhibitory concentrations of both drugs were determined independently and in ratios (SMX:TMP) of 20:1, 10:1, 5:1, and 1:1. The medium used was Oxoid CM 261 broth supplemented with 5% lysed horse blood added when the medium was at 50°–60 °C. A heavy inoculum of the organism was used and the cultures were evaluated after 48 h incubation at 37 °C. These conditions, as later shown by other investigators, were not optimal for detecting a synergistic effect against *Nocardia* spp., and may have been responsible for the equivocal results obtained in this investigation.

A similar evaluation with four isolates of *N. asteroides* and one of *N. brasiliensis* by BEAUMONT (1970), using Oxoid DST agar with 5% lysed horse blood and smaller inocula of the organisms, showed marked synergy with the combination at a 10:1 ratio when the data were plotted as an isobologram. BEAUMONT stressed the importance of appropriate culture medium and a low inoculum in the detection of potential synergy. Using a medium especially prepared for sensitivity testing with TMP/SMX (Wellcotest Agar), BUSHBY (1973) demonstrated excellent potentiation at a ratio of 1:1 with summed fractional inhibitory concentrations of less than 0.5 for 20 of 21 isolates of *Nocardia* spp. Synergy was equivocal for most of these strains at a higher ratio of 9:1. Other investigators have confirmed the importance of the inoculum size and the culture medium employed in evaluating the sensitivity of *Nocardia* spp. TMP/SMX (BACH et al. 1973 b).

Effective treatment of pulmonary nocardiosis with co-trimoxazole has been reported with concurrent in vitro sensitivity determinations on the isolated organisms (H. ADAMS and BROOKS 1977; BEELER et al. 1976; PAVILLARD 1973; MAD-ERAZO and QUINTILIANI 1974; COOK and FARRAR 1978). H. ADAMS and BROOKS (1977) successfully treated five patients with *N. asteroides* pneumonia. In each case SMX/TMP discs (23.75/1.25 µg) gave ≥ 32 mm zones of inhibition at 48 h and "clear-cut synergism" was demonstrated by inhibition patterns using juxtaposed discs. CARROLL et al. (1977) demonstrated in vitro susceptibility at clinically relevant concentrations of the combination with 14 of 14 isolates of *N. asteroides*, 7 of 7 isolates of *N. brasiliensis*, and 6 of 6 isolates of *N. caviae*.

A detailed evaluation of factors affecting the in vitro susceptibility of *Nocardia* spp. TMP/SMX was reported by BENNETT and JENNINGS (1978). These investigators used Mueller–Hinton agar which was pretested for suitability in the assessment of susceptibility to the combination. They evaluated nine isolates of *N. asteroides* and one of *N. caviae*. Determination of potential synergy was based on the fractional inhibitory concentration for each ratio of TMP/SMX against each of the isolates. Demonstration of synergism was found to be critically dependent on the particular isolate, duration of culture, and the ratio of the two drugs. There was no significant difference between the two relatively small inoculum sizes (5 and 170 colony forming units) used in this study. Consistent with earlier reports (BUSH-BY 1973; R. WALLACE et al. 1977), the authors concluded that the commercial formulation of co-trimoxazole does not contain a sufficient amount of TMP to provide significant potentiation of the sulfonamide effect against *Nocardia* spp. They suggested that substantially larger doses of TMP may be needed, and expressed concern with respect to the possible hematologic consequences of the dose that might be required. It is noteworthy, in this regard, that folinic acid, which can be used to treat or prevent potential hematologic changes, does not interfere with the in vitro susceptibility of *Nocardia* spp. to the combination (PAVILLARD 1973).

Since the introduction of the drug, numerous case reports have been published alleging successful therapy of infections due to *N. brasiliensis* and *N. asteroides* with TMP/SMX. A comprehensive review of the treatment of nocardiosis and actinomycetoma with the combination was published by HAVAS (1975) and of actinomycotic mycetoma caused by *N. brasiliensis* by LOPES (1976a). Both authors concluded that there was substantial evidence of the effectiveness of co-trimoxazole in the treatment of infections caused by *N. brasiliensis*, and HAVAS stated that further studies were justified in nocardiosis caused by *N. asteroides*. A survey of the articles reviewed by HAVAS (1975) and LOPES (1976a) as well as more recently published reports (Table 2) supports essentially the same conclusion now, i.e., that there is substantial demonstration of efficacy against actinomycetoma and superficial infections caused by *N. brasiliensis*, and that further studies are justified in nocardiosis caused by infection with *N. asteroides*.

There are no published controlled studies comparing the efficacy of TMP/SMX with other modes of therapy such as long- or intermediate-acting sulfonamides alone, or the combination of tetracycline or minocycline with erythromycin in the treatment of nocardiosis. Furthermore, the propensity for relapse of the disease has been stressed by recent investigators, calling attention to the need for longer periods of observation than have often been reported. The potential value of TMP/sulfonamide could be established by demonstrating a more rapid and certain cure or a decreased likelihood of relapse with the combination. Additional clinical stud-

Table 2. Reported cases of nocardiosis treated with TMP/SMX

Reference	Country	No. of patients	*Nocardia* species	Results[a]
Peniche et al. (1969)	Mexico	13	*N. brasiliensis*	9VG, 3G, 1F
Escalona (1969)	Mexico	8	*N. brasiliensis*	4VG, 3G, 1F
Ochoa and Tamayo (1969)	Mexico	14	*N. brasiliensis*	6VG, 7G, 1F
Marcovitch and Norman (1970)	England	1	*N. asteroides*	1VG
Baike et al. (1970)	Tasmania	1	*N. asteroides*	1VG
Lopes et al. (1971)	Mexico	2	*N. brasiliensis*	2VG
Adams et al. (1971)	Australia	1	*N. asteroides*	1G
Evans and Benson (1971)	Australia	1	*N. brasiliensis*	1VG
Ochoa (1971)	Mexico	1	*N. brasiliensis*	1VG
Mahgoub (1972)	Sudan	1	*N. brasiliensis*	1VG
Kremer (1972)	Australia	1	*N. asteroides*	1F
Pinkhas et al. (1973)	Israel	1	*N. asteroides*	1G
Pavillard (1973)	Australia	6	*N. asteroides*	5VG, 1F
Van Beers and Yourassowsky (1974)	Belgium	1	*N. asteroides*	1VG
Hamal (1974)	England	1	*N. asteroides*	1F
Sierra et al. (1974)	Columbia	1	*N. asteroides*	1G
Maderazo and Quintiliani (1974)	United States	1	*N. asteroides*	1VG
Maibach et al. (1975)	United States	1	*N. brasiliensis*	1VG
Beeler et al. (1976)	United States	2	*N. asteroides*	2VG
Nitidandhaprabhas and Sittapairochana (1975)	Thailand	1	*N. asteroides*	1VG
Frazier et al. (1975)	United States	1	*Nocardia* sp.	1VG
Sher et al. (1977)	United States	1	*N. asteroides*	1F
H. Adams and Brooks (1977)	United States	5	*N. asteroides*	5VG
Katz and Fanci (1977)	United States	1	*N. asteroides*	1G
Leelarasamee et al. (1977)	Thailand	1	*N. asteroides*	1VG
Cook and Farrar (1978)	United States	3	*N. asteroides*	3VG
Peterson et al. (1978)	United States	1	*N. caviae*	1F
Saksun et al. (1978)	United States	1	*N. madurae*	1G
Geiseler et al. (1979)	United States	1	*N. asteroides*	1F
May (1979)	United States	1	*N. asteroides*	1G
Satterwhite and Wallace (1979)	United States	3	*N. brasiliensis*	3VG
Satterwhite and Wallace (1979)	United States	1	*N. asteroides*	1VG
Poirier et al. (1979)	France	1	*N. asteroides*	1VG
Rodriguez et al. (1979)	Spain	1	*N. asteroides*	1VG
Gottlieb and Chatterjee (1979)	United States	1	*N. asteroides*	1F

[a] VG = very good; G = good; F = failure

ies with concurrent in vitro sensitivity data are eagerly awaited. Special circumstances, such as the treatment of patients with infection of the central nervous system, may warrant the use of the combination, even in the absence of controlled comparative studies. Otherwise, the use of TMP should be limited to patients who fail to improve on SDZ or another long- or intermediate-acting sulfonamide alone.

E. Atypical Mycobacteria

Several species of mycobacteria in addition to *Mycobacterium tuberculosis* and *M. leprae* have been implicated in a variety of human infections. These have been variously classified according to colony pigmentation and growth rate of the organism in vitro. These classifications, however, do not correspond to any epidemiologic or chemotherapeutic characteristic of the organism. The diseases caused by the atypical mycobacteria include pulmonary granulomas, meningitis, lymphadenitic granulomas with or without necrosis, septic arthritis, and skin infections.

Among the more common of these distinctly uncommon human pathogens are the "rapid growers," *M. fortuitum* and *M. chelonei*. Similarity of these organisms to *Nocardia* spp. prompted J. WALLACE et al. (1980) to investigate their responsiveness in vitro to TMP and SMX. SMX alone was moderately active against 31 of 32 isolates of *M. fortuitum* with inhibition at 32 µg/ml or less and 5 of 8 of *M. chelonei*, with inhibition at 64 µg/ml or less. All of the isolates were resistant to 64 µg/ml TMP, and there was no enhancement of sulfonamide activity by TMP at a 1:20 ratio of TMP:SMX. A number of investigators have reported similar negative results in vitro with a variety of species including *M. fortuitum*, *M. chelonei*, *M. kansasii*, *M. smegmatis*, *M. scrofulaceum*, *M. phlei*, *M. flavescens*, *M. vaccae*, *M. diernhoferi*, and *M. peregrinum* (SWENSON et al. 1980; DALOVISIO and PANKEY 1978; LASZLO and EIDUS 1978; HOKAMA 1976).

In contrast to these results, HILSON et al. (1971) found that while TMP had no activity against *M. tuberculosis* or *M. leprae*, it was moderately active in vitro against *Mycobacterium marinum*. The latter organism, *M. marinum*, has been identified as the cause of cutaneous granulomatous ulcers in swimmers and of fatal infections in tropical fish. BARROW and HEWITT (1971) reported successful treatment of one such skin infection acquired from a tropical fish tank with 160 mg TMP + 800 mg SMX twice daily for 6 weeks. In vitro susceptibility of this isolate was also demonstrated by the disc diffusion method. In a letter published in the *Archives of Dermatology* 4 years later, TURNER et al. (1975) acknowledged the results of BARROW and HEWITT and claimed similar success in six additional patients with *M. marinum* infections. These six patients were later reported in detail by KIRK and KAMINSKI (1976). Six additional cases have since been reported in some detail; one each by KECZKES (1974), WOOLFSON et al. (1976), and KELLY (1976) and three by BLACK and EYKYN (1977). All of these patients apparently acquired their infections from tropical fish tanks. All were treated successfully with TMP/SMX, in some cases after unsuccessful therapy with other antimicrobial drugs, such as tetracycline and clindamycin. Because of the frequency with which this indolent skin infection is associated with handling tropical fish, it has been suitably dubbed "fish tank granuloma." It has, however, also been reported in epidemic form in freshwater swimmers.

The reports of these several investigators combined with in vitro evidence that this organism is susceptible to TMP/SMX (HILSON et al. 1971) suggest that this drug should be considered for the treatment of fish tank granulomas since the organism is generally resistant to conventional antimycobacterial and other antimicrobial agents. However, CUNNINGHAM et al. (1978) reported a patient with fish tank granuloma due to infection with *M. marinum* which was insensitive to TMP/SMX in vitro. Their patients was reported to be responding well to treatment with erythromycin.

With the possible exception of *M. marinum*, TMP/SMX does not appear to be indicated for the treatment of infections with atypical mycobacteria. The observations of J. WALLACE et al. (1980) suggest the need for further evaluation of the role of sulfonamides in the treatment of patients with *M. fortuitum* and *M. chelonei* infections. Enhancement of activity by the addition of TMP appears unlikely, though assessment of ratios other than the 1:20 reported in their abstract may be of some interest in view of recent findings in *Nocardia* spp. (BENNETT and JENNINGS 1978).

F. Mycoses

Of the various mycotic infections of humans, only a few have been suggested as potential targets for treatment with TMP/sulfonamide. They are histoplasmosis, paracoccidioidomycosis (South American blastomycosis), phycomycosis due to infection with *Basidiobolus haptosporus* and related fungi, and chromomycosis.

I. Histoplasmosis

Microconidia of *Histoplasma capsulatum* are found in soil from many parts of the world. They are especially common where soil is heavily contaminated with bird droppings. These small spores are able to reach the alveoli of human lungs by inhalation and there they are transformed to active, budding yeast forms. The primary infection is mild or asymptomatic in the majority of cases. Patients who develop chronic fibronodular pulmonary histoplasmosis or disseminated histoplasmosis require therapy since these are uncommon, but potentially fatal, manifestations of the disease. Prolonged treatment with amphotericin B is associated with a cure rate of approximately 50%.

MACLEOD (1970) first reported successful treatment of a patient with chronic histoplasmosis with co-trimoxazole when the patient refused therapy with intravenous amphotericin B. This patient, whose manifestations included chronic fibronodular pulmonary disease of 10 years duration, adrenal insufficiency, and a chronic oropharyngeal ulceration, was later described in detail by *Macleod* et al. (1972). He had been treated originally with streptomycin and isoniazid for a presumptive diagnosis of tuberculosis. When the patient was first seen, culture of a tongue ulceration yielded *H. capsulatum* resistant in vitro to 500 µg/ml amphotericin B and 50 µg/ml sulfadoxine. He was treated nevertheless for 11 months with sulfadoxine and for 7 months with sulfadimidine with no effect on the tongue lesion which actually progressed during treatment. Subsequent therapy will TMP 160 mg + 800 mg SMX twice daily resulted in almost complete healing of this lesion after 10 months.

A similar case in which amphotericin B could not be used was reported by JONQUIERES et al. (1975). Their patient, with an antecedent history of pulmonary emphysema, but no evidence of acute pulmonary histoplasmosis, presented with a nasal mucosal ulceration and hepatosplenomegaly. The diagnosis of histoplasmosis was made when *H. capsulatum* was cultured from a biopsy of the nasal lesion. Following unsuccessful treatment with sulfadoxine, complete healing of the nasal ulceration and involution of the enlarged liver and spleen occurred during 3 months treatment with co-trimoxazole.

A third patient with an oral mucosal lesion due to infection with *H. capsulatum*, but without evidence of disseminated disease, was also effectively treated with co-trimoxazole following unsuccessful therapy with oral fluorocytosine by JAYAREEWAL et al. (1975). Their patient required almost 3 months therapy. Two Nigerian children with well-documented disseminated histoplasmosis were described by SERIKI et al. (1975). One, a 5-year-old boy, remained febrile while on amphotericin B and the other, a 10-year-old boy, developed a severe pancytopenia while on the same drug. Both were successfully treated with TMP/SMX and rifampicin.

NEGRONI et al. (1977) reported a series of 18 patients, 3 with chronic pulmonary histoplasmosis with cavitation and 15 with chronic disseminated histoplasmosis. Multiple organ involvement was documented in most cases and all diagnoses were confirmed by identification of *H. capsulatum*. Two of these patients relapsed following previous therapy with sulfonamides and amphotericin B. Treatment of these 18 patients for periods varying from 1 month to 2 years with TMP 160 mg + SMX 800 mg twice daily resulted in a clinical cure in all but one case. The one patient who was not cured was a 19-year-old woman with chronic lymphocytic leukemia who was intolerant of the drug. The treatment regimen was otherwise well tolerated by most of the patients and the authors considered the combination to be very useful in the treatment of histoplasmosis because of its "high efficacy and low toxicity." Two additional cases of disseminated histoplasmosis from Malaysia were reported to have been cured following treatment with co-trimoxazole as the sole antimicrobial drug (GANESAPILLAI et al. 1978).

A deep cutaneous and systemic mycosis indigenous to parts of Central and East Central Africa is caused by *Histoplasma duboisii*. This organism is similar morphologically and biochemically to *H. capsulatum*. Treatment generally consists of surgical drainage of the deep cutaneous abcesses and administration of amphotericin B for disseminated infection. Response of this infection to TMP/SMX has also been reported (K. BROWN et al. 1974; EGERE et al. 1978). In both cases, prior treatment included amphotericin B or 5-fluorocytosine, response to which was unsatisfactory. The patient of K. BROWN et al. was felt to have impaired immunity due to coexistent lepromatous leprosy.

II. Paracoccidioidomycosis

South American blastomycosis is a systemic mycosis indigenous to Mexico, Central America, and parts of South America, caused by infection with the fungus *Paracoccidioides brasiliensis*. The infection is generally thought to be acquired by inhalation of spores, and commonly presents with indurated oral mucosal ulcers and signs of pulmonary involvement. Severe infections require treatment with intravenous amphotericin B, often followed by prolonged administration of oral sulfonamides.

The first observations of successful therapy with TMP/SMX in patients with sulfonamide-resistant South American blastomycosis were reported by Lopes and Armond (1968). They reported that treatment with TMP alone was ineffective, but a good response was obtained in three of four patients with sulfonamide-resistant *P. brasiliensis* using the combination. Barbosa and Vasconcelos (1973) reported the treatment of 33 patients infected with *P. brasiliensis* with co-trimoxazole for periods varying from 18 to 60 days. Clinical characteristics of their patients were described in detail with 14 of 33 showing evidence of visceral involvement, and all having documented infections from 1 month to 2 years duration. They ranged in age from 12 to 68 years. A uniform dose regimen of TMP/SMX was used, consisting of 240 mg TMP + 1,200 mg SMX twice a day for 20 days followed by 160 mg TMP + 800 mg SMX twice daily for an additional 20 days and finally 80 mg TMP + 400 mg SMX twice daily for the last 20 days. Most patients tolerated the drug well. Results of treatment were reported as excellent (complete remission of lesions within 20 days) or very good (complete remission of lesions within 35 days) in all but one patient. Barbosa and Vasconcelos noted the rapidity of response in the patients, who improved concluding that in their opinion TMP/SMX was the best available treatment for South American blastomycosis.

A similar group of 16 patients were treated by Furtado et al. (1975) with a twice daily regimen of 160 mg TMP + 800 mg SMX for periods varying from 90 to 410 days. Response was excellent in eight, good in six, fair in one, and poor in one. These authors were also quite impressed with the safety and efficacy of the combination in this disease, but cautioned that a further period of observation was required before a final conclusion could be reached. A less favorable conclusion was reached by Pedrosa et al. (1974) who compared treatment with amphotericin B, sulfadoxine, or TMP/SMX in 23 patients with paracoccidioidomycosis. In five patients treated with the combination, the response was good in two, fair in two, and poor in one. These authors concluded that TMP/SMX offered no particular advantage over treatment with sulfadoxine alone in their patients, but noted that the former regimen was especially well tolerated for periods varying from 28 to 710 days.

Lopes (1976b) reviewed the cases reported by Barbosa and Vasconcelos (1973), Pedrosa et al. (1974), and Furtado et al. (1975) as well as nine of his own treated with TMP/SMX for paracoccidioidomycosis. Results in his nine patients were excellent with treatment varying from 83 to 190 days. In his conclusion, Lopes recommended the combination as the treatment of choice, especially for sulfonamide-resistant cases of South American blastomycosis.

III. Phycomycosis

A group of invasive mucocutaneous mycoses known individually as mucormycosis (*Rhizopus* and *Mucor* spp.), entomophthoromycosis *(Basidiobolus haptosporus)*, and rhinoentomophthoromycosis *(Conidiobolus coronatus)* are referred to collectively as the phycomycoses. All are capable of causing extensive soft tissue invasive disease. Amphotericin B is recommended for the treatment of these infections, though potassium iodide and co-trimoxazole have been reported to be effective in the latter two infections. Fomufod and Antia (1971) first reported successful therapy with TMP/SMX in two children from Nigeria with entomophthoromycosis. Both were cured following therapy for 1 and 4 months respectively. Previous treatment in one of these children with potassium iodide and amphotericin B had been unsuccessful. The next report of successful treatment of this disease with co-trimoxazole was from Thailand (THIANPRASIT 1978). Successful treatment of 15 cases confirmed by culture was briefly described, using tablets containing 80 mg TMP + 400 mg SMX each, four tablets a day in adults and two tablets a day in children for 6–8 weeks. GREENHAM (1979) described in some detail four patients with severe invasive infections with *Basidiobolus* spp. from Kenya. Three were cured of their infection with co-trimoxazole therapy, though one also required amputation of the hand. The fourth patient died of severe pelvic involvement and obstructive uropathy. The author alluded to other patients he had cured by administration of co-trimoxazole for periods of 6–8 weeks.

Rhinophycomycosis or conidiobolomycosis due to infection with *Conidiobolus coronatus* is a severe invasive mycosis, predominantly of the upper respiratory tract. MARTINSON (1971) first reported successful treatment with TMP/SMX of two patients with this infection resistant to treatment with potassium iodide. Similar results were reported in a patient from India (SINGH et al. 1976) who was intolerant of amphotericin B and unresponsive to treatment with potassium iodide alone. This patient responded promptly when treated with co-trimoxazole for 8 weeks. Failure of severe infections with *Conidiobolus coronatus* to respond to amphotericin B, potassium iodide, or TMP/SMX were described by KAMALAM and THAMBIAH (1978) and GRATEAU et al. (1975). In both cases there was severe lymphatic involvement, leading one of the authors to describe the clinical presentation as an "elephantiasic" form of the disease.

IV. Chromomycosis

This chronic granulomatous infection of the skin is characterized and diagnosed by the presence of brown septate hyphae in the lesion. Two patients with this infection from Malaysia were described as responding to treatment with TMP/SMX by GANESAPILLAI et al. (1978) in a review of the use of the combination for the treatment of deep cutaneous and systemic mycoses.

The severity of most of the invasive and systemic mycoses of humans, and the established efficacy of amphotericin B and potassium iodide in some cases, indicate that these should remain the treatment of choice for most of these patients, despite the acknowledged toxicity of the former agent. Fluorocytosine also seems to have a role in the therapeutic armamentarium against many mycotic infections. Nevertheless, the striking success of several investigators with co-trimoxazole, especially in the treatment of basidiobolomycosis, paracoccidioidomycosis, and in some cases of histoplasmosis indicate that additional studies with this drug are warranted. This is particularly of interest in those cases where intolerance to amphotericin B and resistance to potassium iodide and fluorocytosine are observed.

G. Pseudomonas Infections

A variety of species of *Pseudomonas* other than *P. aeruginosa* have been reported to be susceptible to TMP alone or in combination with SMX. These include particularly *P.pseudomallei*, *P.cepacia*, and *P.maltophilia*. These are natural sapro-phytes, capable of causing infection in humans as opportunistic pathogens. The clinical setting generally involves either a massive inoculum or a compromised host.

I. Pseudomonas pseudomallei

Melioidosis is a disease of humans with a clinical spectrum varying from a chronic inapparent infection to an acute fulminant course, frequently with a fatal outcome. It is caused by infection with *P.pseudomallei* which most commonly gains access to the host by soil contamination of a skin abrasion or wound. The disease is en-demic in South-East Asia, but has been reported throughout the world. The most common serious form of the disease is a pneumonitis, with or without septicemia. Mortality in patients with septicemia is greater than 50%, even with appropriate antimicrobial therapy. *P.pseudomallei* is resistant in vitro to most antimicrobial drugs, with the following important exceptions: tetracyclines, chloramphenicol, kanamycin, SDZ, and TMP/SMX. Depending on the severity of the infection, vig-orous therapy with one or a combination of two of these drugs is recommended.

The first demonstration of antimicrobial synergy with TMP/SMX against *P.pseudomallei* was reported by BEAUMONT (1970). Seven isolates were sensitive in vitro to a 1:5 combination with minimum inhibitory concentrations (MICs) of 1 μg TMP + 5 μg SMX or less, including three isolates which were resistant to one or the other of these drugs alone. These results were confirmed by BASSETT (1971) using a 1:20 combination with 14 additional isolates of *P.pseudomallei*. The MIC for one of these, however, was 4 μg/ml TMP + 80 μg/ml SMX. In vitro susceptibil-ity of 33 isolates of this organism, also to a 1:20 combination, was reported by EVERETT and KISHIMOTO (1973). Many of these isolates were quite resistant to one or both drugs alone, but most were inhibited by the combination at clinically achievable levels, and synergy was demonstrable in all of them.

The first case of melioidosis treated successfully with TMP/SMX was reported by I. MORRISON in 1970. This patient, a 37-year-old man, had a 4-year history of fever, splenomegaly, and a draining sternal sinus. He had been treated unsuccess-fully with chloroquine, p-aminosalicylic acid, streptomycin, and antimony. Cul-ture from the sternal sinus grew *P.pseudomallei*, and subsequent splenectomy and treatment with TMP/SMX resulted in an "uneventful recovery."

The next reported case of melioidosis treated with the combination was a 5-year-old child in Papua, New Guinea, whose illness was more acute than that of I. MORRISON's patient but who also lacked pulmonary involvement (DE BUSE et al. 1975). This patient, who presented with a toxic febrile illness, had an abdominal abscess and multiple cutaneous abcesses from which *P.pseudomallei* and *S.aureus* were cultured. Following unsuccessful therapy with chloroquine (for suspected malaria), methicillin, and gentamycin, the child responded promptly to treatment with kanamycin and TMP/SMX.

Successful treatment of a patient with pulmonary melioidosis with the com-bination was reported by JOHN (1976). This patient, a 21-year-old U.S. Air Force mechanic, presented with a 2-week history of fever, chills, anorexia, weight loss, and a nonproductive cough. A chest X-ray showed a cavitary lesion in the left upper lobe, and multiple sputum cultures grew *P. pseudomallei*. Following unsuccessful therapy with parenteral penicillin and kanamycin, the patient responded promptly to treatment with 160 mg TMP + 800 mg SMX administered twice daily. Therapy was continued for 8 weeks, though the abscess cavity had resolved after only 19 days. The patient remained asymptomatic 7 months after discontinuing the drug.

A more recent case with a very similar clinical presentation described by FULLER et al. (1978) required much larger doses of the combination administered continuously for 7 months. It was also their impression that concurrent use of other drugs (tetracycline, chloramphenicol, and kanamycin) along with TMP/SMX resulted in antimicrobial antagonism. In a subsequent letter to the same journal, TANPHAICHITRA et al. (1979) refuted this concept, advocating multiple drug therapy for patients with disseminated melioidosis. The reported successful therapy in seven patients with *P. pseudomallei* septicemia by means of TMP/SMX in various combinations with chloramphenicol, kanamycin, tetracycline, levamisole, human lymphocyte transfer factor, and amikacin. One of these patients was reported elsewhere in greater detail by TANPHAICHITRA (1979). Finally, R. MORRISON et al. (1979) reported an interesting patient with chronic prostatitis due to *P. pseudomallei*. Following unsuccessful therapy over a period of several years with a number of antimicrobial drugs to which the organism was susceptible in vitro, the patient was apparently cured of his infection by prolonged treatment with TMP/SMX.

II. Pseudomonas cepacia and Pseudomonas maltophilia

Two additional species of *Pseudomonas* with broad antimicrobial resistance are *P. cepacia* and *P. maltophilia*. These are opportunistic human pathogens. Infections generally occur in compromised invidivuals or following a heavy inoculum. They have been reported as contaminants of intravenous solutions and commonly in endocardial vegetations of heroin additcs. The in vitro sensitivity of *P. cepacia* and *P. maltophilia* to TMP and SMX, and the high degree of synergy exhibited by the combination are amply documented in published reports. TAPLIN et al. (1971) reported antimicrobial susceptibility data for a large number of isolates of *P. cepacia* obtained from between the toes of U.S. Army troops during swamp training. These were uniformly resistant to all of the drugs tested except chloramphenicol, novobiocin, and TMP/SMX. All 14 isolates were inhibited in vitro at concentrations of 0.25 µg/ml TMP + 5 µg/ml SMX or less. NORD et al. (1974a) found this combination to be synergistic for 18 of 18 isolates of *P. maltophilia* and 8 of 8 isolates of *P. cepacia*. Others have reported similar results with isolates of these two organisms from a variety of sources (BUSHBY 1973; MOODY and YOUNG 1975; PATRICK et al. 1975; EKSTRÖM et al. 1979, HOLMES et al. 1979; FELEGIE et al. 1979; YU et al. 1979), though occasional resistant isolates have been described (NORD et al. 1974b; TOMIOKA et al. 1978).

BASSETT et al. (1970) reported successful treatment of a *P. cepacia* wound infection with TMP/SMX. The first successful treatment of two patients with endocarditis due to *P. cepacia* with this combination was described by PHILLIPS et al. (1971). Several investigators have subsequently reported similar cases, most of whom were also treated successfully with TMP/SMX, occasionally in combination with other antimicrobial drugs such as kanamycin or polymyxin B (SPELLER 1972; SELIGMAN et al. 1973; RACHAL et al. 1973; NEU et al. 1973; HAMILTON et al. 1973). Isolates of *P. cepacia* have also been described from sputum or bronchial washings of patients with cystic fibrosis (LARAYA-CUASEY et al. 1977; BLESSING and LEWISTON 1976). Most of these have proved to be susceptible in vitro to TMP/SMX and clinical response to treatment was reported to be good (LARAYA-CUASEY et al. 1977).

Patients with endocarditis due to *P. maltophilia* have also been treated successfully with oral TMP/SMX. The first such patient was a 35-year-old man with severe rheumatic heart disease who became febrile 3 weeks after mitral valve replacement (FISCHER 1973). Growth of *P. maltophilia* was observed in blood cultures. He failed to respond to treatment with gentamycin and carbenicillin, but improved rapidly when therapy was changed to 160 mg TMP + 800 mg SMX administered orally twice daily. This treatment was continued for 3 months and the patient remained well during the reported 15 months follow-up. Three additional patients with *P. maltophilia* endocarditis were described by YU et al. (1978). All were treated successfully with TMP/SMX plus various combinations of polymyxin B, carbenicillin, and kanamycin.

An additional patient with a catheter-associated urinary tract infection due to *P. maltophilia*, also treated successfully with TMP/SMX, was described by WISHART and RILEY (1976). Other patients with similar infections were treated successfully by these investigators with sulfadimidine alone (four patients) or kanamycin alone (two patients). The successful use of an intravenous formulation of TMP/SMX to treat a small number of patients infected with *P. cepacia*, *P. maltophilia*, or *P. putrefaciens* has also been described (SCHMIDT et al. 1980). The latter organism, *P. putrefaciens*, has been shown to be sensitive in vitro to TMP/SMX, and the combination has been used to treat patients with skin ulcers infected with this organism (DEBOIS et al. 1975; DEGREEF et al. 1975; APPELBAUM and BOWEN 1978).

The occurrence of infections with these multiresistant opportunistic human pathogens remains a clinical problem. Most isolates have proved to be resistant to the majority of antimicrobial agents that are readily available, the only consistent exceptions being chloramphenicol and TMP/SMX. Because of the nature of these infections, a prolonged period of therapy is frequently deemed advisable. It is fortunate, in that case, that TMP/SMX is effective when administered orally and well tolerated in most cases during a prolonged treatment regimen. Whether used alone or in combination with other antimicrobial drugs, co-trimoxazole would appear to be the treatment of choice for infections with *P. pseudomallei*, *P. cepacia*, and *P. maltophilia*.

H. Other Infections

The topics in preceding sections of this chapter were selected on the basis of the abundance of preclinical and clinical data suggesting that TMP alone or in combination with a sulfonamide may provide effective therapy in human infections, though well-controlled clinical studies in most cases were not available. There are many other examples of human diseases treated with these drugs which appear only as isolated reports, favorable or unfavorable. A few of these warrant brief mention.

I. Bubonic Plague

Bubonic plague, a legendary disease shared by humans and the many rodent species with which they have long cohabitated, is caused by infection with the bacillus, *Yersinia pestis*. Like the organism of brucellosis, *Y. pestis* is readily ingested by macrophages in which it survives following inoculation by the bite of an infected flea. Though far less common today than during the historic pandemics of earlier centuries, plague is still seen regularly in many parts of the world. Successful treatment and chemoprophylaxis of plague has been recorded with several antimicrobial drugs including sulfonamides, tetracycline, streptomycin, and chloramphenicol. The case mortality rate of 50%–60% untreated can be significantly reduced by proper chemotherapy, though many fatal cases with pneumonic, septicemic, or menigitic involvement still occur.

The sensitivity of *Y. pestis* to TMP/SMX was reported by VAN-AI et al. (1972a) who also reported successful chemoprophylaxis of the infection in mice. These authors later reported successful therapy of *Y. pestis* infection in 12 patients with bacteriologic confirmation in 6 (VAN-AI et al. 1972b, 1973). Therapy with two tablets (160 mg TMP + 800 mg SMX) administered twice daily was continued for 11–15 days in uncomplicated cases and for 15–17 days in three patients with septicemia. The response was prompt with abatement of fever within 5 days in all but one case. Prior experience with streptomycin, chloramphenicol, and tetracycline was associated with a mortality of 0.5%–15%, leading the authors to urge further evaluation of the efficacy of co-trimoxazole in the treatment of bubonic plague.

BUTLER et al. (1974) reported similar evidence of in vitro sensitivity and synergy with the combination against an isolate of *Y. pestis* from a patient who was subsequently cured with TMP/SMX as the sole antimicrobial drug employed. BUTLER et al. (1976) later reported additional patients with bubonic plague treated successfully with the combination, though noting that patients treated with streptomycin had a shorter mean duration of fever. Other investigators have also confined the in vitro sensitivity and synergy of TMP/SMX against *Y. pestis* (DA SILVA et al. 1975; CROWNGOLD 1977). These results indicate that, while further clinical studies are eagerly awaited, TMP/SMX may be very effective therapy for patients with bubonic plague.

II. Rickettsiosis

Microbes of the family Rickettsiaceae are capable of causing human disease adventitiously when humans enter the cycle of insect vector to mammalian reservoir normally inhabited by these organisms. The single exception is louse-borne typhus in which humans are the principal reservoir. The Rickettsiaceae are obligate intracellular organisms, the various species of which are widely distributed throughout the world. They are typically divided into three groups: the spotted fever group, the typhus group, and Q fever. With the exception of Q fever, human ricketsial infections are characterized by an abrupt febrile illness with a diffuse vasculitis causing headache and skin rash.

1. Boutonneuse Fever

TMP/SMX is not generally regarded as effective in the treatment of rickettsioses of the spotted fever (STEIGMAN 1977) or the typhus (HUYS et al. 1973) groups, though PORTO (1978) reported 32 patients with boutonneuse fever *(Rickettsia conorii)* treated with co-trimoxazole, two tablets every 12 h, who became afebrile within 3.8 days. It has been suggested that treatment with sulfonamides alone, and possibly in combination with TMP, may actually worsen the course of Rocky Mountain spotted fever (STEIGMAN 1977).

2. Q Fever

Infection with *Coxiella burnetii* causes an acute illness in humans, characterized by fever, headache, myalgia, and frequently pneumonitis. Endocarditis has also been reported. The organism is unique among the rickettsiae in that there is no arthropod vector and no rash associated with the disease. The disease, referred to as Q fever (so named by DERRICK in 1937 – "Q" for "query") is transmitted by inhalation of the organism. The first case of Q fever endocarditis treated with TMP/SMX was described by FREEMAN and HODSON (1972). The patient, a 45-year-old woman, responded to treatment with the combination as well as tetracycline, both of which were administered for 4 months. A second patient, a 22-year-old man with pericarditis, also successfully treated with co-trimoxazole, was later described by CAUGHEY (1977). Two additional patients with Q fever endocarditis treated with TMP/SMX in addition to tetracycline have been reported in detail more recently (WILLEY et al. 1979; KIMBROUGH et al. 1979). Though the fact that tetracycline was used in these patients makes it difficult to discern the role of TMP/SMX, G. BROWN (1973) indicated in a review of the disease that treatment of patients with endocarditis due to Q fever with tetracycline alone is generally not sufficient, and recommended concurrent use of co-trimoxazole.

III. Legionella pneumophila and Pittsburgh Pneumonia Agent Infections

Among the newly described bacterial infections causing pneumonitis, two have had in vitro sensitivity determinations which included TMP/SMX; *Legionella pneumophila* and the "Pittsburgh pneumonia agent" (PPA). The former was reported to be quite sensitive in vitro to the combination (THORNSBERRY et al. 1978; SARAVOLATZ et al. 1979), while the latter appeared quite sensitive in an embryonated egg culture (MYEROWITZ et al. 1979). Erythromycin has been clearly established as the treatment of choice for patients with *L. pneumophila* infections. The role of TMP/SMX in the treatment of patients with pneumonitis due to PPA has not been established, though at least one patient was successfully treated with the combination as the only antimicrobial drug given (MYEROWITZ et al. 1979).

IV. Isospora belli Infections

Coccidia are single-cell organisms responsible for chronic intestinal infections of domestic and wild animals, and only rarely in humans. Two such cases, due to infection with *Isospora belli*, were reported as responding to treatment with TMP/

SMX administered for a period of 3 weeks (SYRKIS et al. 1975; WESTERMAN and CHRISTENSEN 1979). The patient of WESTERMAN and CHRISTENSEN also had *Giardia lamblia* identified in the stool specimen. However, diarrhea and weight loss continued, despite therapy with metronidizole and tetracycline. Diarrhea "subsided dramatically" within 48 h of starting treatment with co-trimoxazole. Another patient with chronic diarrhea due to *Isospora belli*, who was also allergic to sulfonamides, failed to improve when treated with trimethoprim alone, 200 mg twice daily (C.M. MANSBACH II, 1980, personal communication; see also Chap. 17).

V. Malakoplakia

Malakoplakia is a rare disorder, generally of the urinary tract, thought to be due to an abnormality of intracellular digestion of bacteria in macrophages. The disease is characterized by a histiocytic infiltration of the bladder wall, prostate, ureters, or retroperitoneum. The macrophages are identified by the presence of intracellular concentrically lamellated structures called Michaelis–Gutmann bodies. One patient with progressive retroperitoneal involvement and a urine culture which grew *Escherichia coli* responded well to treatment with TMP/SMX after failure to respond to ampicillin, clindamycin, or gentamycin (MADERAZO et al. 1979). The authors speculated that the effectiveness of the combination was related in part to its ability to gain access to intracellular bacteria in macrophages, analogous to its activity against infections with *Y. pestis* and *Brucella* spp.

VI. Pediculosis

Finally, among the more novel uses of the combination which have been reported since its introduction is that described by SHASHINDRAN et al. (1978). These authors reported successful treatment of several patients with pediculosis capitis. Following an incidental observation of relief from infestation with head lice in a 12 year-old girl being treated for a respiratory infection, the investigators systemically evaluated the efficacy of the combination and the two components, TMP and SMX alone, in 20 additional patients. Only the combination was effective. A second 3-day course of treatment was required about 10 days after the first, because of the lack of any effect on the nits which persisted and hatched at that time. The same investigators (SHASHINDRAN et al. 1979) later reported that the combination was not effective in patients with scabies. They attributed the difference to the fact that *Pediculus humanis capitis* var. lives on blood meals from the host whereas *Sarcoptes scabiei* ingests mainly tissue debris. It is possible, in the former case, that the antimicrobial agent interferes with bacterial digestion of blood in the parasite's gut.

References

Adams AR, Jackson JM, Scopa J, Lane GK, Wilson R (1971) Nocardiosis. Diagnosis and management with a report of three cases. Med J Aust 1(13):669–674

Adams HG, Brooks GF (1977) *In vitro* sulfamethoxazole-trimethoprim activity against *Nocardia asteroides*: efficacious therapy in five patients with *Nocardia* pneumonia. Abstr, 17th ICAAC, October 1977. Obtainable from: American Society for Microbiology, Washington, DC

Alberola V, Marin J, Abellan MT, Bori JV, Pascual-Leone A (1969) A study of the antibacterial association of trimethoprim and sulfamethoxazole in sundry infections. Med Esp 62(368):382–387

Appelbaum PC, Bowen AJ (1978) Opportunistic infection of chronic skin ulcers with *Pseudomonas putrefaciens*. Br J Dermatol 98(2):229–231

Ariza J, Gudiol F, Rufi G, Priu R (1977) Tratamiento de la brucelosis aguda con trimetoprim-sulfametoxazol. Med Clin (Barc) 69:437–441

Arroyo D, Noriega AR (1976) Experience with trimethoprim-sulphamethoxazole in the treatment of chronic brucellosis. In: Williams JD, Creddes AM (eds) Proc 9th Int Congr Chemother, London, M-629 (Abstr). Plenum, New York

Bach MC, Monaco AP, Finland M (1973a) Pulmonary Nocardiosis: Therapy with minocycline and with erythromycin plus ampicillin. JAMA 224:1378–1381

Bach MC, Sabath LD, Finland M (1973b) Susceptibility of *Nocardia asteroides* to 45 antimicrobial agents in vitro. Antimicrob Agents Chemother 3:1–8

Baikie AG, MacDonald CB, Mundy GR (1970) Systemic nocardiosis treated with trimethoprim and sulfamethoxazole. Lancet 2:261

Barba G, Merlo N (1972) L'associazione trimetoprim-sulfametossazolo nel trattamento della infezione brucellare. G Mal Infett Parassit 24(2):79–84

Barbosa W, Vasconcelos WMP (1973) Acao da sulfametoxazol associada ao trimetoprim na terapeutica da blastomicose Sul-Americana. Rev Patol Trop 2(3):329–339

Barnett M, Bushby SRM (1970) Trimethoprim and the sulfonamides. Vet Rec 87:43–51

Barrow GI, Hewitt M (1971) Skin infection with *Mycobacterium marinum* from a tropical fish tank. Br Med J 2(5760):505–506

Bassett DJ (1971) The sensitivity of *Pseudomonas pseudomallei* to trimethoprim and sulfamethoxazole in vitro. J Clin Pathol 24:798–800

Bassett DCJ, Stokes JJ, Thomas WRG (1970) Wound infection with *Pseudomonas multivorous*. A water-borne contaminant of disinfectant solutions. Lancet 1:1188–1191

Beaumont RJ (1970) Trimethoprim as a possible therapy for Nocardiosis and Melioidosis. Med J Aust 2:1123–1127

Beeler BA, Wann LS, Bushby SRM, Brooks GF (1975) Sulfamethoxazole-Trimethoprim (SMX-TMP) in the treatment of pulmonary nocardiosis. In: Williams JD, Geddes AM (eds) Proc 9th Int Congr Chemother, London, M-637 (Abstr). Plenum, New York

Bennett JE, Jennings AE (1978) Factors influencing susceptibility of *Nocardia* species to trimethoprim-sulfamethoxazole. Antimicrob Agents Chemother 13:624–627

Bertaggia A (1975) The parenteral (intravenous and intramuscular) use of trimethoprim-sulfamethoxazole. Clin Ter 75:611–633

Billi O, Frongillo RF (1971) Clinical trials with a new bactericidal preparation: the trimethoprim sulphamethoxazole association. Riforma Medica 85(14):378–384

Black MM, Eykyn SJ (1977) The successful treatment of tropical fish tank granuloma *(Mycobacterium marinum)* with co-trimoxazole. Br J Dermatol 97(6):689–692

Black WA, McNellis DA (1970) Sensitivity of *Nocardia* to trimethoprim and sulfamethoxazole in vitro. J Clin Pathol 23:423–426

Blessing J, Lewiston NJ (1976) Pseudomonas in cystic fibrosis sputum: sensitivity to oral antibiotics. Am Rev Respir Dis 113(4):37

Brown GL (1973) Clinical aspects of Q fever. Postgrad Med J 49:539–541

Brown KGE, Molesworth BD, Gjalt-Boerrigter FG, Tozer RA (1974) Disseminated *Histoplasmosis duboisii* in Malawi: Partial response to sulfonamide/trimethoprim combination. East Afr Med J 51(5):584–590

Bushby SRM (1973) Trimethoprim-sulfamethoxazole: in vitro microbiologic aspects. J Infect Dis [Suppl] 128:442–462

Butler T, Bell WR, Link NN, Tiep ND, Arnold K (1974) *Yersinia pestis* infection in Vietnam. I. Clinical and hematologic aspects. J Infect Dis [Suppl] 129:S78–S84

Butler T, Levin J, Link NN (1976) *Yersinia pestis* infection in Vietnam. II. Quantitative blood cultures and detection of endotoxin in the cerebrospinal fluid of patients with meningitis. J Infect Dis 133(5):493–499

Calonghi GF, Signorini C, Fassio PG (1973) Ulteriori indagini sulla sensibilità *in vitro* di ceppi di brucella umana e bovina all'associazione sulfametossazolo-trimetoprim. G Mal Infett Parassit 25(2):129–131

Calonghi GF, Goglio A, Marchiaro G, Fassio PG, Auriemma L, Gavazzeni G (1978) On the treatment of acquired toxoplasmosis with co-trimoxazole. G Mal Infett Parassit 30(2):204–206

Cantalamessa S, Russo N, Vetrano A (1972) Esperienze cliniche sull'uso del trimethoprim-sulfametossazolo nella brucellosi. G Mal Infett Parassit 24(12):905–907

Carroll GF, Brown JM, Haley LD (1977) A method for determining in vitro drug susceptibilities of some nocardia and actinomadurae. Results with 17 antimicrobial agents. Am J Clin Pathol 68:279–283

Caughey JE (1977) Pleuropericardial lesion in Q fever. Br Med J 1(6074):1447

Cellesi C, Barberi A, Terragna A (1973) Activity of the trimethoprim-sulfamethoxazole combination in the mouse (Histochemical study). Boll Ist Sieroter Milan 52(1):70–76

Chalhoub ES (1976) Brucellosis: its treatment with co-trimoxazole. J Kuwait Med Assoc 10:51–53

Colonnello F, Calonghi GF, Signorini C (1970) Sensibilità in vitro di ceppi di brucelle isolate dall'uomo e dai bovini all'associazione trimetoprim-sulfametossazolo. G Mal Infett Parassit 22:481–482

Cook FV, Farrar E (1978) Treatment of *Nocardia asteroides* infection with trimethoprim-sulfamethoxazole. South Med J 71:512–515

Crowngold T (1977) Susceptibility of *Yersinia pestis* to trimethoprim and sulfamethoxazole, singly and in combination, as well as to amoxicillin. S Afr J Med Lab Technol 23(2):15–18

Cunningham MJ, White PM, Samman PD (1978) Co-trimoxazole resistant *Mycobacterium marinum*. Br J Dermatol 99(5):597

D'Alessandro L, Faenza L, Di Palma D, Russo P (1974) L'associazione TM-SMX nel trattamento della brucellosi. Minerva Med 65(41):2350–2356

Daikos GK, Papapolyzos N, Marketos N, Mochlas S, Kastanokis S, Papasteriadis E (1973) Trimethoprim-sulfamethoxazole in brucellosis. J Infect Dis [Suppl] 128:731–733

Dalovisio JR, Pankey GA (1978) Antibiotic sensitivity profile of *Mycobacterium cheloni* and *Mycobacterium fortuitum*. Clin Res 26:27 A

Da Silva YPS, Nunes MP, Suassuna I (1975) Estudo, In Vitro, sobre a susceptibilidade de *Yersinia pestis* isoladas no Brasil as sulfonamidas, tetraciclinas, aminoglicosideos, penicilinas e esitromicinas. Rev Assoc Med Bras 21(7):204–206

Debois J, Degreef H, Vandepitte J, Staepen J (1975) *Pseudomonas putrefaciens* as a cause of infection in humans. J Clin Pathol 28(12):443–446

DeBuse PJ, Henderson A, White M (1975) Melioidosis in a child in Papua New Guinea: Successful treatment with kanamycin and trimethoprim-sulphametoxazole. Med J Aust 2(12):476–478

Degreef H, Debois J, Vandepitte J (1975) *Pseudomonas putrefaciens* as a cause of infection of venous ulcers. Dermatologica 151:296–301

Derrick EH (1937) "Q" fever, a new fever entity: clinical features, diagnosis and laboratory investigation. Med J Aust 2:281–283

Domart A, Robineau M, Carbon C (1973) La toxoplasmose acquise: une nouvelle chimiothérapie: l'association sulfamethoxazole-trimethoprime. Nouv Presse Med 2(5):321–322

Egere JV, Gugnani HC, Okoro AN, Suseelan AV (1978) African histoplasmosis in eastern Nigeria: report of two culturally proven cases treated with Seprin and Amphotericin B. J Trop Med Hyg 81(11):255–229

Ekström B, Fellner H, Forsgren U, Magni L, Ortengren B (1979) Antibacterial activity of co-trimazine in vitro and in vivo. Infection 7(2):74–80

Escalona E (1969) Micetoma actinomicosico, su tratamiento con trimetoprim-gantanol. Rev Med Hosp Gen Mex 32:827–833

Evans RA, Benson RE (1971) Complicated nocardiosis successfully treated with trimethoprim and sulfamethoxazole. Med J Aust 1(13):684–685

Everett ED, Kishimoto RA (1973) In vitro sensitivity of 33 strains of *Pseudomonas pseudomallei* to trimethoprim and sulfamethoxazole. J Infect Dis [Suppl] 128:S 539–S 542

Eyles D, Coleman N (1953) Synergistic effect of sulfadiazine and Daraprim against experimental toxoplasmosis in the mouse. Antibiot Chemother 3:483–490

Feldman HA (1973) Effects of trimethoprim and sulfisoxazole alone and in combination on murine toxoplasmosis. J Infect Dis 128(S):S 774–776

Felegie T, Yu VL, Rumans LW, Yee RB (1979) Susceptibility of *Pseudomonas maltophilia* to antimicrobial agents, singly and in combination. Antimicrob Agents Chemother 16(6):833–837

Fiori GP, Poggio A, Marchesi E (1978) Co-trimoxazole and human brucellosis: a clinical and therapeutic evaluation. G Mal Infett Parassit 30(2):173–176

Fischer JJ (1973) *Pseudomonas maltophilia* endocarditis after replacement of the mitral valve: a case study. J Infect Dis [Suppl] 128:S 771–S 773

Fomufod AK, Antia AV (1971) Successful treatment of subcutaneous phycomycoses with trimethoprim-sulfamethoxazole (Septrin). Trop Geogr Med 23:208–211

Frazier A, Rosenow EC, Roberts GD (1975) Nocardiosis. A review of 25 cases occurring during 24 months. Mayo Clin Proc 50(11):657–663

Freeman R, Hodson ME (1972) Q fever endocarditis treated with trimethoprim and sulfamethoxazole. Br Med J I(5797):419–420

Frezzotti R, Terragna A, Rossolini A, Bardelli AM, Cellesi C, Figura N (1978) Attinità del co-trimoxazolo nella toxoplasmosi studio sperimentale e clinico. G Mal Infett Parassit 30(2):199–204

Fuchs F, Kimball AC, Kean BH (1974) The management of toxoplasmosis in pregnancy. Clin Perinatol 1:407–422

Fuller PB, Fisk DE, Byrd RB, Griggs GA, Smith MR (1978) Treatment of pulmonary melioidosis with combination of trimethoprim and sulfamethoxazole. Chest 74(2):222–224

Furtado T, Marcos AR, Maia FAA (1975) Treatment of South American blastomycosis by trimethoprim-sulfamethoxazole combination. Folha Med 71(3):275–279

Gambarella A, Caporale L, Molinaro F (1978) Trimethoprim-sulfamethoxazole in the treatment of lymphonodal toxoplasmosis. Policlin Sezione Med 85(2):124–130

Ganesapillai T, Rajagopalan K, Kannan-Kutty M (1978) Trimethoprim-sulfamethoxazole as an additional drug for the deep cutaneous and systemic mycoses. Dermatol SE Asia:76–81

Geddes AM, Goodall JAD, Boosey CM (1973) Studies with intravenous trimethoprim. In: Daikos GK (ed) Proc 8th Int Congr Chemother, vol 2. Hellenic Society of Chemotherapy, Athens, pp 225–228

Geisler PJ, Check F, Lamothe F, Anderson BR (1979) Failure of trimethoprim/sulfamethoxazole in invasive *Nocardia asteroides* infection. Arch Intern Med 139(3):355–356

Giunchi G, de Rosa F, Fabiani F (1971) Trimethoprim-sulfamethoxazole combination in the treatment of acute human brucellosis. Chemotherapy 16:332–335

Giunchi G, de Rosa F, Fabiani F (1972) The treatment of acute brucellosis in humans with the trimethoprim-sulphamethoxazole combination. G Mal Infett Parasit 24(2):77–79

Gottlieb LS, Chatterjee SN (1979) Disseminated nocardiosis in a compromised host. Dial Transplant 8(4):342–343

Grateau P, Pons J, Rigaud A, Pasturel A, Thuing S (1975) Rinoentomophtoromycose: à propos d'une nouvelle observation. Med Armees 3(4):291–310

Greenham R (1979) Subcutaneous phycomycosis: not always benign. Lancet 1:97–98

Grossman PL, Remington JS (1979) The effect of trimethoprim and sulfamethoxazole on *Toxoplasma gondii* in vitro and in vivo. Am J Trop Med Hyg 28(3):445–455

Grossman PL, Krahenbuhl JL, Remington JS (1978) In vivo and in vitro effects of trimethoprim and sulfamethoxazole on *Toxoplasma* infections. In. Siegenthaler W, Lüthy R (eds) Proc 10th Int Congr Chemother, vol 1. Am Soc Microbiol, Washington DC

Hamal PB (1974) Primary pulmonary nocardiosis: case report. Thorax 29(3):382–386

Hamilton J, Burch W, Grimmett G, Orme K, Brewer D, Frost R, Fulkerson C (1973) Successful treatment of *Pseudomonas cepacia* endocarditis with trimethoprim-sulfamethoxazole. Antimicrob Agents Chemother 4(5):551–554

Hassan A, Erian MM, Farid Z, Hathout SD, Sorensen K (1971) Trimethoprim-sulfamethoxazole in acute brucellosis. Br Med J 3:159–160

Havas L (1975) The treatment of some deep mycoses (South American blastomycosis, nocardiosis and actinomycetoma) with a combination of sulfamethoxazole + trimethoprim (bactrim, septrin) – literature review. Mykosen 18(6):263–273

Hilson GRF, Banerjee DK, Holmes IB (1971) The activity of various antituberculosis drugs in suppressing experimental *Mycobacterium leprae* infection in mice. Int J Lepr 39(2):349–353

Hokama S (1976) In vitro sensitivity of the sulfonamides against atypical mycobacteria. Tuberculosis 51(7):287–291

Holmes B, Lapage SP, Easterling BG (1979) Distribution in clinical material and identification of *Pseudomonas maltophilia*. J Clin Pathol 32:66–72

Huys J, Freyens P, Kayihigi J, Van den Berghe G (1973) Treatment of epidemic typus. A comparative study of chloramphenicol, trimethoprim-sulfamethoxazole and doxycycline. Trans R Soc Trop Med Hyg 67(5):718–721

Jaffe JJ, McCormack JJ, Meymarian E (1972) Comparative properties of schistosomal and filarial dihydrofolate reductases. Biochem Pharmacol 21:719–731

Jayareewal FRB, Attopatu M, de Fonseka I, Ratnaike VT (1975) Case report; histoplasmosis of the buccal cavity. Ceylon Med J 20:45–47

John JF Jr (1976) Trimethoprim-sulfamethoxazole therapy of pulmonary meloidosis. Am Rev Respir Dis 114(5):1021–1025

Jonquieres EDL, Bena JL, Negroni R (1975) Systemic histoplasmosis successfully treated with trimethoprim-sulfamethoxazole. Arch Argent Dermatol 25(1):95–97

Kamalam A, Thambiah AS (1978) Lymph node invasion by *Conidiobolus coronatus* and its spore formation in vivo. Sabouraudia 16(3):175–184

Katz P, Fanci AS (1977) *Nocardia asteroides* sinusitis. Presentation as a trimethoprim-sulfamethoxazole responsive fever of unknown origin. JAMA 238(22):2397–2398

Kean BH (1972) Clinical toxoplasmosis – 50 years. Trans R Soc Trop Med Hyg 66:549–571

Keczkes K (1974) Tropical fish tank granuloma. Br J Dermatol 91:709

Kelly R (1976) *Mycobacterium marinum* infection from a tropical fish tank: Treatment with trimethoprim and sulfamethoxazole. Med J Aust 2(18):681–682

Keri J, Telegdy L (1975) Experience gained in the treatment of human brucellosis. Orv Hetil 7:375–379

Kimbrough RC, Ormsbee RA, Peacock M, Rogers WR, Bennetts RW, Raof J, Krause A, Gardner C (1979) Q fever endocarditis in the United States. Ann Intern Med 91(3):400–402

Kirk J, Kaminski GW (1976) *Mycobacterium marinum* infecton. Aust J Dermatol 17(3):111–116

Kouba K, Nevarilova A, Rajlichova J (1978) Septrin in the treatment of human toxoplasmosis. Cesk Epidemiol Mikrobiol Immunol 27(3):175–178

Kremer EP (1972) Pulmonary and cerebral nocardial abscess. Med J Aust 2(10):538–540

Ktenidou KS, Papaikonomou K, Papapanagiotou J (1974) Sensitivity of *Brucella melitensis* to chemotherapeutic agents. Acta Microbiol Hell 19(5):314–313

Kuschnaroff TM, Takeda AK, Galvao PAA, Pessoa MC, Lomar AV (1973) Nota prévia a respeito de nova droga usada no tratamento de toxoplasmose. Folha Med 67(4):617–621

Lafrenz M, Ziegler K, Sanger R, Budde E, Naumann G (1973) Neue Aspekte bei der Behandlung der Toxoplasmose. Muench Med Wochenschr 115:2057–2061

Lal S, Modawal KK, Fowle ASE, Peach B, Popham RD (1970) Acute brucellosis treated with trimethoprim and sulfamethoxazole. Br Med J 3(5717):256–257

Laraya-Cuasey LR, Lipstein M, Huang NN (1977) *Pseudomonas cepacia* in the respiratory flora of patients with cystic fibrosis (CF). Pediatr Res 11(4):502

Laszlo A, Eidus L (1978) Inhibition of fast growing mycobacteria with trimethoprim (TMP). J Antimicrob Chemother 4(6):582–583

Leelarasamee A, Vanichakarn S, Aswapokee P, Aswapokee N, Nilvarangkur S, Jaroonvesma N (1977) Disseminated nocardiosis after pulmonary collapse: a case report. Southeast Asian J Trop Med Public Health 8(4):558–562

Lopes CF (1976a) Associacáo sulfametoxazol-trimetoprim do tratamento do micetoma actinomicotico por *Nocardia brasiliensis*. Folha Med 73:89–92

Lopes CF (1976b) Treatment of South American blastomycosis with the sulfamethoxazole-trimethoprim combination. An Bras Dermatol 51(3):207–213

Lopes CF, Armond S (1968) Ensaio terapêutico em casos sulfa-resistentes de blastomicose Sul-Americana. Hospital (Rio de J) 73:1245–1255

Lopes CF, Cisalpino EO, Armond S, Porto RV, Maia FAA, Peixoto V (1971) Dermatoses tratadas por associacáo sulfametoxazol e trimetoprim. Folha Med 62(2):167–172

Lopez TS, Alonso EC, Estevez IF, Gonzalez RA (1976) Brucellosis: consideraciones clinicas y terapéuticas. Revisión de 50 casas. Rev Clin Esp 141(2):131–137

Lyons C, Owens CR, Ayers WB (1943) Sulfonamide therapy in actinomycotic infections. Surgery 14:99–103

Machado O, Dantos A, Silva S, Gomes JFR (1967) Observacóes sóbre a atividale do sul-fametoxazol no tratamento da toxoplasmose. Rev Inst Med Trop Sao Paulo 9:346–349

Macleod WM (1970) ... and histoplasmasis. Lancet II:363

Macleod WM, Murray IG, Davidson J, Gibbs DD (1972) Histoplasmosis: a review, and account of three patients diagnosed in Great Britain. Thorax 27:6–17

Maderazo EG, Quintiliani R (1974) Treatment of nocardial infection with trimethoprim and sulfamethoxazole. Am J Med 57:671–675

Maderazo EG, Berlin BB, Morhardt C (1979) Treatment of malakoplakia with trimetho-prim-sulfamethoxazole. Urology 13(1):70–73

Mahgoub ES (1972) Treatment of actinomycetoma with sulfamethoxazole plus trimetho-prim. Am J Trop Med Hyg 21:332–335

Mahgoub ES (1977) Mycoses of the Sudan. Trans R Soc Trop Med Hyg 71:184–188

Maibach HI, Gorham W, Aly R (1975) Nocardia brasiliensis mycetoma: treatment with co-trimoxazole. Arch Dermatol 111:656

Maier W von, Piekarski G (1976) Experimentelle Untersuchungen über die Wirksamkeit der Kombination Sulfamoxol/Trimethoprim (CN 3123) auf die Toxoplasma-Infektion der weißen Maus. Arzneim Forsch (Drug Res) 26(42):620–622

Marcovitch H, Norman AP (1970) Treatment of nocardiosis. Lancet 2:362–363

Martinson FD (1971) Chronic phycomycosis of the upper respiratory tract. Am J Trop Med Hyg 20(3):449–455

May J (1979) Disseminated nocardiosis in an immunosuppressed host. Response to trimethoprim-sulfamethoxazole. Rocky Mt Med J 76(3):133–134

Minoprio JL (1976) Relazione su un'epidemia di brucellosi nella regione de Huanacache (Mendoza) debellata mediante l'associazione trimethoprim-sulfametossazolo. Clin Ter 11(3):217–221

Mössner G (1970) Klinische Ergebnisse mit dem Kombinationspräparat Sulfamethoxa-zol + Trimethoprim. In: Umezawa H (ed) Proc 6th Int Congr Chemother, vol 1. University Park Press, Baltimore, pp 966–970

Moody MR, Young VM (1975) In vitro susceptibility of Pseudomonas cepaciai and Pseu-domonas maltophilia to trimethoprim and trimethoprim-sulfamethoxazole. Antimicrob Agents Chemother 7(6):836–839

Morrison IM (1970) Chronic melioidosis. Proc R Soc Med 63:289–290

Morrison RE, Young EJ, Harper WK, Maldonado L (1979) Chronic prostatic melioidosis treated with trimethoprim-sulfamethoxazole. JAMA 241:500–501

Myerowitz RL, Pasculle AW, Dowling JN, Pazin GJ, Puerzer M, Yee RB, Rinaldo CR, Hakala TR (1979) Opportunistic lung infection due to "Pittsburgh pneumonia agent." N Engl J Med 301(18):953–958

Negroni R, Rubinstein P, Gonzalez-Montaner J (1977) Tratamiento de la histoplasmosis crónica con sulfimetoxazol-trimetoprima. Med Cutan Iber Lat Am 1:71–76

Neu HC, Garvey GJ, Beach MP (1973) Successful treatment of Pseudomonas cepacia endo-carditis in a heroin addict with trimethoprim-sulfamethoxazole. J Infect Dis [Suppl] 128:S 768–S 770

Nguyen BT, Stadtsbaeder S (1975) In vitro activity of cotrimoxazole on the intracellular multiplication of Toxoplasma gondii. Pathol Eur 10:307–315

Nguyen BT, Stadtsbaeder S, Horvat F (1978) Comparative effect of trimethoprim and py-rimethamine, alone and in combination with a sulfonamide, on Toxoplasma gondii: In vitro and in vivo studies. In: Siegenthaler W, Lüthy R (eds) Proc 10th Int Congr Chemother, vol 1. Am Soc Microbiol, Washington DC, pp 137–140

Nitidandhaprabhas P, Sittapairochana D (1975) Treatment of nocardial mycetoma with trimethoprim and sulfamethoxazole. Arch Dermatol 111:1345–1348

Nord C-E, Waldstrom T, Wretlind B (1974b) Sensitivity of different *Pseudomonas* species and *Aeromonas hydrophila* to trimethoprim and sulfamethoxazole separately and in combination. Med Microbiol Immunol (Berl) 160(1):1–7

Nord C-E, Wadstrom T, Wretlind B (1974a) Synergistic effect of combinations of sulfamethoxazole, trimethoprim, and colistin against *Pseudomonas maltophilia* and *Pseudomonas cepacia*. Antimicrob Agents Chemother 6(4):521–523

Norrby R, Eilard T, Svedhem A, Lycke E (1975) Treatment of toxoplasmosis with trimethoprim-sulfamethoxazole. Scand J Infect Dis 7:72–75

Ochoa AG (1971) Trimethoprim and sulfamethoxazole in pregnancy. JAMA 217:1244

Ochoa AG, Tamayo L (1969) Tratamiento del micetoma actinomicético por *N. brasiliensis* con Ro 6-2580/11. Comunicacion preliminar. Med Rev Mex 49:473–476

Oomen LJA (1976) Human brucellosis in Kenya. Trop Geogr Med 28:45–53

Paradisi F, Cristiano P, Cioffi R (1976) Un caso di toxoplasmosi acquisita trattata con cotrimossazolo. G Mal Infett Parassit 23(12):719–722

Paschetta G (1972) Sulfametossazolo-trimetoprim e vàccinoterapia nella cura della brucellosi. G Mal Infett Parasit 24(5):386–388

Patrick S, Hindmarch JM, Hague RV, Harris DM (1975) Meningitis caused by *Pseudomonas maltophilia*. J Clin Pathol 28(9):741–743

Pavillard ER (1973) Treatment of Nocardial infection with Trimethoprim/Sulfamethoxazole. Med J Aust [Suppl] 1:65–69

Peabody JW Jr, Seabury JH (1960) Actinomycosis and nocardiosis. Am J Med 28:99–115

Pedrosa PN, Wanke B, Coura JR (1974) Emprego da associação sulfametoxazol + trimetoprim no tratamento da paracoccidioidose (blastomicose Sul-Americana). Rev Soc Bras Med Trop 8(3):159–165

Peniche J, Minor A, Lavalle P (1969) El tratamiento de los micetomas actinomiceticos con gantanol-trimetoprim (Ro 6–2580). Resultadas en 15 pacientes. Dermatologia (Mex) 13:309–317

Peterson DL, Hudson LD, Sullivan K (1978) Disseminated *Nocardia caviae* with positive blood cultures. Arch Intern Med 138(7):1164–1165

Philippon A, Kazmierczak A, Névot P (1972) Traitement de la brucellosis de la souris par les antibiotiques (tetracycline, ampicilline, triméthoprime-sulfaméthoxazole) en association avec *Corynebacterium parvum*. Ann Inst Pasteur 123:349–362

Phillips I, Eykyn S, Curtis MA, Snell JJS (1971) *Pseudomonas cepacia (multivorans)* septicemia in an intensive-care unit. Lancet 1:375–377

Pilet C, Monteil JC (1972) In vitro study of the combination of sulfamethoxazole and trimethoprim against different strains of *Brucella*. Bull Assoc Fr Vet Microbiol Immunol Spec Mal Infect 11:43–52

Pinkhas J, Oliver I, de Vries A, Spitzer SA, Henig E (1973) Pulmonary nocardiosis complicating malignant lymphoma successfully treated with chemotherapy. Chest 63:367–370

Poirier R, Colognac-Chapelon R, Kleisbauer JP, Peloux Y, Laval P (1979) Broncho-pneumopathies à *Nocardia asteroides*. Nouv Presse Med 8(20):1693

Porto A (1978) The treatment of rickettsial Boutonneuse fever with cotrimoxazole. 14th Ann Meet Int Soc Interim Med Rome 1978, NO 354. Karger, Basel

Porto A, Barreto A, Mauricio H (1974) Comparacào de dols esquemas terapêuticos da brucelose aguda. J Med (Porto) 88(1627):148–149

Rachal JJ, Simberkoff MS, Hyams PJ (1973) *Pseudomonas cepacia* tricuspid endocarditis: treatment with trimethoprim, sulfonamide and polymyxin B. J Infect Dis [Suppl] 128:S762–767

Remington JS (1976) Trimethoprim-sulfamethoxazole in murine toxoplasmosis. Antimicrob Agents Chemother 9:222–223

Rigatos GA, Polyzos AK, Kappos-Rigatou I (1975) Die Trimethoprim-Sulfamethoxazol-Kombination zur Behandlung der Brucellose. Muench Med Wochenschr 117(22):961–962

Rivera JV, Perez JB (1957) Pulmonary nocardiosis treated with chloramphenicol. Arch Intern Med 100:152–156

Robertson L, Farrell ID, Hinchliffe PM (1973) The sensitivitiy of *Brucella abortus* to chemotherapeutic agents. J Med Microbiol 6(4):549–557

Rodriguez JAG, Luengo FM, Galán JLV (1979) Nocardiosis pulmonar: descripción de un
caso. Med Clin (Barc) 73:73–76

Roux J, Van Lam N, Andriambololona L (1974) Sctivité antibactérienne de l'association
sulfaméthoxazole-triméthoprime. J Med Montp 9(4):162–167

Saksun JM, Kave J, Schachter RK (1978) Mycetoma caused by *Nocardia madurae*. Can
Med Assoc J 119(8):911–914

Sander J, Midtvedt T (1970) The effect of trimethoprim an acute experimental toxoplasmosis in mice. Acta Pathol Microbiol Scand [B] 78:664–668

Saravolatz LD, Pohlad DJ, Quinn EL (1979) In vitro susceptibility of *Legionella pneumophila*, serogroups I–IV. J Infect Dis 140(2):251

Satterwhite TK, Wallace RJ (1979) Primary cutaneous nocardiosis. JAMA 242(4):333–336

Schmidt U, Sen P, Kapila R, Levy F, Lange M, Middleton J, Louria DB (1980) Clinical
experience with intravenous trimethoprim-sulfamethoxazole (SXT) for serious infections. In: Nelson JD, Grassi C (eds) 19th Intersci Conf Antimicrob Agents Chemother,
Boston, Oct 1–5, 1979. Am Soc Microbiol, Washington DC

Seah SKK (1975) Chemotherapy in experimental toxoplasmosis: comparison of the efficacy
of trimethoprim-sulfur and pyrimethamine-sulfur combinations. Am J Trop Med Hyg
78(7):150–153

Seligman SJ, Madhavan T, Alcid D (1973) Trimethoprim-sulfamethoxazole in the treatment of bacterial endocarditis. J Infect Dis [Suppl] 128:S754–S761

Seriki O, Aderele WI, Johnson A, Smith JA (1975) Disseminated histoplasmosis due to
Histoplasma capsulatum in two Nigerian children. J Trop Med Hyg 78(12):248–255

Shashindran CH, Gandhi IS, Krishnasamy S, Ghosh MN (1978) Oral therapy of pediculosis
capitis with cotrimoxazole. Br J Dermatol 98(6):699–700

Shashindran CH, Gandhi IS, Lal S (1979) A trial of cotrimoxazole in scabies. Br J Dermatol
100(4):483

Sher NA, Hill CW, Eifrig DE (1977) Bilateral intraocular *Nocardia asteroides* infection.
Arch Ophthalmol 95(8):1415–1418

Sierra F, Restrepo A, Moncada LH (1974) Nocardiosis pulmonar. Antioquia Med 24(1):65–
69

Singh D, Kochhar RC, Seth HN (1976) Clinical records: rhinoentomophthoromycosis. J
Laryngol Otol 90(9):871–875

Speller DCE (1972) *Pseudomonas cepacia* endocarditis treated with co-trimoxazole and
kanamycin. Br Heart J 35:47–48

Stadtsbaeder S, Calvin-Preval MC (1973) L'association trimethoprim + sulfamethoxazole
au cours de la toxoplasmose experimentale chez la souris. Acta Clin Belg 28(1):34–39

Steigman AJ (1977) Rocky Mountain spotted fever and the avoidance of sulfonamides. J
Pediatr 91(1):163–164

Sueri L (1972) Prime osservazioni sul trattamento della brucellosi con l'associazione trimethoprim-sulfametossazolo per via orale ed endovenosa. G Mal Infett Parassit 24(1):3–7

Sueri LA (1973) Further observations on the treatment of brucellosis with the combination
trimethoprim-sulphamethoxazole by oral and intravenous routes. G Mal Infett Parassit
25(1):65–67

Sueri L, Ielasi G (1974) The treatment of various infectious diseases by intravenous administration of the trimethoprim-sulfamethoxazole combination (slow infusion). G Mal Infett Parassit 26(6):672–678

Sueri L, Vaglia A, Ciammaruchi R (1978) Terapia della brucellosi con Co-trimoxazolo. G
Mal Infett Parassit 30(2):168–171

Swenson J, Thornsberry C, Silcox V (1980) Susceptibility of rapidly growing mycobacteria
to 33 antimicrobial agents. In: Nelson JD, Grassi C (eds) Proc 11th ICC and 19th
ICAAC, Boston, Oct 1–5, 1979. Am Soc Microbiol, Washington DC

Syrkis I, Fried M, Elian I, Pietrushka D, Lengy T (1975) A case of severe human coccidiosis
in Israel. Isr J Med Sci 11(4):373–377

Szaflarski J, Sokola A, Herman ZS (1974) Tentative treatment of experimental toxoplasmosis in mice. IX. Effect of trimethoprim, sulfomethoxazole and their combination Seprin.
Acta Parasitol Pol 22:261–263

Tanphaichitra D (1979) Acute septicaemic melioidosis with pulmonary hilar prominence: a case report with a unique chest radiographic pattern. Thorax 34(4):565–566

Tanphaichitra D, Vanwari S, Siristonpun Y, Promjunyakul K (1979) Melioidosis. Therapy with multiple antimicrobial agents and cellular immunity. Chest 75(5):646–647

Taplin D, Bassett DC, Mertz PM (1971) Foot lesions associated with *Pseudomonas cepacia.* Lancet 2(7724):568–571

Telegdy L, Kéri J (1976) Treatment of human brucellosis with doxycycline and trimethoprim-sulfonamide. In: Williams JD, Geddes AM (eds) Proc 9th Int Congr Chemother, London, vol 6. Plenum, New York, pp 379–382

Terragna A, Rossolini A, Cellesi C, Figura N, Barberi A (1973) Activity of the combination trimethoprim-sulfamethoxazole on experimental toxoplasmosis. Arzneim Forsch 23(9):1328–1331

Terragna A, Cellesi C, Rossolini A, Figura N (1974a) Attività dell'associapione trimethoprim-sulfamethossazolo (TM-SMZ) nella toxoplasmosi sperimentale del topo. G Mal Infett Parassit 26(7):861–867

Terragna A, Rossolini A, Cellesi C, Figura N (1974b) L'associazione trimethoprim-sulfametossazolo (TM-SMZ) nella toxoplasmosi sperimentale del topo. Gaz Med Ital 133:330–336

Thianprasit M (1978) Successful treatment of basidiobolomycosis with trimethoprim and sulfamethoxazole. Dermatol SE Asia (SEAMEO):82–83

Thiermann E, Apt W, Atias A, Lorca M, Olguin J (1978) A comparative study of some combined treatment regimens in acute toxoplasmosis in mice. Am J Trop Med Hyg 27(4):747–750

Thornsberry C, Baker CN, Kirven LA (1978) In vitro activity of antimicrobial agents on Legionnaires disease bacterium. Antimicrob Agents Chemother 13(1):78–80

Tomioka S, Kobayashi Y, Uchida H (1978) Susceptibilities of glucose-nonfermentative gram-negative rods to antimicrobial agents. In: Siegenthaler W, Lüthy R (eds) Proc 10th Int Congr Chemother, Zurich, Sept 18–23, vol 1. Am Soc Microbiol, Washington DC, pp 440–442

Turner T, Burry JN, Kirk J, Reid JG (1975) *Mycobacterium marinum* infection. Arch Dermatol 111(4):525

Van-Ai N, Duc-Hanh N, Van-Dien P, Van-Lè N (1972a) Effets in vitro et in vivo du triméthoprime-sulfaméthoxazole sur *Yersinia pestis*. Bull Soc Pathol Exot Filiales 65(4):759–764

Van-Ai N, Duc-Hanh N, Van-Dien P, Van-Lè N (1972b) Peste bubonique et septicémique traitée avec succès par du triméthoprime-sulfaméthoxazole. Bull Soc Pathol Exot Filiales 65(6):770–780

Van-Ai N, Duc-Hanh N, Van-Dien P, Van-Lè N (1973) Co-trimoxazole in bubonic plague. Br Med J 4(5884):108–109

Van Beers D, Yourassowsky E (1974) Traitement d'une nocardiose pulmonaire par le co-trimoxazole. Etude clinique et microbiologique. Med Mal Infect 4(3):139–144

Wallace JR, Bigby T, Septimus EJ (1980) The activity of sulfonamides against *Mycobacterium fortuitum* and *Mycobacterium cheloni*. In: Nelson JD, Grassi C (eds) Proc 11th ICC and 19th ICAAC, Boston, Oct 1–5, 1979. Am Soc Microbiol, Washington DC

Wallace R, Septimus EJ, Musher DM, Martin RR (1977) Disc diffusion susceptibility testing of *Nocardia* species. J Infect Dis 135:568–575

Werner H, Egger I (1975) Vergleichende chemotherapeutische Untersuchungen über die Wirksamkeit von Bactrim und anderen Kombinationspräparaten auf die Proliferative- und Zystenbildungsphase von *Toxaplasma gondii* in NMRI-Mäusen. Zentralbl Bakteriol [B] 231:349–364

Westerman EL, Christensen RP (1979) Chronic *Isospora belli* infection treated with co-trimoxazole. 91(3):413–414

Willey RF, Matthews MB, Peutherer JF, Marmion BP (1979) Chronic cryptic Q-fever infection of the heart. Lancet II(8137):270–279

Williams H (1977) Toxoplasmosis in the perinatal period. Postgrad Med J 53(624):614–617

Wishart MM, Riley TV (1976) Infection with *Pseudomonas maltophilia* hospital outbreak due to contaminated disinfectant. Med J Aust 2(19):710–712

Woolfson H, Saunders KE, Meade G (1976) Fish tank granuloma. Br J Clin Pract 30(5):122, 127

Yu VL, Rumans LW, Wing EJ, McLeod R, Sattler FN, Harvey RM, Deresinski SC (1978) *Pseudomonas maltophilia* causing heroin-associated infective endocarditis. Arch Intern Med 138(11):1667–1671

Yu VL, Felegie TR, Yee RB, Pasculle AW (1980) In vitro synergism with the use of three antibiotics simultaneously against *P. maltophilia*. In: Nelson JD, Grassi C (eds) 19 th Intersci Conf Antimicrob Agents Chemother, Boston, Oct 1–5, 1979, No 587. Am Soc Microbiol, Washington DC

Subject Index

Acedapsone
  as a repository form of dapsone 30
  pharmacokinetics and metabolism 38
  water solubility and half-life 35
Acetylpyridine-NADPH
  as substrate for DHFR 66
Acinetobacter calcoaceticus 247
Adenine
  reversal of sulfonamide activity 41
Adenosine Diphosphate
  product of thymidylate synthesis 15
Adenosine Triphosphate
  in thymidylate synthesis 15
S-Adenosylmethionine 15
Adenlyate Cyclase 357
Aerobacter aerogenes
  prostatitis from 383
Agranulocytosis
  adverse effect of TMP/SMX 209, 218, 219, 224
Albumin 223, 224
Amethopterin (see Methotrexate)
Amikacin
  in melioidosis (Pseudomonas pseudomallei infection) 427
p-Aminobenzoic acid, pABA 44, 45
  displacement by sulfonamides 1, 18, 19, 31, 41, 43, 76, 218
  hyperproduction of 45, 244
  in de novo synthesis of dihydrofolate 16, 40, 43
  reversal of sulfonamide activity 26, 39, 43, 137, 155, 158
  use by sporozoa 306
  as a substrate for dihydropteroate synthase 40
p-Aminobenzoylglutamate, pABG
  as a substrate for dihydropteroate synthase 43
  difficulty of transport into microorganisms 17
Aminoglycosides
  in Yersina enterocolitica infections 374
4-Aminoimidazole Ribonucleotide, AIR 16

Aminopterin 109
  active transport into Streptococcus faecium 17
  fetal toxicity 197
2-Amino-4-hydroxy-6-hydroxymethyldihydropteridine
  intermediate in folate biosynthesis 40
5-Amino-4-imidazole carboxamide ribonucleotide, AICAR
  accumulation in sulfonamide-inhibited cultures 41
  folate cofactors and 14
Amoxicillin
  in bronchitis 400–402
  in non-typhoidal salmonella infections 361
  in sinusitis in adults 312
  in typhoid fever 364
  in urinary tract infections 268, 270
  treatment of typhoid carriers 6, 360
Amphotericin B
  in chromomycosis 425
  in histoplasmosis 422, 423
  in paracoccidioidomycosis 423, 424
  in rhinoentomophthoromycosis 424
  treatment of phycomycosis 424, 425
Ampicillin
  adverse effects 407
  concentration in plasma and prostatic fluid 387, 388
  effect of treatment on postgonococcal urethritis 351
  in bronchitis 400–402, 407
  in gonorrhea 349, 350
  in Hemophilus influenzae infections 309–314
  in Malakoplekia 431
  in non-typhoidal salmonellosis 320, 361, 367, 368
  in shigellosis 321, 322, 368–371
  in sinusitis 312
  in typhoid fever 321, 360, 362–364
  in urinary tract infections 268, 270, 333
  in Yersinia enterocolitica infections 375, 376

Ampicillin
  minimum inhibitory concentration in H.
    influenzae 309; in gonorrhea 349, 350
  physicochemical characteristics 387
  prophylaxis of Hemophilus influenzae
    313
  prophylaxis of UTIs 316
  resistance to 5, 283, 309, 310, 321, 322,
    333, 349, 350, 360, 363, 364, 367, 369,
    370, 375
  treatment of typhoid carriers 6, 360
Ampiclox
  in bronchitis 400–402
Anaphylaxis
  adverse effect of TMP/SMX 209
Angioneurotic oedema
  adverse effect of TMP/SMX 209, 211
Anhydroleucovorin, see 5,10-
    methenyltetrahydrofolate
Antimetabolites
  theory of 26, 55
Aplastic Anaemia
  adverse effect of sulfonamides 219
Azathioprine
  interaction with TMP/SMX 223

Bacillus pumilus 178
Bacteroides
  insensitivity of TMP 78, 90
Basidiobolus 425
  haptosporus 422, 424
5-Benzyl-2,4-diaminopyrimidines 112–
  116
  as single agents 94–96
  assay methods 177–179
  biologic effects 59
  commercially distributed analogs 107
  comparative antibacterial activity and
    DHFR inhibition 113
  differential binding to DHFRs 59
  fractional inhibitory concentration 80
  resistance to 87–90
  synergy with sulfonamides 80
  6-substituted derivatives 115
  substitution of a heterocyclic ring for the
    benzene moiety 116
  6-unsubstituted derivatives 112
  variations in the bridge between the
    pyrimidine and benzene rings 116
Blastomycosis
  South American (see
    paracoccidioidomycosis)
Bordetella pertussis 262, 403
Boutonneuse Fever 430
Bratton-Marshall Surveillance Method
  177, 179

Bronchiectasis
  prophylaxis of 404–406
  treatment 397, 403
Bronchitis 5
  chronic 5, 397–402, 404–406
  prophylaxis of 404–406
  treatment of 397–402
  treatment with TMP/SMX 5, 397–402,
    406
Brucella
  abortus 411, 412
  insensitivity of TMP 78
  melitensis 411, 412
  sensitivity to TMP/SMX 90
  suis 411
Brucellosis 411–414
  treatment with tetracycline 412–414
  treatment with TMP/SMX 412–414
Bubonic Plague 411, 429

Calcium Folinate 404
Campylobacter fetus 92
Candida albicans 386, 405
Candidiasis 210, 320
Carbenicillin
  in Pseudomonas maltophilia infections
    428
  in urinary tract infections 272
  in Yersinia enterocolitica infections 375
  resistance to 375
Cefaclor
  prophylaxis of Hemophilus influenzae
    infections 313
Cellulitis 320
  periorbital 312
Cephalexin
  in bronchitis 400–402
  in spina bifida cystica 315
  in urinary tract infections 268–270, 315
Cephalothin
  concentration in plasma and prostatic
    fluid 387
  in Chancroid 353
  in Yersinia enterocolitica infections 375
  physicochemical characteristics 387
  resistance to 375
Chancroid 343, 352–354
Chest Infections 397–409
Chlamydia
  in children 316–318
  psittaci 316–318
  trachomatis 266, 343, 348, 350–352, 391
Chloramphenicol
  adverse effects 219, 247, 365
  concentration in plasma and prostatic
    fluid 388
  in brucellosis 414

in bubonic plague 429
in cholera 372, 373
in melioidosis (p. pseudomallei
    infection) 426, 427
in Nocardiosis 418
in non-thypoidal salmonella infections
    320, 361
in P. cepacia and P. meltophilia
    infections 427, 428
in paratyphoid fever 360
in sinusitis 312
in thyphoid fever 320, 321, 360–366
in Yersinia enterocolitica infections 374
resistance to 1, 5, 321, 360, 363, 364,
    369, 370
toxicity 360
Chloroguanide
    chemical structure 293
    in malaria 297, 300, 302, 304
7-Chlorolincomycin
    concentration in plasma and prostatic
        fluid 388
Chloroquine
    in malaria 299, 305
Chlorpromazine 219
Chlorpropamide
    interaction with TMP/SMX 224
Cholangitis 324
Cholera 357, 371–373
Chromomycosis
    treatment with TMP/SMX 411, 422,
        425
Citrobacter 247
    freundii 262
Citrovorum Factor, see 5-
    formyltetrahydrofolate
Clindamycin
    adverse effects 210
    in M. Marinum infections 421
    in Malakoplekia 431
    resistance to 363, 364
Clostridium
    botulinum 92
    difficile 92, 210
    insensitivity to TMP 78, 92, 261, 262
    perfringens 261, 262
Cloxacillin
    in Yersinia enterocolitica infections 375
    resistance to 375
Coccidiosis 306, 358, 359
Colitis 210
Conidiobolus coronatus 424, 425
Conjunctivitis
    in children 317
Corynebacterium diphtheriae 262
Coumarin 238

Counter-immunoelectrophoresis (CIE)
    318, 319
Coxiella burnetii 430
Creatinine 168, 216, 217, 235, 236, 264
Crystalluria 217
Cycloguanil 112
Cystic Fibrosis 405
Cystitis 264, 266, 267

Dapsone
    antimalarial activity 30
    antimalarial use 304, 305
    important characteristics of 35
    in treatment of leprosy 29
    mechanism of action 44
    pharmacokinetics and metabolism 38
    present status in therapeutics 46
Deamino-NADPH
    as substrate for DHFR 66
Deoxyuridine Monophosphate
    in thymidylate synthesis 15
Dermatitis
    adverse effect of TMP/SMX 211–216
Diabetes 275
Diaminodiphenylsulfoxide 44
2,4-Diaminopyrimidines 94
    as single agents 94–96
2,4-Diamino-5-p-chlorophenoxypyrimidine
    chemical structure 293
Diaminodiphenylsulfone (DDS) (see
    Dapsone) 158
Diaveridine 107, 306
Dihydrofolate, FAH$_2$ 1, 87, 133, 191, 218
    as substrate for DHFR 56
    cooperative binding to DHFR 57
    de novo synthesis in bacteria 18, 40
    DHFR K$_m$ values 58
    mode of binding to DHFR 15
    orientation for binding to DHFR 67
    product of thymidylate synthesis 12, 13,
        15
    reduction of synthesis of by
        sulfonamide 86
    stereochemistry of reduction 121
    structure 11
    synthesis of cell-free extracts 43
Dihydrofolate Reductase, DHFR 55–70
    amino acid sequences 63, 120
    assay and kinetic studies 56
    Asp-27 in inhibitor binding and
        catalysis 65
    basis of selectivity 58–67
    conformation and cooperativity 62
    first isolation 40
    genetics 69
    hyperproduction of 69
    hysteretic behavior of 62

Dihydrofolate Reductase, DHFR
  in the development of resistance to
    TMP 246, 248
  in the mechanism of action of
    trimethoprim 3, 18, 156, 218, 280,
    281
  inhibition of by TMP/SMX 158, 197–
    199
  inhibitor binding analysis 59
  inhibitors of 16, 17, 107–122, 293, 407
  interconvertible forms of 63
  isozymes of 63, 65
  kinetic studies of 58
  mechanism of action 57
  molecular weight of 58
  plasmid-coded reductases 68
  protozoal 294, 295, 303
  role in cellular metabolism 11–20
  selective inhibitors of 107–122
  stabilization by methotrexate 69
  stereochemistry of reduction 67, 121
  synergism with sulfonamides 45
  three-dimensional structures of 65–67,
    120
  turnover number of 58
  two NADPH binding sites 62
  X-ray studies 15
Dihydrofolate Reductase Inhibitors 107–
  122
  antimalarial use 296
  as antiprotozoal agents 293–306
  5-benzyl-2,4-diaminopyrimidines 112
  bicyclic analogs of the
    diaminopyrimidines 117
  comparative binding of 60
  concept of specificity of 111
  1,2-dihydro-1,3,5-triazines 117
  historical perspective of 109
  penetration into bacterial cells of 60,
    111
  5-phenyl-2,4-diaminopyrimidines 111
  structure-activity relationships 107
  use in combination with sulfonamides
    against malaria 303–305
Dihydrofolate Synthetase
  function in folic acid metabolism 40
Dihydropteridine pyrophosphate 155
Dihydropterin Pyrophosphokinase
  function in folic acid synthesis 40
Dihydropterinsulfonamides 44
Dihydropteroate
  biosynthesis of 40, 294
  synthesis in cell-free extracts 43
Dihydropteroate Synthase 1, 86, 158, 245,
  294
  altered sensitivity to sulfonamides 45
  function and isolation of 40

  inhibition by
    dihydropterinsulfonamides 44
  sulfonamide inhibition of 31
Dihydropteropterine pyrophosphate 44
Dihydropteroyloligo-gamma-L-glutamates
  as substrates for DHFR 57
1,2-Dihydro-1,3,5-triazines
  anthelmintic activity of 117
Dimethylchlortetracycline
  in bronchitis 400–402
Doxycycline
  concentration in plasma 388
  concentration in prostatic fluid 388
  in bronchitis 400

Enterobacter
  antibody against 391, 392
  prostatitis from 379, 380, 383, 386
  resistance of 266
  resistance to amplicillin 310, to
    sulfonamides 243, 244, 266; to
    tetracycline 333; to trimethoprim 95,
    247, 250–252, 266, 283
  sensitivity to TMP 6, 233, 262, 264
  thymine-dependent mutants of 89
  UTI from 264, 333–335, 385
Enterococci
  prostatitis from 379, 380, 383
  use of exogenous folates 87
Entomophthoromycosis 424
Erythema
  Multiforme 211, 214–216, 224, 277
  Nodosum 211
  Toxic 210, 212–215
Erythromycin
  concentration in plasma and prostatic
    fluid 387, 388
  in chlamydial infection 318, 351
  in L. pneumophila infections 430
  in M. marinum infections 422
  in Nocardiosis 419
  in Yersinia entercolitica infections 375
  physicochemical characteristics 387
  prophylaxis of Hemophilus influenzae
    313
  resistance to 349, 375
Erythromycin/ampicillin
  in Nocardiosis 418
Escherichia coli
  antibody against 385
  diarrhea 357, 358
  effect of SMX and TMP/SMX on
    generation rates of 131–158
  effect of TMP metabolites on 173
  enteropathogenic 357
  enterotoxigenic 357
  in chronic bronchitis 399

in malakoplakia 431
in meningitis 314
prostatitis from 380, 383, 385, 388, 392
resistance to sulfonamides 86, 245, 266
resistance to trimethoprim 96, 246, 247, 251, 282, 283, 363
resistant strains 3, 4, 87, 249, 367, 370
sensitivity to TMP 76, 87, 262, 334
sensitivity to TMP/SMX 90–92
thymineless mutants of 89, 246
UTIs from 315, 334
Exanthemata 210, 211

Flavin Adenine Dinucleotide
in methionine biosynthesis 41
Fluorocytosine
in chromomycosis 425
in histoplasmosis 423
in mycoses 425
Folate
as substrate for DHFR 57
antagonism of 293
chemical synthesis of 39
deficiency 191, 218, 280
de novo synthesis 80, 86
depletion of 133, 137, 337
functions in cellular metabolism 11–20
in reversal of dapsone activity 44
metabolism of 6, 39, 42, 76, 223
occurrence of 11
orientation for binding to DHFR 67
origins of 16
polyglutamate derivatives 40
reduction of 40
stereochemistry of 15
stereochemistry of reduction 67, 121
structure 11
structure elucidation of 43
transport into bacteria 18
transport systems 17
Folate Reductase
inhibition of by TMP 191, 200
Folic Acid (see Folate)
Folinic Acid (see 5-Formyltetrahydrofolate)
5-Formamido-4-imidazole carboxamide ribonucleotide 14
Formiminoglutamic Acid
excretion of 13, 280
5-Formiminotetrahydrofolate, 5-Formimino-FAH$_4$
as formate equivalent 12
conversion to 5,10-methenyl-FAH$_4$ 13
Formylglycinamide ribonucleotide 14
5-Formyltetrahydrofolate, 5-Formyl-FAH$_4$, Folinic Acid
antagonism of aminopterin toxicity 55

antagonism of TMP toxicity 280–282
antagonism of TMP/SMX toxicity 6, 87, 417, 419
as formate equivalent 12
chemical synthesis of 13
conversion to 5,10-methenyl-FAH$_4$ 13
enzymatic conversion to 10-formyl-FAH$_4$ 40
reversal of feto-toxic effect of TMP/SMX 198, 199
transport into bacteria 17
use during treatment of toxoplasmosis 305, 415
10-Formyltetrahydrofolate, 10-Formyl-FAH$_4$
as cofactor in purine biosynthesis 14
as formate equivalent 12
in folic acid metabolism 40
10-Formyltetrahydrofolate Synthetase 12
Friend erythroleukemia virus 280
Furazolidone
in cholera 372
in shigellosis 370

Garnerella vaginalis (haemophilus) 92
Gas Liquid Chromatography 178
Gastrointestinal Disorders 280
lower 210
upper 209, 210
Genital Infections 343–354
Gentamicin
in chest infections 405
in Malakoplekia 431
resistance to 283
Giardia lamblia 431
Glossitis 208, 209
Glucose-6-phosphate dehydrogenase (G6PD) deficiency 365
Glucuronides 235
Glycinamide Ribonucleotide 14
Glycinamide Ribonucleotide Transformylase 13
Glycine 14, 80, 82, 83
reversal of sulfonamide activity 41
Gonococcal Urethritis 344–346
Gonorrhea 93, 343, 346
Gram's Stain 353
Granulomatous Disease 324
Guanine
reversal of sulfonamide activity 41
Guanosine Triphosphate 16
in folic acid metabolism 39
Guanylate Cyclase 357

Haematuria 217
Haemolytic Anaemia 220

Haemophilus   89
    chronic bronchitis from   397–400, 402,
        403, 405–408
    dissemination of   312–314
    resistance to TMP   250
    thymine-dependent mutants of   89
    ducreyi   343, 353
    in children   309
    influenzae   5, 262, 312, 314
    resistant strains   407, 408
Hexamethylentetramine   238
High Pressure Liquid Chromatography
    178, 180
Histoplasma capsulatum   422, 423
    duboissii   423
Histoplasmosis   411, 422, 423
Homocysteine
    in the biosynthesis of methionine   15
Horse Blood
    in medium   75, 76
Hydroxymethyldihydropterin   31
Hyperbilirubinaemia   221

Inosinic Acid
    biosynthesis of   14
Isoleucovorin, see 5,10-
    methenyltetrahydrofolate
Isospora belli   306, 358, 359, 430, 431
Isospora belli Infections   358, 359, 411,
    430, 431
Ito-Reenstierna Skin Test   353

Kanamycin
    concentration in plasma and prostatic
        fluid   387
    in chancroid   353
    in melioidosis (P. pseudomallei
        infection)   426, 427
    in P. Cepacia infections   428
    in P. maltophilia infections   428
    in prostatitis   389
    physicochemical characteristics   387
Kernicterus   221
Klebsiella
    aerogenes   81, 363
    meningitis   314
    pneumoniae   89, 90, 92, 262, 264
    in chronic bronchitis   399, 400, 406
    resistance to TMP and TMP/SMX   90,
        92, 244, 247, 251, 252, 283
    resistant strains   3, 4
    prostatitis from   383
    thymine-dependent mutants of   89

Lactobacilli   243
Lactobacillus casei   280, 293
Legionella pneumophila   430

Leucopenia   218, 219, 223
Leucovorin, see 5-Formyltetrahydrofolate
Levamisole
    in melioidosis (Pseudomonas
        pseudomallei infection)   427
Lincomycin
    adverse effects   210
    concentration in plasma and prostatic
        fluid   388
Listeria monocytogenes
    resistance to TMP   250
Lyell's Syndrome (toxic epidermal
    necrolysis)   208, 211–216, 224, 277
Lymphogranuloma venereum   343, 352

Malakoplakia   411, 431
Malaria   293–305
    life cycle of the parasite   295, 296
    treatment with pyrimethamine   294,
        295, 297–303
    treatment with pyrimethamine/
        sulfonamide   303–305
    treatment with TMP   281, 295
Mastoiditis
    in children   310, 312
Mecillinam
    in E. coli diarrhea   358
Megaloblastic anemia   6, 218, 222, 280
Melioidosis   426, 427
Meningitis   232, 309
    in children   310, 314, 315
Mesenteric Adenitis   323, 324
Methenamine hippurate
    prophylaxis of UTIs   274, 275
    resistance to   284
5,10-Methenyltetrahydrofolate, 5,10-
    Methenyl-FAH$_4$
    as cofactor in purine biosynthesis   14
    as formate equivalent   12
    formation from 5-formyl- and 5-
        formimino-FAH$_4$ 13
    in folic acid metabolism   41
Methenyltetrahydrofolate cyclohydrolase
    12
Methicillin   217
Methionine   80, 82, 83
    biosynthesis of   15
    reversal of sulfonamide activity   41
Methotrexate   6, 17, 18
    cooperative binding to DHFR   62
    development of   110
    DHFR binding site   15, 65, 121
    DHFR Ki values of   119
    DHFRs resistant to   68
    effect of 4-amino group on DHFR
        binding   65
    fetal toxicity   197

inhibition of dihydrofolate reductase
55, 60
interaction with TMP   281
interaction with TMP/SMX   238
non-selective binding to DHFRs   59
stabilization of DHFR   69
synthesis of   55
5,10-Methylenetetrahydrofolate, 5,10-
Methylene-FAH$_4$ 12, 13
absolute configuration   67
as formaldehyde equivalent   14
depletion of   20, 299
in folic acid metabolism   41
in thymidylate synthesis   15
Methylenetetrahydrofolate
dehydrogenase   12
x-Methylfolate   55
5-Methyltetrahydrofolate, 5-
Methyl-FAH$_4$ 17
as principal reservoir of FAH$_4$ in
mammals   15
formation from 5,10-methylene-FAH$_4$
14
in folic acid metabolism   41
Metronidazole
in Isospora belli infections   359, 431
Michaelis-Gutmann bodies   431
Minocycline
in Nocardiosis   419
Mucor spp.   424
Mucormycosis   424
Mueller-Hinton Medium   96
Mycobacterioses   411, 421, 422
Mycobacterium
atypical   421, 422
chelonei   421
diernhoferi   421
flavescens   421
fortuitum   421
insensitivity to TMP   78, 261
kansasii   421
leprae   421
marinum   421
peregrinum   421
phlei   421
scrofulaceum   421
smegmatis   421
tuberculosis   78, 262, 421
vaccae   421
Myelomeningocele   314

Nafcillin   217
Nalidixic Acid
concentration in plasma and prostatic
fluid   387
in shigellosis   368
physicochemical characteristics   387

resistance to   247
Neisseria
catarrhalis   311
gonorrhoeae   76, 262, 343, 350
insensitivity to TMP   78, 261
meningitidis   262, 314
prostatitis from   391
sensitivity to TMP/SMX   90
Neomycin
in non-typhoidal salmonella infections
361
Nephritis (Acute Interstitial)   217
Nicotinamide adenine dinucleotide,
NADH   14
as substrate for DHFR   57
Nicotinamide adenine dinucleotide
phosphate, NADPH
as substrate for DHFR   56, 66
binding site in lactic dehydrogenase   66
cooperative binding to DHFR   62
DHFR binding site of   65, 66
DHFR K$_m$ values of   58
in reduction of dihydrofolate   13, 40
Nitrofurantoin
adverse reactions   275
concentration in plasma and prostatic
fluid   387
in diagnosis of bacterial prostatitis   382,
383
in urinary tract infections   268, 269, 270,
334, 336, 387
physicochemical characteristics   387
prophylaxis of UTIs   274, 275, 316
resistance to   285
Nocardia
asteroides   262, 417–420
brasiliensis   417–420
caviae   417–420
insensitivity to TMP   78, 261
madurae   420
sensitivity to TMP/SMX   90
Nocardiosis   93, 411, 417–420
Novobiocin
in P. cepacia and P. maltophilia
infections   427

Ocular Trachoma   317
Oleandomycin
concentration in plasma and prostatic
fluid   387
physicochemical characterisitcs   387
Ormetoprim   107, 115
Osteomyelitis   234, 324, 359
Otitis Media   5, 309, 320
in children   310, 311
Oxacillin   217

Oxolinic Acid
  in shigellosis   368
  in urinary tract infections   268, 270, 272,
    274, 275
Oxytetracycline
  concentration in plasma and prostatic
    fluid   387
  physicochemical characteristics   387

Pancytopenia   6, 220
Pantothenic Acid   16
Paracoccidioides brasiliensis   423, 424
Paracoccidioidomycosis   411, 423, 424
  treatment with TMP/SMX   422
Paratyphoid Fever   359, 360
Pediculosis capitis   411, 431
Pediculus humanis capitis   431
Pediococcus cerevisiae
  growth requirements   17
Penicillin   28
  concentration in plasma and prostatic
    fluid   387
  effect of treatment on postgonoccal
    urethritis   350, 351
  in Chancroid   353
  in gonorrhea   343
  physicochemical characteristics   387
  resistance to   348–350, 353, 403
Pentamidine Isothionate
  in P. carinii pneumonia   5, 319, 404
Phenylbutazone   219
Phenytoin
  interaction with TMP/SMX   223, 238
Photodermatitis   211
Phycomycosis   411, 424, 425
  treatment with TMP/SMX   422
Pilocarpine   386, 387
Pittsburgh pneumonia agent (PPA)   430
Pivampicillin
  effect of treatment on postgonoccal
    urethritis   350, 351
Plasmids
  in development and transference of
    resistance   1, 4, 87, 245, 332, 333, 363,
    367, 370
Plasmodium   293
  berghei   293, 296, 303, 418
  falciparum   297, 298, 300–302, 304, 305
  gallinaceum   296, 303
  malariae   296–298
  ovale   296
  vivax   296, 298, 300, 302, 303
Pneumococci
  resistance to sulfonamides   245
  resistance to TMP   250
Pneumocystis carinii   403, 404
  diagnosis of   319

  in children   318–320
  treatment with TMP/SMX   5, 281, 306,
    318–320, 403, 404
Pneumocytosis   5
Pneumonia   320, 402–404
  diagnosis of pneumocystis carinii   319
  pneumocystis carinii   318–320, 403, 404
  treatment with TMP/SMX   402–404,
    406
Pneumonitis
  in children   317
Polymyxin   261
Polymyxin B
  concentration in plasma and prostatic
    fluid   387
  in P. cepacia infections   428
  in P. maltophilia infections   428
  physicochemical characteristics   387
Potassium Iodide
  in chromomycosis   425
  in mycoses   425
  in phycomycosis   424, 425
  resistance to   425
Primaquine   302
Probenecid
  effect of treatment on postgonoccal
    urethritis   350, 351
Proctitis   348
Proguanil   112
Promin
  in the treatment of leprosy   29
Prontosil
  discovery of   25
  reduction of sulfanilamide   26
Prostate   380
  antibacterial effect of fluid   385, 386
  persistence of bacteria in   389, 390
  pH of fluid   388–390
  transurethral resection of   390
Prostatectomy   390
Prostatis   379–392
  bacterial   379–390
  classification of   379, 381
  diagnosis of bacterial   382–386
  granulomatous   384
  immunoglobulins in prostatic fluid in
    384, 385, 391, 392
  incidence of   380–382, 384
  nonbacterial   379–381, 390–392
  pH of prostatic fluid in   390
  prostatodynia   379–381
Prostatodynia   379–381
Proteinuria   210
Proteus
  in chronic bronchitis   399
  in vitro growth   398, 399
  mirabilis   251, 252, 383, 392

morgani 283, 383
prostatitis from 383, 392
resistance to TMP and TMP/SMX 247,
251, 252, 283
sensitivity to TMP 262
thymine-dependent mutants of 89
vulgaris 76, 81, 84, 85, 87
Providencia 247
Pruritus 210
Pseudomonas
aeruginosa 78, 91, 249, 262, 425
antibody against 391, 392
cepacia 426–428
in chronic bronchitis 399, 405
in vitro growth 398, 399
insensitivity to TMP 78, 261, 262
maltophilia 426–428
prostatitis from 379, 380, 383, 392
pseudomallei 426, 427
putrefaciens 428
resistance to TMP 3
resistant strains 389, 390
Pseudomonas Infections 425–428
response to TMP/SMX 425–428
Pteridines
pKA 117
Pteroic Acid
polyglutamates of 40
Pteroyl-gamma-L-glutamates 57
Purine 80, 82, 83, 157
Pyelonephritis 264, 267
Pyrexia 211
Pyrido(2,3-d)pyrimidines 118
Pyrimethamine
absorption 300
adverse effects 415, 417
antimalarial use 294, 295, 297, 299–304
chemical structure 293
clinical trials 297, 298
disadvantages of 298, 299
effect on DHFR hysteresis 62
half life 301, 416
in coccidiosis 30
in combination with dapsone 30
in combination with sulformethoxine
29
in toxoplasmosis 18, 30, 415–417
inhibition of DHFRs 60
interaction with TMP/SMX 222
pharmacokinetics 300, 301
plasmodial resistance to 46
resistance to 301, 303, 304
slowness of schizonticidal effects 299
synergy with sulfonamides 151, 152,
303–305
uptake mechanism for 17

use in combination with sulfonamides
against toxoplasmosis 305
Pyrimethamine/Sulfadiazine 303, 304
in P. carinii pneumonia in children 319

Q fever 411, 430
Quinacrine 297
Quinazolines 118

Rhizopus spp. 424
Riboflavin 16
Ribonucleotide Diphosphate Reductase
246
Ribose-1-phosphate 20
Rickettsiaceae 429, 430
Rickettsiosis 429, 430
Rifampicin
in chlamydial infections in children 318
in histoplasmosis 423
in Yersinia enterocolitica infections 374
prophylaxis of Hemophilus influenzae
313, 314
resistance to 282
synergy with TMP 261
treatment of typhoid carriers 6, 365
Rocky Mountain Spotted Fever 430

Salmonella
choleraesuis 359
enteritidis 359, 360, 365, 368
flexneri 369
heidelberg 360
in children 314, 320, 321
meningitis 315
oslo 366
paratyphi 359, 365
resistance to trimethoprim 247, 251,
363
resistant strains 363, 366
schottmuelleri 87
sensitivity to TMP 262
sonnei 369, 370
thymine-dependent mutants of 89
typhi 5, 320, 321, 359, 361, 365
typhimurium 87, 201, 360, 365, 367, 368
Salmonella Infections 359–368
Salmonellosis 359–368
in children 320, 321
Sarcoptes scabiei 431
Serine
in the biosynthesis of 5,10-methylene-
FAH$_4$ 14
reversal of sulfonamide activity 41
Serratia
marcescens 90
resistance to trimethoprim 244, 247
thymine-dependent mutants of 89

Shigella   321, 322, 368–371
    boydii   368, 370
    diarrhea   357
    dysenteriae   368–370
    flexneri   5, 386, 371
    resistance to sulfonamides   1
    resistance to TMP   247
    sensitivity to TMP   262
    sonnei   5, 368, 371
Shigellosis   5, 321, 322, 368–371
Sinusitis   320
    in children   311, 312
Spectrofluorometry   177, 235
Spectrophotometry   179
Spina bifida cystica   315
Staphylococcus
    aureus   76, 84, 324, 405
    effect of TMP metabolites on   173
    epidermidis   315, 383
    in chronic bronchitis   399, 405, 406
    lung abscess from   403
    prostatitis from   385
    pyogenes   262, 399, 403
    resistance to sulfonamides   245
    resistance to TMP   250, 283
    sensitivity to TMP   262
    thymine dependent mutants of   89
Stevens-Johnson Syndrome   208–211,
    213–216, 224, 277
Streptococcus
    effect of TMP metabolites on   173
    faecalis   91, 243, 244, 316
    faecium   6, 201
    in chronic bronchitis   397, 399, 400, 402,
        403, 405, 406, 408
    pneumonia   5, 87, 310, 314, 397, 399,
        400, 402, 403, 405, 406, 408
    pyogenes   87, 92, 332
    resistance to TMP   250
    resistance to TMP/SMX   4
    resistant strains   408
    sensitivity to TMP   262
    zooepidemicus   85
Streptomycin
    in brucellosis   412
    in bubonic plague   429
    resistance to   1, 245, 247, 251, 363, 364,
        370
Sulfacetamide   28
    important characteristics of   35
Sulfadiazine   32
    absorption   163, 164
    assay methods   179, 180
    concentration in plasma and tissues
        164, 166–168, in prostatic fluid 167,
        168; in sputum   407
    disposition and metabolism   163–180

effect on renal function   217
elimination of   237, 238
excretion   168
half-life of   28, 170, 171
important characteristics of   35
in Chancroid   352, 353
in lymphogranuloma venereum   352
in melioidosis (P. pseudomallei
    infection)   426, 427
in Nocardiosis   418, 420
introduction in therapeutics   27
metabolism   175–177
pharmacokinetics of   154, 155, 168, 169
physicochemical properties   154, 155,
    164, 165
protein binding of   164, 165
synergy with pyrimethamine   304
synergy with trimethoprim   81, 94
use with chloroguanide as an
    antimalarial   303
Sulfadimethoxine
    glucuronide derivative of   38
    half-life   29
    important characteristics of   35
Sulfadimethyloxazole (SDMO)   148, 150,
    154, 155
Sulfadimidine
    concentration in plasma and prostatic
        fluid   387
    in histoplasmosis   422
    in P. maltophilia infections   428
    in shigellosis   370
    physicochemical characteristics   387
Sulfadoxine
    in histoplasmosis   422, 423
    in malaria   305
    in paracoccidioidomycosis   424
    resitance to   367, 422
Sulfaguanidine
    in regard to ionization theory   34
Sulfalene   94
Sulfamerazine
    assay   180
    half-life of   28
    important characteristics   35
    introduction in therapeutics   27
Sulfamethazine
    assay   180
    important characteristics of   35
    introduction in therapeutics   27
Sulfamethizole   27
    absorption   229
    important characteristics of   35
    in urinary tract infections   268, 270
Sulfamethoxazole
    absorption   163
    acute toxicity studies   186

and impaired renal function 235
antagonistic effect on TMP action 151
assay methods 179, 180
concentration 2, 164, 166–168, 264; in
    amniotic fluid 233; in bile fluid 233; in
    breast milk 232; in cerebrospinal fluid
    232; in erythrocytes 234; in lung tissue
    234; in plasma 387, 388; in prostatic
    fluid 167, 168, 233, 387, 388; in sputum
    399, 400, 406, 407; in vaginal fluid 233
disposition and metabolism 163–180
effect on renal function 217
elimination of 235–237
excretion 168
fetal toxicity tests 189, 197–199
half-life 29, 170, 171, 235
important characteristics of 35
in atypical mycobacterial infections 421
in chlamycial infections in children 317,
    318
in chlamydia trachomatis infections 351
in cholera 372, 373
in combination with trimethoprim, see
    trimethoprim/sulfamethoxazole
in gonorrhea 343
in meningitis 232
in shigellosis 369
in toxoplasmosis 415, 416
in urinary tract infections 268, 270–273,
    315
in Yersinia enterocolitica infections 374
inhibitor of development of resistance to
    TMP 283, 286
interaction with Warfarin 223
lag in effect on growth 80
LD$_{50}$ 187
mechanism of action 1–3, 141
metabolic incorporation of 44
metabolism 174, 175, 235
metabolites of 235
minimum inhibitory concentration
    77–79, 81–84, 318, 349, 400
pharmacokinetics 229–238
physicochemical properties 154, 164,
    387
prophylaxis of UTIs 316
protein binding of 164, 165, 232
renal clearance of 236
reproductive toxicology 197–201
resistance to 348–350, 369, 370, 389
stability 97
synergy with trimethoprim 81, 318
teratogenic effects of 222
thyroid studies 195, 196
use in TMP/SMX 92–94
volume of distribution in plasma 231
water solubility 97

Sulfamethoxydiazine
    half-life of 29
    important characteristics of 35
Sulfamethoxypyrazine
    antimalarial activity of 30
    half-life of 29
    important characteristics of 35
Sulfamethoxypyridazine
    haematologic effects of 219
    half-life of 28, 39
    important characteristics of 35
Sulfamethoxytyridazine
    in Chancroid 353
    penetration into aqueous humour 232
Sulfametral
    in combination with TMP 94
Sulfamoxole
    half-life of 29
    in combination with TMP 94
Sulfanilamide
    important characteristics of 35
    ionization of 33
    prontosil conversion to 25
    reversal of activity by p-aminobenzoic
        acid 41
    substitution in the benzene ring of 32
Sulfanilic Acid 43
Sulfaphenazole
    glucuronide derivative of 38
    half-life of 29
    important characteristics of 35
Sulfapyrazine
    half-life of 39
Sulfapyridine
    in the treatment of pneumonia 27
Sulfaquinoxaline 306
Sulfasalazine
    haematologic effects of 219
Sulfathiazole 32
    assay 180
    in lymphogranuloma venereum 352
    in pneumonia 27
Sulfisomidine (SIMD) 38, 154, 155
Sulfisoxazole 27
    concentration in plasma and prostatic
        fluid 387
    important characterisitics of 35
    in Chancroid 352, 353
    in chlamydial pneumonia in children
        318
    in otitis media 311
    in urinary tract infections 28, 268, 270,
        272, 387
    physicochemical characteristics 387
    prophylaxis of UTIs 316
    resistance to 353
    water solubility of 34

Sulfonamides   16, 25–47
  N$_4$-acetyl derivatives of   34, 36, 37
  adverse effects   277, 353, 366
  agranulocytosis from   219
  antagonism by pABA   76
  antimalarial use in combination with
    pyrimethamine   294
  antimicrobial spectrum of   30
  aplastic anemia from   219
  assay methods   179, 180
  assay of   26
  bactericidal activity of   80
  bacteriostatic activity   132
  concentration in plasma and prostatic
    fluid   386
  development of   26–31
  effect on generation rates of E. coli   130–
    133
  effect on renal function   217
  fractional inhibitory concentration   80
  goitrogenic activity   195
  haemolysis from   220
  half-life of   38
  important characteristics of   35
  in bubonic plague   429
  in Chancroid   352, 353
  in chlamydial infections in children   318
  in combination with pyrimethamine   30
  in genital infections   343–354
  in granulomatous disease in children
    324
  in lymphogranuloma venereum   352
  in M. foruitum and M. chelonei
    infections   422
  in malaria   294, 303–305
  in Nocardiosis   418, 419
  in paracoccidioidomycosis   423
  in prostatitis   380
  in urinary tract infections   270–273, 337,
    338
  influence of concentration on synergy
    with TMP   145–151
  inhibition of folic acid synthesis by   43
  inhibitor of development of resistance to
    TMP   3, 87, 283–286, 338
  interaction with sulfonylurea drugs   224
  kernicterus induced by   221
  kinetics of antibacterial effects   131–133
  lag phase of   131, 133
  lipid solubility of   36
  long-acting   28–30, 36, 38
  mechanism of action   19, 25, 39–46
  mechanisms of acquired resistance to
    244, 245
  medium suitable for   75
  metabolic incorporation of   44
  minimum inhibitory concentration   243

  mode of action   155, 156
  mutational resistance to   244, 245
  organisms resistant to   243
  parasite resistance to   45
  pABA antagonism of   41
  pediatric use   309–324
  pharmacokinetic studies of   26
  pharmacokinetics and metabolism of
    37
  physicochemical properties and
    antimicrobial activity of   32–35
  physicochemical properties   164, 165
  plasmid-mediated resistance   4
  present status in therapeutics   46
  prophylaxis of Hemophilus influenzae
    313
  prophylaxis of UTIs   274, 275
  protein binding of   36, 37, 164, 165
  R factor-mediated resistance to   245
  resistance to   1, 86, 243–245, 266, 270,
    271, 331, 332, 338, 350, 353, 363, 364,
    366, 424
  reversibility of action   137
  selection criteria for combination with
    TMP   151–155
  selectivity of action   44
  skin reactions from   214, 216
  structure-activity relationships of   25,
    31–39
  synergism with dihydrofolate reductase
    inhibitors   45
  synergy with benzylpyrimidines   80
  synergy with pyrimethamine   151, 152
  synergy with TMP in UTIs   337, 338
  thrombocytopenia from   220
  tissue distribution   164
  water solubility   34
p-Sulfonamidobenzeneazo-
  dihydrocupreine   25
Sulfones
  antimalarial use   303
  antimicrobial spectrum of   30
  development of   26
  in combination with pyrimethamine   30
  mechanism of action   41, 44
  pharmacokinetics and metabolism of
    38
  physicochemical properties and
    antimicrobial activity of   32, 34, 35
  present status in therapeutics   46
  resistance to   46
  structure-activity relationships   31
  treatment of leprosy   29
Sulfonylurea   238
Sulformethoxine
  antimalarial activity of   30
  antimalarial use   304

half-life of   29
important characteristics of   35
Sulphafurazole
   in nongonococcal urethritis   351
Susceptibility Testing
   disc diffusion method   96, 97
   serial dilution method   96–98
Syphilis   354

Tetracycline
   concentration in plasma and prostatic
      fluid   386, 387
   effect of treatment on postgonococcal
      urethritis   351
   in brucellosis   412–414
   in bubonic plague   429
   in Chancroid   353
   in chlamydial infections   318, 343, 351
   in cholera   372, 373
   in chronic bronchitis   400–402, 404
   in Isospora belli infections   359, 431
   in M. marinum infections   421
   in melioidosis (P. pseudomallei
      infection)   426, 427
   in Nocardiosis   418, 419
   in Q fever   430
   in shigellosis   368
   in urinary tract infections   333
   in "whooping cough"   403
   in Yersinia enterocolitica infections
      374, 375
   physicochemical characteristics   387
   resistance to   1, 332, 333, 349, 353, 354,
      357, 363, 364, 367, 369, 370
Tetrahydrofolate, FAH$_4$ 3, 11–20, 80, 82,
   87, 133, 157, 299, 337
   functions of   40
Tetroxoprim   107
   absorption   163
   activity in comparison with
      trimethoprim   78–80
   chemical structure   143, 174
   disposition and metabolism   163–180
   excretion   168
   half-life   170, 171
   in combination with sulfadiazine in
      bronchitis   407
   metabolism   173, 174
   minimum inhibitory concentration
      78–80
   pharmacokinetics   154
   physicochemical properties   154, 164,
      165
   plasma and tissue concentrations   166,
      167
   protein binding of   164, 165
   resistance to   143

tissue distribution   164
Tetroxoprim/Sulfadiazine   94
   adverse effects   407
   in bronchitits   407
Thin Layer Chromatography   177–179
thio-NADPH
   as substrate for DHFR   66
Thrombocytopenia   220, 224
Thrombocytopenia/Pancytopenia   209
Thymidine   4, 76, 80, 83, 87, 88, 92, 96, 98,
   157, 246, 363, 366, 367
Thymidine-dependent Organisms   4
Thymidine Phosphorylase   4, 20, 76, 96, 98
Thymidylate   299
   biosynthesis of   13, 15, 19
   hydrolysis of   20
Thymidylate Synthetase   12, 15, 19, 20, 88,
   246, 295
Thymine   76, 82, 92, 98, 246, 332, 367
   in reversal of sulfonamide activity   41
   in thymineless death   20
Thymineless Bacteria   249
Thymineless Death   80, 83, 137
Thyroid-Stimulating Hormone (TSH)   196
Thyroxine   196
   penetration into aqueous humour   232
Tolbutamide
   interaction with TMP/SMX   224
Toxoflavin   16
Toxoplasma gondii   414–416
Toxoplasmosis   305, 411, 414–417
   treatment with TMP/SMX   411, 412,
      414–417
Triampterene
   cooperative binding to DHFR   57
Trigonitis (acute urethra syndrome)   266
Triiodothyronine   222, 233
Trimethoprim   18, 19
   absorption   163, 229
   administration to patients in acute
      megaloblastic states   218
   adverse reactions to   277–279
   4-amino-3,5-disubstituted analogs   114
   as single agent   94–96, 261–286
   assay methods   177
   bacterial strains sensitive to   262
   bacterial uptake mechanism for   17
   bactericidal activity of   80
   biphasic inhibition of growth   138–142
   chromosome-mediated resistance   3, 4
   concentration   2, 93, 164, 166–168, 262–
      265; in amniotic fluid 233; in bile fluid
      233; in bone 234; in breast milk 232; in
      cerebrospinal fluid 232; in lung tissue
      234; in plasma 261, 386–390; in
      prostatic fluid 167, 168, 233, 386–390;

Trimethoprim
    in sputum 399, 400; in vaginal fluid
      233; in erythrocytes 234
    cooperative binding and its effect on
      DHFR selectivity 119
    cooperative binding to DHFR 57
    dermatologic reactions to 277, 280
    development of resistance to 142, 143
    DHFR binding site 121
    DHFR inhibition assay 56
    DHFRs resistant to 68
    3',5'-dimethoxy-4'-OR substituted
      analogs 114
    disposition and metabolism 163–180
    effect of antagonist on 141
    effect on DHFR hysteresis 62
    effect on generation rates of E. coli 133–
      135
    effect on renal function 216, 217, 224
    elimination of 235–237
    elimination of with impaired renal
      function 235–237
    epidemiologic overview of resistance to
      250–252
    excretion of 168, 264
    gastrointestinal reactions to 280
    half-life 170, 171, 235, 261, 416
    half life in renal insufficiency 264
    hematologic reactions to 280, 281
    in chlamydial infections in children 317,
      318
    in Chlamydia trachomatis infections
      351
    in cholera 372
    in E. coli diarrhea 358
    in genital infections 343–354
    in gonorrhea 343
    in Isospora belli infections 431
    in malaria 295
    in meningitis 232
    in paracoccidioidomycosis 424
    in prostatitis 388–390
    in pseudomas infections 425–428
    in rhinoentomophthoromycosis 424
    in shigellosis 369
    in typhoid fever 366
    in urinary tract infections 6, 95, 96,
      264–273, 333, 335–338
    in Yersinia enterocolitica infections 374
    influence of concentration and inoculum
      size on bactericidal effect 135–137
    inhibition of DHFRs 60
    intramuscular administration 196
    kinetics of antibacterial effects 133–143

    lag in effect on growth 80, 133
    LD_{50} 187
    mechanism of acquired resistance to
      245–248
    mechanism of action 1–3, 141, 142, 156,
      157
    medium suitable for 76
    metabolism 169–173, 234, 235
    metabolites of 234, 235
    minimum inhibitory concentration
      76–79, 81–84, 243, 264, 265, 282, 283,
      318, 366, 389, 390, 400
    mutagenicity studies 201, 202
    mutational resistance to 245–247
    NMR studies of DHFR binding 67
    organisms resistant to 244, 286
    overdosage with 281
    pediatric use 309–324
    pharmacodynamic activity 185, 186
    pharmacokinetics 93, 154, 229–238,
      262, 281, 334
    physicochemical properties 154, 164,
      165, 387
    plasmid-mediated resistance 4, 247,
      251, 252, 332
    prophylactic use in immunosuppressed
      patients 275, 276
    prophylaxis of UTIs 273–275
    protein binding of 164, 165, 232, 261
    renal clearance of 236
    reproductive toxicology 197–201
    resistance to 4, 87–90, 94–96, 142, 143,
      151, 243–252, 266, 267, 282–286, 331,
      333, 348–350, 358, 363, 366, 367, 369,
      370, 389, 408, 421
    reversal of activity 87, 137, 138
    selective binding to DHFRs 59, 61
    selectivity and the 4'-methoxy group
      114
    skin reactions from 216
    species insensitive to 78
    stability 97
    6-substituted derivatives 115
    substitution of a heterocyclic ring for the
      benzene moiety 116
    synergism with sulfonamides 45
    synergy with sulfadiazine 81
    synergy with sulfamethoxazole 81, 318
    synergy with sulfonamides in UTIs 337,
      338
    teratogenic effects of 221, 222
    the 4'-isopropenyl derivative 113
    thyroid studies 196
    tissue distribution 164
    toxicity of 275
    toxicity tests 185–202

transference of resistance markers to
   248
6-unsubstituted derivatives   112
use alone in bronchitis   6
use alone in chest infections   407–409
use alone in toxoplasmosis   416
use during pregnancy   281
use in Finland   277, 282, 283
variations in the 3'- and 5'-substituents
   114
variations in the bridge between the
   pyrimidine and benzene rings   116
volume of distribution in plasma   231
water solubility   97
X-ray structure of E. coli DHFR
   complex   67
Trimethoprim/Sulfadiazine
concentration in urine   237, 238
elimination of   237, 238
in bronchitis   407
in non-gonococcal urethritis   352
intramuscular administration   196
in urinary tract infections   6, 268, 270
toxicity tests   193, 194
Trimethoprim/Sulfadoxine
intramuscular administration   196
Trimethoprim/Sulfafurazole
toxicity tests   193
Trimethoprim/Sulfamethoxazole, TMP/
   SMX, Co-trimoxazole   1–7, 16, 29
administration to patients in acute
   megaloblastic states   218
administration to women breast-
   feeding   232
adverse effects   6, 207–224, 365, 397,
   402, 404, 406
agranulocytosis from   209, 218, 219, 224
anaphylaxis from   209
and impaired renal function   217, 224,
   231, 235, 237, 314
angioneurotic edema from   209, 211
antibacterial activity   75–99
approved indications in U.S.   5
bacteriostatic synergy of   82
chromosome-mediated resistance   3, 4
comparison with trimethoprim alone in
   treatment of chest infections   408, 409
concentration   2; in amniotic fluid 233;
   in bile fluid 234; in bone 234; in breast
   milk 232; in cerebrospinal fluid 232,
   314; in lung tissue 234; in plasma 230,
   231, 390; in prostatic fluid 233, 390; in
   sputum 400; in vaginal fluid 233
cross-resistance with penicillin   349, 350
demonstration of synergy by disc
   diffusion method   82, 83, 96, 97

dermatitis from   211–216
effect of medium on synergy of   82
effect of treatment on postgonococcal
   urethritis   350, 351
effect on generation rates of E. coli   143–
   145
effect on renal function   197, 217
fertility tests   198–200
fetal toxicity tests   189, 197–199
folic acid deficiency from   218
half life of   230, 231, 412
immunosuppressive effect   196
in ascending cholangitis in children   324
in atypical mycobacterial infections
   421, 422
in boutonneuse fever   430
in bronchiectasis   397, 403–406
in bronchitis   5, 397–402, 404–406
in brucellosis   412–414
in bubonic plague   411, 429
in chest infections   397–409
in chlamydial infections   317, 318, 350–
   352
in cholera   373, 374
in chromomycosis   425
in Chancroid   353, 354
in entomophthoromycosis and
   rhinoentomophthoromycosis   425
in E. coli diarrhea   357, 358
in genital infections   343–354
in gonococcal pharyngitis   348
in gonococcal urethritis   344–346
in gonorrhea   343–351
in histoplasmosis   422, 423
in human coccidiosis   306
in Hemophilus influenzae infections
   310–314
in Isospora belli infections   359, 431
in lung abscess due to Staphylococcus
   pyogenes   403
in lymphogranuloma venereum   352
in L. pneumophila infections   430
in melioidosis (P. pseudomallei
   infection)   426, 427
in meningitis   232
in meningitis in children   314, 315
in mycoses   425
in Malakoplekia   431
in M. marinum infections   421
in non-gonococcal urethritis   351, 352
in non-typhoidal salmonella infections
   361, 366–368
in Nocardiosis   418–420
in osteomyelitis   324
in otitis media   310, 311
in paracoccidioidomycosis   424

Trimethoprim/Sulfamethoxazole
  in phycomycosis   424, 425
  in pneumonia   402–404
  in prostatitis   385, 388–390
  in pseudomonas infections   425–428
  in Pediculosis capitis   431
  in Pneumocystis carinii infection   306
  in PPA ("Pittsburgh pneumonia agent")
    infections   430
  in P. carinii pneumonia   319, 404
  in P. cepacia and P. Maltophilia
    infections   427, 428
  in P. putrefaciens infections   428
  in Q fever   430
  in rickettsiosis   430
  in shigellosis   322, 368–371
  in sinusitis   312
  in syphilis   354
  in toxoplasmosis   412, 414–417
  in typhoid fever   5, 360–366
  in urinary tract infections   73, 265, 267–
    273, 315–318, 331–339
  in "whooping cough"   403
  in Yersinia enterocolitica infections
    323, 324, 374, 375
  incidence of strains resistant to   249
  interaction with Azathioprine   223
  interaction with methotrexate   6, 238,
    281
  interaction with phenytoin   223, 238
  interaction with pyrimethamine   222
  interaction with Warfarin   223
  interactions with other drugs   238
  intravenous use   314, 404
  jaundice from   208, 209, 221, 224
  kinetics of antibacterial effects   143–158
  LD$_{50}$ 187
  leucopenia from   218, 219, 223
  mechanism of action   18
  minimum inhibitory concentration of   3,
    82, 84, 97, 98, 133, 134, 318, 349, 350,
    389, 390, 412, 426
  mode of action   158
  mutagenicity studies in humans   201,
    202
  optimum ratio of TMP and SMX in
    82–84, 93, 97, 145–151
  overtreatment of UTIs   334, 335
  parenteral use in cancer patients   6
  parenteral use in pneumonia and
    bronchitis   406
  pediatric use   309–324
  pharmacokinetics   229–238, 367
  plasmid-mediated resistance   4
  prophylactic use in immunosuppressed
    patients   275, 276, 319, 320

  prophylaxis of chest infections in patients
    with cystic fibrosis   405
  prophylaxis of chronic bronchitis   404–
    406
  prophylaxis of Hemophilus influenzae
    313
  prophylaxis of P. carinii pneumonia
    319, 320, 404
  prophylaxis of UTIs   274, 275, 316
  reproductive toxicology   197–201
  resistance to   248, 249, 282–286, 321,
    331, 336, 338, 348–350, 360, 363, 364,
    366, 367, 369–371, 389, 408
  sensitivity of bacteroides to   90
  skin reactions from   215, 216
  spectrum of activity of   90–92
  synergy   3, 84–87, 145, 158, 248, 249,
    318, 337, 412, 415, 416, 418, 419, 426
  thrombocytopenia from   220
  thyroid studies   195, 196
  toxic erythema from   214, 215
  toxicity   339
  toxicity tests   185–202
  treatment of typhoid carriers   360, 364,
    365
  urinary recovery of   236
  use against sulfonamide-resistant
    strains   248, 249
  use against TMP-resistant strains   249
  use during pregnancy   221, 222, 224, 281
  use in Finland   282, 283, 338
  volume of distribution in plasma   231
Trimethoprim/Sulfamethoxypyrazine
  acute toxicity studies   187
  LD$_{50}$ 187
  reproductive toxicity studies   201
  toxicity tests   195
Trimethoprim/Sulfamoxole
  in chronic bronchitis   406
  LD$_{50}$ 194
  pharmacodynamic activity   186
  reproductive toxicity studies   200
  toxicity tests   194
Trimethoprim/Sulfamoxazole
  in chronic bronchitis   406
Trimethoprim/Sulfisoxazole
  in urinary tract infections   272
Typhoid Fever   320, 321, 359–364

Ureaplasma urealyticum   351, 391
  prostatitis from   391
Urethritis
  nongonococcal   351, 391
  postgonococcal   350, 351
Uridine   76
Uridine Diphosphate   246

Uridylate   8
Urinary Tract Infections   5, 249, 250, 331–
   339
   association with prostatitis   379
   clinical studies of the use of TMP in
      266–273
   complicated, recurrent, or chronic   271–
      275
   in children   315–318
   incidence of   380
   lower (cystitis)   267
   prophylaxis   273
   uncomplicated   267
   upper (pyelonephritis)   267
   use of TMP alone against   264–270

Urticaria   211–213, 216

Vancomycin   210
Vasculitis   211
Vibrio cholerae   247, 262, 371–373

Warfarin
   interaction with TMP/SMX   223

Xanthopterin   16

Yersinia enterocolitica   373–375
   in children   322–324
Yersinia pestis   429